Sustainable Education and Development

Joseph N. Mojekwu · Wellington Thwala ·
Clinton Aigbavboa · Lawrence Atepor ·
Samuel Sackey
Editors

Sustainable Education and Development

Springer

Editors
Joseph N. Mojekwu
University of Lagos
Lagos, Nigeria

Clinton Aigbavboa
Faculty of Engineering and the Built Environment
University of Johannesburg
Johannesburg, South Africa

Samuel Sackey
Kwame Nkrumah University of Science and Technology
Kumasi, Ghana

Wellington Thwala
Department of Construction Management and Quantity Surveying
University of Johannesburg
Johannesburg, Gauteng, South Africa

Lawrence Atepor
Cape Coast Technical University
Cape Coast, Ghana

ISBN 978-3-030-68835-6 ISBN 978-3-030-68836-3 (eBook)
https://doi.org/10.1007/978-3-030-68836-3

This Springer imprint is published by the registered company Springer Nature Switzerland AG
The registered company address is: Gewerbestrasse 11, 6330 Cham, Switzerland

Contents

The Implication of Societal Perception and Value on Quality Education: The Nigeria Example, 1999–2019

A. D. Famoye(✉)

Department of History and International Studies, Adekunle Ajasin University, Akungba-Akoko, Ondo State, Nigeria

Abstract. The job of a researcher can be broadly categorised into two aspects. The first aspect involves the conduct of his research with the goal of making ground-breaking discoveries or at least making distinct contributions that will expand the frontiers of existing knowledge. The second phase has to do with the transfer of these discoveries inform of knowledge to the students. However, since the researcher does not operate outside the society, his success or failure at all of these stages is considerably determined by the perception and the value that the society ascribes to education. Society in this context involves several human classes, but the government, parents, guardians and the students as the most influencing sets. It is on the above background that this paper examines the relevance of the societal view and value of education to the development and attainment of quality education in Nigeria between 1999 and 2019. The paper relies heavily on empirical evidence. This was supplemented with existing secondary source materials and a few national newspapers. The paper argues and concludes that the nonchalant attitude of the public towards education were major banes of quality research and education in Nigeria during the twenty years under review. It is opined that since the societal perception and value are fundamental to the development of education, there is an implication, therefore, that the Nigerian education may not develop beyond its current state until there is a change in the way the society perceives, values and approaches the sector.

Keywords: Researcher · Society · Perception · Value and quality education

1 Introduction

In 1999, when the country returned to democracy, after fifteen years of uninterrupted military rule, expectations were high as the citizens looked forward to the civil rule to bring about good governance and other dividends of democracy. Like all sectors of the national life, there were expectations in the education sector too. It was believed that the new system of government would transform the nation's education such that it would be able to compete internationally. Among other things, it was expected that the new Nigeria would prioritise education as a way of facilitating national development.

J. N. Mojekwu et al. (Eds.): *Sustainable Education and Development*, pp. 1–9, 2021.
https://doi.org/10.1007/978-3-030-68836-3_1

However, after twenty years into the democratic rule, it appeared that the hope that had greeted democracy had been dashed as education and research activities were continuously neglected by the successive government. This was demonstrated in the budgetary allocations for education, which was not only below the recommendation of the United Nations Educational Scientific and Cultural Organisation (UNESCO), but also continued to reduce on annual. The government was disinterested in all matters that were capable of stirring the quality education (Matthew 2016). Generally, there appeared to be a discouraging societal perception and value of education. This was established in wide national lack of concern in research and quality education by the general public, especially the three major stakeholders- government, parents/guardians and students.

It is on the above viewpoint that this paper examines the implication of the societal perception and value of education on the attainment of quality education in Nigeria between 1999 and 2019. In other words, the paper seeks to understand to what extent the general importance or value that the Nigerian society placed on education affected the development of Nigerian education in terms of research and quality of education provided within the period under review.

The paper is built on empirical evidence. A total number of 50 (face-to-face and phone) interviews were conducted. These involved carefully selected individuals, who were well informed on the subject-matter. In addition, 300 questionnaires were roughly distributed to people across the focus social groups- government, parents/guardians and students. Further insights were, however, provided by secondary source materials and local newspapers.

2 Theoretical Framework for Analysis

The Systems Theory is used as the theoretical framework for the analysis in this paper. System theory opines that an entity is a system made up of components (Mele et al. 2010). This was propounded in the 1940s by Ludwig von Bertalanffy and furthered promoted by Ross Ashby and George Bateson (Wilkinson 2011). Therefore, when applied socially, it implies that the society is an arrangement made up of complex elements, such as individual, groups, agencies and so on, relating as a whole with their actions and interactions affecting or influencing the overall performance of the society. In other words, the society is more or less a product of combined functions of its integrated parts. Thus, it can be deduced that the society can only be understood by first understanding the nature, working, contributions and interrelation process of its parts or segments since the society is only a reflection of the complimentary efforts of such subdivisions.

The application of the System Theory as a framework for studies in education has been around for a while. For instance, (Oyebade 2001) emphasises the importance of the theory in the search for genuine and long lasting solution to student conflict or violence in Nigeria's tertiary institutions. It is argued that for the tertiary institutions in the country to enjoy peace, they must, in the working principles of the theory, acknowledge that all units from the administration to the students union is relevant to the scheme of peace. And more importantly, all the units must be ready to embrace the use of compromise as an important means of settling their differences.

Also, (Gupta and Gupta 2013) examines how the systems approach can help improve the productivity of the school. It is argued that if all components or persons involved in education or school system, including the students, parents, teachers, education inspectors and so on, are fully aware of how complex learning situations are and diligently play their roles, the school will operate and deliver effectively on its mandate. Similarly, (Dahiru et al. 2018), engages in how social system theory, a variation of the System Theory, can be practically used to enhance an effective school system. It argues that while the theory can be used to identify fundamental factors that influence effectiveness in the school, it can also help in improving on such factors such that they will enhance productivity in school.

However, in what seems like a breakaway from the above focuses, this paper engages the System Theory in a historical manner to understand to what extent the perceptions and value that the Nigerian government, parents and students placed on education influenced or affected the delivery of quality education in the country between 1999 and 2009. Thus, the paper sees education in Nigeria as a system and the concerned social groups as the components of the system, which determined the functions and the level of development of the system (education).

3 Conceptual Clarification

3.1 Society

The term 'society' originates from a Latin word, socius, meaning companionship or friendship (Zerihum 2005). And like many social science concepts, it has been accorded several meanings, depending on the context of the users. For instance, while a society is generally viewed as a human group with a relatively large population and autonomy in the organisation of their social relations, a sociologist or an anthropologist may see the term as a complex pattern of norms of interactions existing among members of a given space or territory. Thus, while the former is concerned with the inhabitants of a territorial space, the latter pays more attention to the nature of interactions evolving among the inhabitants of the environment.

However, for the purpose of our analysis, the paper adopts Mayhew's (1968) definition, which sees 'society' as a social population, with clearly identified inhabitants interacting with each other and occupying a definite territorial space. In other words, the society is a group of humans in a particular environment with an organised social life. Thus, it includes the government, parents, guardians, students, and other groups of human decision-makers that, in one way or the other, have the potentials to influence policies in such a society.

3.2 Societal Perception

According to the Oxford Advanced Learners Dictionary (2005), 'perception involves an idea, a belief or an image you have as a result of how you understand something'. (Qiong 2017) also says that 'in 'philosophy, psychology, and cognitive science, perception is the process of attaining awareness or understanding of sensory information'. Since perception is ones' viewpoint on a particular object or subject, it can be deduced societal perception represents a general or popular thought and viewpoint of a society about a particular thing or idea in relations to their belief or experiences over a period of time.

3.3 Societal Value

According to (Thome 2015), value includes an enduring belief or conception that construes something as preferable or desirable. Thus, value does not only guide actions, it also influences perceptions and feelings. In a broad sense, value may be considered as attitude-related attribute that are projected upon people, objects and situations. Value like perception usually motivates towards a given goal. Thus, a societal value involves the importance that a society ascribes to a particular thing, which is cable of influencing their actions or inaction towards such things. Also, it can be deduced from the foregoing that perception and value are closely interacting, with the former influencing the latter and vice versa. For example, while the value one places on something may influence one's way of thinking and attitude towards it, so also can one's thought and attitude toward same thing influence one's value towards it.

Based on the above, this paper examines how the general viewpoint and value that the Nigerian society placed on education influenced the development or attainment of quality education in the country during the period under review.

4 The State of Education in Nigeria Between 1999 and 2019

Prior to the transition from the military rule to the democratic system in 1999, education in Nigeria can be said to be in bad condition, considering challenges such as poor funding, lack of research facilities, inadequate or unqualified teaching staff, wrong policies, and so on (Odia and Omofonmwan 2007). So, when democracy was restored in May 1999, expectations were very high as the citizens hoped that the new system of government would lead to a socio- economic transform of the country and emergence of policies that would guarantee quality and affordable education. However, twenty years after, it seemed that all hope had been dashed as the country's education became worse for it.

While there are lot of things to be said concerning the condition of the Nigerian education during the period under consideration, the paper is, however, of the opinion that the best way to describe the state of the nation's education as at that time is to focus on two major factors, which were funding and physical facilities made available for research and teaching. It is strongly believed that other factors were largely the offshoots of these two factors. In other words, these two best demonstrated the general state of things as far as education in the county was concerned.

From 1999 to 2019, Nigeria was under four administrations- Obasanjo, Yar'Adua, Jonathan and Buhari. A look at the budgetary allocations for education by these administrations shows that Nigeria did not meet up with UNESCO prescription of 26% of national budget for education. In fact, such records show a sequence of decline in the allocations on yearly basis (Matthew 2016). From primary to tertiary institutions, paucity of fund was a major phenomenon. Although the government created a number of intervention agencies such as the Tertiary Education Trust Fund (TETFUND), Industrial Training Fund (ITF), Petroleum Technology Development Fund (PTDF), Universal Basic Education (UBE) (Ogunbenle and Edogiawere 2016), such efforts were only able to bring little succour as the long time starvation of fund had created more problems that these agencies could exclusively handle. More importantly, the systemic corruption involving government official and school administrators ensured that the significant part of such intervention funds were mismanaged or ended up in private pockets (Egbefo 2012).

Across all levels of education, academic unions such as the Nigerian Teachers Union (NUT), College of Education Academic Union (COEASU), Academic Staff Union of Polytechnics (ASUP) and Academic Union of Universities (ASUU) had to embark on several industrial actions, at the state and national levels, to compel the government to release more fund for fundamental projects and arrears of salaries and allowances. While many have condemned the industrial actions on the basis that they were also counterproductive to education, the government's failure to do the needful until the industrial actions were activated was a strong proof that strike was the only potent weapon that the labour unions had to make the government do the right thing.

Closely related to funding was physical infrastructure. Due to inadequate funding, Nigerian education across all stages was confronted with the challenge of inadequate or dilapidated physical facilities. Primary and secondary schools appeared to have suffered more. In many cases, the pupils had no proper classrooms and had to learn under dilapidated buildings or trees with no or inadequate desks. In such situations, many had to sit on the floor in overcrowded rooms (Olawoye 2020).

Tertiary institutions were not spear too with inadequate offices for teachers and insufficient lecture theatres for learning. Aside the fact that many libraries were not well equipped with current and relevant books and online facilities, there was also a trend of increasing number of moribund laboratories (Arogundade 2010). In many instances, lecturers and students were largely left with the option of independently funding their research works. Consequently, effective research and teaching activities were considerably hindered.

It can be deduced from the foregoing that Nigerian education during the period under assessment was deprived of basic necessities that could encourage quality research and teaching capable of stirring desired national socio-economic development. The education sector continued to take the back stage as far as government attention was concerned and as such the country's education could not even rank among the first one hundred in Africa (Ademola-Olateju 2019). As the purported 'giant of Africa', one would have expected the country to live to that responsibility by dominating and providing directions in education in Africa, however, due to the familiar problems, a lot of Nigerian students began to seek education outside the country, even in countries that were less developed than Nigeria. Similarly, but with more consequence, a great number of Nigeria academics, who should have made immense contributions to the development of the country's education and overall national development through their inventions in science and technology had to migrate to countries with better education structures and welfare packages, and where their impact on the society would be duly acknowledged.

5 The Relevance of the Societal Perspective and Value to the State of Education Nigeria, 1999–2019

While the government has been largely held responsible for the bad state of the country's education, it can, however, be argued that the overall perception and value that the Nigerian society placed on education was more responsible for the falling standard of education in the country between 1999 and 2019. In other words, the paper opines that the long time neglect suffered by education in the country was as a result of the fact that the major stakeholders in the society did not prioritise quality education. Based on this background, the next section of the paper examines how the perception and value that the major stakeholders, government, parents/guardians and students, placed on education was relevant to the development of education in Nigeria during the period under review.

5.1 Government

Like their predecessors, the four successful administrations between 1999 and 2019 invested very little in education. Their attitude towards education seemed to suggest that, education in their own perspective, was not crucial to the citizens and national development. It is hard to explain how government that claimed to be passionate about national development would for two decades continuously under fund its education (Onyekwena et al. 2016). Even when, they consistently provided bailouts to order sectors such as the aviation and power, education which was central to the sustainability of such sectors was grossly neglected.

The government was disinterested in education, except it was possible to use it to score political marks. Thus, education was so much attached to politicking that making of irrelevant and counterproductive policies by the government almost became a norm. For instance, while it was widely expected that Goodluck Jonathan, a Ph.D. holder and most educated president in the country, would use the wealth of his knowledge, experience and informed position about Nigerian education to transform the sector, he, however, chose to establish more universities and polytechnics across the country in a bid to score cheap political marks tilted toward his winning the presidential election of 2015 (Erunke 2017). There were similar incidents too at the state level. For example, in Ondo State, the administrations of Olusegun Agagu (2003–2009) and Olusegun Mimiko (2009–2017), for obvious political reasons, established universities in their home communities, even when the pre-existing state owned university and polytechnic, Adekunle Ajasin University and the Rufus Giwa Polytechnic, were begging for funding just to survive. While the former established the Ondo State University of Science and Technology at Okitipupa, the latter established the University of Medical Sciences in Ondo Town. Consequently, the institutions became more financial burdens to the state government such that they could not be properly maintained. Despite the public outcry about the condition of these tertiary institutions and call for a merger as the most effective cost saving method that would ensure appropriate maintenance of the institutions, Akeredolu's administration, which succeeded Mimiko's administration, seemed to have lacked the political will to do that.

5.2 Parents/Guardians

In a country where education scholarship was scarce and education loan was not in existence, Nigerian parents or guardians solely shouldered the responsibility of sending their children to schools from the elementary to tertiary level. Having been perpetually denied access to basic social amenities such as good road network, stable electricity and so on, one would ordinary have expected the Nigerian parents or guardians to have at least agitated for quality education for their children. However, most Nigerian parents and guardians appeared not to have bothered about the falling standard of education. It seemed that education to them was not more than act of mastering ‘reading and writing’. Thus, this section of the society did not only fail to demand for quality education, but sometimes also blamed the academic unions for embarking on industrial actions that were meant to press for their welfare and better funding of education (Ben TV 2013).

A larger population of Nigerian parents and guardians seemed unperturbed by the continuous falling standard of the country’s education. Generally, they seemed not to value or understand the importance of quality education as they appeared to be more interested in the certificates their children acquire than the worth of education they received.

However, it needs to be stressed that the involvement of the parents and guardians in falling standard of education was not only through their passive roles. There were instances where they had been actively involved in destroying the system too. For example, there were reports of parents’ involvement in examination malpractices (Omonijo and Fadugba 2011). They did this just to ensure that their children passed their examinations, not minding the immediate and future implications of this negative interference on education and the overall development of the country. Generally, it can be said that the perception and value that this section of the society attached to education were considerably narrow and unintelligible and as such the group was more of a weak link in the quest for quality education in Nigeria.

5.3 The Students

From the available records, it is evident that the overall perception of the students was not significantly different from that of the parents or guardians. This was severally demonstrated in increase number of examination practice cases, violent protest, lackadaisical attitude towards learning, disinterest in supervised research, increasing involvement in internet fraud and other social vices like cultism (Odia and Omofonmwan 2007). It is also important to mention the place of student unionism. Ordinarily, student unionism was supposed to be about the welfare of the students, with the most important goal being provisions of environment conducive enough for research and learning. However, many student union leaders appeared to be more interested in how they could use such privileged positions to amass personal wealth or negotiate their future politically or professionally.

It will be recalled that, even when it was obvious that the students would benefit more, student union leaders usually opposed the academic unions’ industrial actions meant to compel the government to be alive to its responsibilities. For example, when ASUU embarked on a nationwide strike in 2013 in its demand for increment in funding of the public universities by the government, the students unions on several occasions accused ASUU of fighting for its personal interests and also threatened to take legal actions against the academic union if the industrial action was not suspended (Premium Times 2013). One would have expected that, as the most important stakeholders in the education sector, the students should have led the struggle for quality education in the country. However, they largely seemed to see nothing wrong with the existing structure as long as they could graduate and obtain their certificates on record time.

So, like the Systems Theory operates, the condition of education in Nigeria between 1999 and 2019 should be seen as a product of the actions and inactions of different human components or social groups in the society, most especially the government, parents and students. Thus, while the government was reluctant in providing the necessary resources that could bring about quality education in the country, other important stakeholders largely represented by the parents and students could not mount the needed pressure on the government and even in some instances caused more damage through their negative interference in the system. This was because their perception, understanding and value of education fell short of what can be properly regarded as quality education. The result of this process of interactive or interrelated human actions and inactions was that research activities and quality teaching or learning suffered: quality education largely eluded the Nigerian society.

6 Conclusion

The paper has examined how the societal perception and value of education was relevant to the attainment of quality education in Nigeria between 1999 and 2019. It is observed that the perception and value that the major stakeholders in the country attached to education had more to do with attendance and obtaining of certificates from schools. It appeared, therefore, that the issue of quality education was secondary and unimportant to them. Government clearly failed in its responsibility of funding, provision of equipment and making of relevant policies to ensure quality education for the citizens. Parents/guardians and the students themselves did not only fail to make the government accountable or live up to its responsibilities, they also through some of their activities such as examination malpractice, cultism and so on contributed to the falling standard of education. Consequently, quality education largely eroded the nation during the period under review, not because the government failed in its duties, but because the society was docile and conducive enough to accommodate and celebrated such act of ineptitude from the authorities. By and large, the implication is that Nigerian education, either now or in the future, can only be salvaged from its current bad state and the nation's chances to enjoy quality education will only come through, when the major stakeholders in the country understand and value the purpose of quality education to national development.

References

Ademola-Olateju, B.: The Largest University System in Africa, and the Worst, The Premium Times (2019)

Afolayan, F.O.: A holistic review of public funding of primary education in Nigeria. IOSR J. Res. Method Educ. **4**(6), 68–74 (2014)

Arogundade, A.B.: Problems of facilities in south-west Nigerian universities and the way forward. J. Educ. Adm. Policy Stud. **2**(2), 39–43 (2010)

Akintunde, B.: Inside the Broken Schools in Nasarawa Where Pupils Sit on Floor to Learn. The Premium Times (2019)

Ben TV. 'ASUU Strike: Our Losses, Frustrations, by Students, Parents, Businessmen' (2013)

Dahiru, A.S., Basri, R., Aji, A.A., Asimiran, S.: Modelling social system for school effectiveness. Int. J. Acad. Res. Bus. Soc. Sci. **8**(12) (2018)

Egbefo, D.: Corruption in the Nigerian education system: its implication in manpower and development in age of globalization. J. Arts Educ. **6**(2), 149–266 (2012)
Erunke, J.: 12 varsities established by Jonathan have only 3,765 academic staff- Panel. The Vanguard (2017)
Eze, J.: New Universities Established by Jonathan face Probe. The Premium Times (2016)
Gupta, S., Gupta, A.: The systems approach in education. Int. J. Manag. **1**(1), 52–55 (2013)
Hornsby, A.S.: The Oxford Advanced Learners' Dictionary of Current English. Oxford University Press, Oxford (2005)
Matthew, I.A.: Financial allocation to education: trends issues and way forward in Nigeria. J. Plus Educ. **9**(1), 227–242 (2016)
Mayhew, L.H.: Society. In: Sills, D.L. (ed.) International Encyclopaedia of Social Science, vol. 577. Crowell, Collier and Macmillan, New York (1968)
Mele, C., Pels, J., Polese, F.: A brief review of systems theories and their managerial applications. Serv. Sci. **2**(12), 126–135 (2010)
Odia, L.O., Omofonmwan, S.I.: Educational system in Nigeria problems and prospects. J. Soc. Sci. **14**(1), 81–86 (2007)
Ogungbenle, S.K., Edogiawere, M.N.: Budgetary allocation and development in Nigeria tertiary institutions. Igbinedion Univ. J. Account. **2**, 377–407 (2016)
Olawoye, D.: Pupils in School Attended by Ondo Deputy Governor Sit on Bare Floor, Learn in Classrooms with Leaky Roof Despite N13bn Education Expenditure. The Sahara Reporter (2020)
Omonijo, D.O., Fadugba, O.A.: Parental influence on wards in escalation of examination misconduct in Nigeria. Eur. J. Soc. Sci. **19**(2), 297–307 (2011)
Onyekwena, C., Uzor, E., Okoro, T., Adeniran, A.: Financing basic education in Nigeria: what are the feasible options? In: Centre for the Study of the Economies of Africa (CSEA) (2016)
Oyebade, S.A.: Applying the general systems theory to students' conflict management in Nigeria's tertiary institutions. Lagos J. Educ. Adm. Plan. **1**(1), 36–49 (2001)
Qiong, O.: A brief introduction to perception. Stud. Literat. Lang. **15**(4), 18–28 (2017)
The ICIR. 'NANS Threatened Legal Action against ASUU over Strike'. www.icirnigeria.org, Accessed 13 June 2020
Thome, H.: Values, Sociology of James D. Wright (editor-in-chief). In: International Encyclopedia of the Social & Behavioral Sciences, 2nd ed., pp. 47–53 (2015)
Wilkinson, L.: Systems theory. In: Goldstein, S., Naglieri, J.A. (eds.) Encypclopedia of Child Behaviour and Development. Springer, Heidelberg (2011)
Zerihum, D.: Introduction to Sociology. Ethiopia Public Health Training Initiative (2005)

Impact of TETfund Intervention on Quality Assurance of Basic Education in Plateau State, Nigeria

T. I. Oke(✉)

Department of Educational Foundations(Administration/Planning Unit), Faculty of Education, University of Jos, Jos, Nigeria

Abstract. This study focused on the impact of TETfund intervention on the quality assurance and development of Basic Education in Plateau state. The study employed the use of cross sectional survey design, while stratified and simple random sampling techniques were used for selecting 30 schools out of the 402 upper basic institutions in the state and proportional to size sampling technique was used to select 600 respondents for the study. Three research questions were raised and answered. A questionnaire called TETfund Intervention and Quality Assurance of Basic Education Questionnaire ((TIQABEQ) developed based on 4-point Likert- like scale was used as instrument for data collection. The instrument was validated by experts and the reliability coefficient of 0.78 was obtained. The study used mean, and standard deviation in answering research questions with 2.50 as the criterion mean. Thus, the results of analysis revealed that TETfund has contributed a lot to the development of Basic Education Institutions in the state and that its contributions covered areas such as infrastructure, staff development and other instructional materials and this has significantly improved the quality of students educational attainment in basic institutions. Based on these findings, the study concluded that TETfund has intervened in the development of Basic education institutions in the state and recommended that government should allocate more funds to enable it deliver on its mandate, management of TETfund should embark on needs assessment before executing projects and that TETfund should increase its yearly allocations to institutions among others.

Keywords: Impact of TETfund · TETfund intervention · Quality assurance · Basic education · Plateau state

1 Introduction

Quality management and assurance of educational provision has become one of the central issues accorded priority in the recent educational reform going on worldwide, and quality assurance is seen to be one of the mechanisms used in achieving it. However, the understanding of quality and the possible ways and means of assuring quality in education varies. Quality assurance is the meeting or conforming to generally accepted standards as defined by quality assurance bodies or appropriate academic and professional committees (Awogwugwu 2009).

J. N. Mojekwu et al. (Eds.): *Sustainable Education and Development*, pp. 10–20, 2021.
https://doi.org/10.1007/978-3-030-68836-3_2

The notion of quality varies from that of providing a distinctive, special or even exclusive product or service, to meeting or conforming to predetermined specifications or standard, to value for money or to fitness of purpose. According to Whiteley (2011), quality assurance in education has become an all-embracing concept that includes all policies, processes and actions through which the quality of education provided is developed and maintained.

Education quality can be viewed as a set of elements that constitute the input, process and output of the education system, which provides services that completely satisfy both internal and external strategic constituencies by meeting their explicit and implicit expectations. If basic education is viewed as a system, then any quality management programme must therefore assess inputs, process and outputs of education program (Peter 2005; Oke 2018).

Quality management in education is a vital milestone in the development of the modern and future Nigeria. Being an indicator for organization performance, the quality of education should be the primary goal of all educational institution. Quality management includes all the activities that managers carryout in an effort to implement their quality policy. These activities include quality planning, quality control, quality assurance and quality improvement (Akpan 2011).

Quality Management is defined as a management approach that aim to achieve and sustain long term organizational success by encouraging employee feedback and participation, satisfying customers needs and expectations respecting societal values, beliefs and obeying government statutes and regulations in order to achieve continual improvement in education, managers should ensure that Quality management is carried out.

Quality assurance is the concern that certain accepted criteria of minimum standards of quality should be achieved in the production of goods and services. It involves putting in place certain techniques and procedures that ensure the quality of product Fadipe (2000). Ekong (2008) described the concept of quality assurance as involving all the policies, systems and processes directed to ensuring the maintenance and enhancement of the quality of educational provision within an institution. In the basic school system, quality assurance is the guarantee of confidence and certainty that standard and quality of a program run by the educational institutions are being maintained and enhanced. To achieve this, quality assurance system has to be established.

2 Statement of Problem

It is a known fact that most of our educational facilities are in their state of decay, particularly those in basic institutions. For instance dilapidated school plants, buildings, lack or inadequate library and laboratory facilities, overcrowded classrooms and limited examination halls as can be seen during examinations as examination malpractice is always high in our various institutions of learning particularly basic institutions.

Closely related to the decay of educational facilities in our institutions is the area of staff development where most of staff members are grossly under developed due to deficiency insubject mastering emanating from lack of in-service training programme, on the job training, seminars, conferences, and workshops to enable them update their knowledge to face the current educational challenges. Most of our institutions have no adequate and conducive classrooms, no ICT facilities and the problem of power failure.

The decay of infrastructural facilities in our educational institutions and inadequate staff development experience is as a result of inadequate funding to raise the standard of present structures and facilities. If fund is made available more ICT facilities will be provided, examination halls, hostel accommodation and more classrooms will be built, likewise library and laboratory with equipment will equally be provided to ease teaching and learning. On the other hand, in-service training programmes, on- the- job training, conferences, workshops and seminars can be best organized for staff development if funds made available.

However, when TETfund was set up, it was the believed of stakeholders in the state that the fortunes of all educational institutions will be redeemed going by its mandate. The big question however, is that going by the pervading outcries on the fall in the standard of education in Plateau state; can the TETfund really and effectively justify its existence so far? Are there correlations between the funds made available by the TETFund to institutions and the projects on ground?

This paper is set to: (1) assess the extent of TETFund intervention on the quality educational development and achievement in Basic Institutions in Plateau state (2) ascertain the extent to which TETFund has contributed to quality infrastructural development in Basic Institutions in Plateau State, and (3) examine the extent to which TETFund has contributed to quality staff development in basic institutions in Plateau State.

3 Research Questions

The following research questions were raised to guide the study:

1. What is the extent of TETfund intervention in the quality educational development and achievement of basic institutions in Plateau State?
2. To what extent has TETFund contributed to quality infrastructural development in basic institutions in Plateau State?
3. What is the extent of TETFund contributions to quality staff development in basic institutions in Plateau State? State?

4 Theoretical Framework

The study on impact of TETfund intervention on quality assurance of basic education development is anchored on the Public Goods Theory put forward by Samuelson (1954). The theory states that Public goods are consumed by everybody in need of it. It states that goods that are collectively consumed are non-rival and non-excludable. He sees public good as having inherent quality of which requires public production he gives education and military as examples of public goods. This theory was further improved upon by Holcombe (1996) in his book “Public Finance: Government Expenditure and Revenue in United State Economy”. Proving that the largest redistribution programs in US is social security and education which redistributes regardless of need. Resources (human and material), infrastructures and instructional facilities provided therewith in Basic institutions in Plateau state, Nigeria are like public goods to be consumed by citizens (pupils and students) in need of it, they can be consumed by additional consumers at no additional cost. A public good is good produced by government, and it is generally made available for the benefit of its citizens.

5 Conceptual Discuss on TETFund Intervention and Quality Assurance of Basic Education in Nigeria

The Universal Basic Education (UBE) that advocates for free and compulsory education came as a replacement for Nigeria's Universal Primary Education Scheme (UPE) of the 6-3-3–4 system of primary education. The 9-3-4 system of education was designed in conformity with the Millennium Development Goals (MDGs) and Education For All (EFA) (Oke 2018). The UBE involves 6 years of Primary School and 3 years of Junior Secondary School, culminating in 9 years of Free, compulsory, uninterrupted schooling, and transition from one class to another is automatic but assessed through continuous assessment. This scheme is monitored by the Universal Basic Education Commission (UBEC), and State Universal Basic Education Board (SUBEB) and has made it free and a right of every child. Therefore, the UBEC law Section 15 defines UBE as early childhood care and education. The law stipulates a 9-year formal schooling, adult literacy and non-formal education, skill acquisition programmes and the education of special groups such as nomads and migrants, girl child and women, Al-majiri, street children and disabled group (Fadipe 2000).

The need to assess quality in educational provision is now generally accepted as one of the tools of educational reforms. Quality assurance as stated earlier refers to the 'planned and systematic actions [deemed] as necessary to provide adequate confidence that a product or service will satisfy given requirements for quality' (Jackson 2008).The resources needed for teaching and learning process in basic institutions include personnel, (teaching and non-teaching) classrooms, laboratories, workshops, staff offices and libraries. Others are hostels, staff quarters, students and staff recreation centres, sports and games facilities, roads, electricity and water supply, these must be of high qualities (Oke 2011a: 2011b). There are two trends in the provision and availability of these facilities in Nigerian educational institutions. There was steady improvement in the physical plans from the 60s and 70s to the mid-80s of the educational institutions that were established during this period. The major phases of the master plans were implemented. Good classrooms, libraries, laboratories, workshops and staff offices are part of the facilities earlier available in adequate numbers. These institutions were able to support comfortable residential accommodation for students where laundry was free, rooms were well laid out and three -course meals were served (Jagaba 2008).

The collapse of oil boom in the early 80s made it difficult for educational institutions established since this period to compete with the pre-boom era ones in terms of quality and quantity of resources availability. The second trend is the decay in the facilities in all our educational institutions, regardless of its proprietorship. This decay is so terrible that it has been a source of frequent condemnation by the parents and students (Popoola 2001). One of the various attempts to provide remedy to the menace of inadequate provision in educational sector was the establishment of Educational Tax Fund (ETF).

Education Tax Fund (ETF) was established as an intervention agency under the Education Tax Act No. 7 of 1993, and amended by Education Tax (Amendment) Act No. 40 of 22nd December, 1998 with project management to improve the quality of education in Nigeria. The Promulgation of Education Tax Act was necessitated by the widely recognized decline in educational standards and the deep rot in infrastructure and other facilities at all levels of the Nigerian educational system, Plateau State inclusive. Education Tax Fund is a product of funding crises that arose in the educational sector as a result of the introduction of the Structural Adjustment Programme (SAP) introduced in the Nigerian economy in the 1980s when funding of education became a huge challenge (Ayodele 2006). The argument by Academic Staff Union of University (ASUU) then was that government alone cannot fund educational activities; hence the need to introduce public tax funding that culminated in the establishment of Education Tax Fund (ETF) then, today known as TETFund (Adavbiele 2016).

The present Board of the Fund was however inaugurated in 2009 and to enable the Fund achieve its noble objectives, the Act imposes two percent (2%) Education Tax on the assessable profit of all registered companies in Nigeria. In furtherance of this, the Federal Inland Revenue Service (FIRS) was empowered by the Act to assess and collect the Education Tax from all registered companies in the country. The Fund, in return, administers the tax imposed by the Act, and disburses the funds to educational institutions at the federal, state and local government levels. It also monitors the projects executed with the funds allocated to the beneficiary institutions.

The mandate of the Fund as provided in Sections 5(1)(a)–(g) of the Act No. 7 is to administer and disburse the amount generated to government educational institutions, including basic and post basic schools, specifically to the following areas: Work centres and prototype development; staff development and conference attendance; library systems at the different levels of education; research equipment procurement and maintenance; Education Book Development Fund and execution of the nine-year compulsory basic education programme. Also, providing funding for educational facilities and infrastructural development;

Emphasis was placed on science and technology, due to the expensive nature of training of resource persons and equipment required within the country. The funding was increased from N60 million in 2008 to N80 million in 2009 for each federal and state university on equality basis. From 2008 to 2011, higher institutions have received N240 million each for staff training alone. While a total of N17bn was disbursed to all Primary and Secondary schools during this period (Tahir 2009). "Virtually, all the capital projects seen in many of the state institutions (Basic, Post- Basic and Tertiary) certainly, are ETF funded, and there is no public institution in this country, where there are no ETF projects" (Rufai 2012).

Other ancillary funding that the agency has undertaken include the Graduate Teachers Training Scheme, the Academic Publishing Scheme, the National Research Fund, the Almajiri Education Programme, and the Textbooks Distribution Projects for Primary and Junior Secondary Schools(Basic schools). The provision of needed infrastructure for learning at the basic education level is one of the major achievement recorded by TETFund. Today, TETFund had drawn the attention of government to the yearning needs of our educational institutions, and the global ranking of our universities have as well improved (Rufai 2012).

6 Methodology

The research design that was adopted by the researcher for the study was the cross sectional descriptive survey type. The population of the study was 6,140 with 5,231 teaching staff, and 909 non-teaching staff respectively in 402 upper basic institutions in Plateau State The population comprised of male and female respondents from all the upper basic institutions in Plateau State. A sample of 600 respondents was randomly selected using simple random sampling technique. A closed-ended questionnaire titled: TETfund Intervention and Quality Assurance of Basic Education Questionnaire ((TIQABEQ) developed by the researcher was used for data collection.

The instrument was meant to collect data from academic staff, non-academic staff. The instrument had two sections, ‘A’ and ‘B’. Section ‘A’ was made up of respondents bio-data while section ‘B’ contained the twenty six(26) items designed on the basis of 4-point Likert like scale of strongly agree(SA), agree(A), disagree(D) and strongly disagree(SD) and scored as 4,3,2 and 1 respectively. The validity of the instrument was ascertained and reliability and internal consistency of the instrument was established through the use of Cronbach Alpha method on 20 respondents as sample for the pilot study. The procedure yielded a reliability coefficient of 0.75 which shows that, the instrument was good and reliable.

A face-to- face method was used for data collection, while the study employed the use of descriptive statistics in analyzing the data. The descriptive statistics of mean and standard deviation was used to answer research questions and Statistical decisions on the research questions were taken using the cumulative and criterion mean (2.50) for each question.

7 Results

Research Question One: What is the extent of TETfund intervention in the development of Basic institutions in Plateau State?

Table 1. The extent of TETfund Intervention in the development of Basic institutions

Items	Mean	Std. deviation	Decision
TETfund provided instructional facilities in our institutions	3.68	1.67	Agree
TETfund contributed little in development of our institutions	2.36	0.85	Disagree
There are TETFund projects in our institutions	3.37	0.63	Agree
TETfund intervention has been beneficial to our institutions	3.58	0.90	Agree
TETfund intervention is not necessary in our institutions	2.30	0.89	Disagree

Cumulative mean = 3.06
Criterion mean = 2.50

Table 1 above showed that the cumulative mean of the items computed as 3.06 is greater than the criterion mean of 2.50 used for statistical decision. This implies that the respondents agreed that TETfund has intervened in their institutions as according to them, the body has provided infrastructural facilities, which have been of benefits to the institutions and that there are TETfund projects in their schools. However, it was discovered also that respondents disagreed strongly on the position that there are no TETfund projects in their institutions, and that TETfund intervention is not necessary since the respective mean rating for the items was 2.36 and 2.30 respectively, which are less than the criterion mean.

Research Question Two: To what extent has TETfund contributed to infrastructural development in basic institutions in Plateaus state?

Table 2. TETfund intervention and Infrastructural Development in Basic institutions

Items	Mean	Std. deviation	Decision
There was serious decay in the area of accommodation in institutions before the introduction of TETfund	3.40	0.66	Agree
Enhances Structural development in institutions	3.18	0.74	Agree
There was total collapse of infrastructures in institutions before the introduction of TETfund	3.14	1.93	Agree
Provision of enough e-libraries in institutions	3.26	0.69	Agree
Provision of enough seats in lecture halls	3.38	0.67	Agree
Construction of better roads and drainage system	3.30	0.74	Agree

Cumulative mean = 3.28
Criterion mean = 2.50

Table 2 revealed that TETfund interventions in the area of infrastructural development in basic institutions in the state include provision of accommodation(X = 3.40), seats to halls(X = 3.38), laboratory materials(X = 3.35), and better roads and drainages(X = 3.30) among others. However, since the cumulative mean value of 3.28 computed is greater than 2.50 used as the criterion mean, it implies that all the items are areas that TETfund has intervene in basic institutions in the state.

Research Question Three: To what extent has TETfund contributed to Staff development in Basic institutions in Plateaus state?

The findings from Table 3 showed a cumulative mean of 3.34 and a criterion mean of 2.50. This means that the criterion mean is less than the cumulative mean. Based on this, we conclude that all the items are ways in which TETFund has intervened in the area of staff development in basic institutions in the state. Thus, the findings revealed that the intervention has helped in enhancing teachers skills acquisition(X = 3.76) and that it has benefited both academic and non-academic staff of the institutions(X = 3.38) and others.

Table 3. Summary of Mean Rating of TETfund Intervention and Staff Development

Items	Mean	Std. Deviation	Decision
Staff development and training	3.19	0.84	Agree
Bridges the gap between lectures and modern technology	3.12	0.71	Agree
Provided home and abroad in-service training for lecturers	3.27	0.74	Agree
Benefits to both academic and non-academic staff	3.38	0.63	Agree
TETfund has enhances skills acquisition	3.76	0.68	Agree

Cumulative mean = 3.34
Criterion mean = 2.50

8 Discussion of Findings

The finding revealed that TETfund has intervened in basic institutions in the State as there are TETfund projects in all the schools. Buttressing this view, Peter (2015) opined that TETFund intervention has significant effect on research and infrastructural development in educational institutions in Nigeria. This has significant impact on the quality of educational delivery in basic institutions.

Also, the findings revealed that there was total collapse of infrastructures facilities in basic institutions in the state before the emergence of TETFund. The results identified the contributions of TETfund on infrastructural development to include the provision of Seats in the classrooms, school library materials, structures, laboratory equipment, accommodations and the construction of roads and good drainages in the institutions among others. This agreed with the view of Bogoro (2015) that TETFund uses its funds mainly for the general improvement of education in Federal and States educational institutions.

Similarly, the findings from the analysis of research question revealed that members of staff, academic and non – academic staff have benefited from TETfund in areas such as in–service training, skills acquisition and ICT training programmes among others. It added that a good number of the teachers have been trained both at home and abroad courtesy of TETfund intervention. This finding is in line with the view of Oke (2018) that an average of ten academic staff benefits from international training programmes of TETFund sponsorships every year. This also supports the view of Bogoro (2015) who asserted that TETfunds are expected to facilitate research activities that will impact positively on the competitiveness of the country on the global scientific milieu, and build up the research capacity of Nigerian researchers to contribute to the national development efforts as well as tackle global challenges.

Therefore, with more intervention by TETfund, more Staff of the basic institutions in the State will benefit from training programmes. This concurred with the findings of Udu and Nwekede (2014) in their study on TETfund intervention in Ebonyi State University that by 2000 when EBSU started receiving allocations from the TETFund, situations started improving gradually and that EBSU has been able to experience a boost in infrastructural development; many academic staff have also received research grants; many have been sponsored to local and international seminars and conferences in addition to TETFund sponsored oversea training and retraining of academic staff.

9 Conclusion

The findings from this study revealed that TETfund intervention in basic institutions in the state cut across all the institutions, and that areas such as infrastructural development, staff development and research activities have received a boost in institutions in the state since its inception. The study found that TETfund activities have gone a long way in improving the quality of both academic and non-academic staff of the institutions owing to the multi-faceted nature of its services and activities.

TETfund has contributed immensely in the development of basic institutions in Plateau State and to ensure better service, TETfund should be supported by stakeholders in education, and its funding arrangement should be improve upon to enable the body deliver on its mandate of promoting research and innovations and in curbing the menace of infrastructural deficit in basic institutions, and supporting human capital development programmes for quality assurance in basic institutions in the State.

10 Recommendations

Based on the findings of this study, the following recommendations have been made:

i. The management of TETFund should always embark on needs assessments before embarking on project execution.
ii. TETfund should ensure that all monies released to institutions are used for the purpose for which they have been budgeted for before further demands are made to enhance transparency in the institutions.
iii. TETFund management should put in place mechanisms to evaluate all abandoned projects in basic institutions in Plateau State and also guide against diversion of TETFund monies.
iv. There is need for more enlightenment for teachers in basic institutions by TETFund desk officer on procedures for accessing the funds.
v. Non-governmental agencies and other individuals should be encouraged to assist in the provision of physical infrastructure and other needs of basic institutions for quality outputs.
vi. Government should ensure that more funds are allocated to the education sector in line with the 26% UNESCO requirement.

References

Academic Staff Union of Universities (ASUU). TETFUND: An Intervention Agency Bastardized? (2013). Accessed 23 June 2019, https://asuu-ng.org/test/nuctetfundscam.pdf

Adavbiele, J.A.: Impact of education trust fund (ETF) on basic institutions in Nigeria: J. Res. Method Educ. **6**, 18–25 (2016). www.iosrjournals.org

Akpan, C.P.: Quality assurance management in higher education. In: Bassey, S.U., Bassey, U.U. (eds.) Management of Higher Education in Africa Uyo, Nigeria Abaam Publishers (2011)

Awogwugwu, G.N.: Management of secondary schools for qualitative education: the anambra state case. In: Olagboye, A.A., Fadipe, J.O. (eds.) Management of Nigeria Education: Law Structure and Responsibilities. Nigeria, NIEPA (2009)

Ayodele, O.O.: Tax policy Reforms in Nigeria. Longman Nigeria Plc, Lagos (2006)

Bassey, S.U.: Universal Basic Education: its Funding (2004). https://www.nesu.Edu/aern/bassey./him/, Accessed 28 June 2019

Bogoro, S.E.: Sustainability of higher institutions in Nigeria: challenges and prospects. In: TET-Fund, Abuja. Paper presented at 44thAir Force Institute of Technology Convocation Lecture on August 18 (2015)

Education Trust Fund. Education Tax Fund at a Glance. ETF, Abuja (2000)

Ekong, D.: Quality: trends from UNESCO regional consultation on higher education. In: Paper of Synthesis of Regional Conference, UNESCO, Paris (2008)

Fadipe, J.O.: Efficiency indicators for quality control in Nigerian school system. In: Fadipe, J.O., Gedele, O.K. (eds.) Management of Nigerian Education Personnel Administration and Quality in Education. NIEPA, Nigeria (2000)

Jagaba, M.M.: Crisis in the management and funding of primary education in Nigeria, I960 to Date. In: Sokoto Educational Review. Faculty of Education and Extension Services, Usmanu Danfodiyo University, Sokolo, Nigeria (2008)

Oke, T.I.: Management of Primary and Secondary Education in Nigeria: Theory and Practice. University of Jos Publisher Ltd., Jos (2011a)

Oke, T.I.: School Plant Management: Principles and Practice. University of Jos press, Jos (2011b)

Oke, T.I.: Entrepreneurship education: a remedy for the menace of unemployment in Nigeria. Int. J. Educ. Stud. **1**(4), 91–99 (2013)

Oke, T.I.: Higher education policy and entrepreneurship development in Nigeria: a critical analysis. In: Studies in Educational Planning and Administration,(SEPA) Ondo, NIEPA (2018)

Omooba B.T.: Challenges of universal basic education (UBE) in Nigeria in the 21st century. In: Being a Paper Presented at the 3rd National Conference of the Federal College of Education, Katsina, 26th–29th July 2004 (2004)

Peter, N.C.: Assessment of the government funding programmes in tertiary education institutions in Nigeria South East zone. (Unpublished thesis ph.d) Ebonyi State University Abakaliki (2015). http://www.handle.net/1234678/649

Peters, R.S.: The meaning of quality in education. In: Beaby, C.C. (ed.) Qualitative Aspects of Educational Planning. UNESCO, HEP (2005)

Popoola, P.O.: Nigerian universal basic educational scheme: learning from universal primary education experience. J. Educ. Thought **1**(2) (2001)

Rufai, R.A.: Federal government allocates N25 billion to Tertiary institutions. National Universities Commission, Abuja (2012)

Samuelson, P.A.: The pure theory of public expenditure. Rev. Econ. Stat. **36**(4), 387–389 (1954)

Tahir, G.: UBE Disburses N17bn to schools. Daily Trust, p. 5 (2009)

TETFund. Allocations Abuja (2016). https://www.vanguard.ngr.com

Udu, T., Nkwede, J.O.: Tertiaryeducation trust fund interventions and sustainable development in Nigerian Universities: Evidence from Ebonyi State University, Abakaliki (2014)

UNESCO. Basic Education, Emerging Issues, Challenges and Constraints. In: The Stale, of Education' in Nigeria. UNESCO Office, Lagos (2005)

Universal Basic Education. UBE Programme: Annual Report (2003). UBE, Abuja (2004)

Universal Basic Education Commission. Basic Information on Universal Basic Education. UBEC, Abuja (2005)

Whiteley, P.: Quality assurance: its centrality to the administration of caribbean tertiary lebel. Caribbean Educ. Ann. **VI**, 13–24 (2001)

World Bank. World Bank Press Release on Education for All (2004). www.worldBank.Org/education/efa.asp, https://www.web.worldbank.org, Aug 2019

Multiculturalism, Multidisciplinarity and Inclusivity in African Education and Healthcare

J. I. Unah(✉)

Department of Philosophy, Faculty of Arts, University of Lagos, Lagos, Nigeria
junah@unilag.edu.ng

Abstract. The central problem addressed by this paper is tripartite in nature: the poor governance of diversity by political actors in developing African multiethnic and multicultural societies, the evident lack of synergy amongst academic disciplines in tertiary institutions that vitiates the capacity of their graduates to be adequately equipped for the world of work in these countries and the frequent abridgement of inclusiveness in the practice of medicine that negatively impact efficient and sustainable healthcare service to the African people. The objective is to clarify the interconnected concepts of multiculturalism, multidisciplinarity and inclusivity with a view to demonstrating how understanding of these concepts could help to resolve the problems that vitiate the capacity to govern diversity, of the difficulties besetting higher education institutions in producing graduates with problem solving skills and wealth creation capabilities and of a healthcare delivery industry that effectively addresses the health and wellness needs of the people. The three interrelated concepts are based on the theoretical framework of existential ontology of inter-subjectivity and Edmund Husserl's phenomenology of consciousness. Multiculturalism is a description of a socio-cultural situation in which identities of different cultures coexist in a geopolitical space or the characteristics of the disparate entities coexisting in a culturally diverse society. Multidisciplinarity is the practice whereby experts from different academic disciplines pool aspects of their subjects together to form a new subject of study to address a new problem or respond to emerging issues in knowledge production; which separate disciplines, working independently of each other, could not resolve. Likewise, inclusivity is the practice and advocacy of allowing that the diverse entities in an environment be harnessed for peaceful coexistence, participatory and problem solving education and teamwork practice of medicine for efficient healthcare service. The paper deploys the qualitative research methodology of critical analysis and clarification of new and existing concepts to illuminate the subject-matter and enhance understanding. This understanding will assist in setting multi-sectoral goals for the achievement of peaceful inclusive societies, sound, participatory and inclusive education, and effective, efficient, and inclusive healthcare system.

Keywords: Multiculturalism · Multidisciplinarity · African education · Inclusive healthcare

J. N. Mojekwu et al. (Eds.): *Sustainable Education and Development*, pp. 21–31, 2021.
https://doi.org/10.1007/978-3-030-68836-3_3

1 Introduction

Cultural diversity has been described as cogent and as brutally real as biodiversity (UNESCO 2001, art. 1). Cultural diversity is governed by political multiculturalism. Multiculturalism could be defined as a description of all the identities—ethnic, cultural, religious, gender, minorities, et cetera—and the characteristics of the entities warehoused in a diverse universe; it describes a situation in which entities of distinct natures and disparate cultures find themselves cohabiting or coexisting in the same environment. When properly analyzed and calibrated, multiculturalism domiciles inclusivity as its operative tool. By the same token, multidisciplinarity is "the practice in which people of different disciplines collaborate, with each drawing on the knowledge of their specialty or discipline; a practice of integrating knowledge and methods from different disciplines, forging or foisting a real synthesis of approaches or perspectives". Inclusivity is the exercise of "inviting, accommodating and integrating" elements of different traditions with the objective of achieving a desirable synthesis or a positive social purpose. Evidently, both the principles and practices of multiculturalism and multidisciplinarity domicile the doctrine of inclusivity in achieving lofty standards and people-friendly objectives for the advancement of the cause of human civilization.

Multidisciplinarity, sometimes called interdisciplinarity, is the name of what is aimed at by the inclusivity discourse; especially, as it relates to reviewing the curriculum of university education in Nigeria in general, and the healthcare discipline and industry in particular; with the conviction that 'The synergy of diverse disciplines can lead to a sweet pot" or produce a fruitful, wonderful and sustainable result in the healthcare industry (Mastro 2014).

2 Inclusivity in Multuculturalism and Multidisciplinarity

In political philosophy, multiculturalism has come to mean an understanding of the way human societies are assumed or structured to respond and possibly adapt to cultural and religious differences; often involving a whole range of issues in what has been described as "identity politics", "politics of difference", and "politics of recognition" (Song 2016); which is also about, but not limited to, economic interests and power politics in the allocation or distribution of resources adjudged to be a commonwealth or resources belonging to all (Song 2016). Multiculturalism is not only about the recognition of identities and the differences obtaining amongst them for which mutual respect and mutual cooperation becomes imperative, it is also about the recognition and respect for 'diversity within diversities' in such a way that appeal to cultural rights must never be used as an excuse to persecute ethnic and religious minorities, the different others or persons with disability, or persons with different sexual orientations (UNESCO 2005, art. 2).

It is on account of considerations of these sorts that UNESCO 2001 (art. 1) made a declaration recognizing diverse ethnicities, practices and orientations of humans across the globe as elements in the definition of multiculturalism in these words: 'Culture takes diverse forms across time and space. This diversity is embodied in the uniqueness and plurality of the identities of the groups and societies making up humankind. As a source of exchange, innovation and creativity, cultural diversity is as necessary for humankind as biodiversity is for nature. In this sense, it is the common heritage of humanity and should be recognized and affirmed for the benefit of present and future generations." UNESCO makes the point that a fully developed consciousness or understanding of the import of multiculturalism implies that it is the only available guarantor of peace, security and social cohesion, and a springboard of development, as well as an "ethical imperative, inseparable from respect for human dignity" (UNESCO 2001, art. 4). This is the understanding of multiculturalism or expression of cultural diversity that works.

3 Uses and Applications

The positive use and application of multiculturalism is that deriving from the nature, meaning and imperatives of cultural diversity which demands the recognition and acceptance of identities and their differences [be they groups or individuals] within a universe of multiplicities. This understanding allows for distinct and disparate identities [individuals or groups] within a society, especially a society put together by imperial power for administrative convenience, to retain their uniqueness by self-expression and self-determination in socio-cultural and economic activities within their jurisdictions or natural habitats, while maintaining cordial relations and cooperation with contiguous other groups or individuals; either by geographical proximity or political affiliation with some distant entities. This way of understanding cultural diversity or multiculturalism fosters the spirit of inclusiveness. Cultures are defined by the self-expression and self-determination of groups and of individuals within them; even as they collaborate and cooperate with people of other cultures. This means that the principle of inclusivity warehouses three internal sub-principles namely, Self-expression, Self-determination, and Cooperation. What this means is that in any major activity affecting all the groups, each group is entitled and required to participate with equal recognition, on the basis of equality. This is the meaning of inclusiveness; of which the contrary practice will breed discord, mutual distrust, inter-group antagonism, hate speech, and strife. Thus, inclusivity means and demands,

[i] The practice of self-expression, whereby cultural identities use their language for the transmission of the knowledge of nature and culture, including but not limited to, traditions, customs and values, religious beliefs and practices, et cetera; while conceding similar rights to other identities or groups including the individuals within the larger collectivity;

[ii] The practice of self-determination, whereby individuals and groups within a cultural identity or ethnicity explores and exploits the resources available in their natural environment or habitat and contribute to the larger collectivity as defined by their operating manual or article of association usually called the constitutions of state, and

[iii] The practice of intergroup cooperation because each cultural group or identity is assured and guaranteed its duties, obligations and rights.

Evidently, the concept of inclusion, inclusiveness or inclusivity, as it is interchangeably used, is intertwined with the concept of multiculturalism or cultural diversity; where larger or dominant groups and state actors understand the latter [cultural diversity] as the existence of diverse cultural groups with natural, inalienable, rights to self-expression and self-determination which must be respected by other groups and individuals within the larger collectivity. Consequently, for any multicultural society, such as Nigeria, seeking to achieve the peace necessary for development and the realization of enlightened self-interest and prosperity by individuals and groups domiciled in its territorial jurisdiction, the following should constitute some critical agenda for immediate attention:-

1. The law-making assembly should uphold and issue a declaration that ethnic and religious identities or groups have inalienable right to self-expression, in whatever form they deem fit within the confines of the law of the land; including but not limited to the right to exist in their natural habitat devoid of molestation, harassment, dislocation, assaults and forceful eviction from and occupation of their ancestral lands;
2. The legislature should direct that executive action[s] should guarantee safety of life and property of all citizens, as provided for in the country's constitution;
3. The legislature should declare and direct that migrant populations from other parts of the country should also be protected against unwarranted discriminations and attacks by host communities where they carry on the economic activities of pastoralism and nomadism; provided that they too respect the rights of their hosts to practice farming occupation and their farmlands and belongings protected from destruction by the activities of cattle herding;
4. That the law assembly should direct the executive arm to make adequate provisions for herders in parts of the country with adequate facilities to accommodate them peacefully, while exploring a more durable option of assisting them to improving husbandry occupation in accord with global best practices; such as commercial ranching.
5. That the issue of security threats arising from the upsurge in violent banditry and kidnapping, now assuming epidemic proportions across the country, should be tackled with commitment and professionalism by the security forces, by directing and funding community policing for effectiveness, and allowing the military to concentrate on tackling the insurgency in the north eastern part of the country, and
6. That there is a need for the power structure of the country to provide for sustainable inclusive opportunity for self-determination of the cultural identities comprising the union.

The point in all of this is the application of the principle of inclusion inherent in cultural diversity in addressing the problem of insecurity in the country with insistence on community policing; which commonsense and global best practice dictate; the resolution of the herders-farmers crisis by assisting both parties to be fully involved in taking part in conversations and decisions that would not encroach on each other's rights, and in the protection of the expression of cultural rights in verbal, religious, artistic, and traditional practices; including the rights of the different others, as well as ethnic and sexual minorities, and disadvantaged identities.

Where multiculturalism or cultural diversity is used as a veil for domination and a tendency to ethnic cleansing or where it is used to surreptitiously impose a monolithic culture or 'describe a narrative in which the need for the protection of the rights of native dwellers against the invasion of domineering migrant populations seeking to impose their life ways or culture on aboriginal communities and peoples,' such as present day Nigeria, there would be a tendency to disintegration. This is because where the desire to dominate is strong on the part of the domineering group, in an arrangement originally put together by colonial fiat, there is often a tendency to separatism, and multiculturalism can't work as an integrative policy. The quicker the separation of the distinct groups into autonomous communities or independent republics, the greater the possibility of sub-regional peace. And any country or nation state where sustainable inclusive societies cannot be guaranteed, separation is the best option for peaceful coexistence; not genocide. This is because the tendency to domination and the imposition of monolithic culture in a diverse nation is utterly antithetical to the ethos of cultural diversity, and it has been responsible for genocidal activities in sub-Saharan Africa. Olanrewaju et al. (2017) and Udebunu (2011) have all agonized over the pretentious and idiosyncratically wayward multiculturalism or its subversion for the advancement of monolithic agenda by some state actors in Nigeria. And this tendency to subvert the ethos of cultural diversity has been clearly identified as the veritable source of the internecine conflicts warned about in the UNESCO Universal Declaration on Cultural Diversity; amply referenced in the United Nations Report on Cultural Rights (UN Report 2018).

On positive multiculturalism, Canada readily comes to mind as a country that authentically practices cultural diversity; but the historical context is different from that of Nigeria; as it had no history of forced coexistence or amalgamation of culturally disparate identities. A combination of the factors of sociology of mixed colonial experience [French and English], an initially assimilated nativity, and the fact of migrant influx produced an ingenious multiculturalism that has become the apple eye of Europe and the envy of nearby America and the world. Canada's cultural diversity was passed into law by parliament in 1988; making the country the first in recorded history to pass a multiculturalism law as official political policy of integration; which is second to none in practical terms, owing to its unpretentious and unwavering application of inclusivity principle in welding a culturally heterogeneous society into what has been described, not as a 'melting pot' or 'sweet pot' or 'salad bowl', but as a "cultural mosaic" (Brosseau and Dewing 2018). The idea of a cultural mosaic is intended to suggest a form of multiculturalism, different from other systems such as "melting pot", often used to describe the United States' much touted assimilationist policy (Gibbon 1938).

In any event, it does not appear the American melting pot or the Canadian cultural mosaic would work in Nigeria. Intersubjective or consensual multiculturalism is the type that may work in Nigeria; given the history and antecedents of its people. Now, what does consensual or intersubjective multiculturalism mean?

The brute reality of sparse migration regardless, most African societies are autochthonous communities; with historically entrenched cultural value systems that they seek enabling infrastructure to develop for use and export to the world. Is it the Edo, the Yoruba, the Hausa/Fulani, the Biron, the Igala, the Ika, the Igbo, the Tiv, the Gboko, the Isoko, the Urhobo, the Kalabari, the Ibibio, and a host of other identities too numerous to exhaustively mention here, with their deeply seated cultural values that anybody or any group can coercively assimilate? What they all seek is the genuine political space to participate, develop their cultural confidence and contribute to the pool of mankind's heritage. They all seek to be brought to the front burner by inclusion to express their reality and determine the way they want to be. This innate desire can only be actualized in a consensual multicultural space in which no groups or individuals are harassed or traumatized in freely choosing their way of being.

4 Theoretical Framework of Intersubjective Multiculturalism

The concept of intersubjective or consensual multiculturalism avers that every identity and historical entity has a title to legitimacy and space for the free expression of the human spirit, and for creativity and innovation, and for further development of capacities and capabilities; and that every individual or group has a unique contribution which it is destined to make from its subjectivity and cultural specificity to advance the cause human civilization. Intersubjective multiculturalism proceeds from the basic assumption of existential ontology that truth about anything springs from human subjectivity, which finds expression in and corroboration with other subjectivities (Unah 1996, pp, 214–215). It builds on the phenomenological theory of the intentionality of consciousness, espoused by Edmund Husserl, which maintains that thought or consciousness is free and always about something, real or imagined (Husserl 1970, pp. 8–24). It also avers that whatever it is that consciousness is about can lead to the creation of values; or the discovery of new ways of doing, new epistemologies, for the promotion of happiness and human flourishing. It asserts that every creation, every system of values, is a product of culture, and that all cultures in a universe represent diverse ways of self-expression of identities, of groups, of individuals, cohabiting a geopolitical space; and complementing each other for the production of peaceful and sustainable inclusive societies. Unarguably, therefore, wherever there are diverse identities creating multiple cultures, inclusion or inclusivity becomes an organizing principle. Thus, inclusion arising from intersubjective consensus is the tool of diversity in propelling peaceful coexistence and prosperity of nations. Collectivities of diverse cultures that fail to integrate their members inclusively will forever remain in turmoil or disintegrate.

5 Inclusivity in Education

Multidisciplinarity or interdisciplinary approach to learning is implied by, aims at, and thrives on inclusivity or the practice of inclusion; a development that has become necessary in tertiary education to assure synergy in practice or overcome the threats of disciplinary irrelevance or a desire to fill identified knowledge gap. The design or creation of inclusive courses or programmes becomes imperative when disciplines or courses fail to attract sustainable students' enrollment or subscription or when practice is repeatedly pointing in the direction of broader knowledge capacity of its workforce; or where recruiting organizations are continually seeking employees that can multitask or who possess capacities and capabilities for broad based understanding, instead of graduates of narrow specialties.

The practice of inclusivity in the multidisciplinary approach to learning happens when leaders or experts of traditional disciplines come together to select and integrate relevant courses from different disciplines to create a new programme or programmes for the expansion of knowledge production or to answer to the demands of industry and society. New programmes have emerged in the Nigerian university system to integrate or synergize existing disciplines. Geophysics or Geosciences have been created by integrating elements of geography, geology and physics, for instance; and courses in architecture, geography, and management have been synergized to form new programme[s]. Courses in history, law, philosophy and sociology can be integrated to form a programme in refugee studies. Courses in philosophy, education, sociology and law can be synergized to create a programme or course of study in public ethics. And courses in medicine, clinical sciences and ethics [philosophy] can be or has been integrated to form a programme in public medicine. I tried to get philosophy, political science and economics to create a public service discipline; after its popular brand in Oxford University, the PPE programme; but that has not happened, and the Obafemi Awolowo University, Ile-Ife, has taken the initiative and has mounted the programme already. And because of the way it has positively impacted public service in Britain, the PPE is one of the most popular programmes at the University of Oxford; being that it has produced a large number of British prime ministers, parliamentarians, and journalists (Beckett 2017).

Inclusion and interdisciplinarity in university education in Nigeria can mean integrating industry practice with the curriculum; already begun by the incumbent University of Lagos Management, with its partnership with 20 business organizations for its Entrepreneurship Education programme; a vision to prepare University of Lagos graduates for job and wealth creation! Incidentally, this is the model practiced in South Korea, perhaps, in several other Asian countries; adjudged already as quite impactful to society and very successful. Unfortunately, time will not allow me to elaborate on this.

However, an expanded version of the South Korean model can be proposed for experimentation. This expanded model demands that the admission policy of universities should require prospective candidates to pre-register with any vocational practice as apprentices for skill acquisition while pursuing a degree programme. The objective is to ensure that university students are allowed by regulation to engage with any vocation while studying for their degrees to ensure that they acquire a skill before graduation. This is already being practiced by some students who are thinking ahead. Making it into a policy will encourage more students to do it, especially if one full lecture-free day and half day of Saturdays every week is allowed for such an undertaking. In doing this, all relevant agencies and stakeholders should be involved and carried along.

6 Anticipating and Addressing Challenges

But since the practice of inclusion in university education is essentially multidisciplinary; which can be perceived to mean the poaching of traditional disciplines to create 'salad bowl' courses or programmes that may become more popular than the parent courses, there is need for caution; as this often goes with a whittling down of the quality and potency of disciplinary contents; usually attracting snide comments and scathing criticisms from leaders of the traditional courses or disciplines. So, inclusion and multidisciplinary approach to learning are not without difficulties and challenges; which demands frequent engagement with the stakeholders to identify genuine fears, misgivings, and misunderstandings, and address them.

Accordingly, inclusivity and interdisciplinarity mean inclusive faculty and collaborative effort in selecting courses and designing programmes involving an amalgam of cognate and diverse disciplines; it means designing programmes that increase the diversity of leaders, teachers, learners, and other categories of staff. Inclusive faculty will be identified with the principles of belongingness, being recognized and being valued. Inclusive faculty should be conscious of the impact of inclusion on 'engagement, recruitment and retention,' and on productivity and performance. Above all, inclusive faculty will be recognized by its responsiveness to how people perceive inclusion and a willingness to introduce changes that resonate with stakeholders (Chaudhry and Higgins 2003).

Exploring the idea of inclusive and integrative curriculum approaches in teaching which, he thinks, promotes active learning, Odeh, entertains a somewhat different notion of inclusion or multidisciplinarity, as he speaks of three different curriculums—multidisciplinary, interdisciplinary, and transdisciplinary curriculums; each with a distinctive slant to inclusivity. The first entails studying a topic from the perspective of more than a single discipline "and solving a problem using a different disciplinary approach", a position that he attributes to Klaassen (2018), (Odeh 2018); the second is about fostering an understanding of theories that cut across disciplines and "highlighting the process and meaning rather than" forging a synthesis of different disciplinary contents. This is to be found in Odeh (2018), and the third approach which he characterizsed as "removing the boundaries between the core disciplines" and blending them to form an entirely new context of "real-world themes" thus introducing a different stream course altogether; a curriculum structure that Odeh attributes to Doyle and Bozzone (2018). These different curriculum structures are the forms that inclusive education takes in many modern universities; the University of Lagos inclusive. Now, what about inclusion in the health care industry?

7 Inclusion in Healthcare Industry

In several healthcare journals, inclusion is more or less construed as the fostering of the congenial or conducive conditions including multidisciplinary teamwork necessary for efficient and successful delivery of health care services to patients or members of the public. In other words, inclusive healthcare is conceived as multidisciplinary teamwork in healthcare delivery. Quoting the introductory of William Mayo's Inaugural address delivered in 1910 to the Rush Medical College, Charlotte Hughes writes: "It has become necessary to develop medicine as a cooperative science; the clinician, the specialist, and the laboratory workers uniting for the good of the patient, each assisting in elucidation of the problem at hand, and each dependent upon the other for support" (Hughes 2018). Admitting that healthcare is, by nature and design, a multidisciplinary profession whereby doctors, nurses, and health professionals from diverse specialties are brought together to work as a team, engaging each other frequently in conversations, and sharing resources together; Hughes identified two clear conditions of a successful inclusive delivery of health services, namely:

[i] That health teams must be in a position to make a comprehensive evaluation of a patient's illness or disease, and follow it up with a full-fledged plan of treatment, and
[ii] That the team should possess a capacity to collaborate to "create and promote health initiatives for diverse communities and to provide education to instill disease-prevention behaviors amongst patients" (Hughes 2018).

Hughes goes further to draw up an ethic for better outcomes; being that the factors of complex and specialized clinical care, 'aging populations and the increase of chronic diseases such as diabetes, heart disease, cancer', et cetera, and the challenge of managing and caring for patients with multiple health issues have combined forces to render inclusive multidisciplinary teamwork inevitable. She lists inclusive work ethics as,

[a] Respect and trust among members
[b] Efficient use of skill mix within the team
[c] Endorsed clinical governance structures by the team, and
[d] Endorsed systems and protocols by the team for communication and interaction among team members.

And citing *The AMA Journal of Ethics*, Hughes (2018) identifies three core competences of sustainable inclusive teamwork as [i] maximizing collective intelligence [ii] inclusive collaboration, and [iii] open communication (Hughes 2018); all of which are enhanced by constant instructions and training. Reinforcing this perspective, Mayo and Woolley (2016) aver that "Teams are smartest when everyone feels free to speak up and function best when leadership is inclusive and patient focused."

Added to the foregoing is the fact that internet and digital technology have opened up frontiers and opportunities for exploring and realizing the full potentials and benefits of multidisciplinary care [MDC]; indicating that inclusive collaboration beckons in the healthcare industry to the extent that increased knowledge of patients about the nature of their disease and the therapeutic options available to them means that more and more patients are eager to participate in therapeutic decisions (Fuentes-Afflick 2018).

8 Recommendations and Conclusion

It does appear that the integration of African herbal medicine as part of the multidisciplinary health [MDC] programme for a holistic healthcare system is inevitable. Inclusion should not be advocated and promoted only in the context of orthodox [western] medicine. The way for integration and inclusion to work seamlessly is for all brands of practice of medicine to be recognized, promoted, valued and supported; just as orthodox medicine is recognized, promoted, valued and supported. Leaders, experts and practitioners of orthodox western medicine should be wooed and won over by proponents of the inclusivity project; for they are the stakeholders that would ultimately recommend funding for research and development of African herbal medicine. Perhaps, we may begin by referring patients and clients not responding to clinical treatment to some registered traditional African healthcare practitioners for participation in healthcare service delivery. There are reported cases of ailments not successfully treated or that defied orthodox medicine which had been competently handled by herbal practitioners. Inclusive multidisciplinary healthcare can bring more of such cases into the public domain. Test results from medical laboratories of some diseases explainable in the vernacular could also be frontloaded to the qualified or registered herbal practitioners for treatment.

Funding support for investigative research of aspects of traditional medicine practice is another way that experts and scholars in academic medicine can promote inclusion of alternative medicine; just as the Chinese and other cultures have done to develop their indigenous medicine.

More importantly, inclusivity project in the health industry should frontally deal with issues of discrimination against gender; against neglected, relegated, underserved, disadvantaged persons and groups; as well as the different others and stigmatized sexual minorities, and integrate them into the nation's public healthcare delivery system; to midwife a holistic and inclusive sustainable healthcare delivery regime and culture.

There is a need for the practitioners of the inclusivity project to encourage their stakeholders to subscribe to courses in ethics offered in the Departments of Philosophy nationwide; that is, for students in medicine, law, architecture, education, business, political science, et cetera to offer relevant courses in ethics, aesthetics, epistemology, and ontology; to broaden their outlook and capacity for critical moral judgment and rigorous logical thinking.

Pre-tertiary pupils and students, at the primary and secondary levels of education, require pre-university orientation and training in moral character, and the principles of creative, imaginative, and critical, logical thinking; all of which fall within the mandate of philosophy to provide. The inclusivity project should join forces with philosophy in propagating the teaching of moral character and cognate subjects at the basic levels of education to equip and fortify them with the Ubuntu morality of a "We" rather than an "I" to prepare the ground for the emergence of a new generation of Nigerian citizenry that would subscribe to university education ready to unleash their creative, disciplined, understanding of the meaning of the principles of diversity and inclusion in the pursuit of higher knowledge and learning, to emerge after graduation as young men and women of learning and character.

In congruence with the principles of inclusivity and multidisciplinary education, undergraduate students should be assisted to connect properly with industry, acquire entrepreneurial skills and competencies for job creation and wealth creation; and their teachers involved in the teaching of the new inclusive curriculum should be sufficiently engaged not to allow any room for occupation by unwholesome thoughts, and thus, render ineffectual the generational curse of suicide-committing students and faculty. With well-thought out inclusive education curriculum, university undergraduates and their lecturers should be adequately preoccupied with engaging scholarship to make the thought of joining their ancestors forcibly and prematurely unattractive. Inclusive and multidisciplinary education, when properly understood and executed, should put an end to the boring, frustrating and, sometimes, purposeless engagements that make teaching and learning a nightmarish endeavour.

Finally, the analysis of the concept of multiculturalism indicates that it is the political expression of cultural diversity or ethnic pluralism in the literature. Cultural diversity is such a brute reality that a mono-cultural society is inconceivable. Diversity implies inclusiveness for the sustenance of peaceful coexistence in human societies.

References

Beckett, A.: PPE: the Oxford degree that runs Britain. theguardian.com (2017)

Brosseau, L., Dewing, M.: Canadian Multiculturalism (2018). Background Paper: 15 Sept 2009, Revised on: 03 Jan 2018, No. 2009-20-E. https://www.canada.ca>services>culture

Chaudhry, A.S., Higgins, S.: On the need for a multidisciplinary approach to education for knowledge management. Libr. Rev. **52**(2), 65–69 (2003). https://doi.org/10.1108/00242530310462134

Doyle, M., Bozzone, D.: Multidisciplinary teaching providing undergraduates with the skills to integrate knowledge and tackle “big” questions. J. Cent. Interdisc. Teach. Learn. **7**(1), 12–17 (2018)

Fuentes-Afflick, E.: Promoting Inclusion in Academic Medicine. JAMA Netw. Open **1**(4), e181010 (2018). https://doi.org/1001/jamanetworkopen.2018.1010

Gibbon, J.: The Canadian Mosaic. McClelland & Stewart Limited (1938). www.definitions.net. Accessed 01 Sept 2019

Hughes, C.: Multidisciplinary Teamwork Ensures Better Healthcare Outcomes (2018). https://www.td.org/insights/multidisciplinary-teamwork-ensures-better-healthcare-outcomes

Husserl, E.: The Paris Lectures. Translated by Petter Koestenbaum. Martinus Nijhoff, The Hague (1970)

Klaassen, R.G.: Interdisciplinary education: a case study. J. Eng. Educ. **43**(6), 842–859 (2018)

Mayo, A.T., Woolley, A.W.: Teamwork in health care: maximizing collective intelligence via inclusive collaboration and open communication. AMA J. Ethics **18**(9), 933–940 (2016). https://doi.org/10.1001/journalofethics.2016.18.9.stas2-1609

Mastro, V.A.: A Cornucopia of Multidisciplinary Teaching (2014). Edutopia. Accessed 8 Aug 2014

Odeh, S.: Multidisciplinary teaching: an approach to active learning (2018). https://learningandteaching-navitas.com/multidisciplinary-teaching-approach-active-learning/. Accessed 24 Sept 2018

Olarenwaju, I.P., Loromoke, E.R., Adekoye, R.A.: Multiculturalism, value differences and cross-cultural conflicts in Nigeria: surgery on a centenarian. J. Afr. Union Stud. **6**(1), 39–62 (2017)

Song, S.: Multiculturalism. Stanford Encyclopedia of Philosophy: plato.stanford.edu (2016)

Udubunu, C.: Nigeria and the dialectics of multiculturalism. Ogirisi: New J. Afr. Stud. **8**(1), 1–15 (2011). https://doi.org/10.4314/og.v8i1.1

Unah, J.I.: Phenomenology. In: Unah, J. (ed.) Metaphysics, Phenomenology and African Philosophy. Hope Publications, Ibadan (1996)

UN Report on Cultural Rights: Universality, Cultural Diversity and Cultural Right (2018). https://undocs.org/en/A/43/227

UNESCO: UNESCO Convention on the Protection and Promotion of the Diversity of Cultural Expressions. Article 2, 2005 (2005)

UNESCO: Universal Declaration on Cultural Diversity. Articles 1 & 4, 2001 (2001)

The Challenges of Girl Child Education in Sokoto State, Nigeria and Its Implications for National Development

M. J. Haruna(✉) and A. Nafisa

Department of Education Foundation, Shehu Shagari College of Education, Sokoto, Sokoto State, Nigeria

Abstract. The study investigated the challenges of Girl Child Education in Sokoto State, Nigeria and its implications for National Development. The population of the study is One Thousand, Five Hundred and Twenty one (1,521) lecturers drawn from Shehu Shagari College of Education, Sokoto and Alhaji Umaru Ali Shinkafi Polytechnic, Sokoto. A sample size of three hundred and six (306) was used for the study. A thirteen items structured questionnaire of strongly Agree, Agree, Disagree, Strongly Disagree and Undecided was used for data collection on the assumed variables of the challenges of Girl Child Education and its implications for National Development. Descriptive statistics of frequency count and percentages was employed to determine the level and percentage responses of the respondents to the questionnaire items. The findings of the study revealed that majority of school age girls in Sokoto state are out of school as indicated by 67% of the respondents on the statement made on this variable and that most of the respondents agreed that dropout syndrome is one of the major challenges affecting the development of Girl child education in the state. It was also discovered that majority of girls passing out from secondary schools in Sokoto state have low aspiration for higher education as well as the study of science and technology courses. Religious misconception by parents and economic problems also largely contributed to the factors affecting the development of Girl Child Education. Based on the findings of the study appropriate recommendations such as need for improved funding on education, establishment of more Centres for Continuing Education and introduction of Empowerment Programme that will help to improve the economic well being of parents were advanced.

1 Introduction

Education is a fundamental tool for national development. This explains why Mangvwat as cited in Haruna (2004) describes education as one of the indicators of level of social development of a nation. The role of female education to this effect is particularly important because they are partners in progress and play important roles on child bearing and rearing, home maintenance, to mention but a few. In a study of two hundred Countries conducted by King and Hill (1992) they found that there is relationship between a nation's economic development and female education where countries with a large gender gap measured as a ratio between past male and female school enrolment will have lower

J. N. Mojekwu et al. (Eds.): *Sustainable Education and Development*, pp. 32–42, 2021.
https://doi.org/10.1007/978-3-030-68836-3_4

economic productivity than another country with the same amount of capital stock and labour force but smaller gender gap in education. It is thus not amazing that several global interventions towards girls' right to education such as UNESCO, the education for All (EFA), the United Nations Girls Initiative (UNGEI) etc. have stressed the need for enhancing girl child education.

In Sokoto state, Nigeria, female education is surrounded by numerous challenges relating to large stock of girl that are out of school, school withdrawal syndrome, low attitude towards the study of science and technology among others. Hence the need for finding out the causes of this phenomenon with a view to providing necessary suggestion on how to address the problem in order to give the female folk in the state necessary opportunity(ies) to meaningfully participate and contribute to national development.

2 Conceptual Definition of Terms

The following terms as used in the write up are hereby defined as follows:-

Girl Child: The girl child may be described as an offspring from birth to eighteen (18) Years of age Haruna (2004). This is in agreement with Dashen and Dushen (2004) description that girl child falls within the framework of the eighteen years.

National Development: National development refers to the sum total of positive changes that a country puts forward to attain over a period of time which will have positive impact on the nation's citizenries. This is normally achieved through various efforts of the nation's citizens – groups and individuals. This is in line with the opinion of Chiaknaan and Ahmad (2009) that changes which are positively inclined and which occur for the interest of the entire society is what is referred to as national development.

Challenges: This refers to the different forms of hindrance to the development of girl child education and thereby placing the girl child to the disadvantaged position of being able to meaningfully and effectively contribute to the issue of national development.

3 Statement of the Problem

Sokoto state of Nigeria according to Ibrahim et al. (2019), Haruna and Yabo (2009) is considered as one of the educationally backward states in Nigeria especially in the area of girl child education. This, for instance, explains why female education in the state appears to be characterized by the phenomena of low aspiration for higher education, less interest in the study of science and technology subjects/courses, school dropout for school syndrome as well as low turnout for school by the girl child (Ibrahim et al. 2019). The causes of these problems include, among others, religious misconception, poverty and socio-cultural perception to mention but a few. Since education is the strongest tool for effective national development, this situation undoubtedly and grossly affects the females' role in national development. This is so because it hinders them from actualizing their human and intellectual potentialities, which limits their chances of gainful employment, political participation in the nation's body polity among others. There is no gain saying that females are partners in progress and no nation can fully develop without the factor of females. Hence, the needs for a research work on the challenges being faced by the girl child in the educationally backward state of Sokoto, Nigeria and which affects their ability to contribute to National Development. In essence, this research was intended to link the issue girl child education with national development contrary to other researches which only viewed girl child education from such perspectives as academic achievements, socio cultural view point and attitude to school learning/education (Haruna 2004, Ibrahim et al. 2019, Hashimu et al. 2017 and Kebbi and Sifawa 2017). The objectives of the study are to identify the challenges of girl child education in Sokoto state vis a-vis the issue of National Development; to find out the effects of the challenges of girl child education in Sokoto state on national development and to determine the solution to the challenges being faced by the girl child education in Sokoto.

4 Theoretical Framework

The Phenomenon of female marginalization and existence of educational gap between the male and the female folk has long been a source of concern to educationists and researchers (Haruna 2004, Haralambos and Holborn 2008 and Haruna and Yabo 2009) to mention but a few. This scenario may not be unconnected with numerous problems surrounding the development of female education among many communities in Nigeria and in Sokoto State in particular and which affects the latter's chances to effectively contribute to National Development. In view of the importance attached to the female education, the issue of gender educational gap has been viewed from different theoretical perspectives such as the structural functionalists, the symbolic interactionism and the social conflict. The social conflict theory according to Macionis (1989) is a theoretical framework based on the view that society as a system is characterized by social inequalities and social conflict that generate social change. Against this background, this Research was based on the premise of the conflict theoretical framework. This theory attempts to challenge the humanly caused social inequalities among social groups and individuals as is the case with the social status of Girl Child Education in Sokoto state which placed the Girl Child on the disadvantaged position when compared with their male counterpart in terms of general response and access to western type of school education and this no doubt affects their national development.

5 The Concept of Girl Child Education

The girl child according to Offorma (2009), is a biological female offspring from birth to eighteen (18) years of age. In the same vein, Dashen and Dashen (2004) as previously used talked of the girl child as falling within the framework of age eighteen years. This according to them suggests that it is a formative age which coincides with the primary and secondary education levels of education. At this age parents play significant role in upbringing the girl child. The education of the girl child of recent has become a bone of contention for individuals, governments and non-government organizations which according to Maisaje (2011) is due to the mixed feelings attached to the girl child education. This according to him is based on some social and cultural practices that were inimical to giving formal education to the girl child.

Girl Child Education and National Policy on Education (NPE): The position of the Nigeria's National Policy on Education on the importance attached to the girl child education is very categorical and clear. For instance, the NPE (2013) says "Education is compulsory and a right for every Nigerian irrespective of gender, social status, religion, ethnic background and any peculiar individual challenges". Furthermore the NPE emphasizes "provision of equal access to qualitative educational opportunities for all citizens at all levels". Thus, the NPE is not discriminative on the issue of girl child education and this may not be unconnected with the feeling that girls (if educated) will be better prepared and equipped to effectively contribute to national development.

Importance of Girl Child Education for National Development: A popular adage maintains that when you educate a girl you educate a nation and society but when you educate a man, you educate an individual and a single soul. This assertion according to Haruna (2011) recognized the role of female folk as mothers, home makers as well as their role (if educated) in the social, economic and political development of a nation. Against this background, the importance of gild child education to National Development has been variedly described and confirmed by scholars, educationists and researchers. Razaq (2006), for instance, maintain that "whether in technology, industry or science education helps to ensure adequate supply of human resources needed for national development". Hence if educated the girl child will according to Audu (2011) greatly enhance National Development. This is so because girls have potentials which need to be unfolded or helped to develop through education and training. Politically, every nation depends on enlightened citizenry to arrive at meaningful decisions that will guide it to achieve its various programmes policies and agendas. Thus education according to Haruna (2011) helps enhance the females' political participation and development. Research conducted in Nigeria and elsewhere have also confirmed the existence of relationship between female education and economic development of a nation. For instance, King and Hill (1992) in their study of two hundred (200) countries discovered that there is correlation between female education and economic development of a nation. Their findings revealed that a country with a large gender gap measured as a ratio between past male and female school enrolment with lower will have economic productivity than another country with the same amount of capital stock and labour force but smaller gap in education.

From the foregoing it is evident that the importance of female education for national development cannot be overemphasized.

Factors Affecting the Development of Girl Child Education in Sokoto State: In spite of the importance of the girl child education as previously discussed, the issue of girl child education in Sokoto state is still lagging behind and this in no doubt is affecting the Nigeria's national development in general and Sokoto state in particular. A number of factors are responsible for this scenario. These factors include among others low enrolment, poverty, dropout syndrome, religious and socio-cultural misconceptions, unemployment problem, low morale towards the study of science and technology as well as low aspiration for higher education.

The global figure for out of school according to Abdulrahman (2016) is estimated at 121 million, 65 million being girls and over 80% of these girls live in sub Sahara Africa (Daily Sun: July 25: 15), In the same vein, UNESCO (2000) states that 40% of Nigerian children aged 6–11 do not attend primary school with the Northern Nigeria region (where Sokoto state falls under) recording the lowest school attendance rate in the country particularly for girls.

The factor of poverty remains a major impediment to the growth and development of girl child education in Nigeria generally and in Sokoto state in particular. The poverty level in the Nigeria's rural areas has from 1980–1996 rose from 18%–70% and Momoh (2002) notes that over 50% of Nigerians are poor and live below one American Dollar per day. This situation affects the development of the girl child education in no small measure as many parents and families cannot afford meaningful support for the education of their wards especially the girl child. This explains cases of the phenomenon of school dropout rate as confirmed by Offorma (2009) and UNICEF (2003).

Religion and social cultural misconception contributes a lot to the low state of girl child education in Sokoto state. Western Education was synonymous with Christian religion in those days and Islam predated Christianity in the Northern part of Nigeria (where Sokoto state falls under). Hence people from this part of the country were and many are still skeptical about western education which allows free interaction of boys and girls and as Christianity inclined education system. Hence, many parents according to Haruna (2004) perceives it as capable of exposing girls to moral laxity and which according to UNICEF (2001) parents use to justify early marriage for their female wards. It is however pertinent to note that Islam as a religion is not against the girl child education because the first verse revealed to Prophet Muhammad (PBUH) says "Read in the name of thy Lord" which means go to school and acquire knowledge. In line with this, the daughter of a renowned Islamic Scholar, reformist and Jihadist, Usman Bn Fodio by name Nana Asmau played a lot of role in the promotion of the female education in the then Sokoto Caliphate during her time.

6 Research Methodology

The research design for this study was descriptive survey. Accordingly, the data collected from the respondents to the research questionnaire were analyzed using descriptive frequency percentage count in which the responses were respectively grouped into positive and negative categories. The positive category covers all responses that fall under strongly agree and agree options while the negative category fall within the strongly disagree and disagree options as provided in the questionnaire.

7 Population

The population size for this study is one thousand, five hundred and twenty one (1,521) lecturers drawn from Shehu Shagari College of education (SSCOE) Sokoto and AlhajiUmaru Ali Shinkafi Polytechnic (AUASP) Sokoto. The breakdown of this population is made up of eight hundred and ninety three (893) lecturers from SSCOE and six hundred and twenty eight (628) lecturers from AUASP. The choice of these institutions and their lecturers was based on the premise that the two higher institutions of learning are respectively the oldest and the biggest institutions owned by the state. The lecturers from these institutions are mostly state indigenes and were drawn from the three senatorial districts (East, Central and West) of the state and include both male and female. Hence, these lecturers are in good position to provide representative information on the existing status of girl child education in different parts of the state.

8 Sampling Technique and Sample Size

Simple random sampling method was adopted to select a sample size of three hundred and six (306) respondents comprising of two hundred and six male lecturers and one hundred female lecturers respectively were used for this study. Accordingly, one hundred and eighty (180) lecturers were drawn from SSCOE while one hundred and twenty six (126) lecturers were drawn from AUASP. And in both cases male and female lecturers were used.

9 Instrumentation

A self-designed questionnaire titled The challenges of Girl Child Education Questionnaire (TCGEQ) of five options of strongly agree, agree, disagree, strongly disagree, undecided (Likert Scale) was employed to collect relevant information from the options offered for the respondents on the assumed variables on the challenges of girl child education in Sokoto state and its implications for national development.

10 Validity of the Instrument

To ensure the validity of the instrument, the questionnaire was validated by three experts from the Departments of educational foundations, curriculum and instruction and educational psychology and counseling, Shehu Shagari College of education, Sokoto.

11 Reliability of the Instrument

Reliability is a measure of degree to which instruments will yield constant results offer repeated trials. To achieve this, the instrument was pilot tested and a reliability coefficient of 0.76 was obtained (Table 1).

Table 1. Challenges of girl child education

S/N	Statement	Scores	% Positive scores	% Negative score	Total percentage
1	Majority of girls of school age in Sokoto state are out of school	712/1065	67	23	100%
2	Drop syndrome is not one of the challenges affecting the development of girl child education in Sokoto state	713/1065	23	67	100%
3	Most girls passing out from secondary schools in Sokoto state have high aspiration for higher education	704/1065	34	66	100%
4	Female students in Sokoto state have high morale towards the study of science and technology subjects/courses	692/1065	28	72	100%
5	Low response towards education by females in Sokoto state can be party associated with inadequate sensitization on the importance of education	769/1065	72	28	100%
6	Parents low morale towards the education of their female wards is not in any way related to the earlier's low income	699/1065	35	65	100%
7	Religious misconception partly influences the poor altitude of parents towards the education of their female wards	692/1065	64	26	100%
8	Inadequate funding for education by the Sokoto state government grossly improves the development of female education	872/1065	26	74	100%

(continued)

Table 1. *(continued)*

S/N	Statement	Scores	% Positive scores	% Negative score	Total percentage
9	Socio-cultural misconception and perception about the social roles of female in the society party influence parents' high morale altitude towards the education of their female wards in Sokoto state	742/1065	76	24	100%
10	Inadequate Centers for Continuing Education in Sokoto state adversely affects the development of female education	812/1065	74	26	100%
11	Unemployment problem does not affect females' interest in pursuance of school education in Sokoto state	620/1065	42	58	100%
12	The consequences of females' poor response to school education in Sokoto state affects their role in National development in the following ways:	3125/4260	73	27	100%
13	The following measures can help in addressing the challenges being faced by female education in the state and better prepare them for national services/development:-	3431/4260	80	20	100%

The findings from the above indicated that 67% of respondents agreed that majority of girls of school age in Sokoto state are out of school while 23% disagreed. Responses to item two indicates that, 67% of the respondents disagreed that dropout syndrome is not one of the challenges affecting girl child education in Sokoto state and 23% agreed that it is not one of the challenges affecting the development of girl child education in the state. Responses to item 3 indicates that 66% of respondents disagreed that girls passing out from secondary schools have high aspiration for higher education while 34%

agreed on this. On response to item four 72% of the respondents disagreed that female students in Sokoto state have high morale towards the study of science and technology courses while 28% of them agreed that they have high aspiration. Responses to item five indicates that inadequate sensitization on the importance of education was not considered as one of the factors affecting the development of girl child education by 28% of the respondents while 72% agreed. In the same vein 65% of respondents to item six disagreed that parent's low morale towards the education of their female wards is not related to the earlier's low income and 35% of them agreed with this supposition on the item. Responses to item seven reveals that 71% of the respondents agreed that religious misconception partly influences the poor attitude of parents towards the education of their female wards in Sokoto state and only 29% disagreed. Sequel to response to item eight that inadequate funding on education by Sokoto state government grossly improves the development of girl child education was disagreed by 64% of the respondents while 36% of them agreed that inadequate funding improves the development of female education in Sokoto state. It was also discovered that, 76% of the respondents disagreed that socio-cultural misconception and perception about the social roles of female in the society partly influences parents' high morale attitude towards the education of their female wards in Sokoto state and 24% agreed to this statement. Inadequate centers for continuing education in Sokoto state adversely affects the development of female education in Sokoto state was agreed by 74% of the respondents and only 26% disagreed. 58% of the respondents disagreed that Unemployment problem does not affect female's interest in pursuance of school education in Sokoto state and 42% of the respondents agreed to this statement on item eleven. The findings against item twelve reveals that 73% of the respondents agreed that the stated consequences of female's poor response to school education in Sokoto state affect their role in national development and only 27% disagreed. On the measures suggested to improve the development of female education in Sokoto state which include adequate funding, sensitization and empowerment programme were agreed by 80% of the respondents and only 20% disagreed with the measures.

12 Summary of the Major findings

The following problems were positively responded to or agreed by the respondents as challenges militating against the development of Girl Child education in Sokoto state which include:

1. Majority of school age girls in Sokoto state are out of school.
2. Most girls passing out from secondary schools have low aspiration for higher education.

    a. Religious misconception partly influences the poor attitude of parents towards the education of their female wards.
    b. The consequences of females low response to school education limits their role in national development by inhibiting the actualization of their human potentials which affects their roles as home maintainers and child bearers/rearers, political

participation/representation/opportunities as well their level of participation in the civil service

c. Such measures as improved funding, sensitization, empowerment programme as well as the role and support of NGOs, donor nations agencies and international communities can help in reducing the effects of the challenges of girl child education in the state and better prepare them for contribution to national development
d. Inadequate Centre's for continuing education in Sokoto state affect the development of girl child education in Sokoto state.

   It was also equally found that majority of the respondents disagreed that:

   a. Dropout syndrome is not one of the challenges affecting development of Girl Child education
   b. female students in Sokoto state have high morale towards the study of science and technology subjects/courses
   c. Low response towards education by females is due to inadequate sensitization.
   d. Parents' low morale towards the education of girl child is not related to parents' income.
   e. Inadequate funding by Sokoto state government improves the girl child education in the state.

   6, Socio-Cultural misconception does not contribute to the problem of Girl Child education.

e. Unemployment problems does not affect the attitude of Girl Child towards school education
f. Employment opportunities should be provided for females passing out from schools.

13 Conclusion

This paper was rounded off with a conclusion that majority of girls in Sokoto state are out of school and those in schools have low aspiration for high education as well as the study of science and technology courses.

14 Recommendation

Based on the foregoing research findings, the following recommendations were deemed necessary.

1. The state government needs to improve funding for education and encourage the girl child education through provision of scholarships and other financial support for girl child education.

2. There is the need for the establishment of more centers for continuing education where those girls who might have dropped out of school or not have heard the opportunity to start school early can continue with their education.
3. Effective empowerment program need to be introduced so as to reduce the poverty level of parents so as to be able to contribute and support the education of their female wards.
4. Public enlightment on the importance of girl child education need to be intensified by the state government, NGOs, religious leaders and other concerned members of the society.

References

Abdulrahman, S.: Girl Child Education in Zamfara state of Nigeria. Daily Sun Newspaper of June 15 2016 (2016)

Audu, U.D.: Actualizing vision 202020 through girl child education: focus on the secondary school level. J. Women Coll. Educ. (JOWICE) (2011). Akins Press and Services (NIG), Jos

Birnin Kebbi, A.M., Sifawa, A.B.: Attitudes of Muslim Parents towards Girl Child Education among contemporary Muslim in Nigeria: A case study of some selected North western states (2017)

Boyd, P.C, Manheim, P., Bushmer, K.: The Research Advisors. 25, Island Rock, Plymouta, M.A., 02360 (2006)

Chiakaan, J., Ahmad J.I.: Referring public relations profession for national development. LAJAST **1**, 68–74 (2009)

Daily Sun Newspaper, 25 July 2015

Dashen, A.N., Dashen, P.N.: Girl child education as an imperatival for women empowerment. JOWICE **1**(1), 24–30 (2004)

Federal Government of Nigeria: National Policy on Education. NERDC Press, Lagos, Nigeria (2013)

Haruna, M.J.: The role of female education towards the realization of vision 20:2020 in Nigeria. J. Women Coll. Educ. (JOWICE) (2011). Akins Press and Services, Jos, Nigeria

Haruna, M.J.: A study of the relationships between marital status and academic achievements of two hundred level female students of Shehu Shagari college of education, Sokoto (Unpublished M.Ed. Thesis). University of Jos, Jos, Nigeria (2004)

Haruna, M.J., Yabo, I.M.: Towards reducing the effects of class differences in the education. Nigeria Child. Niger. J. Sociol. Educ. **111**(3) (2009). Deka Publications, Jos

Hashimu, S., Balarabe, A., Sulaiman, S.: Factors inflaming female education in Sokoto metropolis: a case study of Umaru Ali Shinkafi Polytechnic. Sokoto. Beam J. Arts Sci. (2017). Umaru Ali Shinkafi Polytechnic Sokoto, Sokoto, Nigeria

Ibrahim, F., Bala, B.H., Gwandu, S.A., Abdullahi, A.: The Impact of Female Education on Socio-economic Development of Sokoto State, A PGE Research Project. SSCOE, Sokoto (2019)

King, E., Hill, M.A.D.: Women Education in Developing Countries: A Review of Barriers, Benefits and Policy (In UNESCO, 2005). UNESCO, Washington (1992)

Maisaje, S.J.:Girl child: key to achievement vision 2020. J. Women Coll. Educ. (JOWICE) (2011). Akins Press and Services (NIG), Jos

Momoh, A.: Privatization in Nigeria: Issues and Experience. The Punch News Paper, 24 April, p. 4 (2002)

UNESCO: World Education Report, 2002 in Nigeria (2002)

UNICEF: Annual Report (2003)

Implementation of Design Thinking and Innovation Strategies by Ghanaian Companies: A Case of CPC

C. K. Okai-Mensah[1](✉), E. K. Howard[2], and M. A. Osei[3]

[1] Department of Fashion and Textiles Studies, Accra Technical University, Accra, Ghana
[2] Department of Industrial Art, College of Art and Built Environment, KNUST, Kumasi, Ghana
[3] Department of Fashion, Blue Crest University College, Accra, Ghana

Abstract. Design thinking is seen as an iterative approach to problem-solving and helps businesses to continuously reposition and think critically about business problems in a more human-centric way. The whole process creates innovative solutions to Prototype and Test, which helps companies set product goals, understand business outcomes, map out user journeys, prioritize Minimum viable product features, and create a future-oriented product roadmap. The Stanford Design thinking Model has been considered as one of the best models that elicit excellent results in both service delivery and product design and innovation businesses. The study sought to establish how design companies in Ghana are adopting design thinking and innovation strategies in their operations using the Stanford Design Thinking Model. A case study approach was employed to evaluate the operation of Cocoa Processing Company through interviews, observation and administration of questionnaire. The study found that almost all the stages of the design thinking process were practiced adequately except the prototyping and testing stages. Research have shown that over 700 new products has shown that approximately 60% of new products fail in the market place because there was no need for the product in the market; the product did not match the market need, poor market research, and poor product positioning. The study recommends that production companies consider implementing the design thinking process to create an exciting culture of innovation, empowers employees to think outside the box, reduce wastes, increase the speed to the market, and improve profitability. Monitoring and evaluation, the performance of the product in the market, as well as reactions to pricing, product quality, and packaging must be key consideration factors in such initiative. This will help proper pricing as well as collate data for future ventures and track the gains made after the introduction of the new, improved products.

Keywords: Design thinking · Design innovation · Stanford design thinking model · CPC-Ghana

1 Introduction

Traditional business methods based on the continuous contraction of cost and boosting efficiency are not limitless and drive to problematic business results and lost competitiveness in the long term (Volkova and Jakobsone 2016). They further suggested that

J. N. Mojekwu et al. (Eds.): *Sustainable Education and Development*, pp. 43–56, 2021.
https://doi.org/10.1007/978-3-030-68836-3_5

concepts such as strategic design, design management, design thinking, and design-driven innovation are notably entering the business environment by conceptually new applications to foster order in external chaos.

Design is now taking a leading position in organizational management and should not be limited to its role as a tool but should be extended to contribute to drawing the company strategy and should be considered in every part of the developmental process (Elmansy 2017). Elmansy suggested that design is now considered a process rather than a tool, and the design thinking process is a customer-centered method that allows for the final product to be liked and meets his expectations. Several design thinking models have been established to build a customer-oriented design, and to pick the best model to follow depends on the complexity of the model and the size of the company (Elmansy 2017).

Design Thinking Ghana Conference was first held at the CEIBS Accra Campus on 19th May, 2017. Over 160 participants had the opportunity to explore how to apply design thinking to their business challenges. The conference was aimed at helping participants better appreciate and comprehend the practice of Design Thinking. It was to equip the participants to discover ways it can be utilized more in the Ghanaian community. The organizers of the conference were Ghana Design Network and the Ashesi D: Lab with the support of partners including CEIBS Accra Campus, Cobalt, Mullen Lowe, Design Thinking Ghana Meetup Group, Ghana Think Foundation, Ghana Netherlands Business and Culture Centre, Design Thinkers Group, Netherlands, IStream, MEST, and GN Electronics ('CEIBS Hosts 1st Design Thinking Ghana Conference' 2017).

The Care Community Hub (CCH) pilot was implemented by Concern Worldwide and Grameen. Foundation in collaboration with the Ghana Health Service as part of the Innovations for Maternal, Newborn and Child Health Initiative (Innovations) funded by the Bill & Melinda Gates Foundation. This case study was one of four in a series that reports on the application of design thinking in MNCH programming in Africa (Lafond and Davis 2016).

The Maternal, Newborn, and Child Health (MNCH) Initiative (Lafond and Davis 2016) developed and piloted innovative mediations to address conjoint barriers to improving the effectiveness of basic MNCH health services in low-resource settings. This was a result of the growing importance among designers, global health practitioners, and sponsors to understand the potential benefits of applying design thinking methods and tools for resolving complex social problems. Research and learning related to the application of design thinking were central to the initiative's overall strategy (Lafond and Davis 2016). Experience Point (2018) posit that Lego, IKEA, Apple, and Microsoft have applied different design thinking models to build customer-oriented products. Companies can improve their innovation capabilities, address complex problems, increase profit, and improve their competitiveness capabilities through the application of design thinking.

According to Powell and Cassill (2006), the amount of risk and associated cost for new product development is usually related to the demands of the market, and new product failure rates are considerable. They again opined that, in recent years, the failure percentage has been increasing and that approximately 40% of all new products failed. Lynn and Reilly (2002) research over 700 new product teams and estimated that approximately 60% of new products fail in the market place. The various reason cited for product failure includes no need for the product in the market, the product did not match the market need, poor market research, and poor product positioning (Powell and Cassill 2006). Elmansy (2017) it has been established that different stages of design thinking can help the designers to think through solutions for problems. Creative tools can be used to find solutions or address the problem differently at various stages. In the Define stage, tools such as Root Cause Analysis Method (RCAM), which includes the 5 Whys, fish borne, bowtie, can be employed to determine the root cause of the customer problems identified. Tools such as the Political, Economic, Social, Technological, Legal, Environmental (PESTLE) analysis, Strengths, Weaknesses Opportunities and Threats (SWOT) analysis (ISO/TS 9002:2016), and Theory of Inventive Problem Solving (TRIZ) can be employed to improve the efficiency of the final product at the strategic level (Elmansy 2017). TRIZ method, according to Elmansy, is a basic tool used to solve challenging business problems and achieve innovation. TRIZ is mostly used during the define and prototype stages to achieve innovation. Other benefits of applying the design thinking process are improving the company's profitability and competitiveness in the market. There is a strong relationship between achieving innovation, profitability, competitiveness, and design thinking (Elmansy 2017). Five options to improve the product or the company's market position have been noted in Dr. Georg Tacke, David Vidal, and Jan Haemer book Profitable Innovation. Top on the list is the introduction of new innovation and differentiated products with 77%.

2 Review of Related Literature

Brown (2019) defines design thinking as "discipline that uses the designer's sensibility and methods to match people's needs with what is technologically feasible and what a viable business strategy can convert into customer value and market opportunity." According to (Hobcraft 2017) describes Design Thinking as a human-centric approach to the innovation drawing on the designer's thought to integrate the needs of the people, the possibilities of technology, and the requirements for business success. He alluded to the fact that Design Thinking has evolved at many organizations as a way to solve user problems in creative and innovative ways. Much of the thinking behind the Design Thinking process focuses on challenging assumptions and redefining problems for products, services, and improved customer experience. Brown (2019) describes design thinking as a solution-focused, problem-solving methodology that helps organizations and individuals alike to get a desired and improved outcome on an inner problem, or to work forward on a future plan. It is useful to tackle challenging problems that are not adequately defined or vague by comprehending the customer needs involved. Re-framing the problem in a customer-oriented way, creating many ideas in brainstorming sessions, and by adopting a hands-on approach in prototyping and testing. Furthermore, design thinking allows the user to have a more structured plan for understanding innovation and to grow more as an organization and to give it a competitive advantage over its peers.

Design thinking can further be described as a cyclic and unending process of problem-solving that helps businesses continuously reposition and think critically about business problems in human-centric ways. It inspires companies to think differently about business objectives and whether or not they are attainable (Dossey, 2019). More importantly, design thinking prompts business stakeholders to analyse their business strategy and how it will translate into a product strategy. Practicing design thinking also offers many strategic advantages and deliverables. The entire process creates innovative solutions to prototype and test, and helps companies set product goals, understand business outcomes, map out user journeys, prioritize most viable product features, and create a future-oriented product roadmap (Dossey 2019).

Brown (2019) suggested that design thinking is scalable and can be applied continually to improve the present plan. These attributes of design thinking promote contribution to different types of innovation, including disruptive, sustaining, and breakthrough innovation.

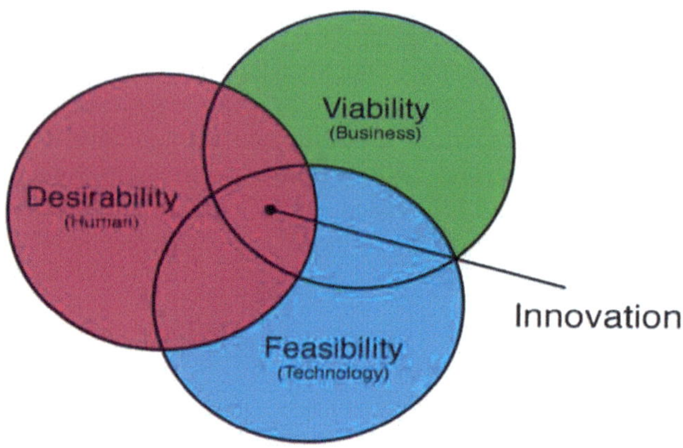

The design thinking fuels innovation (source: modified based on the IDEO).

The nature of the design thinking process fuels innovation in the company. The following considerations: technology, business, and human values have to be considered to achieve innovation. The design process (Lafond and Davis 2016) often starts by using a "desirability lens" that is used to examine the needs, desires, and behaviours of the people that designers want to affect with solutions. This is very important to designers' developing and maintaining empathy for end-users. It increases the probability of fashioning a solution that is responsive to the unmet or hidden user needs and desires. The desirability is used throughout the process. Designers after the desirability bring in the "feasibility lens" and "viability lens" to refine their solutions based on financial, capacity, and other considerations (Lafond and Davis 2016). These strategies are used to ensure product success in the market and to achieve innovation.

According to Elmansy (2017), different models have been introduced to define the design thinking process. Some of the common ones are ZURB Design Thinking, Double-Diamond Design Thinking, and the IBM Design Thinking Processes. He further observed that these models vary based on their approach, number of stages, the relation between stages, and naming of each stage. These models follow similar processes, including determining the problem that needs to be solved, defining the problem, designing the scope, developing the Prototype, designing the final product, and obtaining feedback.

The ZURB Design Thinking Model shares Hasso Plattner Institute of Design at Stanford's simplicity and considers two essential stages: developing the final product and getting feedback. The ZURB model consists of five stages, namely, Define, Ideate, Prototyping, Building, and Analysing. The last two stages represent the building of the final product and analysis of the impact of the product on the market and customer feedback.

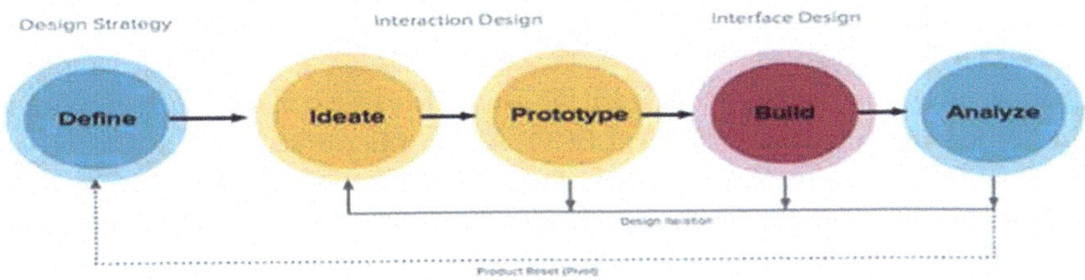

Zurb design thinking model (source: Zurb University).

This model presents two different types of iteration cycles - the design iteration and the product reset (pivot). The first iteration cycle includes the iteration between the stages, namely, Define, Ideate, Prototype, build, and analyse. If things do not go on as planned, the team iterates between the four stages above to identify the problems and solve them to improve the product. The hard reset is the second iteration process. Here it is a significant failure or the product does not meet the requirements, the product resets and returns directly to the Define stage to start the process from beginning to redefine the problem.

The Double Diamond Diagram process was established by the British Design Council in 2005 as part of their in-house research to determine how organisations manage their design processes. The Design Council process has four main stages; namely, Discover, Define, Develop, and Deliver. The project strategy is defined by the first two stages. The executive solution is in line with the third and fourth stages.

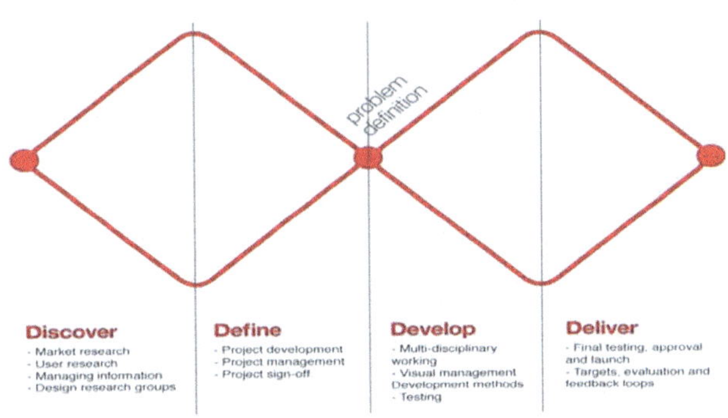

The Double Diamond Diagram by the Design Council (source: Design Council).

This process begins with a trigger point that can be a situation or an idea that requires the attention of the team to "understand" it and research into the current information about the problem to be solved. This is the research stage where research activities such as marketing research, user research, managing information, and design research groups can be conducted. The project objectives and goals are defined during the "Define" stage. Activities such as project development, project management, and project sign-off can be achieved during the "Define" stage.

The "Develop" stage is the second part of the Double Diamond Diagram that consists of developing the Prototype, iterate, and tests the product to ensure it meets the goals of the project. This involves multidisciplinary work such as development methods, visual management, and testing of the Prototype. "Deliver" is the last stage where the final product is finalized and made available to the consumer. Final testing, product approval, evaluation, and feedback are conducted at this stage. The research, including eleven case studies of leading companies such as LEGO, Alessi, Microsoft, Sony, Starbucks, and others, employed the use of The Double Diamond Diagram. Therefore, the model is widely accepted and adopted by a wide range of companies because it was developed based on different types of organizations.

The IBM design thinking is considered one of the recently published design thinking models, IBM in 2013, began a project to inculcate a design-driven culture. It took three years to achieve this, and it involved more than 750 designers and 10,000 employees in the company. The project is aimed at building a design process that hinges on a perfect understanding of the consumer needs and builds empathy. The new model was characterized by a remarked speed and accessibility to meet the demand of modern organisations. The IBM model targeted a larger scale of organisations including large enterprises such as IBM (which has more than 385,000 employees).

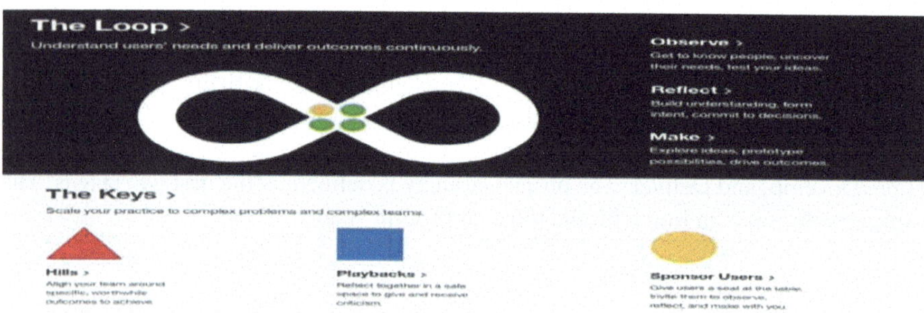
The Loop >
Understand users' needs and deliver outcomes continuously.
Observe >
Get to know people, uncover their needs, test your ideas.
Reflect >
Build understanding, form intent, commit to decisions.
Make >
Explore ideas, prototype possibilities, drive outcomes.
The Keys >
Scale your practice to complex problems and complex teams.
Hills >
Playbacks >
Sponsor Users >

The IBM Design Thinking model (source: IBM).

Nevertheless, the previous models were more biased towards small and medium enterprises (Elmansy 2017).

The IBM design thinking model consists of three stages - Observe, Reflect, Make, which form the so-called "Loop." "Observe," which is the first stage, focuses on monitoring and coming out with a good understanding of the problem at stake. The design team analyses the information to them into the project plan at the "Reflect" stage. The "Make" stage is where the prototypes are developed and delivered to the customer. IBM, in this model, assumes that there is no final product, and all the final products here are prototypes that can be improved in accordance with the eternal flow of the loop with feedback from the end-user. The IBM model is based on three main principles, as represented in the figure above. They focus on consumer satisfaction, multidisciplinary teams, and restless reinvention. The yellow dot in the loop diagram, the user-cantered process, represents the consumer. The multidisciplinary teams from different departments involved in the design process are represented by the green dots, and the restless reinvention refers to the iteration nature of the process. The assumption is that nothing is perfect, and every product is a case for iteration and development.

The IBM model organizes how the process is used among intricate teams through three main keys are Playbacks, Hills, and Sponsor Users in order to ensure the scalability of the design process. The "Hills" are the project goals, the "Playback" are used to put the stakeholders on the same page and ensuring that the different teams are up to date on the progress of the project through manful meetings, and the "sponsored User" ensures the involvement of the customer who is in the heart the process through testing and feedback process. The IBM design thinking model was developed to be accessible to fit in different companies of different sizes, including IBM itself. This is a distinctive advantage comparing the design mentioned above thinking models with other models. This model is still new, and so there is not yet had enough feedback from companies who adopted.

The Hasso-Plattner Institute of Design at Stanford and has continually been used by individuals and firms to innovate their selves better. The 5-stage model is as follows: Empathize, Define, Ideate, Prototype, and Test.

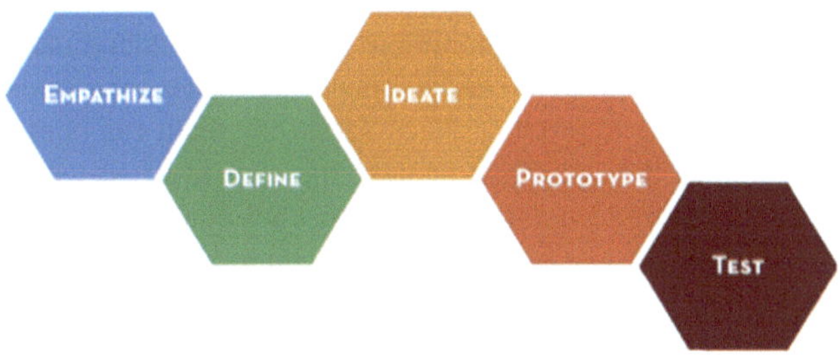

Hasso PlattnerInstitute of Design at Stanford (source: Stanford d. School and Hasso PlattnerInstitute).

Empathize-This stage is used to get a better understanding of the problem that needs to be solved. Activities at this stage include: consulting experts on the matter, engaging farther to better comprehend the problem at hand, and working on the issue through groups to have a deeper understanding of everything that is involved with the problem. Design Thinkers gain insight into the needs regarding the issue along with setting aside their personal assumptions regarding it the problem at this stage. A significant amount of information is collected during this stage and is taken to the next stages to assist in defining the problem and understand how to solve it.

Define-The second stage of Design Thinking is called Define. During this stage, the information gathered at the empathy stage is put together. Mainly, the team analyse data and puts them in order to better concrete the problems that the team has defined to this point. The Define stage will help the team gather great ideas and understand how to use them effectively. From here, the team will start to progress into the third stage of Design thinking, Ideate.

Ideate-The third stage of Design Thinking is called Ideate. Design thinkers, during this stage, start to use the information from the previous stages to generate logical ideas. From here, the team will start to make ideas that may be "out of the box" or perhaps just ideas that may normally be skipped over when not all of the information is presented. This stage allows for an alternative way to solve normalized problems. By the end of this phase, the team should have a few ideas to solve the problem. It is important during this phase that the team could generate many ideas just so they have to choose from when starting the next phase in the Design Thinking process, Prototype.

Prototype-The fourth stage of Design Thinking is called prototype. During this stage, the team will work on creating a number of inexpensive products with specific features. This allows for the Design Thinkers to investigate possible solutions to the problems that were identified in the earlier stages of the Design Thinking process. With each new prototype, the team investigates a different aspect of the problem and explores how each of the prototypes would fix the problem. By the end of this stage, the Design Thinkers should have a better understanding of the constraints they are apparent in the prototype. This is also allowed for the team to the problems that would be created by each prototype, and how they could fix the prototype to make the prototype inherently better.

Test-The Test is the fifth stage of the Design Thinking process. The prototypes are tested during this stage to see how well the problem has been solve/handle. The team is allowed to make alterations and fine-tuning to make the product more appropriate to their needs. The team goes back to the earlier stages and revise their information to get the best outcomes for their end product. Necessarily, the team can continue to do this until they are either solve their problem or until they are satisfied with their product. All the models have different design thinking approaches but share the same strategy to build a user-cantered process.

3 Methodology

The study used the Stanford Design Thinking Model through the Case Study method of the Qualitative research approach to evaluate the extent to which companies in Ghana with specific reference to CPC is implementing Design thinking strategies in its operation. The 5-stage model was initially proposed by the Hasso-Plattner Institute of Design at Stanford and has continually been used by individuals and firms to innovate their selves better. The 5-stage model is as follows: Empathize, Define, Ideate, Prototype, and Test. The straightforwardness of this model is considered both an advantage and a disadvantage. The simple, clear stages allow for designers to understand the different stages of the design thinking process. However, it does not define some important stages, such as the delivery of the product and the feedback. These could be used to solicit information from the user and used to improve the future versions of the designed product or service.

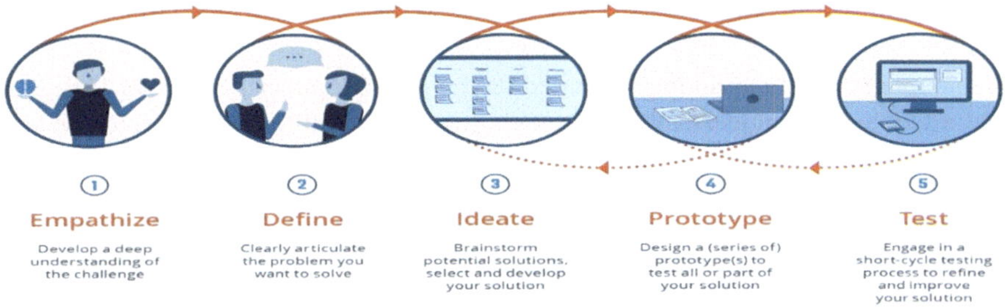

A case study approach is a phenomenon of qualitative research paradigm was used to gain insight into the design thinking approach to research and development at an anonymous company. When the interrogatives such as "how, what, and why" are used as questions, case stud are the preferred method to use. Where the researcher has minimal control over events, and the focus is on a contemporary phenomenon within a real-life context, case studies are used (Yin 2009). Case study research is also appropriate when the boundary between the phenomenon under investigation and its social context is blurred (Yin 2009). A qualitative approach enabled the researchers to take note of Cocoa Processing Company's application of design thinking in its design and development process. A sensemaking approach Basu and Palazzo (2008) was used to provide insight into how people involved in the case though, spoke and behaved in relation to the concepts of design thinking and innovation: as this would help to understand how these ideas influenced the design and development at the Cocoa Processing Company Limited.

Data for the case were collected in two stages: first through desk research based on documents published online by and about Company. Desk research deals with the collection of secondary materials from the internet, internal sources, library agencies, and many others. This was followed by the collection of primary data gained through the administering of the questionnaire to the Product Research and Development Manager. When the questionnaire was received, a semi-structured interview was constructed and conducted with the Product Research and Development Manager, who was a key member in the new product development team of the Company. The desk research on the Company, the interviews, and the data gathered with the questionnaire was used to validate available evidence.

Interviews were critical to the construct of the case study. The interview took the form of guided conversations rather than structured enquiries. As a result of the documentary analysis and the completed questionnaire, the Product Research and Development Manager, were interviewed to provide a better understanding of how CPC is using the concept of design thinking in its design and development of new products. This chain of evidence explicitly links the questions asked, the data collected, and the conclusions drawn. The principle is to allow any reader of the case study to follow the derivation of any evidence from initial research questions to ultimate case study conclusions (Yin 2009). Data from the documentary review and interviews were analysed and compared. The data comprised a mixture of qualitative information, with an emphasis on the written and spoken data. A final draft of the case was sent to the Research and Development Manager, who assessed the historical correctness of the data.

4 Results and Discussion

The interpretation of the findings is based on the Hasso Plattner Institute of Design at Stanford (d. School) model evolving through Empathize, Define, Ideate, Prototype, and Test.

Empathy

CPC has designed and developed Peanut coated with White, Milk, and Dark Chocolate in the past one year. Complaints from customers that the pebble, 'dragees', were too sweet and hard on the teeth necessitated this improved product. Also, customers now prefer chocolate with a higher percentage of cocoa mass (dark chocolate) because they perceive it is healthier. This affirms that CPC is empathising with its customers. Krieger (2010) observed that it is only through contact, observation and empathy with end users that a designer can hope to design solutions that fit into the user's environment. The information collected from CPC's customers was passed on to the Innovative Process and Product Development Team (IPPDT), who are responsible for the innovation process and product improvement and new product development. The IPPDT consists of the Director of Production, Product Research and Development Manager, Chief Accountant, Production Manager, Production Superintendent, Plant Maintenance and Facility Manager, Quality Assurance Manager, and Supply Chain & Logistics Manager.

The following interested parties; IPPDT, customers, target market, regulators such as Food and Drugs Authority, Ghana Standards Authority were contacted for their opinion on the new product. The aim and objectives of the new products were to develop;

1. a new chocolate dragees, product without the external sugar/colour, layer of pebbles
2. less/low sugar
3. more nutrition
4. suitable for adult
5. with more variety (white, dark, milk, chocolates).

The following assumptions were made in the design and developments;

1. The soft exterior will withstand harsh weather to a moderate degree but not like pebbles
2. Price would be slightly higher than pebbles
3. Perform as well as or better than similar products (maltegers on the market).
4. Appeal to the elderly.

Define

The ideas were analysed, and it came out that the market was ready for a product like the new products and was expectant. The Innovation Process and Product Development Team (IPPDT) meetings, through formal, gave an opportunity for all stakeholders to make suggestions regardless of their knowledge of the product. These constructed criticisms were instrumental in the restructuring of the new product.

Ideation

Ideas are first discussed at departmental levels. Representatives from each department present their ideas to the IPPDT meeting for future discussion. Different prototypes agreed on during the brainstorming stage, depending on the product type, may present trial samples to show the team and request their comments on the recipe, intended packaging, and the availability of raw materials.

The following considerations were made during the brainstorming stage;

1. Availability of ingredients, machines, packaging
2. Feasibility of lab trials and pilot studies on the production floor
3. Product distribution
4. competitors

Prototypes

In-house sensory evaluation by the trained panel and hedonic scale sensory test for larger consumer groups are conducted to ensure that the output (that is the product) meets the input requirements. Regulatory permits and certifications are also sourced and included in the marketing report. When the prototypes fail to meet customer requirements, the entire design and department process start again until the desired outcomes are obtained, or there is a review of the aspect of the product that has fallen short for the recommendation.

Testing

The prototypes are tested in two ways; in-house sensory panel. Comment from this Test is sent to the IPPDT meeting who performs statistical tests of significance. Product may be deferred to a later time depending on the nature of feedback gained on the product.

Reduction of waste and production cost was achieved during the bulk production stage because at the design and development phase, issues of rejects, rework, and waste was investigated. Equally, root causes and corrective actions were determined and resolved. This invariably improved the speed to market the product based on the lessons learned. The new products, Peanut coated with White, Milk, and Dark Chocolate, were an improvement on an existing product that the market or consumers have been looking for (low sugar, more nutrition, and suitable for adults, perceived health benefits). Patronage has increased since the products were launched, and production output has also increased. All the new products developed were launched by the company to showcased them to the public. This was not part of Stanford's design thinking model. In my view, as a researcher, I believe it is a necessary action as indicated by the Double Diamond Diagram design process developed by the British Design Council. "Deliver" is the last stage where the final product is concluded and sent to the market. The activities done at this stage involved final testing, product approval, evaluation, and feedback.

Design Thinking Gaps

It can be derived from the information gathered that CPC is implementing almost all the steps or stages of the design thinking process. However, it was found out that after coming out with the prototype, they tested it with the sensory team who were not their major consumers and not the originators of the problem to be solved. Lynn and Reilly (2002) researched over 700 new product teams and estimated that approximately 60% of new products fail in the market place. This was opined by Powell and Cassill (2006) that in recent years, the failure percentage has been increasing and that approximately 40% of all new product failed. The various reasons cited for product failure includes, no need for the product in the market; the product did not match the market need, poor market research, and poor product positioning.

Secondly, it was observed that there was no monitoring and evaluation (Post-launch review) to the product. Monitoring and evaluation (Post-launch review) of a successful product in the market involves reactions to pricing, product quality, and packaging. Monitoring and evaluation also help the company to plan for proper pricing as well as collate data to improve on the product and also for future ventures. This will also help to track the gains made after the introduction of the newly improved products.

The involvement of customers at diverse stages of the new product development process encourages manufacturers to directly bring in their preferences, limiting distortions and filtering effects related to market research and data analysis (Choi et al. 2005). Throneburg finds out what works, not by asking researchers, but by staying in close contact with the customers who buy his product and that he only enters the market if he can design products that the consumer considers beneficial (Choi et al. 2005). In order to effectively enhance new product success, Cooper (2018) suggests that a company may integrate lead users who are innovative companies, organizations, or individuals that are well ahead of market trends and even have needs that go far beyond the average user into the process. They contribute to the anticipation of requirements that will eventually be shared by the mass market to more easily recognized the problems. 'Consumer-focused innovation' can also be adopted. Here customers or users are invited to help the product developer design the next new product and provide many ideas for significant product improvements. Consumers, according to Cooper (2018) are 2.4 times more efficient at developing significant innovations than producers, and much more prolific and efficient product developers when the field is in its early stages.

Okai-Mensah et al. (2020)

Once the product is launched, there must be continuous management of the product over the lifecycle to maintain profitability and brand identity, with both marketing and development (Cooper 2010). The organization-wide generation of market intelligence pertaining to current and future customer needs, dissemination of intelligence across departments, and organization-wide responsiveness to it (Choi et al. 2005). Through proper market orientation, the firms can gain a better understanding of customer needs and wants and great knowledge of competitor's activities and market trends.

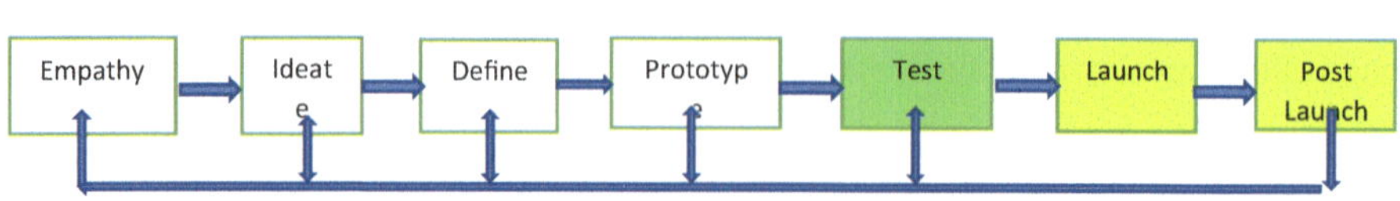

5 Conclusion and Recommendations

The Stanford Design thinking Model has been considered as one of the best models that elicit excellent results in both service delivery and product design and innovation businesses. However, developing a strategy in the mature stage to extend the life of the product requires consideration of each aspect of the product from cost to advertising, distribution, and special consideration at different stages of the product's lifecycle can be included. After the product is launched, there is a need for continuous management of the product over the lifecycle to maintain profitability and brand identity. Monitoring and evaluation (Post-launch review) of the product in the market, as well as reactions to pricing, product quality, and packaging, will also help the company to plan for proper pricing as well as collate data for future ventures. This will also help to track the gains made after the introduction of the new, improved products. The study recommends that production companies consider implementing the design thinking process. This will create an exciting culture of innovation and empowers employees to think outside the box, reduce wastes, increase the speed to the market, and improve profitability. It is also recommended that monitoring and evaluation (Post-launch review) the performance of the production in the market, as well as reactions to pricing, product quality, and packaging to be considered. This will help the company to plan for proper pricing as well as collate data for future ventures and track the gains made after the introduction of the new, improved products.

References

Basu, K., Palazzo, G.: Corporate social responsibility: a process model of sensemaking. Acad. Manag. Rev. **33**(1), 122–136 (2008)

Brown, T.: Change by Design: How Design Thinking Transforms Organizations and Inspires Innovation. Harper Business, New York (2019)

Powell, N.B., Cassill, N.L.: New textile product development: processes practices and products. J. Text. Apparel Technol. Manag. **97**(2), 155–166 (2006)

CEIBS Hosts 1st Design Thinking Ghana Conference (2017)

Choi, W., Powell, N.B., Cassill, N.L.: new product development and its applications textiles. J. Text. Apparel Technol. Manag. **4**(4), 1–28 (2005)

Cooper, R.G.: The drivers of success in new-product development. Ind. Mark. Manag. **76**, 36–47 (2018). https://doi.org/10.1016/j.indmarman.2018.07.005

Cooper, W.D.: Textile and apparel supply chains for the 21st century. J. Text. Apparel Technol. Manag. **6**(4), 1–10 (2010)

Dossey, A.: How design thinking Leads to a Better Minimum Viable Product (MVP) (2019). https://clearbridgemobile.com/how-design-thinking-leads-better-mvp/#Developing_an_Effective_MVP

Elmansy, R.: Design Thinking Guide: What, why, and how (2017). https://www.designorate.com/design-thinking-guide-what-why-how/

ExperiencePoint. The business case for design thinking (2018). https://blog.experiencepoint.com/the-business-case-for-design-thinking

Hobcraft, P.: Improving your business potential for innovation - limitations and criticisms of design thinking organizations have a growing recognition that there is no "plug and play" system for Design Thinking (2017). https://blog.hypeinnovation.com/improving-business-potential-innovation-criticisms-design-thinking.

ISO/TS 9002:2016 Technical Specification: Quality Management Systems – Guidelines for the application of ISO 9001:2015
Krieger, M.: Introduction to design thinking (2010). https://www.slideshare.net/mikeyk/intro-to-design-thinking
LaFond, A., Davis, N.: The Use of Design Thinking in MNCH Programs: A Case Study of the Care Community Hub (CCH) Pilot, Ghana. JSI Research & Training Institute Inc., Arlington (2016)
Lynn, G., Reilly, R.: Blockbusters: The Five Keys to Developing Great New Products. Harper Business, New York (2002)
Volkova, T., Jakobsone, I.: Design thinking as a business tool to ensure continuous value generation. Intell. Econ. **10**, 63–69 (2016). https://doi.org/10.1016/intele.2016.06.003
Yin, R.K.: Case Study Research – Design and Methods, 4th edn. Sag, Los Angeles (2009)

Assessment of Some Management Strategies in Resolving Labour Dispute in Colleges of Education in the North-West Nigeria

M. Magaji(✉), M. J. Haruna, and A. Nafisa

Department of Education Foundation, Shehu Shagari College of Education, Sokoto, Sokoto State, Nigeria

Abstract. This study on the assessment of management strategies in resolving labour dispute in colleges of education in the Northwest Nigeria. The study is guided by three research objectives, three research questions and three research hypotheses. Among the research objectives is to find out if there is any relationship between dialogue strategy and resolution of labour dispute. The research question of the study is there any relationship between dialogue and resolution of labour dispute. The study adopted a descriptive research of correlation type, with 13 colleges of education, 5 federal and 8 state owned colleges of education with a total population of 5,680 which comprises 5180 labour Union members, 60 management staff, 91 deans and 351 heads of department. A sample of 357 was selected which include 255 labour Union members, 23 management staff, 25 deans and 54 heads of department. The study used a self-drafted questionnaire titled "Management Strategies in Resolving Labour Dispute Questionnaire in colleges of education in the North-west Nigeria (MSRLDQ)". The data collected for the study was analysed using descriptive statistics of frequency counts, tables, percentages, mean and standard deviation. The null hypotheses were analysed using Pearson Product Moment Correlation Co-efficient. One of the findings of study indicate that there is positive significant relationship between dialogue, negotiation and mediation strategy in resolving labour disputes in colleges of education in the North-west Nigeria. The study concluded that adoption of dialogue strategy by the college of education management help to resolve labour dispute effectively in Colleges of Education in the North-west Nigeria. The study recommended that when the management of College of Education seem in capable to meet all the demands of labour Unions, both parties should come to dialogue in a round table, and honestly adhere to the terms of any agreement reached. However, if dialogue fail to resolve an issue external intervention like conciliation, arbitration panels, industrial court or elder statement should be allowed in dispute resolution to prevent disruptions of activities in the institution.

Keywords: Labour dispute · Management · Management strategies · Resolution of labour dispute

J. N. Mojekwu et al. (Eds.): *Sustainable Education and Development*, pp. 57–65, 2021.
https://doi.org/10.1007/978-3-030-68836-3_6

1 Introduction

Labour Dispute is a recurring phenomenon in employee: employer relation. In every organization, whether it is unionized or not there will always be disagreement between the employer and employees, either on wages or the general conditions of service of workers. This is evident in all institutions and organizations around the world and in Africa in particular. The complex nature of organization, make labour dispute inevitable in the work environment. Also the pursuance of incompatible goals by the management and employees leads to labour dispute.

Labour Dispute is inevitable in organization because of the need disequilibrium of the workforce and human factors such as multiculturalism, maladministration, greed, inadequate funding, political interfering and atmosphere of distrust. Undoubtedly, every organization is battling with one form of dispute or the other. This is because dispute is unavoidable where two or more persons form a group either as a company, an organization, a religion or an education institution. Every organization constitute a combination of employees from different backgrounds, personality traits dispositions, needs and sense of judgment. Federal and State Colleges of Education in Nigeria cannot be said to be an exception, considering numerous challenges facing them (Ajemole 2017).

2 Statement of the Problem

In most Nigerian Colleges of Education, management and staff members under the umbrella of their respective unions act like opposition parties on issues bothering their different interests. For instance, issues like delay in payment of fringe benefits (allowances) such as overtime, earn and excess workload meant to be enjoyed by College of Education staff often cause disagreement between the two parties, or sometimes between unions and Government such that the Colleges of Education may be closed down for months to the detriment of the innocent students especially in Colleges of Education in Northwest, Nigeria. Labour dispute seems to be one of the commonest challenges militating against Nigeria College of Education. It has made Colleges of Education irregularities such as industrial strike, absenteeism, lockout, overtime ban and work-to-rule. The result of all these include interruption of the smooth running of academic calendar, brain drain of academia, victimization, sack of lecturers, wastage, blackmail and litigation; all of which discredit the College of Education management in North-west Nigeria (Ajemole 2017). The gap the paper want to fill, to bring out the best management strategy in resolving labour dispute in Colleges of education in North-West, Nigeria because other management strategies are not applicable in resolving labour dispute in colleges of education. The objectives of the study is to identify the dialogue strategy in labour dispute resolution in the Colleges of Education in North-West Nigeria; to determine negotiation strategy in labour dispute resolution in the Colleges of Education in the North-West Nigeria and to establish the mediation strategy in labour dispute resolution in the Colleges of Education in the North-West Nigeria.

Research Questions
The following Research questions have been formulated to guide the study

1. What are the dialogue strategy in labour dispute resolution?
2. What are the negotiation strategy in labour dispute resolution in the Colleges of Education in the North-West Nigeria?
3. What are the mediation strategy in labour dispute resolution in the Colleges of Education in the North-West Nigeria?

Research Hypotheses

The following research hypotheses are formulated to guide the study.

Ho_1 There is no significant relationship between dialogue strategy and resolution of labour disputes in the colleges of education in North-West Nigeria.

Ho_2 There is no significant relationship between negotiation strategy and resolution of labour disputes in North-West Nigeria.

Ho_3 There is no significant relationship between mediation strategy and resolution of labour dispute in the colleges of education in North-West Nigeria.

3 Theoretical Framework

The theory that form the basis of this research is Conflict Theory. Historically, societies have been plagued with class struggles and survival of the fittest in the context or situation where oppressors and the oppressed are constantly in opposition. These struggles had caused revolutions, re-constitution of societies and devastations of the gladiators (Martin 2018).

Although, many theories are relevant to this study, the finding was hinged on the conflict theory. This is because labour dispute is a form of conflict in Colleges of Education in Nigeria. In line with conflict theory in the context of labour dispute, the bourgeois (Colleges of Education management) and proletariat (labour unionist). The perceived exploitation of employees by the management could be the probable cause of most labour disputes in Nigerian Federal and State College of Education. Also, the escalation of labour dispute could hinged on the failure of both the parties of capitulate for peace to reign.

4 Conceptual Framework

It deal with management, management strategies and labour dispute.

Dispute can be seen as a disparity between two or more parties on an issue they field to reach compromise or agreement on. Kesterner and Ray (2012) saw dispute as the involvements of two parties (or groups) who incompatibly strive for a goal which can only be reached by one party. It is inevitable. An inevitable outcome of groups and an attendant feature of human interaction (Fatile and Adejuwon 2012).

Dispute can equally be seen as un-avoidable outcome, of peoples interaction as a result of their divergent views, different backgrounds and need dispositions that make individuals uniquely different from the groups organization or institution as a whole, Duetsch and Coleman (2010) opined that dispute is inevitable where there is a meaningful interaction. Micheal (2012) also views it as a serious disagreement that last for long time between groups of people. Adeyemi and Ademilun (2012) described the concept as a destructions behaviour such as demonstration, protests, arguments or aggression that emanate from disagreement, friction to opposition between two or more parties.

Management is the process of mobilizing available scarce human and material resources in an organization to realize stated goals and planned mission. Adeyemi (2010) defined management as the process directed towards maximizing the potentials of peoples and coordinating their efforts to attain some pre-determined goals.

Management strategies are techniques that are used to direct and control an organization to achieved a set, of goals. These include strategies for leadership, administration and business excursion. The following are example of management strategies which include: dialogue, negotiation, mediation. Kazeems (2010).

Dialogue Strategy and Resolution of Labour Dispute

Dialogue Strategy is a mechanism adopted to curtail labour disputes such that management and Labour Union Leaders dialogue on the subject of particular agitation. The influence of dialogue strategy in Resolution of Labour Dispute cannot be over emphasized. According to Ajewole (2014) maintained that, adoption of dialogue strategy by the management used to prevent or manage labour dispute effectively and such adaptation had positive relationship on Resolution of Labour Dispute in Colleges of Education. Particularly if the Colleges of Education management could dialogue with the representative of Labour Unions and adhere to the terms, there is high probability that labour dispute could deescalate. Hence, Resolution of Labour Disputes could be guaranteed.

Negotiation and Resolution of Labour Dispute

Negotiation according to Fatile (2011) sees negotiation as "a structured process of dialogue between conflicting parties about issues in which their opinions differ. Thus, negotiation is a direct process of dialogue and discussion taking place between at least two parties who are faced with a conflict situation or a dispute. By taking to each other solution is achieved. Munck (2012) noted that managing dispute is an extensive and potentially resolved on a common ranging from simple negotiation between two people to international arbitration tribunals involving nations to the traditional adjudicative of each country's legal system. Social dispute such as ethnic, community and special interest group dispute can be managed through the dispute continuum or using third party facilitators to assist the parties in transforming the dispute through problem solving, dialogue and peace building. Third parties to the dispute can involve consultants, educators, Quakers, labour mediators, diplomats, judges and your next door neighbor. As dispute filed matures and continue to gain interest, managing and resolving dispute continues to evolve and multiply perhaps, overwhelming potential participants. For this reason, parties to a conflict will have to decide what negotiation makes the most sense to them, is acceptable to both parties and support positive change.

Mediation Strategy and Resolution of Labour Dispute

Mediation is a process in which an impartial third party helps disputants resolve a dispute or plan transactions, does not have the power to impose a binding solution (Lebarson 2011). Best (2015) identified variety processes mediators can use to achieve results. These include "interest based" approaches and "rights based" approaches. Some mediators are "facilitative," providing only process assistance for negotiation and using interest based approaches. Facilitative, interest-based mediation according to Morris (2012) is taught widely in North America for the purpose of community, family and commercial mediation and trends to foster the avoidance of mediator recommendations or suggestions in order to preserve mediator neutrality and to encourage party control of outcomes. According to Miller (2013) mediation is the voluntary, informal, non-binding process undertaken by an external party that fosters the settlement of differences or demands between directly invested parties (Miller 2013).

The influence of mediation strategy on Labour Dispute Resolution cannot be over emphasise Ajemole (2017) found out that, there is positive relationship between mediation strategy and Labour Dispute Resolution, if the Labour Union Leaders and college of education management could abide by the resolution of a third party such as industrial Arbitration panel, National industrial court or Board of Enquiry. The escalation of labor dispute could be curtailed and the college of education administration could be guaranteed.

5 Research Methodology

The study adopted a descriptive research of correlation type, with 13 Colleges of education, 5 federal and 8 state owned colleges of education, with a total population of 5,680 which comprises labour union members, 60 management staff, 91 deans and 351 Head of Departments (H.O.Ds). A sample of 357 were selected which include 255 labour union members, 23 management staff, 25 deans and 54 HODs were proportionally selected and used for the study. The study used a self drafted questionnaire titled "Management Strategies in Resolving Labour dispute in Colleges of Education in the North-West Nigeria" (MSRLDQ). The data collected for the study was analysed using descriptive statistics of frequency counts, tables, percentages, mean and standard deviation. The null hypotheses were analysed using Pearson Product Moment Correlation Co-efficient PPMC.

Validity of Instrument

With respect to validity of the instrument, the draft questionnaire was given to the expert from measurement and evaluation to make critical observation regarding the contents and its suitability as an instrument for the collection of data.

Reliability of Instrument

The reliability of the instrument was measured first using a pilot study. The pilot study was conducted using other college of education not sampled for the study. Test and re-test method of reliability was applied with an interval of three weeks in order to established reliability of the instrument.

6 Findings

Hypotheses Testing

$\mathbf{H0_1}$: There is no significant relationship between dialogue strategy and resolution of labour disputes in the colleges of education in North-West Nigeria.

This hypothesis was tested by subjecting the score for dialogue strategy and resolution of labour dispute scores to Pearson's correlation analysis as shown in Table 1.

Table 1. Relationship between dialogue strategy and resolution of labour disputes.

Variables	N	Mean	Std. Deviation	r-Cal	*p*-Value	Decision
Dialogue strategy	357	27.96	39.20	.159	.003	H_0 Rejected
Resolution of labour dispute	357	7.633	10.942			

From the result of Table 1, dialogue strategy and resolution of labour disputes was positively related and significant, Pearson's $r(352) = .159$, $p = .003$. This indicates a significant relationship between dialogue strategy and resolution of labour disputes because the *p*-value is less than the .05 level of significance. Therefore, H_{01} which states that there is no significant relationship between dialogue strategy and resolution of labour disputes in the colleges of education in North-West Nigeria was rejected.

$H0_2$: There is no significant relationship between negotiation strategy and resolution of labour disputes in colleges of education in North-West Nigeria.

This hypothesis was tested by subjecting the score for negotiation strategy and resolution of labour disputes scores to Pearson's correlation analysis as shown in Table 2.

Table 2. Relationship between negotiation strategy and resolution of labour disputes.

Variables	N	Mean	Std. Deviation	r-Cal	*p*-Value	Decision
Negotiation strategy	357	16.12	4.174	.223	.000	H_0 Rejected
Resolution of labour dispute	357	7.633	10.942			

From the result of Table 2, negotiation strategy and resolution of labour disputes was positively related and significant, Pearson's $r(352) = .223$, $p = .000$. This indicates a significant relationship between negotiation strategy and resolution of labour disputes because the *p*-value is less than the .05 level of significance. Therefore, H_{02} which states that there is no significant relationship between negotiation strategy and resolution of labour disputes in the colleges of education in North-West Nigeria was rejected.

$H0_3$: There is no significant relationship between mediation strategy and resolution of labour disputes in the colleges of education in North-West Nigeria.

This hypothesis was tested by subjecting the score for mediation strategy and resolution of labour disputes scores to Pearson's correlation analysis as shown in Table 3.

Table 3. Relationship between mediation strategy and resolution of labour disputes.

Variables	N	Mean	Std. Deviation	r-Cal	*p*-Value	Decision
Mediation Strategy	357	21.50	8.070	.323	.000	H_0 Rejected
Resolution of Labour Dispute	357	7.633	10.942			

From the result of Table 3, mediation strategy and resolution of labour disputes was positively related and significant, Pearson's $r(352) = .323$, $p = .000$. This indicates a significant relationship between mediation strategy and resolution of labour disputes because the p-value is less than the .05 level of significance. Therefore, H_{03} which states that there is no significant relationship between mediation strategy and resolution of labour disputes in the colleges of education in North-West Nigeria was rejected.

Summary of Findings

The following are the major findings of the study:

1. Dialogue strategy plays positive part in resolving labour disputes in Colleges of Education in North-West Nigeria.
2. Negotiating strategy is positively related to resolving labour disputes in Colleges of Education in North-West Nigeria.
3. Mediating strategy play a vital role in resolving labour disputes in Colleges of Education in North-West Nigeria.

Discussion of Findings

The data presented in the analysis of hypothesis one to three are further discuss respectively. Result in hypothesis one, which states that there is no significant relationship between dialogue strategy and resolution of labour disputes in the College of Education in the North-West, Nigeria was rejected. This also answered research question one and it is concluded that dialogue strategy is related to the resolution of Labour Disputes in Colleges of education in the North-West Nigeria. This means that dialogue strategy is a mechanism adopted to curtail Labour Disputes such that College of Management and Labour Union leaders dialogue on the subject of particular agitation. The finding was in line with Ajewole (2014) mentioned that adoption of dialogue strategy by the Management used to prevent or manager labour dispute effectively and such adaptation has positive relationship on resolution of labour disputes in colleges of education. Particularly if the College of Education Management could dialogue with the representative of labour unions and adhere to the terms, there is high probability that labour disputes could be deescalate. Hence, resolution of labour disputes could be guaranteed.

The result of hypothesis two which states that, there is no significant relationship between negotiation strategy and resolution of labour in colleges of education the North-West Nigeria was rejected. This means that, there is significant and positive relationship between negotiation and resolution of labour disputes in colleges of education in the North-West Nigeria. This suggested that negotiation seems to have universal application as principle in dispute management base on dialogue. People in all societies and cultures across the world talk and negotiate their interest. The finding was in line with Best (2015) maintained that, negotiation is a direct process of dialogue at least two parties who are faced with dispute situation. Both parties come to realization that they have a problem, and both are aware that by talking to each other can find solution to the problem. Morris (2012) Use a variety of approaches. One is "power negotiation" which involves a negotiators Understanding and strategic use of various sources of power to achieve negotiators bargaining goals. Moreover, Munck (2012) noted that, managing dispute is extensive and potentially resolved on a common ranging from simple negotiation between two people to international arbitration tribunal involving nations to the traditional adjudicative of each Country's legal system. Miller (2013) belief that negotiation involves communication usually governed by pre-established procedures between representatives of parties involves in a dispute.

The results in hypothesis three which states that there is no significant relationship between mediation strategy and resolution of labour dispute in Colleges of Education in the North-West Nigeria was rejected. This indicates a significant and positive relationship between mediation strategy and resolution of Labour Disputes in Colleges of Education in the North-west Nigeria. The finding have agree with Ajemole (2017) who found that, there is positive relationship between mediation strategy and labour dispute resolution. If the labour union leaders and College of education management could abide by the resolution of a third party such as industrial Arbitration panel, National Industrial Court or Board of Inquiry. The escalation of labour disputes could be curtailed and the Colleges of education management could be guaranteed.

7 Conclusion

Consequent upon these finding, the paper concluded that adoption of dialogue, negotiation and mediation strategy by the colleges of education management help to resolve labour disputes effectively in colleges of education in the North-West Nigeria.

Recommendations

On the basis of the Findings and Conclusion drawn from this study, the following recommendations were made:

1- When the management of college of education seem in capable to meet all the demands of labour Unions, both parties should dialogue in a round table, and honesty adhere to the terms of any agreement reached. However, if dialogue fail to resolve an issue, external intervention like a conciliator, arbitration panels, industrial courts or elder statesmen should be allowed in dispute resolution to prevent disruptions of activities in the institutions. Hence, labour union leaders and college of education management should learn to abide by the resolution of a third party.

2- Rather than embark on demonstration or any form of dispute to show grievances to the management of college of education labour unions should always give space for hearing and possible negotiations. However, when a dispute is in evitable, violence should be avoided for peaceful dispute resolution. The goals of college of education and interest of the students should always put in consideration.

3- Appropriation of mediation strategy were found to be effective in resolving labour actions in the sampled colleges of education. The adoptions of these strategy are recommended for the resolution of labour dispute in the public colleges of education. Particularly if college of education management should carry the labour union leaders along in their change process and whenever major policies affecting staff jobs are formulated. The management should also dialogue with the labour union leaders or opt for mediation with the intervention of third party where necessary.

Contribution to Knowledge. The major contribution of the paper discover that, Dialogue, Negotiation and Mediation Strategy are applicable in resolving labour dispute in Colleges of Education in the North-West, Nigeria.

References

Adeyemi, T.O.: Causes of consequences and control of studies crises in public and private Universities in Nigeria. Educ. Res. Rev. **4**, 4 (2010)

Adeyemi, T.O., Ademilun, S.O.: Conflict management strategies and administrative effectiveness in Nigerian universities. J. Emerg. Trends Educ. Res. Policy Stud. (JETERAPS) **3**(3), 368–375 (2012)

Ajemole, I.P.: Labour dispute, management strategies and administrative effectiveness in public Universities in South-West, Nigeria. Ph.D. Thesis University of Ilorin. Kwara State Nigeria (2017)

Ajewole, I.P.: Managing labour unrest in Nigeria Universities. J. Educ. Policy Rev. Conresin Publications **6**(2), 93–107 (2014)

Best, S.G.: The method of conflict resolution and transformation in Shedrac. In: Gaya Best (ed) Introduction to Peace and Conflict to Studies in West Africa Ibadan (2016)

Best, S.G.: The methods of conflict resolution and transformation. In: Best (ed.) Introduction to Peace and Conflict Studies in West African. Ibadan: spectrum books Ltd (2015)

Deutsch, M., Coleman, P.: The Handbook of Conflict Resolution: Theory and Practice. Jossey-Bass, San Francisco (2000)

Fatile, C.: Industrial Relations in Nigeria: Theory and Features, p. 132. Labonn and Coy, Lagos (2011)

Fatile, J.O., Adejuwon, K.D.: Conflict and conflict management in tertiary institutions: the case of Nigerian universities. European Journal of Humanities and Social Sciences, vol. 7, no. 1. Special Issue, titled: Planning, policies and global issue (2011). (ISSN 2220–9425)

Kazeem, K., Ige, O.: Redressing the growing concern of the education sector in Nigeria. Edo J. Counselling **3**(1), 40–48 (2010)

Kesterner, B.P., Ray, L.: The conflict resolution training programme. Leader's Manual. Jossey-Bass: United State of America (USA) (2012)

Lebarson, C.: Cooperate Strategy. Financial Management, London (2011)

Martin, M.: Marx and Engels: The Communist Manifesto, p. 35. Penguin Group, New York (2018)

Michael, B.: Industrial action in school. Strikes and students achievement. Canada labour market and skills research Network (2012)

Miller, C.A.: A Glossary of Terms and Concepts in Peace and Conflict Studies. University of Peace, Geneva (2013)

Moris, C.: Definitions in the field of dispute resolution and conflict transformation London zed books (2012)

Munck, R.: Globalization of Nigeria (2006). The new great transformation times. (London, Zed Books) (2012)

Application of Social Science Theories for Effective Teaching and Learning of History in Nigeria: Example of Dialectical Materialism

A. E. Afe(✉)

Department of History and International Studies, Adekunle Ajasin University, Akungba-Akoko, Ondo State, Nigeria

Abstract. There is an ongoing debate among researchers and teachers of history on how some social science theories can be applied for the purpose of effective teaching of the course/subject in Nigeria. It needs not to be overstressed the fact that the initiative has been strongly opposed by the conservative school of thought, which still holds on to the principle of researching and teaching history without theories. These conservatives have argued that such innovation will only erode the original practice, philosophy and methodology of History, which in the end will lead to inefficiency in teaching and contraction or narrowness of the student's thought and knowledge viewpoint. It is, therefore, against this backdrop that this paper examines, with a special reference to Marxist dialectical materialism, how the social science theories can be effectively and gainfully employed to create quality teaching and lifelong learning opportunities, in relation to the learning and teaching of History. The paper relies on primary and secondary sources subjected to descriptive and textual analysis. The paper argues and concludes that like every other teaching methods; the theoretical methods not without its own shortcomings. However, a systematic and careful application of it to the teaching of the discipline promises not to only effectively impact knowledge into the students, but also deepen and broaden their critical reasoning abilities that will in turn propel the desire for further learning and research.

Keywords: Teaching · Research · Learning · History · Marxist theory of dialectical materialism

1 Introduction

One of the major goals of teachers at the beginning of any lesson involves good understanding or effective learning by the students as this will not only guarantee their passing the assessments very well, but also ensure a long lasting impact of the teaching on the students. As a means of achieving this goal, teachers are always in the habit of creating different techniques for teaching their students. In the recent times, such techniques included the use of social science theories to structure their lecture notes, teach and sometimes even engage the students in field works. However, this teaching technique

J. N. Mojekwu et al. (Eds.): *Sustainable Education and Development*, pp. 66–74, 2021.
https://doi.org/10.1007/978-3-030-68836-3_7

is open to criticism, on the ground that it represents a derailing from the original open-ended method of teaching, and that it may narrow the thought of the students. The effort in this paper is not to join the open debate, rather it is an attempt to show how the use of theories, with specific focus on the Marxist dialectical materialism, can help teachers achieve the aforementioned set goals of the teachers as they interact with their students in a bid to impact knowledge into them.

2 Conceptual Clarification of Marxist Dialectical Materialism

Marxist dialectical materialism is a socio-economic theory attributed to Karl Marx (1818–1883) (Slaughter 1918). Though propounded in the nineteenth century from the economic, political and social presumptions, it has since been reconfigured severally to suit different purposes and conditions. Irrespective of the reconfigurations which have broadened and even made the theory complex, the central viewpoint is, however, still intact. Thus, the theory operates on the belief that human society is built on, and revolves around, the exchanges of economic forces. According to the theory, 'economy is the chief-agent of transformation of the society' (Slaughter 1918). In other words, human society rest solely on production or economy and it is this factor that chiefly determines the transformation of the society. Therefore, for the sustenance of any human society, the society, as a matter of compulsion, must produce at least the basic necessities of life; such as food, shelter, water and so on. Thus, the fortune of the society will be so attached to the economic process so much that instead of controlling the material or economic forces, the society is in turn influenced by the economic forces.

Consequently, the society will be stratified into two major socio-economic classes, which are those that control the means of production, the capitalists or bourgeoisie, and those that work for them, the labour or proletariats. Additionally, human behaviour, including the interactions of the classes with each another, will be shaped in consonance with the mode of production (Mises 2001). Most importantly, the nature of interaction between the two socio-economic classes, those who own the means of production and the labour force, will be a major determinant of the type of society that will evolve thereafter (Mises 2001).

Thus, while it is the sole intention of the capitalists to make profits, the workers are also pre-occupied with the commitment to improve their standard of living. A situation will, therefore, arise whereby for a class to maximally attain its goal, it must deprive the other of its benefits. This process of conflict of interests has been referred to as class struggle (Marx and Engels (ed.) Kamenka 1983). In the face of the struggle to end the continuous oppression of the proletariats, who have population advantage, they will be compelled to revolt against the capitalist group. Eventually, this will lead to the emergence of a classless society (Marx and Engels 1848). In sum, it can be said that Marxist dialectical materialism holds the development or changes in the society, political, social or otherwise, which are motivated by economic forces. Inferentially, other factors or explanations are rated secondary or less fundamental agents of societal transformation (Engels: 1883).

3 Extant Literature on Historical Dialectical Materialism

There are lots of studies, which have discussed historical dialectical materialism. While some seems to understand its historical background, methods and variations, others have attempted comparative analyses of these variants. For example, Khasawneh (2018) attempts a discourse on the validity of historical materialism that considered the economic ties as the basis of the social relations. The study argues that, the over the time, Marx's historical materialism has successfully defined the economic doctrine and the social system of different historical stages of human life. A major weakness, however, is that they reject the idea of any economic and social doctrine that accommodate several different historical roles. Thus, socio-economic factors are recognised as the only causes of history. According to the author, Marx saw the origin of historical conflicts is the difference between the situation of production forces and the patterns of production relations. Marx 'also claimed that the class struggles in societies are only social expressions of the imbalance between production forces on the one hand, and production relations on the other' (Khasawneh 2018). Thus, the theory stresses that it is not the consciousness of the people, which determines their existence, but their social existence that decides their consciousness. From the above and it discussed later this represents a gross violation of historical principle that recognises of multiple factors as causes of historical events. Irrespective of the shortcomings, the author argues that Marxist dialectical materialism has continuously been relevant to our understanding of history.

White (2014) attempts a consideration of Bakhtinian dialogic in an oppositional analysis to that of Vygotsky's dialectic position on education. The author's interest in the subject seemed to have been influenced by several assumptions being made of these positions and applied to the contemporary education system. The author observes, for instance, that although dialectics and dialogism are by no means exclusive to these men, their specific interpretations have continued to influence education across the world today. While both are frequently cited in educational texts internationally, the socio-cultural views of Vygotsky appear to be popular with the contemporary education theories than Bakhtinian dialogism. In order to develop her argument, White made an evaluation of the philosophical bedrocks of the two positions which are fundamental irreconcilable differences that need to be considered if the academic benefits of each are to be fully annexed. It is observed that while Vygotsky's ideas are enclosed in the notion of dialectical materialism, the philosophical tenets of dialogism are already subsumed within the dialectic terrain. Consequently, the opportunities that Bakhtinian dialogism has to present to education are largely misunderstood and unrealised. She argues that dialogism offers a possible way to a wide integration of a philosophy of education, especially as it is more concerned with the life of meaning than science and logic. She, therefore, submits that dialogism holds potential to provide a means of engaging with philosophical ideas in education and possible pedagogies (White 2014).

From the perspective of natural science, Wu and Nan (2020) examines the contemporary values of some viewpoints and hypothesis in Engels' dialectics to the promotion of the construction process of theory and practice of human ecological civilization and sustainable development strategy. According to the authors, dialectics in Engels' viewpoint talks only of not of the ways we observe the world, but also of the properties of its objective nature. Thus, the fundamental perspective of dialectics is to 'regard all things as the process of eternal change and movement in the interaction of universal relations' (Wu and Nan 2020).

In the authors' opinion, several aspects of the dialectic propositions of Engels are in tandem with the pertinent theories of contemporary science world. For instance, universal differences always generate universal interaction because the interactions unavoidably are based on the intermediary. Therefore, the general development of things is characterized by the unending sequence of progression and degeneration like holographic view, which interacts constantly. It is argued that we can reduce and prevent a number of disastrous consequences brought on our world by a re-evaluation of Engel's view stand and propositions since they have the potentials of practical significance and the value of correcting the separation between man and nature, society and nature that have been instituted by our contemporary philosophy of consciousness. It can, therefore, be deduced that the work is pay more attention to the relevance of the theory to science and human development.

. Using the documentary instrument of data generation and the technique of constant comparative analysis, Biereenu-Nnabugwu and Uchendu like Cowling attempts a comparative analysis of Hegel and Marxist views on dialectics. While Hegel and Marx agreed on the central role that dialectics plays in the historical development of society, they, however, differ on the standpoints on certain fundamental issues such as the extent or degree of its involvement in the transformation of the society. This study identifies and examines these significant issues and how they contribute to the development of the two ideas on social transformation. It is submitted by the authors that despite identifiable shortcomings, 'Marxian dialectics remains an option, indeed a useful tool in philosophical analysis of not only how the world works, but a means on how to change it' (Biereenu-Nnabugwu and Uchendu 2017).

Cowling, presents a highlight of the relationship between the dialectics proposed by Hegel and Marx. The author proceeds by dividing Hegel dialectics into four major forms or patterns. These include the dialectic of method; historical development through human intellectual labour, and the conception of the social totality resulting from this; the dialectic of the concrete real, and finally the dialectic of human physical labour. He then takes a look at the major forms of the dialectic in Marx, dividing it into periods as a way of showing the extent to that Marxist dialectic is influenced by that of Hegel. 'It submitted that the only part of Hegel's dialectic which is significant in the older Marx is his dialectic of method', suggesting a scientific method to Marx (Cowling 2016).

Away from these familiar focuses, the present study is pre-occupied with how this popular social science theory can be engaged by teachers of history as a mechanism to effectively teach history in our school. In other word, this paper chooses to contribute to the existing knowledge on the theory, not by venturing into the detailed analysis of its history, meaning, methods and forms, but on how the tenets of the theory can help in history education in the classroom.

4 How the Marxist Dialectical Materialism Can Facilitate Effective Teaching and Learning of History in Nigeria

The disinterest of students in history has continued to increase over the years. Among other factors, feedbacks from students have shown that one of the major reasons for this development is the age-long open-ended style or method of teaching that allows teachers to engage in the teaching of the subject without clearly setting the structure and the objectives of lessons with proper theoretical framework. Thus, everything does not only look compressed, but also uninteresting, boring and tiring to the students. It is against this backdrop that a lot of historians or teachers of history are now applying relevant social science theories to teach their students with the aim of addressing the challenges earlier mentioned. Popular among these theories is the Marxist dialectical materialism. Like every socio-science theory, the theory can be used to prepare the structure and objectives of lectures, such that at every point the student can properly analyse their own world or the contemporary society within the theoretical framework. The connection between historical lectures and the analysis of the current situation within this theoretical framework does not only make learning interesting, but also creates in the students a desire to learn more as it promises them good understanding of the society.

While the above seems to be general to all socio-science theories, it is important to now examine the advantages that are particular to the Marxist dialectical materialism as far as using it to ensure effective teaching and learning of history is concerned. To do this, it is only appropriate to examine the major features or views of the theory and see how these views can be engaged to attain the above goals.

According to Collingwood (1964), the object of history refers to the thing that a study of history centres on or the entity that is being studied. While giving further explanation, Collingwood argues that the object of history is nothing but *resgestae*: action of human beings that have been done in the past. In other words, history as a social science subject focuses strictly on the past activities or actions of human beings. It analyses significant past or historical events (actions of man), the causes or motivations for these actions (why), description or details on these actions (course or how) and the consequences of the actions (implication). Accordingly, there is no place for spiritualism in history. In other words, history sees human being, and not supernatural forces responsible for the societal changes.

Marxist dialectical materialism can be engaged as a tool by the teacher to explain this aspect of philosophy and methodology of history. In tune with the above principle of history, dialectical materialism also places premium on human activities as the object of the event being studied, though it argues that such actions were motivated only or mainly by economic calculations. It, therefore, reminds one of this aspect of the fundamentals or philosophy of history. The theory also strengthens our knowledge on the causes of man's actions, even with several available options, and the consequences of the actions or decisions taken. In the theory, the contest between the capitalists and labour is an action taken by man; it is not the one caused by some supernatural forces. Thus, dialectical materialism theory can be used to constantly refresh students' consciousness and understanding of the meaning of history and its object. Again, the theory can also be used to always alert the students' understanding about the fact that there is no place for spiritual forces in history and that all changes in human societies are products of past actions of human beings. Political, social and economic advancement or retrogression of human societies are inventions of man and not predestined by supernatural forces.

The present level of our development as a nation is not the responsibility of providence, as normally opined even sometime among the academics, but of human choice constructed into actions. The accumulation, embezzlement and personalisation of the societal resources by the capitalists, as shown in the theory, are all human actions. Similarly, the revolt by the oppressed after a long period of suffering is also an action taken by human beings. There is no place, where providence came to play in this interaction. In essence, good society and bad society are manmade: it is all a matter of choice and action. Therefore, theory has the potential to make students understand that the nature of the society's development in the future, as in the past and present, is largely going to be determined by people's present actions.

Another reason why many students and their parents take little or no interest in the study of history hangs on the belief that history has no concrete contribution to make to the development of the society. We live in an age that is driven by science and technology. Therefore, they see no place where history or any other course that is not related to natural science and technology can fit in to national development. They cannot comprehend how studying events that happened century or decades ago can add any value to the present; they believe it is just an art of tales by moonlight. Thus, wasting one time on a study that is not more than '*obaku, oba je*' (kings die, others enthroned) is the most unprofitable exercise that anyone can embark on.

A lot needs to be done to correct this notion. The students and their parents need to understand that like science and technology, history is relevant to the development of the contemporary society. The fact is that all fields of study, including the natural sciences and technology, have their history documented and the practitioners do not joke with such historical accounts as they are full of information about the evolution, discoveries, inventions, and transformations of the fields of study from the original practices to the contemporary stages. Talking about societal development, it is apparent that it comes in phases, but with strong connections of these phases with one another. For example, the present stage of our advancement and the attending challenges as a nation is a product of past human activities. And until we understand why and how we come to be where we are, we may not properly fit into the contemporary scientific and technological oriented world.

Dialectical materialism also recognises and can be used to explain the importance of stages or phases in history. The classless society, which is the end stage of the society according to the theory, does not just emerge. The society travels in stages up to the labour's violent reactions phase that eventually produces the classless phase of the society. Just like in biological science, no organism man included; takes its final shape at last emerging level. It has to go through a lot of developmental processes known as growth before its final and complete shape. However, every stage of the development is crucial as it does not only represent the past, but also forms important raw materials for the next phase of development.

Dialectical materialism, if handled carefully, can be used to enlarge students' knowledge and understanding of the philosophy 'causation' or causes of actions in history as it also takes into account the importance of reason(s) for human activities. For instance, the actions of the bourgeoisie and proletariat as illustrated by the theory are propelled largely by their interests. The accumulation of wealth and maximisation of profits at the expense of the workers are responsible for unfriendly labour policies such as low wages, bad working condition, proscription of labour union, implementation of obnoxious taxation, and so on, by the capitalists. Subsequently, the intention to resist the above condition is responsible for the agitation of the workers. In other words, these interests were the causes of the activities of the groups. The importance of this is that it reminds historian that all activities of man are driven by certain interests. That is why, according to Carr (1969), history is a study of causes, which explains why historians usually ask the question 'why'.

Notwithstanding the above, Marxist dialectical materialism falls short of professional historical standard in further relations to causation in history. Although the theory reminds us that human actions are not without reasons, it, however limited the reasons for such actions to economic factors. In contrary, history does not accept mono causal events. Carr argued that the historian's approach to the problem of cause is that he will commonly assign several causes to the same event. Therefore, 'people must be warned off by every possible means from considering the action of any one cause without taking account of the others whose effects are commingled with it' (Carr 1969). In fact, after the compilation of the causes, the historian is expected to further arrange them 'to establish hierarchy of causes which would fix their relation with one another, perhaps to decide which cause, or which category of causes, should be regarded as the ultimate causes, the cause of all causes' (Carr 1969). Thus, the more the questions asked the closer the historian gets to the past. The investigation of the causes of an event from different perspectives such as political, economic, religious, social, strategic, etc., has the potential of giving the historian insights into the past. Consequently, a historian who investigates the cause of an event through the mono causal approach will on a large scale deny himself/herself the opportunity of getting close to what actually happened.

While in some instances, economy could have been a major cause of an event, let us say a war, the occurrence of such events can hardly be limited to it. The Yoruba Interstate Wars (1793–1893), the French Revolution (1789–99), the Crimean War (1853–56), World Wars I (1914–18) and II, The Cold War (1939–45) and the Nigerian Civil War (1967–70), all had economic factors as their causes; even though there were other reasons or causes. Thus, teachers can still catch in on this shortcoming of the theory to teach and ensure a long time learning effect. To successfully do this, it is important to let the students understand that economy only does not drive the society. There are many other causes of societal movement- political, social and so on. More importantly, the teachers must be careful with the teaching method to be used in exposing the students to these causal factors. In this respect, a most appropriate teaching method may be the 'guided discovery learning method'. According to Westwood (2008), guided discovery learning method implies a teaching and learning method where students actively participate in the study such that the discovery and knowledge are largely made by them with a little guide from the teacher. This method helps facilitate deep learning on the part of the students. The process allows the students to view and resolve problems from the multiple perspectives available to them. With little guidance, the students can form hypothesis and create knowledge or add to existing one. Most importantly, the method have been found to promote long time learning as the discoveries made by the students themselves tend to remain with them longer than what they are told (Westwood 2008).

Another great value of history is the ability to predict the future that it gives to anyone, who dedicated to its study. Though no single event has the ability to reproduce itself the same way, certain human actions, over time, have always produced similar results. The fall of great pre-colonial African empires have shown similar pattern and results of overwhelming internal and external socio-political, economic and security challenges as major causes. It is important to note that Marxist dialectical materialism has also proved to be highly relevant in enhancing students' understanding of predictions as a strong value of history. In consonance with historical events, the theory gives an insight into the emergence of revolutions across the continents, as they were usually in form of a protest by the oppressed against the oppressor.

However, it should be noted that while Marxist dialectical materialism reminds one of predictions as an important value of history, its prediction style, however, falls short of the historical standard. Marxist dialectical materialism's prediction is more of prophecy. For example, the theory affirms that human societies will undergo the same process of transformation from classed to classless as capitalism will metamorphose to socialism and thereafter to communism (Marx and Engels 2005). However, no human society can boast yet of being classless. Also, in different parts of the world, societies have continuously exhibited social, economic and political stratifications and in all, though with some differences, the political class, have dictated the policies of government and enjoyed the economic proceeds of the societies more than any other class. Furthermore, the spread of capitalism globally at the expense of socialism since the late 1980s have opened Marxist predictions to serious criticisms. Even in Eastern Europe, the professed headquarters of socialism, there are increasing number of people and states calling for capitalism. It is for reasons like this that history makes predictions that can be termed probable-predictions.

Indeed, the fusion of history and theory may not make the students to predict the exact or specific course, nature or impact of future events, but they will be able to offer useful advice to the society. The application of the theory helps to take the understanding of the students from the classroom experience relevant to the real world, as they are provided an insight into the future. Consequently, they do not only understand the present through the knowledge of the past, but like every true historian, they are privy to the future, and that puts them in good position to even predict it.

Meanwhile on the general basis, the theory's explanation on class struggle has continued to be relevant to our understanding of human societies, the interactions and negotiation of group interest and the place of these factors in the history or development of the society. Although in the theory, class struggle is limited to the economic realm as it plays out between the employers of labour and the proletariat being oppressed (Ollman 1968), its application to historical issues such as ethnicity in multi-ethnic states such as Nigeria, Libya, and so on promises to give good insights into the past and better understanding of the present. The fact that all societies, past and present, have existed based on political, socio-economic or cultural class makes the theory a relevant tool for the study of class or race history.

5 Conclusion

This paper has examined how Marxist dialectical materialism can ensure effective and long time learning in the students. It is observed that the theory, like most social science theories, has the ability to organise lesson in simple and meaningful ways such that teaching will not be boring to the students. Also, the theory has the ability of connecting the lectures to the reality of the students which in turn does not only create good understanding but allows what is taught to sink deeper and last for a long time. Most importantly, if combined with appropriate teaching methods such as the guided discovery method, the theory would encourage and empower the students to form hypothesis and make discoveries by themselves. Thus, on a large scaling, learning will not have only taken place, but also the knowledge acquired can tend last long with the students, who make the discoveries themselves.

References

Biereenu-Nnabugwu, M., Uchendu, P.C.: Dialectics and social transformation in modern political thought: a comparative study of Hegel and Marx. Afr. J. Polit. Sci. Int. Relat. **11**(2), 13–20 (2017)

Carr, E.H.: The October Revolution: Before and After. Knopf, New York (1969)

Collingwood, R.G.: The Idea of History. Oxford University Press, London (1964)

Cowling, M.: The Dialectic in Marx and Hegel–an Outline, paper was presented at the Marxism Panels of the PSA Annual Conference, Brighton, 21–23rd March 2016

Hay, C.: Marxism and the State. In: Gamble, A., Marsh, D., Tant, T., (eds.), Marxism and Social Science. Palgrave, London (1999)

Khasawneh, A.J.: The historical validity of Marx's theory of historical materialism'. Hist. Res. Lett. **46**, 1–8 (2018)

Marx, K., Engels, F.: The Portable Karl Marx, E. Kamenka (ed.). Penguin Books, New York (1983)

Marx, K., Engels, F.: Manifesto of the Communist Party. Progress Publishers, Moscow (1848)

Marx, K., Engels, F.: The Communist Manifesto and Other Writings. Barnes and Noble Books, New York (2005)

Mises, L.: Theory and History: An Interpretation of Social and Economic Evolution. Ludwig von Mises Institute, Alabama (2001)

Ollman, B.: Marx's use of class'. Am. J. Soc. **73**(5), 573–580 (1968)

Slaughter, C.: Marxism, Ideology, and Literature. Macmillan, London (1918)

Westwood, P.S.: What Teachers Need to Know About Teaching Methods. Australia, ACER Press, Adelaide (2008)

White, E.J.: Bakhtinian dialogic and Vygotskian dialectic: compatibilities and contradictions in the classroom? Educ. Philos. Theory **46**(3), 220–236 (2014)

Wu, K., Nan, Q.: The contemporary value of engels' dialectics'. Int. J. Syst. Sci. Appl. Math. **5**(2), 12–19 (2020)

Women Perceptions on Factors Contributing to Job Transition in Higher Learning Institutions in Tanzania: A Phenomenological Approach

M. A. Tambwe[1](✉), M. Y. Mazana[2], and M. A. Mapunda[1]

[1] Department of Marketing, College of Business Education, P. O. Box 1968, Dar es Salaam, Tanzania
m.tambwe@cbe.ac.tz

[2] Department of Mathematics and ICT, College of Business Education, P. O. Box 1968, Dar es Salaam, Tanzania
y.mzomwe@cbe.ac.tz

Abstract. Women job transition issue became important phenomenon, as the transformative agenda called for in the 2030 agenda for Sustainable Development adopted by the United Nations in 2015. However, there is an empirical gap on the factors contributing to women job transition. This study aims to explore the factors of women job transition in Tanzania. A phenomenological qualitative research design using an in-depth interview and documents review were applied. Data were collected from sixteen women working in service sector such as education. A purposive sampling followed by snow-ball sampling technique were used. The data were analyzed using thematic analysis techniques. From participants perspectives the following factors contributing to women job transition in Tanzania; Family matters, Remuneration issues, poor working environment and the need for new exposure. This study reveals the need for employers and policy makers to consider family stability, improvement of remuneration, improvement of the working environment and managers' professionalism to ensure women stay in their job. This information will assist policy makers to come up with new policies or amend the existing ones to create conducive environment for women job satisfaction.

Keywords: Job transition · Women · Phenomenology · Tanzania

1 Introduction

Over the recent decade, globally, there has been a significant decrease in women working as contributing family workers and, in many countries, labour force participation rates gaps have been somewhat diminishing (ILO 2016). Yet, several gaps persist and more needs to be done to address them. Global statistics show that female labour force participation rate stands at 49%, compared to male which is 76% (World Bank 2019). The data for Tanzania on the female labour force participation from 1990 to 2018 shows the average value of 83.73% with a maximum of 87.02% in 2006 and a minimum of 79.39% in 2018 (Tanzania: Female labor force participation 2019). Despite the statistics which

J. N. Mojekwu et al. (Eds.): *Sustainable Education and Development*, pp. 75–88, 2021.
https://doi.org/10.1007/978-3-030-68836-3_8

shows increase of Female Labor Force Participation Rate (FLFPR) globally, Tanzania is also faring well in regards to FLFPR, although the percentage is declining (From 87.02 in 2006 to 79.39 in 2018). These data show that gaps in labour force participation and employment have narrowed and women are shifting away from contributing family work and moving to the services sector, however, the factors leading to women's jobs transition decision remains a matter of concern.

Job transition or mobility can be defined as intra and or inter organizational transitions in the people's work of life (Ng et al. 2007). Due to life changes, economic conditions and competitions, people become more flexible, and self-directed about transition from one job to another. Further, Job transition enhances individual's job satisfaction, knowledge diffusion, innovation, and technology development which will stimulate growth and economic development as well as gender equality. Empirical evidences show that women have shifted from contributing as family workers into wage employment or own account work (self-employment) (Klasen et al. 2019). Statistics show that, the reduction in women contributing family work in favor of wage and salaried employment has increased from 30.4% in 1995 to 40.9% in 2015. Globally, there is higher proportion of women transition from informal to formal economy (ILO 2016). As a result, women job transition issue became an important phenomenon, due to the transformative plan called for in the 2030 agenda for Sustainable Development adopted by the United Nations in 2015.

Realizing the importance of women job transition various studies (Klasen et al. 2019; Afridi et al. 2018; Afande 2015) have been conducted to identify factors contributing to this shift. Nevertheless, these studies are few and have used macro data which do not unfold empirically the factors contributing to women job transition. Furthermore, this field is dominated by quantitative studies which downplay individuals' experiences and personal understanding. Based on these prior studies there is a limited exploration of the factors contributing to women job transition in Tanzania. Therefore, this study aims to explore factors contributing to women job transition decision in Tanzania using a first-hand information through a phenomenological approach. This study is important due to the fact that a better understanding of factors contributing to women job transition is crucial, as it will help policy makers to come up with new policies or amend the existing ones to create conducive environment for women job satisfaction. Generally, the study had the following objective; to explore the factors contributing to women's job transition in Tanzanian Higher Learning Institutions. Specifically, the following objectives were developed; to identify the experiences of women in shifting from one job to another; to understand the reasons for shifting and to recommend measures to ensure women stay in their job.

2 The Theoretical and Conceptual Framework

The current study focuses on the link between women perceptions on the job and the factors contributing to women job transition as phenomenological research seeks to discover how individuals construct meaning of human experiences. Similarly, as the study is qualitative in nature it has to develop a broad foundation of knowledge through inductive discovery (Schuemann 2014). The knowledge obtained were used in navigating patterns and themes that emerge through analysis of data. The study attempts to investigate how women perceive the factors contributing to job transitions in Tanzania Higher Learning institutions based on the previous literatures as indicated in Fig. 1. For that case, this study is grounded on two theoretical pillars: Role Congruity Theory and Decision-Making Theory.

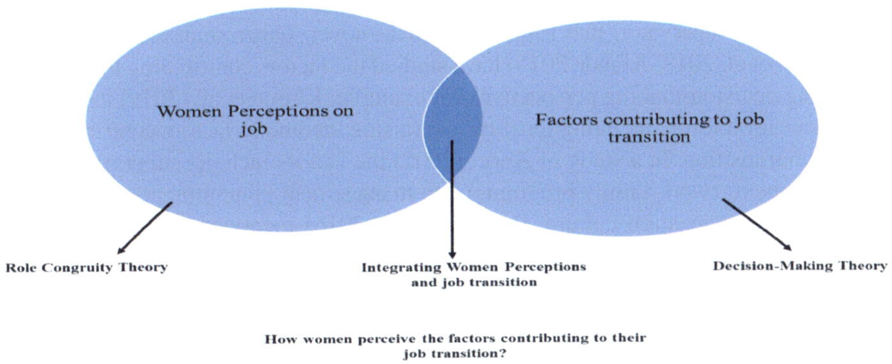

Fig. 1. Conceptual and theoretical framework

Role Congruity theory was propagated by Eagly and Karau (2002) extending on Eagly's social role theory of gender variances and resemblances into new ground (Eagly et al. 2000). It clarifies that gender-role congruent actions are more favorably evaluated than gender-role incongruent actions. For example, traditionally people perceive women and men to behave differently in work settings. These prospects are assumed to be grounded on gender stereotypes that "stem from the traditional roles that men and women have historically occupied" (Rudman and Phelan 2010 p. 192). Previous studies have investigated the factors affecting women on career advancement (Dikkers et al. 2010; Weng et al. 2010). For instance, Dikkers et al. (2010) studied on the effect of ambition on job level and career satisfaction, found that the number of work hours, and the use of work–home arrangements satisfied women. In another study by Weng et al. (2010) on organizational career growth in a sample of Chinese workers found an association between gender and remuneration growth as factors. Another study held interviews among British nurses discovered that opportunities for promotion also contributes to women job transition (Whittock et al. 2002).

On the other hand, Sullivan and Al Ariss (2019) identified five theoretical perspectives on career transitions including career stage, Decision making, adjustment, relational and identity perspective. For this study, decision-making perspective fits well as it explains why people stay or why people make a career transition which is the focus of this study. The key focus of this perspective is determining what factors influence the decision-making process of individuals faced with the opportunity to make a career transition (Sullivan and Al Ariss 2019).

While the rational decision-making approach is still used, current study has combined the existence of chance events (Kindsiko and Baruch 2019) and emotions into the decision-making process (Singh and Greenhaus 2004). Chance incidences, both positive, such as an unanticipated job offer, and negative, such as an employing organization's achievement by a company with different values and goals, have been examined (Forrier et al. 2009; Hirschi 2010; Peake and McDowall 2012). In addition to examining chance incidences, researchers started to reflect how emotions impact the decision to engage in various career transitions. For example, Maertz and Campion (2004) found that some job leavers act impulsively, quitting a job without an alternative position. These workers may have experienced a highly emotionally charged situation, such as an interaction with an abusive supervisor, that triggered their turnover. Other studies (Klasen et al. 2019; Afridi et al. 2018; Afande 2015) have studied the factors contributing to this transition using decision-making perspective. For example, Klasen et al. (2019) mentioned raising education level, declining fertility, and raising income as factors contributing to women job transition. In a study of Knorr (2005) the factors include: supportive working environment, (work-family programs), top management commitment, training and development, organization culture. Dimova et al. (2016) mentioned job stability and job satisfaction as contributing to women job transition. In another study by Afande (2015) the factors are: higher paying employment offers, fewer working hours, family commitment, occupational stress, sexual harassment at work, and lack of promotion opportunities. From these theoretical stances and empirical evidences, this study used the obtained variables in navigating patterns and themes that emerge through analysis of data.

3 Methodology

3.1 Research Approach and Design

As the present study is focusing on the perceptions and understanding of job transition from the women experiences, it leads itself to a qualitative, interpretivist approach through phenomenological design. The term 'phenomenology' is defined by Patton (2002 p. 104) as interpreting "how participants perceive a phenomenon, describes it, feel about it, judge it, remember it, make sense of it, and talk about it with others". The choice of the qualitative approach was based on our interest to capture the lived experiences of women regarding how they interpret job transition phenomenon as Creswell (2014) provided the rationale for the use of qualitative research as a suitable research to interpret experiences of individual(s). For that case, understanding the experiences will provide an opportunity to reflect on the factors contributing to women job shift in order to improve working environment.

3.2 Population, Sampling and Sample Size

The target population of this study was women, especially those who have experienced a phenomenon of shifting from one job to another. This study employed a purposive sampling technique in which rich data from the participants with similar experiences were obtained. Purposive sampling was used to select the first three participants then followed by snow-ball sampling technique which was applied to get the next participant. A snow-ball technique was used to get more contacts for data collection through interviews (Loh et al. 2011).

The study's sample comprised of 16 women in which four were lecturers, three academic staffs, four librarians and five secretaries. The size of the sample in qualitative research is still debatable. Creswell (2014) emphasized that even a sample of ten can represent a reasonable size, as the most important thing in a qualitative research is the quality not the quantity. Furthermore, Leedy and Ormrod (2010) suggested the number of sample size in phenomenological research should range from five to 25. In this study Sixteen participants were within the suggested range of the sample size. The sample size of sixteen was reached when data saturation occurred and new data ceased to emerge from interview.

3.3 Data Collection and Ethics

Data were collected from experienced self and wage employed women in service sectors especially higher education. Our choice of service sector is based on the evidence that globally service sector employs a highest number of women and men. Global statistics show that women employment in services has increased from 41.1% to 61.5% (ILO 2016). Data were collected by means of face to face interview sessions. All interviews were guided by an interview guide, but when the participant's answer to a question necessitated a follow-up question the interviewer probed further. Sometimes prompts and checks were used to ensure the correctness of the captured data (Denscombe 2010). The interviews were conducted at the interviewees' offices, and lasted up to 45 min. The interviews guide consisted of three main questions that are described in Table 1.

Table 1. The interview guides

The interview question	Description
What experiences do women have in shifting from one job to another?	The question aimed at finding out the women feelings and opinions about their past and present job
Why women shift from one job to another?	The question aimed at finding out the factors contributing to women job shift
What do you think should be done to ensure women stay in their job?	To identify measures to correct the problem of frequent women job shifting so as to stimulate growth and economic development

The interview guide was prepared in English language, then translated into Swahili which is a common spoken language in Tanzania. The interviews were audio recorded and transcribed verbatim for subsequent data analysis. The interviewed transcriptions were written in Swahili and the then text extracts translated into English were used to support the findings. In the study all ethical issues were adhered to as participants were asked for their consent and voluntary participation. Anonymity were ensured to protect participant's identity.

3.4 Data Analysis and Trustworthiness

Data were analyzed using qualitative techniques through content analysis, in which themes were generated and illustrated using participants' quotes. At first each data transcript was read from the beginning to the end. Then, the transcripts were re-read this time highlighting text that appeared to be related to, for example, feelings or opinions of women about their present and past job, and writing a keyword or phrase that seemed to capture issues related to women job transition. After coding of five transcripts, preliminary codes were identified which were then used to code all the remaining transcripts, including re-coding of the five transcripts used to generate the initial codes. The codes were then reviewed to ascertain the relationship with the original data while allowing new ones to emerge. The final codes were used to describe major issues describing factors contributing to women job transition. Finally, quotations were presented verbatim to present a true reflection of the voices of the participants to better understand the phenomenon. Trustworthiness was ensured through member check by requesting three participants to read the transcribed data files to check if the transcriptions match the intended meaning of the participants quotations were presented verbatim to present a true reflection of the voices of the participants.

4 Results and Discussion

4.1 What Are the Women Experiences Regarding Their Past and Present Job?

Women raised a number of issues concerning their experiences and opinions regarding their past and present job. Their responses fall into three major themes namely, the link between professionalism and job performance, the working environment, and the customers served. The themes are explained below:

The Link Between Professionalism and Job Performance: Three sub-themes emerged including; the level of education, mastering of works and colleagues' assistance.

The level of education; Women had opinions that the level of education is a cause to their job shift. Their feelings and opinions revolved around the notion that, when one has little education level led to do clerical works under close supervision but after acquiring high level of education led to do a more professional work under minimum supervision or self-directed. During the interview one woman said, "... *library work we used to rotate but initially I was very much on the bags checkpoint but after having a bachelor degree I got into other jobs that are a little bit more professional, like these research you do will move around but then when it comes to me I will take it to content on the CBE website on information system*" (Interviewer 3, 14 years working experience). Another woman said, "... *when I was a secretary I was ordered and directed to do everything, but as I changed and now, I am an academic officer I became more self-controlled (many things I managed myself) and supervise others* (Interviewer 12, 20 years working experience).

Mastering of works; some women expressed their feelings that in their past job they had little education but after acquiring higher education level, they have mastered their works and become experts in their field as evidenced by one woman during the interview, "... *After working for about a year as the library attendant, the job which I was advised by management … I accepted to study for a librarian. When I returned, I was recategorized and until now I am working as a professional librarian. Now I am an expert (she laughed) … it takes me a few seconds to get a book from a shelf*" (Interviewee 1, 10 years working experience).

Colleagues' assistance; women opined that colleagues' assistance is very important aspect in growing someone's profession and performance. The ones who received assistance from colleagues were happy and improved their performance as said by one interviewee, "… *but Mr. XXX did a great job of teaching me he did extra work to teach me, when I was struggling, I asked him, my brother I don't understand … until I went back to school.* (Interviewee 1, 10 years working experience).

The Working Environment: Six sub-themes were identified. These include; Types of job, working hours, Differences in salary, payment mode, availability of opportunity to advance career and poor cooperation between management and staff.

Types of job performed: women views revolve around the types of job they do. During the interview one woman explained, "… *in business the problem was capital, … though data entry depended on the availability of the job because it was temporary …. if it's not available you stay at home*" (Interviewee 6, 5 years working experience). Similarly, another interviewee said "…*In my previous job I was an instructor I dealt directly with students, I teach, I give them practicing questions. But here I deal indirectly with students, only those with problems*" (Interviewee 14, 5 years working experience).

Working hours; some women expressed their feelings based on long working hours in private sector as opposed to the public sector. This is evidenced by the interviewee's narration, "*I used to report at 7 am and leave at 6 pm but the wages are low, and if you do not go to work then your salary is reduced according to the days you were unable to work*" (Interviewee 10, 16 years working experience). In addition to that, another woman said "… *in my first job I was having a tight schedule, I didn't have time to rest or do other social activities. This second job at least I can schedule other things … so it's more flexible with this new job*" (Interviewee 16, 1 year working experience).

Differences in salary, women describe their experience of the past and present job based on the difference in salary obtained as evidence from this quote from the interviewee, "…*in my first job the salary was little but when I changed my job the salary and other benefits increased*" (Interviewee 12, 20 years working experience).

Payment mode, some women expressed their feelings and experiences in their past job in terms of payment mode, that they were paid depending on the hours they worked. This is evidenced by one woman's narration "… *If you do not go to work your salary is cut … you fail to participate in social activities…*" (Interviewee 10, 16 years working experience).

Availability of opportunity to advance career; few interviewed women said that, in their past job they did not get an opportunity to pursue further studies which could enable them to advance their career, but the present job gives them an opportunity to advance their career. The following quote supports the finding, "… *being employed here it gives me the opportunity to aspire to do something else since I came in as a secretary with certificate but because of the opportunity there are evening lessons that I have the opportunity to develop myself as an employee by pursuing bachelor degree and pay half the fees…*" (Interviewee 10, 16 years working experience).

Poor cooperation between management and staff; Women expressed their relationship experience with their boss by comparing past and present job. During the interview one woman had this to say, "*... if there is a conflict between her and the management one sees we don't have to argue then she declares to leave ...*" (Interviewee 5, 3 years working experience).

The Customers Served: Women raised their concerns about customers served in their past and present job. Their responses led to two sub-themes such as types of customers and the number of customers served.

Types of customers served; women said that the type of customers they serve are different from their past job and the present job. The following quote supports the finding, "*... At the bank you cater to a variety of business people, employees and multinationals. There is a challenge in serving such people because they feel they have a right. You need to be humble. The difference here is students, they are like your children, they are submissive even though they are all customers*" (Interviewee 15, 20 years working experience). Similarly, another interviewee's narration supports the results, "*... in practice there are differences in the manner of college students and secondary and primary students. College students are adults with sufficient understanding as compared to children*" (Interviewee 2, 10 years working experience)

Number of customers served; the experience of women on the number of customers served in their past and present job were revealed as evidenced in the following quotes from the interviewee, "*... reception I met many people many times (talk more), being secretary, I meet few people – most of the time I work on computer, e-mail, files ...*" (Interviewee 8, 6 years working experience). In the same perspective, another interviewee's quote supports the result, "*... as a telephone operator I met few clients and I was alone in that office, but now as a professional officer I receive many clients and I am with another colleague in the office whom we assist each other ...*" (Interviewee 9, 27 years working experience).

These findings mean that women's feelings on the past and present job were based on the link between professionalism and job performance, the differences in the working environment and the differences of the customers served. In the past studies, they have not explored women experiences regarding their past and present jobs. Looking at the issues raised some are similar to factors that lead to job transition as report in previous studies, but others are new findings. For instance, Knorr (2005) findings reported among other factors, working environment, training and development leads to job shift. In view of our findings we suggest that despite the working environment and training, the customers served and the new professions acquired by staff make them prefer to do other jobs.

4.2 Why Women Shift from One Job to Another?

Initial coding of this question resulted in ten categories. In the next round, some categories were merged which resulted into four major themes. These themes were: Family matters, Remuneration issues, poor working environment and the need for new exposure.

Family Matters; Two sub-themes have emerged namely multiple roles and men jealousy

Multiple roles, women as family care takers are shouldered with many responsibilities such as being pregnant, giving birth, taking care of the family and so on. These responsibilities make them aspiring to get jobs which will give them some time to fulfil these roles. One of the interviewed women narrated, "… *what made me to shift was birth problems - my baby had a little problem* …" (Interviewee 4, 3 years working experience). Other woman said, "*I was expecting a second child so I have to opt out of work and have a good time to raise the baby*" (Interviewee 15, 20 years working experience). In the perspective, another woman's quote supports the finding, "*Another factor that causes a person to move may be that the woman is married and her husband is not in the area so the wife has to move to follow the husband*" (Interviewee 3, 14 years working experience).

Men jealousy, some women opined that men jealous could be another factor contributing to women job shift as narrated in the following quote, "*Some leave because of a husband, coming home late made their husband to be dissatisfied due to jealous', he orders a wife to leave work, becomes a housewife or opens a business for her*" (Interviewee 15, 20 years working experience).

Remuneration Issues; The interviewed women reported that low salary and lack of allowances contribute to women job shift. One woman had this to say, "… *people really look for better paying jobs, by comparing where I go and where I come from because we look for green pastures*" (Interviewee 11, 16 years working experience). Another interviewee's quote supports the result, "*But another reason why women shift from one job to another is wage difference including salaries and benefits because people are looking for better remuneration*" (Interviewee 9, 27 years working experience).

Poor Working Environment: Women raised their concerns about the impact of poor working environment contribution to women job shift. Their responses led to five subthemes such as lack of appreciation, stigma, tight working schedules, distance from home to work, misunderstanding between management and staff,

Lack of appreciation, interview results reveal that lack of appreciation cause women to shift from one job to another. Some women's opinions exhibited that other cadre like secretaries are not appreciated as evidenced from the following narration, "*Some people see us as worthless, but if you think someone who is worthless is the one who caused you to get there, … this led me to study something else because you see me as worthless*" (Interviewee 5, 5 years working experience).

Stigma, majority of women in this study indicated that they have been stigmatized in different ways which make them feel bad and leave the job. The findings from the interview exhibited some elements of sexual harassment, suppression and despise that caused women to shift jobs. During the interview women have this to say, "*Someone sees here I am being stigmatized, maybe a co-worker wants you for sex and you have no way to avoid him, you decide to look for another job*" (Interviewee 3, 14 years working experience). Another interviewee added, "*some people are very disapproving our cadre, there are people you talk to and they despise secretaries … I don't know maybe another cadre, the secretary usually decides to go to another cadre to avoid this*" (Interviewee 6, 5 years working experience).

Tight working schedules, it was found in this study that women shift job due to long working hours and tight schedules which cause them to fail to attend family and other social activities. This is evidenced by the following interviewee's quote, "... *in other work environments it is more difficult to participate in family or other social activities while in other institutions she is free to carry out her own work responsibilities but also to participate in family and other social activities*" (Interviewee 10, 16 years working experience).

Distance from home to work, the findings of this study indicate that distance from home to work is another factor contributing to women job shift. Most of the women aspires to work near home as evidenced by the following narration from the interviewee, "*one sees the distance where she lives and the work is far away so maybe finding another place to work nearby will be worth it*" (Interviewee 3, 14 years working experience).

Misunderstanding between management and staff, regarding the relationship with the boss women had mixed opinions. Some were of the view that misunderstanding between the superior with the subordinates lead to women job shift while others opined the situation to depend how the subordinate handle it. The interviewee's narration shows, "*it can happen misunderstanding occurs between the boss and the secretary... you know we spend a lot of time in the office, now if you are stressed or uncomfortable, ... why should I stay, I look for a place where I will be comfortable*" (Interviewee 12, 20 years working experience). Another interviewee had this to say, "... *I didn't find it very difficult that made me regret my job... I had good relationships with my bosses. He being fierce I become gentle*" (Interviewee 7, 14 years working experience).

Need for New Exposure; This led to two sub-themes namely, to advance career and search for new challenges

To advance career, women shift from one job to another in order to look for opportunities which will allow them to advance their career. The following quote supports the finding, "*Often someone wants to go and promote their career as I personally shift because I want to grow my career...*" (Interviewee 8, 7 years working experience). Similarly, another interviewee said, "... *some women shift in search of opportunities for further development...*" (Interviewee 4, 3 years working experience).

Search for new challenges, other interviewed women explained that their job shift was caused by their need for new challenges and exposure. This is evidenced by the following interviewee's quote, "... *Others perhaps shift because they want to get more exposure and experience ...*" (Interviewee 2, 10 years working experience). Another interviewee had this to say "... *I've stayed in this job seven years since 2012 now I wish I could grow my career to find new challenges, get to know new people, you never know. and I have been here ...*" (Interviewee 8, 7 years working experience).

The findings from this study corroborates other studies findings (Afande 2015; Klasen et al. 2019; Knorr 2005). Afande (2015) reported on higher paying employment offers, family commitment, occupational stress and fewer working hours as factors contributing to job shift. While Klasen et al. 2019 findings revealed raising educational level, declining fertility and raising income. This study's results came up with new factors from women experiences that, new exposure also contributes to women job shift. However, in previous studies some themes are similar but, interstingly in this study some aspects are peculiar. For instance, the issue of men jealous, lack of appreciation, distance from home to work. These issues might occur in developing contries than developed countries.

4.3 What Should Be Done to Ensure Women Stay in Their Job?

Coding of this question, initially resulted into eight categories. In the next round, some categories were combined leading into four major themes namely family stability, improvement of remuneration, improvement of the working environment and consideration of managers' professionalism.

Family Stability, this theme was captured in terms of husband's job transfers which leads to family instability as wife has to shoulder double responsibilities as a result woman decide to relocate to their husband's job station. Supporting this result one interviewee said, "*... if a woman is with her family in one place can relax... but if I am in Dar es Salaam and the husband is probably in Dodoma, I will panic and struggle to look for another job ... if we were both in Dar Es Salaam I will stay in my job but if we are separate, I have to follow my husband*" (Interviewee 1, 10 years working experience).

Improvement of Remuneration; within this theme, three sub-themes emerged, notably the issue of motivation, salary harmonization and timely promotion.

The issue of motivation; women expressed their experiences on the measures to ensure women stay in their job. Among the measures, the issue of motivation surfaced. Some interviewees considered motivation in terms of appreciation, better salaries and other fringe benefits. From their opinion appreciation can be even through just verbal acknowledgement. This is evidenced by the following interviewee's narration, "*Institutions should try to motivate people, people are leaving to pursue better salaries, management should focus on the problem of why people move away from work it seems things are not right ... putting it right people will not think of leaving their work*" (Interviewee 6, 5 years working experience). In addition, another interviewee said, "*... to retain employee you should motivate them, ... how do you motivate them, even by verbal appreciation or acknowledgement, you don't have to give money eh!*" (Interviewee 12, 20 years working experience).

Salary harmonization; the interviewees proposed that, there is a need for salary harmonization in public institutions so as to ensure women stay in their job as commented by one woman, "*... public institutions should have the same level of salaries scales ... for example, all with bachelor degree should have the same starting salary scale ... there is no reason for government institutions' salary to differ*" (Interviewee 9, 27 years working experience).

Timely promotion and recategorization; the results from the interviewee indicated that, timely promotion is another criterion of concern for women to stay in their job. Others opined that timely promotion can be in terms of recategorization as long as the person meets the required criteria. Supporting this result one interviewee said, "*... the person should be promoted on time ... as long as the person's promotion time is due*" (Interviewee 6, 5 years working experience). Another woman explained, "*... transitioning from one cadre to another ... upon graduation also perhaps a qualified HR person should be given the opportunity to try and even do the HR tasks and not stay there as a receptionist, changing them in terms of recategorization*" (Interviewee 8, 7 years working experience).

Improvement of the Working Environment; With regard to this theme, three sub-themes emerged, particularly, provision of clear job description and scheme of service, communication, *Equality*, regarding equality issue women have different perceptions and experiences. Some women had the opinion that, equal treatment among staff could satisfy women to stay, while others thought that equal representation especially in top positions in the organization could be the reason to women job satisfaction and hence, make them stay. Women proposed that if the top position is held by a man, under him should be a woman and vice versa. The following quote supports the finding, "*I see as they do in parliament fifty-fifty, even in institutional leadership, they have to look for the capable women and give them leadership posts…*" (Interviewee 3, 14 years working experience).

Provision of clear job description and scheme of service, from the conducted interviews, women suggested that a clear job description and scheme of services could make women stay in their job, as evidenced in the following quote, "*The scheme of services should be open to everyone to know their responsibilities*" (Interviewee 5, 3 years working experience). Another woman added, "*… there are should be grounds to be followed that Georgina's work is so and so, and she will do this and this… yes job description*" (Interviewee 2, 10 years working experience).

Communication, women suggested that communication with staff in terms of dialogue through meetings, suggestion box. Also, Human Resource (HR) officers should be a link by trickling down the information from the government to staff. The following quotes support the finding, "*HR at the institution should be the advocate for their people, if something is done in the service then they should be the first to tell their people and not hide the information from above that is beneficial to employees*" (Interviewee 7, 14 years working experience). "*… talking through joint or technical forums, for example, today I want to listen to women employees' challenges … but it is also possible through the sessions some shy away to speak, so there should be suggestion box so that one can write her grudges …*" (Interviewee 10, 16 years working experience).

Consideration of the Managers' Professionalism; In this theme, some women had proposed that managers are made so they have to learn and practice managerial roles. It has been reported in the study that staff retainment function is not efficient, so it was suggested that managers' professionalism should be insisted. "*In the past, someone before you became a manager or a leader in an institution you were trained, that's why in the past, Mzumbe University was a management college where people were trained as managers … you will find in an institution the person is shifting the job, the manger is happy and just sign the letter … they must learn to retain staff in the institution*" (Interviewee 12, 20 years working experience).

The results of this study are in line with Afande (2015) findings on the aspect of giving equal opportunities in training and development as well as supporting women leaders due to their multiple roles. However, it was noted that most of the previous reviewed studies have not proposed solutions to the women job shift. This is the contribution made in our study.

5 Conclusion and Implication

This study aimed to explore the factors contributing to women job transition in Tanzania. Specifically, the study finds the experiences of women regarding their past and present job, the factors contributing to women job transition and the measures to revert the situation. From the discussion of the results the study concludes that professionalism, working environment and the customers served are the critical areas of concern which differentiates one job and the other. It was observed that despite the working environment and training, the customers served and the new professions acquired by staff make them prefer to do other jobs. Factors contributing to women job shift include; family issues, remuneration issues, poor working environment, and need for new exposure. The measures proposed to ensure women stay in their job were; family stability, improvement of remuneration, improvement of working environment and consideration of managers' professionalism.

These results have revealed various factors causing women job transition which have a lot of implications for employers to create conducive environment for women job satisfaction. Job transition leads experienced and competent staff to shift and necessitate the organization to hire new employees who might not have the required competencies. New staff have to be trained and might take time to adopt the organization culture. The staff employment process is costly. Based on these implications, organizations have to ensure improvement of remuneration, improvement of working environment and consider managers' professionalism in order to retain staff and improve work performance.

This study has contributed to the extension of decision-making theory by adding other factors which were not mentioned like, family matters, remuneration, poor working conditions and need for new exposure. Similarly, the study recommended measures to ensure that women stay which was not in the theory.

This study is limited to service sector specifically public higher learning institutions, future study can focus on other service sectors. In addition to that, this study applied qualitative approach, future studies can use quantitative or mixed methods which might provide more insights into the factors and allow the use of large sample which can be generalized.

References

Afande, F.O.: Factors affecting career development of women employees in the banking industry in Kenya. Res. Hum. Soc. Sci. **5**(5), 1–36 (2015)

Afridi, F., Dinkelman, T., Mahajan, K.: Why are fewer married women joining the work force in rural India? a decomposition analysis over two decades. J. Popul. Econ. **31**(3), 783–818 (2018)

Creswell, J.W.: A Concise Introduction to Mixed Methods Research, 4th edn. SAGE Publications, Thousand Oaks (2014)

Denscombe, M.: The Good Research Guide: for Small-Scale Social Research (4th ed ed.). McGraw Hill, New York (2010)

Dikkers, J., Jansen, D., de Lange, A., Vinkenburg, C., Kooij, D.: Proactivity, job characterisitics and engegement: a longitunal study. Career Dev. Int. **15**(1), 60–77 (2010)

Dimova, R., Elder, S., Stephan, K.: Labour market transitions of young women and men in the Middle East and North Africa. Geneva: International Labour Organization, 39 November 2016

Eagly, A.H., Karau, S.J.: Role congruity of prejudicetoward female leaders. Psychol. Rev. **109**, 573–598 (2002)

Eagly, A.H., Wood, W., Diekman, A.H.: Social role theory of sex differences and similarities: a current appraisal. Dev. Soc. Psychol. Gend, **12**, 123–174 (2000)
Forrier, A., Sels, L., Stynen, D.: Career mobility at the intersection between agent and structure: a conceptual model. J. Occup. Organ. Psychol. **82**(4), 739–759 (2009)
Hirschi, A.: The role of chance events in the school-to-career transition: the influence of demographic, personality and career development variables. J. Vocat. Behav. **77**(1), 39–49 (2010)
ILO.: Women at work: Trends 2016. Geneva: ILO (2016)
Khan, S.: Qualitative research method - phenomenology. Asian Soc. Sci. **10**(21), 298–310 (2014)
Kindsiko, E., Baruch, Y.: Careers of PhD graduates: the role of chance events and how to manage them. J. Vocat. Behav. **112**, 122–140 (2019)
Klasen, S., Pieters, J., Santos Silva, M., Tu, N., Thi, L.: What drives female labor force participation? comparable micro-level evidence from eight developing and emerging economies (2019)
Knorr, H.: Factors that contribute to women's career development in organizations: a review of the literature. Online Submission, 38–45 (2005)
Leedy, P.D., Ormrod, J.E.: Practical research: Planning and design. Merrill, Upper Sadle River, New Jersey (2010)
Loh, J.C., Restubog, S.L.: Words that Hurt: a qualitative study of parental verbal abuse. J. Interpersonal Violence **26**(11), 2244–2263 (2011). https://doi.org/10.1177/0886260510383031
Maertz, C.P., Campion, M.A.: Profiles in quitting: integrating process and content turnover theory. Acad. Manage. J. **47**(4), 566–582 (2004)
Marshall, C., Rossman, G.B.: Designing Qualitative Research. Sage publications, Thousand Oaks
Neuman, W.L.: *Social* Research Methods: Qualitative and Quantitative Approaches (7th ed ed.). (D. Musslewhite, Ed.) USA: Allyn and Bacon (2011)
Ng, T.W., Sorensen, K.L., Eby, L.T., Feldman, D.C.: Determinants of job mobility: a theoretical integration and extension. J. Occup. Organ. Psychol. **80**(3), 363–386 (2007)
Patton, M.Q.: Qualitative Research and Evaluation Methods. Sage, Thousand Oaks, CA (2002)
Peake, S., McDowall, A.: Chaotic careers: a narrative analysis of career transition themes and outcomes using chaos theory as a guiding metaphor. Br. J. Guidance Counselling **40**(4), 395–410 (2012)
Rudman, L.A., Phelan, J.E.: The effect of priming gender roles on women's implicit gender beliefs and career aspirations. Soc. Psychol. (2010)
Schuemann, K.B.: A Phenomenological Study into How Students Experience and Understand the University Presidency. Michigan: Western Michigan University (2014). https://scholarworks.wmich.edu/dissertations/261
Singh, R., Greenhaus, J.H.: The relation between career decision-making strategies and person–job fit: a study of job changers. J. Vocat. Behav. **64**(1), 198–221 (2004)
Sullivan, S.E., Al Ariss, A.: Making sense of different perspectives on career transitions: a review and agenda for future research. Hum. Res. Manage. Rev, 100727, 1–17 (2019). https://doi.org/10.1016/j.hrmr.2019.100727
Tanzania: Female labor force participation. (2019). theglobaleconomy.com: https://www.theglobaleconomy.com/Tanzania/Female_labor_force_participation/
Weng, Q., McElroy, J.C., Morrow, P.C., Liu, R.: The relationship between career growth and organizational commitment. J. Vocat. Behav. **77**(3), 391–400 (2010)
Whittock, M., Edwards, C., McLaren, S., Robinson, O.: The tender trap': gender, part-time nursing and the effects of 'family-friendly'policies on career advancement. Soc. Health Illness **24**(3), 305–326 (2002)
WorldBank. Labor force participation rate, female (% of female population ages 15 +) (modeled ILO estimate). Retrieved from The World Bank: (2019, April). https://data.worldbank.org/indicator/SL.TLF.CACT.FE.ZS?locations=TZ

Re-engineering Indigenous Education for Equality and Global Competitiveness of Nigeria Secondary Education

M. O. Ogundele(✉)

Faculty of Education, University of Jos, Jos, Nigeria
ogundele@unijos.edu.ng

Abstract. The study examined the issues relating to re-engineering indigenous education for enhancing equity and global competitiveness of Nigerian secondary education. The concern is due to the problems of decadence on the cultural values and poor value orientations for the technological and vocational skills acquisition among the youths and the products of Nigerian secondary education. The problem therefore viewed the strategies and methods by which the indigenous was used before the advent of western education and the features had significant impacts on the lives of the indigenous people and general society in areas of respect for elders, developing cultural values, skills acquisition and there was equity and access to the education provided. The issue made the write-up to look at the concepts, pedagogical approaches the characteristics of indigenous education and the influence on the life and behaviours of the citizens. The paper however looks at the strategies towards re-engineering the indigenous education programme in Nigeria, in the interest of enhancing equity, access and global competitiveness. The paper viewed strategies for developing equity and access for secondary education program, re-engineering the indigenous education policy for effective secondary education implementation and global competitiveness of the programme was analysed using Analytical method. It was however concluded that the re-engineering of indigenous education will surely develop equity, moral, cultural, technological and vocational orientation values, which will enable the secondary education products to accord respect and be able to compete with the counterparts at the global level. It was however suggested that the principles, methods and ideologies used for training youth traditionally be re-engineered and integrates for effective implementation of Nigerian secondary education programme.

Keywords: Equity and global competitiveness · Re-engineering and secondary education

1 Introduction

Every society have ways of educating her citizens for the benefit of the society. No nation that toyed with education provision to her citizens can be ranked high among other nation at the global level, however before the advent of the western education

J. N. Mojekwu et al. (Eds.): *Sustainable Education and Development*, pp. 89–96, 2021.
https://doi.org/10.1007/978-3-030-68836-3_9

in Africa every society has her own tradition ways of training her offsprings towards becoming a responsible member of the society but, it should be noted that indigenous education is an inclusive Education program which involve the parents and elderly members of the society. However, the community jointly train the children on the ways that the individuals would behave in the society towards becoming relevant in the needs and aspirations of such society. According to Ogundele (2019); indigenous education is a system of education whereby, the cultural values technological knowledge and social norms are transmitted from one generation to the others.

It Should also be noted that in an indigenous education, the parents,elderly members of the society and the environment are responsible for the training of the young ones for the benefit of the indigenous society by the elders. Therefore the required knowledge, society interests and abilities are hereby transmitted to the younger generations, through the following mode: supersitisions, activity oriented, story telling practical efforts and errand message (Owan and Bamanga 1992) however, practical orientation was enforced for the following purpose.

Physical development, Cultural heritage, Respect for elder and people in Authorities, Intellectual skills, Acquisition of specific vocational training and healthy attitude toward honest and dignity of labour and developing sense of belonging and participate in community development.

It is therefore necessary to noted that the society was breeding forth products that are honest, committed and those that have respect and dignity of labor and all these are handed over from one generations to the other generations.

Loius (2018) also stated that the traditional society made use of indigenous languages to train their offsprings so that everyone will be able to have equal right and opportunity delivered to the society, the basic responsibility requires by the society To this end the paper is to examine the need to re-engineer the indigenous education toward developing equitable access to global competitiveness.

2 The Characteristics of the Indigenous Education for Equity and Global Competitiveness

Daramola (2009) identified the basic characteristics of the indigenous education as follows.

Communalism: The training of the young one in the society is a joint effort of every adult member in the traditional society They do everything together for the betterment of the society.Togetherness is a principle of indigenous education.
Skills acquisition: Every elder of the society hand over the baton of a skill acquired to the younger generations of the society to live on in the nearest future.
Respect for elder and people in authority: This is the focus of the traditional education, greetings of the elder people and people of authority are made compulsory aspect of the indigenous education.
Moral upbringing: is a principle of indigenous education the ethical issue are use t train the children right from home and when they go out they would be a good ambassador of their family and the society at large.

Continuity: Indigenous education is the continuous process in all aspects of human endeavors, indigenous education transmit the necessary values to the younger generation which is pass on to others from one generation to the others,without end.
Respects for the culture of the land: The culture of the society are uprightly respected in the indigenous education, respect the culture of the society are transmitted to the children. Such culture are indigenous languages, dressing training and physical mental activities etc.

It should therefore be noted that all things went on smoothly during the traditional societal life. However, with the advent of western education In Nigeria all the issue that brought peaceful co-existence among the traditional society became punctuated such issues like honesty commitment skill acquisition employability, respect for the dignity of labour and respect for the elders and constituted authority,the issues of indigenous education such as practical orientations, technological approach, non-theoretical approach, respect for the cultural value of the land,everyone has equal opportunities and be able to access the various opportunities provided by the indigenous education.

It was interesting to note that the indigenous education was co-ordinated and at free of charge, because the traditional educational system was a joint responsibility of all.

It was also disheartening to noted that the advent and the interference of the missionary education cum colonial education into the life of the indigenous people brought changes to the operating system of the society. It was noted by Abdulkareem (2007) that the colonial education was characterized by theoretica in nature, non-practical orientation,poor skills acquisition and culturally biased. The features of the colonial education however, resulted into series of crises like unemployment, arsons indolence, political thurgry, moral decadence,low respect for the culture of the land dishonesty,war, confusions and contradictions, political instabilities and qualifications without practical skills,global socio- economic crises, population explosion in the labour markets. The basis for this paper therefore, is to examine the strategies for re-engineering the good aspect of indigenous education with current western education so that equity and access to quality education programme can be enhanced especially in Nigerian secondary education.

3 Concepts and Measures of Quality Education in Secondary Education

Quality education can be described as a functional activities that are characterised by the pedagogical approaches in the secondary education system. it is therefore described as a honest, effective and efficient of all the actives in the system which bringforth desirable outcomes of the system.According to Okeke (2001), quality education is described as the adhere to the standard norms that are related to the educational provision such as quality services delivery, quality management potentiality productivity standard, products excellence and outstanding performance. However, quality of secondary Education is described as an extent whereby there is high productivity in the products. So also, it should be noted that the high production of half-baked products in secondary Education constitute a great threats to the high level productivity of Secondary education and the society at large The measure or quality of secondary education include:

High productivity of the graduates and the quality product be reflected in the graduates without compromising the standard through accountability empowerment, partnership and problem-solving techniques, so as to enhance effective quality delivery services of the products.

Transfer of knowledge and innovation of ideas derived from secondary education. This is to say that the gap between the theory and the practical can be bridged in the society through transferring of the knowledge gained and bringing about change and innovation to the ideas that individual come in content with.

Employability of the products from the secondary education system. Quality of secondary education is enhanced in a situation that the product develop in skill that will keep him busy after graduate without joining a labour market that had be felled up by the unemployed graduates.

Achieving desirable goals and objectives with little or no supervison that the products can be work independently towards having high productivity for the society.

Adhere to the standard norms of the society on regular basis is an effective measure to quality products from secondary education. However it should be noted that Secondary Education products should be capable of adhering to the available standard norms of the society as the case may be and at any point in time (Njere 2019).

4 Factors Affecting Quality of Nigerian Secondary Education

The Quality of Secondary Education in Nigeria has been Threatened by Series or Problem.

The Problem Are:

Political Instability: Over the year there are series or change are affecting the secondary policies program and all aspect of the secondary educational programmes, the change in the quality of secondary education provided for e citizens (Manga and Ogundele 2019).

Financial Problem: The financial factor like embezzlement misappropriation of funds inflationary trends economic recession and students and population explosion the problem therefore affect the cost of education equity and access to the secondary education in Nigeria Durosaro (2013).

Dilapidated nature or the infrastructural facilities like classroom building library facilities, technological equipment the problems of over utilization of classroom due to overcrowded classroom are which needs the quality education provision in the secondary education to be affected especially in Nigerian no wonder that many Nigerian secondary education products cannot pass external examination alone unless through their involvement in examination malpractices the problem however affect the global competitiveness of Nigerian secondary education products.

Over dependency on the paper qualification at the expense of the skills acquisition at the practical orientation of the products the problem however constituted threat and the societal disrespects to the secondary education products finally teacher factors constitute problem to quality delivery of the secondary education in Nigerian most of the teacher are not trained in the pedagogical approach some teacher skill morally and ethically found some are not culturally brought up which make them to lack respect to the indigenous cultural values the problem however lead to moral decadence in the society especially in Nigerian.

5 Indigenous Education, Equality and Global Competitiveness of Nigerian Secondary Education.

The issues is that how than the educational integrate the indigenous educational feature to secondary education programmed in Nigeria in the interest of enhancing equality and global competitiveness of the secondary education in Nigeria. However, the integrating strategies are.

The use of indigenous languages by the teachers to teach some basic concept in the school system. Akpan (2019) noted that, the indigenous language can be used to teach basic concept and topic in geography. The use of indigenous language will enhance equitable distribution of ideas on the subject the topic will be adequately related to the environment.

Also, the principle of skills acquisition need to be integrated into the teaching learning process in secondary schools. According to Ogundele et al. (2012) stated that the integration of the principles of traditional education in the area of skill acquisition to secondary education will go along in Nigeria. According to the author, in the traditional society the parent 'would hand over their acquired skills to their upspring and such skill will be transmitted from one generation to others. However the spirit can be adopted and integrated to the secondary school administrators need to integrate the practical training of the student in the entrepreneurial skills acquisition such as tailoring, barbers cabling, hair dressing, printing computer engineering, networking, carpentry building, block melting, and all other skills that individuals can live on after their graduation it shared be integrated to the curriculum and implemented immediately after their secondary school exceptional certificate examinations (2012).

Also, cultural pattern of the society need to be adopted in the school environment culture according to Daramola (2009) in the totality of ways of life and pattern of loving condition in the society. The cultural pattern on the other hand can be reflected in the material and material culture. The author noted that the indigenous society made used of environmental resources and modified theme for the benefit of the society. For instance, the indigenous society recognized their environmental resources such as drainage, climate, soil, vegetation minerals, etc. and modified them for the societal use. However, the material resource within the school environment needed to be used for enhancing effective teaching-learning process in fees school and for the benefit of the society.

The teaching –learning process needed to be activity and practical oriented. For effectiveness and quality secondary, the principles of practical learning whereby the student learn by emigration, participation and executing what they have leant for instance the skill curving chary mailing, dying of cloths, cooking, knitting, home management and the skill are to opened to all and be equality leant in other to develop basic skills knowledge and attitude which were enable individual to live and fraction effectively well within immediate society and at global leveled even with their secondary education certificate Omoregie (2013).

Aspect of functionality education in which the knowledge, skill and attitude imported to the student are made relevant to the socio-economic needs and activity of the individuals and the society. Musa et al. (2015) asserted that since education is provided for the immediate.

Induction into the real life of the society. It should be noted that functionality principles of indigenous education can be integrate in to education to extent that all secondary education students would equally acquired knowledge, skills and values that can be imparted because they are relevant to the socio-economic activities of the society.

The functionality can be in the field of agriculture, building, fishing, iron clothing and marketing etc.

The issues of communication need to be incorporated in the mind of the secondary school students in Nigeria. In the indigenous society the learners acquired a common sprit of togetherness in working. The belief was that the means of production were owned communally. According to Baker and Letendre (2005) in traditional education, the upbringing of any child was the responsibility of the whole community members, for inference according to the authors, if any child misbehaved when their parent on of the community can correct such child on spot. The children belong to the society. It is therefore compulsory for the secondary school to implement the innovative approaches of school based manage communities.

Stakeholders involvement establishment of Parent-Teachers Association in any school and community school-relation. The efforts will aid the Schools in the management of secondary education for equitable provision of quality education in Nigeria.

The spirit of communism will enable the society to gain confident and productive impacts their children learning.

The principles of multiple skills acquisition and multiple specializations adopted by the traditional education 'can be adopted by the secondary school administrators in Nigeria. This is to Say that total quality control must be adhere to during the teaching learning process the total aspect of each areas of specialization need to be taught and acquired y the teacher and the student for the benefit of the individual and the society at large this is say that the practical of subject need to be acquired and the knowledge gained can be inter correlated and transferred to the other subjects in the school system also there is the need to use indigenous language to teach market in schools.

Finally, critical thinking through story telling message and practical orientation and skills acquisition made the and traditional society to be adequately respected in her areas employability and technologically development however the needs for the re-engineering critical thinking and creatively in the encouraged according to Ogundele (2019) noted that the of critical and creative thinking can be integrated into the secondary education through the use of child-centeredness approach practical oriented approach questioning demonstration experimental and educational trip the method according to the author the efforts will aid effective teaching learning process the secondary education quality product that would be proud of by the society at the global level.

6 Conclusion

However, it should be noted that with the integration of indigenous education into the secondary education Programme, the equitable educational provision for glob al competitiveness of secondary education product will be adequately enhance in Nigeria the cultural pattern skill indigenous ideology way of life and norms will be highly respected at the global level it should be noted that the way other people will have them to respect it at the global level.

7 Suggestions

The following suggestion were made to towards effective engineering of the indigenous education for enhancing equity and global competitiveness of secondary education in Nigeria.

The schools need to make use of the local language to teach at the secondary education level the teaching of local language should be give a priority at all level or Nigerian education.

Also education administration should priorities the use of local environmental resources for the improvisation of the instructional material for effective teaching.

Furthermore, activity-based approach and practical skills acquisition should be reinforced among the student using local environmental resources in Nigerian secondary should also community schools relevant need to be institute for effective integrated or indigenous ideology and culture patterns.

Finally, child-centredress approach should always embraced by the teachers for the students to you their local experiences to deal with their classroom situation in the schools.

References

Abdulkareem, A.Y.: Prudency in the Management of Primary Education in Nigeria. Int. J. Educ. Manage. **2**(1), 57–68 (2007)

Akpan, A.U.: Critical rethinking and sustainable national development of technical education in Nigeria a lead paper presentation at forum of benchmarked conference held at university of Uyo on 5th may 2019 (2019)

Akunnubi, P.O.: Integrating information and communication technology to secondary education programmed in Nigeria a conference proceeding Africa conference held at republic of Benin between 13–17 April 2012 (2012)

Baker, D.P., Tende, O.U.: National Differences Global Seminaries Word Culture and Feature of Schooling. Stanford University Press (2005)

Daramola, C.A.: Sociology of Education Ilorin. University Press (2009)

Durosaro, D.O.: Where the show punches the cost of education one hundred insurance lecture presented on 13th August 2013 at University of Ilorin (2013)

Federal Republic of Nigeria. National Policy on Education. NEPDC, Abuja (2013)

Loius, A.: The use of local language for geography teaching in nomachi education programmer problems and present. In: Jimba, D.N., Ogundele M.O., Gyang, T.S. (eds.) Dynamics of Education Planning Policy and Management. Palace Press, Jos (2018)

Manga, S.N., Ogundele, M.O.: Schools Administration. Solace Press, Jos (2019)
Musa, J.M., Jimba, D.N., Ogundele, M.O.: Functional education for transforming teacher education programmer in Nigeria problem and prospect. Educ. Res. Int. **4**(2), 72–82 (2015)
Njere, C.: Adherence to the Standard Norms of the University Basic Education Unpublished Ph.D. Thesis of University of Jos Nigeria (2019)
Ogundele, M.O., Ummi, I.: Toward developing ethical rethinking as creativity of secondary school student in plateau State Nigeria. Prem. J. Educ. **I**(I), 1–0 (2017)
Ogundele, M.O.: Selected Uses in Educational Management. Solace Press, Jos (2019)
Ogundele, M.O, Adegbemi, E.A., Oluwalola, K.: Fundamental of Organizational Behaviors. Ilorin, Ramfix concepts (2012)
Okeke, J.A.: Curriculum transformation for a global competitiveness of Nigerian education. J. Indigenous Educ. **5**(2), 45–53 (2001)
Omoregie, E.O.: Politics and policies in education. In: Omoregie, E.O., Omoike, D. (eds). Educational Administration and Planning. Benin-City Independent Concepts (2013)
Owan, E., Bamangah. O.: Hand Book on Educational Foundation. Jos Jubiee (1992)

The Practice of Industrial and Labour Relations in Higher Learning Institutions: A Case of Mwanza City Council

J. M. Lelo(✉), D. K. Nziku, and A. Mwakolo

Department of Business Administration, College of Business Education, Mwanza Campus, Kangaye, Tanzania
{j.lelo,d.nziku,a.mwakolo}@cbe.ac.tz

Abstract. The specialization of Higher Learning Institutions (HLIs) depends upon the focus which is stated by mission and vision of the institution itself together with professions offered by the particular institution. The HLIs have two specific operation parts which are academic and administrative. Academic part is the core activity of any HLI and employees on this side are called Technical Teachers/Lecture/or academic staff while administrative part is a support cadre which constitute employees termed as technical or supporting staff. Each institution and employers have different motivational approaches as well as leadership style that might encourage or discourage employees at work place depending on the perception of followers, situations and leader as the basic functions of leadership. Employment and Labour Relations Act No. 6 of 2004 owns the minimum employment standards which should be practiced by all organizations in Tanzania (Both Mainland and Zanzibar). The study focused on 12HLIs with a total of 586 employees in which stratified random sampling method was engaged to obtain a sample of 184 respondents. The data were analysed using Statistical Package for Social Sciences (SPSS) of which proper meaning was realised and interpreted. It has seen in the findings, analysis and discussion that in order for the employees to be motivated towards work (Theory Y perspective) the institutions should focus on strengthening industrial relations at workplace so as to make employees think of job only. The return of practicing industrial and labour relations has been approved to have fruitier to the organization, employers, employees, trade unions and the government at a sounding content. The study is constantly reminding HLIs employers to deal with staff fairly as stipulated in the act, so as to reduce number of strikes and turnovers.

Keywords: Industrial relations · Employer · Employee/labour · Higher learning institutions

1 Introduction

1.1 Background of the Practice of Industrial Relations in the Institutions

The survival of any organization in the competitive society lies in its ability to train its human resource to be creative, innovative, inventive who will invariably enhance performance and increase competitive advantage (Vemić 2017; Edralin 2014). Employee

J. N. Mojekwu et al. (Eds.): *Sustainable Education and Development*, pp. 97–108, 2021.
https://doi.org/10.1007/978-3-030-68836-3_10

relations are one of the most pervasive techniques for improving employees' performance enhancing organization performance in the work place (Gupta et al. 2010). Employees are the crucial asset and key element of gaining competitive advantage of any organization and good relations is essential tool for its actualization (Houger 2016). It has further become necessary in view of advancement in modern world to take a critical look at employee relations. Thus the role played by employee relations can no longer be overemphasized. It is also generally agreed that at each level of organizational existence, employee relations is critical to adequately prepare them to meet the goals of the organization. (Houger 2016), if employees are well trained, involved in decision making, and practicing the win-win situation in the organization, its performance and growth will be high.

The thought of organizational consequences of employee relations has become a significant topic in employment relations, human resource management (HRM) and related fields. Indeed over several decades the focus of employee relations has shifted from one of sharing power and improving workers' rights to one of improved organizational efficiencies, performance and other organizational outcomes (Gollan and Wilkinson 2007). Research has identified some links between employee relations and organizational outcomes such as improved occupational health and safety (OHS) outcomes, and better utilization of employees' skills and knowledge for organizational outcomes. The findings of Khattak et al. (2012) also indicated that employee involvement and participation at work has significant positive effect on job satisfaction, leading to improved organizational performance.

The issues in labour management disputes, is not simple and can be solved by power and strength alone. It is arguably that a cooperative attitude is mutually beneficial in terms of output, performance and rewards. It does not assume that conflicts do not exist but effective and proactive collective agreements and grievance procedure exist that can prevent the conflicts from transforming into a crisis. Problems of people in the work place and society in general are the deadly killer diseases, problems of people have stayed long with us in organization because of the missing ingredient of the "personality". Management needs to find new ways of working and thinking. The old principle of command, control, compliance, "of they and we" must be challenged and abandoned. Modern educational institutions are too complex to profitably separate the thinkers and doers (Akuh 2016).

Industrial relations in HLIs have rarely been the focus of academic research, and within an education context have received much less interest than either the school or further education sectors. It is against the backdrop of the relative importance of employee relations in relation to organizational performance that this study addresses. This study is based on the premise that business' and organization's growth is linked to development of the human resources.

Positive outcomes for employees have also been identified from employee relations. This is particularly so with the High Performance Workplace Practices (HPWP) paradigm which identifies employee consequences such as improved job satisfaction, greater skills that can leverage increased pay, and reduced fatigue and stress associated with increased autonomy. The extent of employee outcomes is debated, with some arguing that they are overlooked in favour of organizational outcomes (Boxall and Macky

2014). It appears that when employee relations increases the power of employees, it achieves better outcomes for them (Busck et al. 2010; Hvid and Hasle 2009).

The impact of employee relations on organizational performance has been identified by various scholars and authors to be very crucial to an organization and its effectiveness (Oluoch 2013; Gupta et al. 2010; Aguinis and Kraiger 2009). In the light of the above, organizations are therefore encouraged to build a strong and cordial relationships with their staff to the fullest advantage in order to enhance their effectiveness. Good relations are required for staff to enable them work towards taking the organization to its expected destination. It is against the backdrop of the relative importance of employee relations in relation to organizational performance that this study addresses. This study is based on the premise that business' and organization's growth is linked to development of the human resources. This is due to the fact that for a sustainable organization, there should be a breakthrough in satisfying demand in respect of clients and staff needs. In view of the above, this study research delves into the dynamics of employee relations of the employees of Higher Learning Institution (HLIs) considering intense competition existing in the present institutions and the fact that the retention of quality employees (academic & technical staff) plays a key role in helping organizations to achieve their objectives. The objectives are to identify conditions indicating the existence of industrial relations in Higher Learning Institutions; to examine the practice of industrial and labour relations in Higher Learning Institutions and to determine the effects of practicing Industrial Relations in High Learning Institutions.

2 Theoretical Framework

2.1 Industrial Relations Theory

The theoretical perspective of industrial relations highlighting many different angles of industrial relations which are focusing on three aspects as discussed by two scholars Alan Fox (1966) and Ed Rose (2008). The first theoretical perspective is unitary, which is perceived as an integrated and harmonious whole with the ideal of "one happy family" in which management and other members of the staff share a common purpose by emphasizing mutual co-operation. In this theory a paternalistic leadership approach is seen as paramount components because employees' views are aligning to the objectives of the organization and thus conflict of interest, trade unions and many other misunderstandings have no value in the institutions. This perspective is exercised when the industrial relations in the particular organization is at maximum. Second perspective is Marxist/radical, which is very common when employees are not recognized as potential assets for the development of the organization. Thus this perspective is common in capitalist economic system where there is strong division of interest between capital and labour. In this theory, conflict of interest, trade unions and many other misunderstandings are inevitable in the institutions as a means of creating agreements between management and the employees. The third perspective is pluralism, the institutions are perceived as being made up of powerful and divergent sub-groups namely *management and trade unions where by*, each of them with its own legitimate loyalties and with their own set of objectives and leaders. The role of management would lean less towards enforcing and controlling and more toward persuasion and co-ordination. Trade unions are deemed as legitimate representatives of employees; conflict is dealt by collective bargaining and is viewed not necessarily as a bad thing and, if managed, could in fact be *channeled towards evolution and positive change.* Therefore, for the smooth operations in the institutions, it is suggested that, rulers of the institutions to exercise fairly industrial relations by adapting unitary theory so as to make all the employees happy with the organization for their own betterment.

Diverse terms like "capital-labour relations", 'industrial relations', 'employment relations', 'labour relations' and others like 'workplace relations' and 'employee relations' are rather loosely used interchangeably to mean the same (Venkata 2006). But we can distinguish between some of them. The more commonly used traditional term 'industrial relations' refers to the hoary inter-disciplinary subject derived from parent disciplines such as economics, sociology, psychology and law, which deals rather narrowly with negotiations between employers and unions, industrial action and conflict. By contrast, the less commonly used modern term 'employment relations' conveys "the ubiquitous concern with relationships, individual and collective, arising in and from employment". The broader category of employment relations, which is also considered by some as a more dignified one, thus, includes all aspects of labouring such as; *(i) work organization and worker participation; (ii)nature of employment contracts; (iii)skills, training and motivation*; *(iv) worker organisation, workplace governance and labour-management relations and (v) wages, non-wage benefits and working conditions;*. Some scholars have used "employee relations" to refer to labour-management relations in non-union firms.

The idea of *'work'* is wider than wage employment (formal work), and encompasses self-employment, home working, and domestic work, thus bringing into its real path the wide range of activities in the informal economy. Thus we use the modern terms such as "work and employment relations" or what the industrial relations and labour laws now calls *"labour and employment relations"* as equivalent to the traditional term *"labour relations"* which means all aspects of people at work, formal and informal. It may be noted that sociologists have been in the forefront, more than anybody else, in examining the "tough current world of work in all its shame and glory" alongside investigations into the development of business organizations in the name of "sociology of business". More importantly, as pointed out that, worker needs to be made the central reference point in the subject of industrial relations, in contrast to so much that is written in this field, in which the employee is either completely ignored, or is treated as a regrettable and sometimes troublesome cost of doing business. In this aspect, the dominant theories of work can be tested against the reality experienced by workers.

Employee Relations provides direction and oversight for a variety of non-union staff employment matters, including leaves of absence, staff performance and disciplinary issues, staff employee grievances including formal complaints, investigation of harassment and other workplace misconduct allegations, all anticipated terminations, and unemployment compensation claims. Employee Relations also provides proactive assistance to both employees and supervisors on the interpretation and implementation of policies, procedures, and the staff handbook directives. Employee relations is a study of the rules, regulations and agreements by which employees are managed both as individuals and as a collective group, the priority given to the individual as opposed to the collective relationship varying from company to company depending upon the values of management (Blyton and Turnbull 2004). As such it is concerned with how to gain people's commitment to the achievement of an organization's business goals and objectives in a number of different situations.

2.2 Conceptual Framework Indicating the Relationship Between Key Players of Industrial Relations and Work Performance

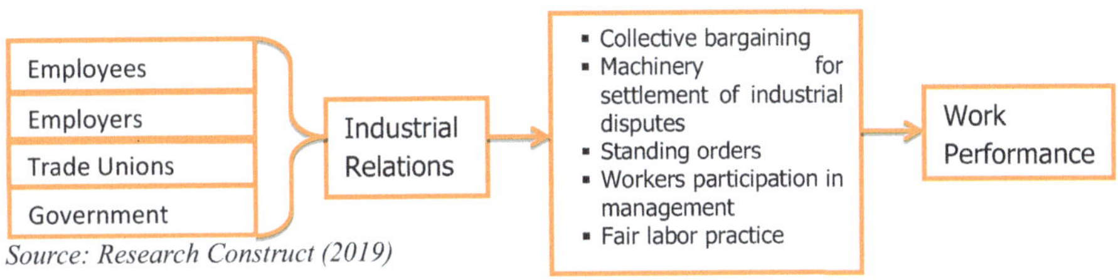

Source: Research Construct (2019)

3 Methodology

3.1 Research Design

Due to the nature of the study, the researchers adopted case study design to make easy during analysis of respondent's ideas. The case study is considered appropriate because it is the best method to describe the characteristics, perceptions and preferences of the organization under study. It also enabled the researchers to critically analyze information gathered from organizations from both personal and professional points of view.

Bryman and Bell (2016), insert that descriptive studies are done when researchers want to establish the relationship of events without interfering with the purpose of reporting facts as they are. Thus, the design was chosen and considered appropriately for this study since it was able to give room for exploratory and descriptive data. This form of data was important in understanding the influence of Employee relations practices on Higher Learning Institutions' (HLI) performance in Tanzania.

3.2 Target Population

The population for the study was mainly made up of Employees of Higher Learning Institutions operating in Mwanza City Council offering Certificate, Diploma, Bachelor Degree and Master Degree. The HLI in Mwanza city have a total number of employees approximately to 1,000. Thus, some of them will be taken randomly to meet the demands of the study.

Mugenda and Mugenda (2012) believe that 5–10% of an accessible population can be selected as a sample for quantitative studies. To achieve the objectives of the study, one hundred (100) workers were selected. The views of the 100 respondents may thus be deemed representative of that of the entire workforce. The respondents were drawn from the HLIs operating in Mwanza city.

3.3 Sampling Techniques

The random sampling technique which is a probability sampling technique was employed in the administration of the research tools for data collection in line with Karlsson (2019). Statement that "though the purposive sampling enables you to use your judgments to select cases which will best enable you to answer your research question and meet your objectives, the random sampling technique presents to the researcher, a more accurate and general perspective of the issue under focus (p. 79)". Finally basing on the concept of Mugenda and Mugenda (2012) reached to take a sample of 100 respondents to fulfil the demand of the study.

3.4 Data Collection Techniques

A standardized questionnaire, capturing the variables under the study was prepared. Kothari and Garg (2014). Defines a questionnaire as a set of questions printed or typed in a definite order or form of or set of forms. They are a list of research questions asked to respondents and they are designed to extract specific information. The questionnaires contained only closed and open ended questions. The closed questions were used to limit the respondents to the variables of the study while the open ended questions enabled respondents to freely give their opinions in a more pragmatic way (Kothari and Garg 2014).

Using a questionnaire, the researchers gathered significant amount of data at a very low cost (Cooper and Schindler 2014). The research instrument was divided into seven parts. Part I covered general information, part II, III, IV, and V, covered questions related to employee relations practices and part VI focused on organizational performance in either private or public HLIs in Tanzania, Part VII gathered information on other factors influencing organizational performance in HLIs. From that perspective, data will be gathered and analyzed accordingly using SPSS as stated in the previously.

3.5 Methods of Data Analysis

Data collected in the course of the research was processed and analyzed using Statistical Package for Social Sciences (SPSS). Descriptive analysis in the form of percentages were used to analyze the data. The data have been analyzed and presented separately, the interpretation or discussions were presented in such a way that, it enabled the researchers to either accept or reject whatever defined idea have about the differences or relationships among variables under study. The main issue was to explore the relationship existing between the process of exercising industrial relations in the HLIs and their performance.

3.6 The Statistical Measurement Model Used in the Analysis

Content analysis was used to test data that was qualitative in nature or aspect of the data collected from the open ended questions. The information was presented by use of bar charts, graphs and pie charts. Multiple regressions were used to determine the predictive power of the factors on organization performance. The study tested the following regression equation.

$$Y = \beta_0 + \beta_1 X_1 + \beta_2 X_2 + \beta_3 X_3 + \beta_4 X_4 + \varepsilon$$

Whereby.
Y - Employee relations.
X_1 - Industrial relations.
X_2 - Employment practices.
X_3- Dispute resolution.
X_4- Employee Communication.
E - Error term (Employees voice).
β_0- Constant.
β_0, β_1, β_2, β_3 & β_4 - Coefficients of independent variables.

The accuracy of data to be collected largely depended on the data collection instruments in terms of validity and reliability. Validity as noted by Robinson (2012) is the degree to which result obtained from the analysis of the data actually represents the phenomenon under study. Validity was censured by having objective questions in the questionnaire. This was achieved by pre-testing the instrument to be used to identify and change any ambiguous, awkward questions and in this study; reliability was censured by pre-testing the questionnaire with a selected sample from one of the departments which was not included in the actual data collection. To ensure a high response rate, frequent follow up visits to the respondents and confidentiality was assured. Diplomatic pleading for response was applied as a response enhancement strategy. Reliability was measured through Cronbach's Alpha which measures the internal consistency. The alpha value ranges between 0 and 1 with reliability increasing with the increase in value. Nunnally and Bernstein stated that reliability of a research instrument can be indicated at a minimal Alpha value of 0.6.

4 Results and Discussion

4.1 Demographics of Respondents

The results of the survey revealed that, out of the sampled 100 respondents, 64% of the respondents were males and 36% were females. The age of the respondents were also considered. With respect to age range of the respondents, the outcome of the study indicates that 25% of the respondents were within the ages of 20–29 years, 45% were within the ages of 30–39, 20% of the respondents were also within the ages of 40–49 years, while 10% of the respondents also fell in 50–59 age range. It can be deduced that majority of the respondents are old enough and fall between 30 to 59 years which means they are experienced and understand the subject matter of study and their field of work. Also, the study considered the number of years that the respondents had worked with the organization. The outcome of the results was that, 10% had worked for 0 to 2 years, 13% had worked 3 to 5 years, 56% had also worked for 6–10 years, and the remaining of 21% had been working for over 10 years. In order to be representative, respondents were selected from, almost all the departments within Higher Learning Institutions. The findings also revealed that the sample was representative of the population of this study in the sense that all the departments are duly represented. The data shows that the respondents were selected from both teaching and non-teaching staff in each academic institution. The current position of the respondents were not left out because, the position in one way or the other affects ones' experience. The result showed that few of the respondents are bosses accounted for 23% of the respondents. Twenty-two (22%) are managers, 40% are other sub-officers while the remaining 15% are officers. This outcome confirms that the respondents were rightly positioned to present their views on the subject matter.

4.2 Conditions Indicating the Existence of Industrial Relations in Higher Learning Institutions

Respondents were the only tool helped the researchers to explore information regarding the existence of elements of industrial relations in higher learning institutions - Mwanza City Council. Likert Scale was used to obtain and to summarize the needful information as tabulated in Tables 1, 2 and 3.

Table 1. Conditions indicating the existence of industrial relations in higher learning institutions

Employees comments	1	2	3	4	5	Total
Fair practice of Trade Unions at workplace	11	10	0	42	37	100
Employees involvement in decision making	10	32	2	30	26	100
Peace and harmony among members of the organization	19	21	10	26	24	100
Proper grievance handling procedures/employees dispute settlement procedures	22	34	1	32	11	100
The existence of unfair labour practices/the presence of any act which threatens the existence of Industrial Relations	21	23	3	33	20	100
Improved salaries/wages of employees at workplace	13	17	6	32	32	100
Proper emphasize to the employees to abide to the organizational standing orders	10	23	3	40	24	100
Each employee is well engaged to own duties and responsibilities	21	29	2	23	25	100
Good socializations among members of the organization	14	19	1	42	24	100
Vesting of a proprietary interest of the workers in the institutions in which they are employed	28	32	17	12	11	100
Fair negotiation of wages and working conditions at workplace	11	23	11	45	10	100

Source: Field Data, 2019.

Various items were identified to obtain information narrating the paramount conditions telling the existence of industrial and labour relations in higher learning institutions. The information was useful to make judgement and to advise the institutions what to do to increase their efficiency and expected level of output. The average of 54.6% of the respondents agreed that, there is an element of existence of industrial relations in higher learning institutions, while the average of 40.3% argued that there is no element of industrial relations. 5.1% were neutral, that means are not able to identify *whether there is or there is no* elements of industrial relations in higher learning institutions.

It is advised to the Higher Learning Institutions' management to practice industrial relations so as to bring happiness to the employees at workplace. It is also observed that, bosses do mostly engage authoritarian management style where the top bosses are the ones to provide directives to the subordinates, but they receive very few advises from the employees, and do not make them part of decision in their operations. It is belied that, when the institutions practice industrial and labour relations numerous benefits as summarized in Table 3 can be realized in the institutions. Thus, it is advisable to the higher learning institutions to exercise industrial and labour relations to enjoy such fruity at great extent.

4.3 The Practice of Industrial and Labour Relations in Higher Learning Institutions

An industrial and labour relation is something complex since it requires creating morale and harmony to the employees at work place. Blyton and Turnbull (2004) asserts that, human nature and behaviour is complex, which is why management has different faces like science, art and professional. The issue here might be difficulty to generalize due to different saturation point of employees' satisfaction in the organization. Various issues identified as indicators for seriousness practice of industrial and labour relations in HLIs were identified as indicated in Table 3 below. Respondents argued depending on what they feel in each measurement; however they were also given a room to air out their views to explore more information. An average of 42.3% of the respondents agreed that there is a practice of industrial and labour relations in HLIs, 46.6% rejected completely while 11.1% remained silent with the situation. It is observed that, there is an element of practicing industrial and labour relation in HLIs however at minimal level with absolute different value of 4.3 between accepted and rejected respondents. From such observation, management of HLIs should invest in the relations to make employees feel part and parcel of the institution. However from employees behavioral theory, it is difficulty for employer to satisfy all the employees at workplace, but they need to build industrial and labour relations at a manageable level.

4.4 The Effects of Practicing Industrial Relations in High Learning Institutions

Some of HLIs are practicing industrial and labour relations in their day to day operations. However employers are always believe that they are practicing industrial and labour relations at great extent. Employers mentioned number of rewards resulted from the practice as indicated in Table 3 above. The average of 9.1% were neutral, 41.8% argued that, there is no any rewards to the HLIs and 49.1% were positive that the institutions are benefiting at maximum in practicing industrial and labour relations at workplace. It is observed that, the variation in response is the indicator of variation in exercising industrial and labour relations at workplace, that is to say HLIs practicing it are the one seeing the benefits and those HLIs not practicing the relations are the one cannot see any benefit at all. It is strongly encouraged to HLIs in Tanzania to exercise industrial relations at great extent so as to uplift their organizations to next higher level and releasing good quality and quantity of their output.

Table 2. The practice of industrial and labour relations in higher learning institutions

Employees comments	1	2	3	4	5	Total
Existence of Trade Unions in the work place	9	9	2	52	28	**100**
Employees involvement in decision making	10	23	30	21	16	**100**
Proper grievance handling procedures /Employees dispute settlement procedures	14	16	9	31	30	**100**
The existence of fair labour practices	23	23	31	12	11	**100**
Fair involvement of employees in Collective bargaining	10	27	17	30	16	**100**
Existence of Machinery for organizational disputes' settlement	44	43	0	9	4	**100**
Employees' abiding to institutional rules and regulations	15	16	0	34	35	**100**
Workers participation in management	32	59	0	2	7	**100**

Source: Field Data, 2019.

Table 3. Effects of industrial relations in higher learning institutions

Employees comments	1	2	3	4	5	Total
The existence of peace and harmony in an organization	21	15	30	24	10	**100**
Good relationship between employer and employee	18	16	2	43	21	**100**
Good relationship among employees	21	19	1	39	20	**100**
Improving good relationship between the organization and customers	22	15	5	28	30	**100**
Improving the working morale among employees	30	45	5	15	5	**100**
Uninterrupted Operations	19	10	7	38	26	**100**
Increased Labour productivity	1	21	12	43	23	**100**
Reduction of industrial disputes	27	20	9	28	16	**100**
Employees' adherence to organizational rules and regulations	10	21	4	45	20	**100**
Good relationship between organizations in the city council	14	21	3	31	31	**100**
High morale of employees at workplace	40	35	4	19	2	**100**
Employees involvement in decision making	11	22	30	27	10	**100**
Improved wages/wages of the employees	16	14	6	42	22	**100**
Economic conditions of the employees are well improved	30	31	9	18	12	**100**

Source: Field Data, 2019.

5 Conclusion and Recommendations

5.1 Conclusion

An industrial and labour relation at workplace is the most paramount practice which enables to streamline the relationship between key players of the employment (employer, employees and trade unions) forming tripartite relationship. Organizations exercising such relationship make the minds of both employers and employees well settled, thinking only about the work and feeling as part and parcel of the organizations. Therefore, the study focused to HLIs for both private and public institutions in Mwanza City Council to explore the inclusion and exclusion of industrial and labour relations at the workplace. In the findings employers were included to air out their voices about the possible benefits realized after proper practice of the relations like; harmony and morale to the employees, uninterrupted productivity, increased productivity, reduction of industrial disputes, and good relationship between members of the organization as few to mention are the fruity consequences. Therefore it can be summed up by persuading HLIs' employers to devote full attention exercising industrial and labour relations in their institutions to garner more benefits as stated and rated in Table 3 of analysis.

5.2 Recommendations

The findings, analysis and discussion of this study has released very paramount lesson that, the value of industrial and labour relations in any organization is relatively high, however its measurements are intangible but its existence can be justified by the devotion of employees towards work commitment. From the study, it can be recommended that, employers have to abide to the Employment and Labour Relation Act No. 6 of 2004 as much as they can because all the elements of industrial and labour relations are centered in it. Furthermore, employers need to understand the issue of exercising industrial and labour relations has more benefits for the organization and can reduce employees' leading force by managers since employees themselves would to be committed toward work.

The practice of industrial and labour relations in higher learning institutions is not just about the utilization of human resources but rather the experience and the expectation of labour at workplace. From the study there will be improvement in bargaining power between employers and employees, in line with enhancing the legal awareness of the rights of each key player. And from both sides they need to establish a sensible organizational arrangement between the parties to engender mutual trust between them, this will easier the practice of the industrial and labour relations and bring total control of a wide variety of human resources across the organization.

References

Aguinis, H., Kraiger, K.: Benefits of training and development for individuals and teams, organizations, and society. Annu. Rev. Psychol. **60**, 451–474 (2009)

Akuh, E.A.: Industrial harmony for academic excellence: An imperative for a productive educational system in Nigeria. Br. J. Educ. **4**(4), 63–71 (2016)

Blyton, P., Turnbull, P.: The Dynamics of Employee Relations. Macmillan International Higher Education (2004)
Boxall, P., Macky, K.: High-involvement work processes, work intensification and employee well-being. Work Employ Soc. **28**(6), 963–984 (2014)
Bryman, A., Bell, E.: Social Research Methods (Fourth Canadian). Don Mills, ON (2016)
Busck, O., Knudsen, H., Lind, J.: The transformation of employee participation: consequences for the work environment. Econ. Ind. Democr. **31**(3), 285–305 (2010)
Cooper, D.R., Schindler, P.S.: Business Research Methods. Data Preparation and Description (2014)
Edralin, D.M.: Precarious work undermines decent work: the unionized hotel workers' experience. DLSU Bus. Econ. Rev. **24**(1), 13–26 (2014)
Fox, A.: Industrial sociology and industrial relations: an assessment of the contribution which industrial sociology can make towards understanding and resolving some of the problems now being considered by the Royal Commission (No. 3). HM Stationery Office (1966)
Gollan, P.J., Wilkinson, A.: Contemporary developments in information and consultation. Int. J. Hum. Res. Manage. **18**(7), 1133–1144 (2007)
Gupta, S., Bostrom, R.P., Huber, M.: End-user training methods: what we know, need to know. ACM SIGMIS Database **41**(4), 9–39 (2010)
Houger, V.P., Roux-Zink, M.R.: Why become a CPT? Perform. Improv. **55**(4), 18–22 (2016)
Hvid, H.: To be in control – v ejentilgodtpsykiskarbejdsmiljølæringog innovation? Tidsskrift for Arbejdsliv **11**(1), 11–30 (2009)
Karlsson, P.S.: Comparative Cross-National Case Study Research: The "Stuff" Research Methods Books Don't Tell You. SAGE Publications Ltd. (2019)
Khattak, M.A., Igbal, N., Bashir, F.: Employee involvement and participation at work: a case study of OTCL after privatization. Int. J. Acad. Res. Bus. Soc. Sci. **2**(6), 469–476 (2012)
Kothari, C.R., Garg, G.: Research Methodology and Techniques New Age (2014)
Mugenda, O.M., Mugenda, A.G.: Research methods dictionary (2012)
Oluoch, J.O.: Influence of best human resource management practices on organizational performance: a case of college of humanities and social sciences university of Nairobi, Kenya. Unpublished Thesis of Master of Arts in Project Planning and Management of the University of Nairobi (2013)
Robinson, D.J.: A Course in the Theory of Groups, vol. 80. Springer, Heidelberg (2012)
Rose, E.D.: Employment Relations: Theory and Controversies (2008)
Vemić, M.B.: A further look at working capital optimization in medium-sized firms: concepts and evidence. In: Optimal Management Strategies in Small and Medium Enterprises, pp. 144–177. IGI Global (2017)
VenkataRatnam, C.S.: Industrial Relations. Oxford University Press, New Delhi (2006)

Time and Cost Model for Road Construction Projects in Nigeria

S. E. Okosun[2(✉)], S. M. Oluwajana[1], N. G. Johnson[2], O. A. Abel[2], and C. A. Olowookere[3]

[1] Department of Quantity Surveying, Obafemi Awolowo University, Ile-Ife, Nigeria
[2] Department of Geography, School of Social Sciences, Federal University Lokoja, Lokoja, Nigeria
[3] Department of Urban and Regional Planning, School of Environmental Studies, The Federal Polytechnic Ado-Ekiti, Ado-Ekiti, Nigeria

Abstract. In recent times, increasing attention of academic and political discussion is directed at issues of time and cost. The incidence of time and cost overruns have always been found to have their attendant cost consequences on construction projects and this has made the problem of time and cost overruns of international concern. Using survey and historical design approaches, this study therefore examines time and cost models for road projects in Nigeria. The purpose of this research was to develop construction model for predicting time and cost performance of road projects in Ondo and Ekiti states. The study adopted purposive/judgmental sampling technique. A total of 131 completed set of questionnaire were retrieved from the construction practitioners out of 188 administered, while archival data on completed road projects executed between 2003 and 2013 were also sourced. Percentile and regression correlation were used to assess cost and time performance of road projects. The results revealed that the average rate of cost overrun of road projects in Ondo state is 2.53% while that of Ekiti state is 1.79%; also time overruns is experienced at the average rate of 26.32% and 19.92% for Ondo and Ekiti states respectively.

Keywords: Construction · Road · Nigeria · Time and cost model

1 Introduction

The construction industry is known to be the prime stimulator of any national economy, the construction industry therefore has a strong linkage with many economic activities and whatever happens to the industry will directly or indirectly influence other industries and ultimately the wealth of the country (Jagboro 2002). The contributions of the construction industry to national economic growth necessitate improved efficiency in the industry by means of cost-effectiveness and timelines which will contribute to the cost savings for the country. Dissanayaka and Kumaraswamy (1999) reveal that time; cost and quality have been identified as the main criteria for measuring the overall success of construction project. Adetola and Ogunsanmi (2006) opine that today's clients are versatile and sophisticated hence, they are conscious of time, cost and quality so therefore,

J. N. Mojekwu et al. (Eds.): *Sustainable Education and Development*, pp. 109–119, 2021.
https://doi.org/10.1007/978-3-030-68836-3_11

clients become unsatisfied when their goal for time, cost and quality are not met thereby hindering them from achieving value for money which is the ultimate desire of any client. In Nigeria, Dissanayaka and Kumaraswamy (1999) explain that time, cost and quality have been identified as the main criteria for measuring the overall success of construction projects, out of these, cost and time tend to be the most critical factors because of their direct economic implications if they are unnecessarily exceeded (Ogunsemi and Jagboro 2006). Similarly, Chan and Kumaraswamy (1996) opine that timely delivery of projects within budget and to the level of quality standard specified by the client is an index of successful project delivery. According to Aje et al. (2014) a project may be delayed in part or whole due to some factors. Time overruns factors include: inclement weather, inaccuracy of materials estimates, inaccurate prediction of craftsmen's production output, inaccurate prediction of equipment production rates (especially in developing countries, where outputs are yet to be standardized), materials shortages, equipment shortages, skill shortages, location project restrictions, inadequate planning, poor labour productivity and design changes. Some of these variables may result in late project completion, whereas others may have no effect on construction time. However, all delays usually cost money. The prime variables of cost overruns have been commonly identified as: unpredictable weather, inflationary material cost, inaccurate materials estimates, complexity of project, contractor's lack of geographical experience, contractor's lack of project type experience, and non-familiarity with local regulations. Therefore, the purpose of this research is to assess time and cost performance of road construction projects in Ondo and Ekiti states, Nigeria. The broad objectives are to identify the background information of respondents (clients, consultants and civil engineers); and assess the **c**ost and time performance of road construction projects.

2 Theoretical Framework

2.1 Time and Cost Performance of Construction Projects

This study considers the feasibility of modeling the duration and final cost of construction using quantitative variable derivable from contract award data i.e. (planned contract duration, actual contract duration, contract sum, completion cost). The study of Ibironke et al. (2011), Shanmugapriya and Subramanian (2013) were based on building projects while this research focuses on civil engineering project i.e. road project. Researchers such as Chan and Kumuraswamy (1995) have carried out studies in the area of time-cost model. Similarly, in Nigeria Aje et al. (2014) have also carried out a study in this area by developing time and cost models for building projects using prequalification and contract award data while this study is based on civil engineering project, specifically road projects. Also many scholars and researchers on time-cost models have not published any work focusing on Ondo and Ekiti states as sample, thereby creating gap for the use of this area. Therefore, the purpose of this study is to assess time and cost performance of road projects with a view to developing model(s) for predicting time and cost performance of road projects in Ondo and Ekiti states.

2.2 Time and Cost Model

Interest in construction time began with pioneering work of Bromilow in 1969 in Australia. In a survey of 370 building projects in Australia, Bromilow (1974) and the subsequent update by Bromilow (1980). The model produced predicted construction duration as follows:

$$T = KC^{B} \tag{1.1}$$

where T is the duration of the construction period from date of site possession to practical completion, in working days. C is the final cost of building in millions of dollars, adjusted to constant labour and material prices; K is a constant describing the general level of time performance for a one million dollar project, and B is a constant describing how the time performance is affected by project size, as measured by cost. The model was summarized as.

$$T = 313C^{0.3} \tag{1.2}$$

Bromilow further made use of mathematical models to show the relationship between cost and time variation and pre-construction time and also analysed overruns on time and cost, which provided a measure of the accuracy of the industry's time and cost prediction. Kumaraswamy and Chan (1995) investigated the effect of construction cost on time with particular reference to Hong Kong; Chan (1999) did a similar research for Malaysian construction industry. All these studies found that the mathematical model presented by Bromilow (1974) holds good for prediction of construction time if the cost of construction is known. A similar work was carried out by Ireland (1983) to predict the construction time of high-rise commercial projects in Australia. Furthermore since most of the studies so far reported dealt with either building or civil engineering projects.

Table 1. Time-cost models developed over the years

Author(s) and year of study	Country	Type
Bromilow (1969)	Australia	Building construction costs
Kaka and Price (1991)	UK	Building and roads
Long and Young (2009)	Korea	Building construction costs
Ogunsemi and Jagboro (2006)	Nigeria	Construction cost
Chen and Huang (2006)	Taiwan	School projects
Chan (1999)	Malaysia	Building construction costs
Ojo (2001)	Nigeria	Construction
Aje et al. (2014)	Nigeria	Building cost and time

Source: Ameyaw et al. (2012)

The studies shown on Table 1 were all conducted in other countries outside Nigeria. The results of the researches may not be suitable for Nigeria. Some of the researches that have been carried out in Nigeria e.g. (Ogunsemi and Jagboro 2006; Ojo 2001; Aje et al. 2014) were carried out on building projects. Also many scholars and researchers on time-cost models have not published any work focusing on Ondo and Ekiti states as sample, thereby creating gap for the use of these areas. Earlier researches in Nigeria were based on time-cost models of building projects with time being the independent variable and cost being the dependent variable while this study is based on time and cost models i.e. models were made for time and separately for cost, hence fill the gap, as none of the studies focuses on civil engineering project i.e. road construction project using cost and time model for Ondo and Ekiti states.

3 Research Methodology

The survey research method was adopted for this study. The study therefore draws its samples from the total number of clients, contractors and consultants who are involved in road construction projects in both Ondo and Ekiti states, Nigeria. A total number of 188 respondents comprising 16 clients, 85 consultants; who are corporate member with their professional body and 87 Contractors registered with the ministry of works in Ondo and Ekiti states were identified. The actual numbers of the respondents were retrieved from information available at Ondo and Ekiti States' Ministries of works. Data on past road construction projects within the study area such as, project type; initial project time, final project time; initial cost and final cost were retrieved. The respondents for this study were Civil Engineers; who are client's representatives and are also corporate members of the Nigerian Society of Engineers and Contractors registered with the Ministry of Works in both Ondo and Ekiti states Nigeria. A total of one hundred and thirty one (131) questionnaires were distributed to 14 clients, 59 contractors and 58 consultants who are involved in road projects in both Ondo and Ekiti states. A total of sixty four (64) copies were returned and certified fit for analysis representing about 48% response rate. On the other hand, for secondary data of past road projects, seventy (70) pro-forma sheets were distributed in Ondo and Ekiti state Nigeria and a total of fifty five (55) were collected and were considered appropriate for analysis. The Statistical Package for Social Sciences (SPSS) version 19 was adopted. Frequency count; distribution, tables and percentages was also used for the study data.

4 Findings

From the general characteristics of respondents (clients, consultants and civil engineers) background, findings reveals that 44.6% of the respondents have higher National Diploma, 43.1% have Bachelor of Science/Bachelor of Technology while 6.2% have Masters Degree in their various field of study. Furthermore, 6.25% of the respondents are fellow members of their respective professional bodies, 31.25% are corporate members and 28.12% are probationer members of their professional bodies. About the year of experience of the respondents, 7.7% of them have less than 6 years experience, 61.5% have above 6 years experience, and 20% have above 10 years experience and 7.7% have above 15 years experience and 1.5% have above 25years working experience in the construction industry. Moreover, 60% have been involved in less than 11 road projects, 23.1% in less than 21 road construction projects, while 4.6% and 9.2% involved in less than 40 and over 40 road projects respectively.

4.1 Cost and Time Performance of Road Construction Projects in Ondo State

The cost and time performance of twenty-six (26) previously executed road projects in Ondo state were assessed and analysis was made based on percentage difference of the initial contract sum and actual completion cost; contract duration and actual completion time. In ondo state, out of the twenty-six past projects surveyed only six did not experience cost overruns (signifying 23%); meaning that 77% experienced cost overruns (see Table 2).

As depicted in Table 2, three out of the twenty-six past projects in Ondo state did not experience time overruns (representing 11%); meaning that 89% experienced time overruns. The sum total of the contract sum of the twenty-six analysed projects is ₦13,727,250,000.00 and the sum total of the Actual completion cost is ₦14,074,830,000.00 and the sum total of the difference in initial and final costs is ₦347, 580, 000.00 which establishes the fact that there were cost overruns. Also the sum total of the contract duration is 454 months and the sum total of the actual completion time is 574 months. The difference in initial and final time is 120 months which shows there was time overruns. The result of the analysis indicates that the rate of cost overrun of road projects in Ondo state is 2.53%. This implies that project performance in terms of cost is about 97%. On the other hand, time overrun is experienced at the rate of 26.32%; the implication is that project performance in term of time is about 74%.

4.2 Cost and Time Performance of Road Construction Projects in Ekiti State, Nigeria

The cost and time performance of twenty-nine (29) previously executed road projects in Ekiti state Nigeria were assessed and analysis were made based on percentage difference of the contract sum and actual completion cost and contract duration and actual completion time (See Table 3). Out of twenty–nine past projects surveyed only nine did not experience cost overruns representing 31%, meaning 69% experienced cost overruns. On the aspect of time overruns only three out of the twenty-nine projects did not experience time overruns i.e. 10% did not experience time overruns and 90% experienced time overruns. Furthermore, the sum total of the contract sum of the twenty-nine analysed past projects is ₦14,995,070,600.00 and the sum total of the actual completion cost is ₦15,263,939,800.00 and the sum total of the difference in initial and final costs is ₦262,869,200.00 which establishes the fact that there was cost overruns. In Ekiti state, the sum total of the contract duration in is 497 months and the sum total of the actual completion time is 595 months, the difference in initial and final time is 99 months which shows there was time overruns. The analysis shown on Table 4 shows that the rate of cost overrun of road construction projects in Ekiti state is 1.79%. The implication is that the average project performance in terms of cost is about 98%. On the other hand, time overrun is experienced at the rate of 19.92% which means that project performance

Table 2. Assessment of cost and time performance of road construction projects in Ondo State, Nigeria

S/N	Contract sum ₦	Actual completion cost ₦	Difference in initial and final costs ₦	Percentage difference	Contract duration Months	Actual completion time Months	Difference in initial and final time	Percentage difference
1	125,750,000.00	126,830,000.00	1,080,000.00	0.86	6	4	−2	−33.33
2	472,000,000.00	358,000,000.00	−114,000,000.00	−24.15	22	25	3	13.64
3	750,000,000.00	820,000,000.00	70,000,000.00	9.33	24	29	5	20.83
4	396,000,000.00	420,000,000.00	24,000,000.00	6.06	10	15	5	50.00
5	472,000,000.00	493,000,000.00	21,000,000.00	4.45	12	18	6	50.00
6	825,000,000.00	865,000,000.00	40,000,000.00	4.85	25	31	6	24.00
7	350,000,000.00	368,000,000.00	18,000,000.00	5.14	24	28	4	16.67
8	572,000,000.00	593,000,000.00	21,000,000.00	3.67	12	18	6	50.00
9	755,000,000.00	835,000,000.00	80,000,000.00	10.60	24	29	5	20.83
10	385,000,000.00	425,000,000.00	40,000,000.00	10.39	10	15	5	50.00
11	825,000,000.00	876,000,000.00	51,000,000.00	6.18	24	31	7	29.17
12	650,000,000.00	662,000,000.00	12,000,000.00	1.85	24	28	4	16.67
13	560,000,000.00	601,000,000.00	41,000,000.00	7.32	18	24	6	33.33
14	961,000,000.00	965,000,000.00	4,000,000.00	0.42	36	43	7	19.44
15	348,000,000.00	356,000,000.00	8,000,000.00	2.30	10	15	5	50.00
16	825,000,000.00	833,000,000.00	8,000,000.00	0.97	24	43	19	79.17

(continued)

Table 2. *(continued)*

S/N	Contract sum ₦	Actual completion cost ₦	Difference in initial and final costs ₦	Percentage difference	Contract duration Months	Actual completion time Months	Difference in initial and final time	Percentage difference
17	420,000,000.00	400,000,000.00	−20,000,000.00	−4.76	12	11	−1	−8.33
18	363,000,000.00	350,000,000.00	−13,000,000.00	−3.58	12	12	0	0.00
19	399,000,000.00	375,000,000.00	−24,000,000.00	−6.02	9	8	−1	−11.11
20	961,000,000.00	965,000,000.00	4,000,000.00	0.42	36	43	7	19.44
21	725,000,000.00	732,000,000.00	7,000,000.00	0.97	24	30	6	25.00
22	348,000,000.00	356,000,000.00	8,000,000.00	2.30	10	15	5	50.00
23	545,000,000.00	601,000,000.00	56,000,000.00	10.28	18	24	6	33.33
24	621,000,000.00	632,000,000.00	11,000,000.00	1.77	24	28	4	16.67
25	18,500,000.00	18,000,000.00	−500,000.00	−2.70	1	1.5	0.5	50.00
26	55,000,000.00	49,000,000.00	−6,000,000.00	−10.91	3	5	2	66.67
	13,727,250,000.00	14,074,830,000.00	347,580,000.00	2.53	454.00	573.50	119.50	26.32

Table 3. Assessment of cost and time performance of road construction projects in Ekiti state

S/N	Contract sum ₦	Actual completion cost ₦	Difference in initial and final costs ₦	Percentage difference	Contract duration	Actual completion time	Difference in initial and final time	Percentage difference
1	508,000,000.00	589,000,000.00	81,000,000.00	15.94	12	12	0	0.00
2	173,000,000.00	175,000,000.00	2,000,000.00	1.16	12	13	1	8.33
3	756,000,000.00	754,000,000.00	– 2,000,000.00	– 0.26	12	14	2	16.67
4	809,000,000.00	810,000,000.00	1,000,000.00	0.12	18	18	0	0.00
5	835,000,000.00	832,000,000.00	– 3,000,000.00	– 0.36	6	7	1	16.67
6	452,000,000.00	471,000,000.00	19,000,000.00	4.20	24	29	5	20.83
7	422,000,000.00	441,000,000.00	19,000,000.00	4.50	12	16	4	33.33
8	326,000,000.00	330,000,000.00	4,000,000.00	1.23	8	10	2	25.00
9	396,000,000.00	420,000,000.00	24,000,000.00	6.06	12	17	5	41.67
10	821,000,000.00	841,000,000.00	20,000,000.00	2.44	36	39	3	8.33
11	350,000,000.00	358,000,000.00	8,000,000.00	2.29	22	25	3	13.64
12	472,000,000.00	493,000,000.00	21,000,000.00	4.45	12	18	6	50.00
13	750,000,000.00	820,000,000.00	70,000,000.00	9.33	24	29	5	20.83
14	396,000,000.00	420,000,000.00	24,000,000.00	6.06	10	15	5	50.00
15	825,000,000.00	865,000,000.00	40,000,000.00	4.85	25	31	6	24.00
16	625,000,000.00	641,000,000.00	16,000,000.00	2.56	36	46	10	27.78
17	451,000,000.00	462,000,000.00	11,000,000.00	2.44	15	24	9	60.00

(*continued*)

Table 3. *(continued)*

S/N	Contract sum ₦	Actual completion cost ₦	Difference in initial and final costs ₦	Percentage difference	Contract duration	Actual completion time	Difference in initial and final time	Percentage difference
18	521,000,000.00	531,000,000.00	10,000,000.00	1.92	24	28	4	16.67
19	392,000,000.00	398,000,000.00	6,000,000.00	1.53	10	14	4	40.00
20	821,000,000.00	842,000,000.00	21,000,000.00	2.56	24	31	7	29.17
21	72,350,000.00	62,990,000.00	– 9,360,000.00	– 12.94	3	5	2	66.67
22	326,000,000.00	300,000,000.00	– 26,000,000.00	– 7.98	18	17	−1	−5.56
23	817,000,000.00	790,000,000.00	– 27,000,000.00	– 3.30	24	22	−2	−8.33
24	81,000,000.00	72,000,000.00	– 9,000,000.00	– 11.11	6	9	3	50.00
25	900,000,000.00	924,000,000.00	24,000,000.00	2.67	18	26	8	44.44
26	858,000,000.00	825,000,000.00	– 33,000,000.00	– 3.85	24	25	1	4.17
27	630,000,000.00	610,000,000.00	– 20,000,000.00	– 3.17	14	14	0	0.00
28	143,000,000.00	120,179,200.00	– 22,820,800.00	– 15.96	24	30	6	25.00
29	66,720,600.00	66,770,600.00	50,000.00	0.07	12	12	0	0.00
	14,995,070,600.00	15,263,939,800.00	268,869,200.00	1.79	497.00	596.00	99.00	19.92

in terms of duration is about 80%. The result of the findings is similar to result of the survey of Ade-ojo and Babalola (2013) which states that cost overruns were at the rate of 0.19% and cost overruns were at the rate of 1.08%.

5 Recommendation and Conclusion

It is evident from the empirical work carried out in this study that there is time and cost overruns effort geared by all stakeholders (clients, contractors and consultants) towards checking this trend and this calls for government at all levels to address the causes of excessive and bottleneck within the bureaucratic structure of the organizations. Therefore, clients and their consultants must ensure they award road contracts to contractors that are competent to handle such projects. The construction stakeholders i.e. clients, consultants and contractors should take necessary steps to mitigate the occurrences of the factors leading to cost and time overruns in order to improve the project performance of road projects. The study concludes that cost and time of road construction projects in Ondo and Ekiti states Nigeria could be determined during tender evaluation. The application of the predictive model from this study will serve as an early warning device for financial and time planning of construction projects, hence fill the existing gaps in review literatures on Time and cost model. It is a belief that a study of this nature will provide information that will enhance appropriate programmes, finances, rethinking the way we construct in communities.

Acknowledgements. The authors wish to acknowledge the contributions of Professor Aje, I. O. at Federal University of Technology Akure, Ondo State, Nigeria for providing the insights, inspiration and authoritative reading materials on road construction models that helped in compiling this paper. The authors also thank the Editor and Reviewers of this Conference/Journal for their help in improving the quality of this paper.

References

Ade-ojo, C.O., Babalola, A.A.: Cost and time performance of construction projects under the due process reform in Nigeria. Int. J. Eng. Sci. **3**(6), 01–06 (2013)

Adetola, A.E., Ogunsanmi, O.E.: Demand for project managers in the Nigerian construction industry. J. Nigerian Inst. Quant. Surv. **54**(1), 12 (2006)

Aibinu, A.A., Jagboro, G.O.: Effects of construction delays on project delivery in Nigerian industry. Int. J. Project Manage. **21**, 261–269 (2002)

Aje, I.O., Adedokun, O.A., Ibironke, O.T.: Time and cost models for building projects using prequalification and contract award data in Nigeria. J. Environ. Des. Manage. **6**(1), 122–131 (2014)

Bromilow, F.J.: Contract time performance – expectations and the reality. Building Forum **1**(3), 70–80 (1969)

Bromilow, F.J.: Measurement and scheduling construction time and cost performance in the building industry. Chartered Builder **10**(9), 57 (1974)

Chan, A.P.C.: Modelling building duration in Hong Kong. Constr. Manag. Econ. **17**(2), 189–196 (1999)

Chan, D.W.M., Kumuraswamy, M.M.: A study of the factors affecting construction duration in Hong Kong. Constr. Manag. Econ. **13**(4), 319–333 (1995)

Chan, D.W.M., Kumuraswamy, M.M.: An evaluation of construction time performance in the building industry. Build. Environ. **31**(6), 569–578 (1996)

Dissanayaka, S.M., Kumuraswamy, M.M.: Comparing contributors to time and cost performance in building projects. Build. Environ. **34**(1), 31–42 (1999)

Ireland, V.: The role of managerial actions in cost, time and quality performance of high rise commercial building, unpublished Ph.D. thesis. University of Sydney, Australia (1983)

Kaka, A., Price, A.D.F.: Relationship between value and duration of construction projects. Constr. Manag. Econ. **9**(4), 384–400 (1991)

Kumuraswamy, M.M., Chan, D.W.M.: Determination of construction duration. Constr. Manag. Econ. **13**(3), 209–217 (1995)

Odusami, K.T., Olusanya, O.O.: Client's contribution to delays on building projects. Quant. Surv. **30**, 30–33 (2000)

Ojo, G.K.: Relationship between contract period and tender sum of construction projects in south-western Nigeria, M.Sc. thesis, Obafemi Awolowo University, Ile-ife (2001, unpublished)

Okosun, S.E., Olujimi, J.A.B.: The role of local government areas and community based development associations in the prevision and maintenance of infrastructural facilities in Ilawe-Ekiti, Nigeria. The Just City: Poverty, Deprivation and Alleviation Strategies, Federal University of Technology Akure, Nigeria, pp. 487–495 (2018)

Ogunlana, S.O., Promkuntong, K., Jearkjirm, V.: Construction delays in a fast-growing economy: comparing Thailand with other economics. Int. J. Project Manage. **14**(1), 37–45 (1996)

Ogunsemi, D.R., Jogboro, G.O.: Time-cost model for building projects in Nigeria. Constr. Manag. Econ. **24**, 253–258 (2006)

Oyewobi, L.O., Ibironke, O.T., Ganiyu, B.O., Ola-Awo, A.W.: Evaluating rework cost- a study of selected building projects in Niger State, Nigeria. J. Geogr. Reg. Plann. **4**(3), 147–151 (2011)

Shanmugapriya, S., Subramanian, K.: Investigation of significant factors influencing time and cost overruns in Indian construction projects. Int. J. Emerg. Technol. Adv. Eng. **3**(10), 734–740 (2013)

Impact of Work-Based Conditions on Labour Productivity of Construction Workers in Ghana

E. Bamfo-Agyei[1(✉)], D. W. Thwala[2], and C. O. Aigbavboa[2]

[1] Department of Building Technology, Cape Coast Technical University, Cape Coast, Ghana
emmanuel.bamfo-agyei@cctu.edu.gh

[2] Department of Construction Management and Quantity Surveying, University of Johannesburg, Johannesburg, South Africa

Abstract. The aim of this research is to develop a work - based conditions framework for estimating the optimal Construction labour Productivity for labour-intensive works in the Ghanaian construction industry. The objectives of the study are to identify the factors influencing work based condition on labour productivity in Ghanaian construction firms; to determine the level of labour productivity on labour - intensive works in Ghanaian construction firms and to the examine the extent to which the construction labour productivity framework fits into the identified factors the Ghanaian construction firms. Stratified sampling technique was used, based on the diverse nature of the population. Records available at the Ghana Social Opportunity Project (GSOP) indicated that there are 920 professionals involved in labour-intensive works and these comprised 200 Contractors; 200 Site Engineers; 200 Facilitators; 200 Time Keepers; 60 District Engineers and 60 Ghana Social Opportunity Project (GSOP) desk officers. Since not all the district offices were handling road construction projects, purposive sampling technique was used to select 40 districts that were in labour-intensive road construction projects under the GSOP programme. Of the 40 districts, 560 respondents were sampled for the study. The data obtained from the study were analysed and presented in tables and diagrams. The findings established that there were four components that contributed to work based conditions and these: Task system; Beneficiary knowledge of task; Work Expectation and Wage system. It was established that there was low productivity on sites and these were as a result of overcrowding of beneficiaries and the use of more aged in the work since the programme is a social intervention programme to support the poor in the community government encouraged many beneficiaries to be recruited for the programme hence do not follow the work study schedule to determine the required number of beneficiaries for a given task.

Keywords: Productivity · Labour intensive · Road · Construction industry · Ghana

1 Introduction

Unfortunately, the lack of reliable means for evaluating the efficiency of labour-intensive construction operations seems to make it more difficult for the construction industry to

J. N. Mojekwu et al. (Eds.): *Sustainable Education and Development*, pp. 120–130, 2021.
https://doi.org/10.1007/978-3-030-68836-3_12

improve productivity. There is also little mention made of how the differences in the workers' abilities in terms of knowledge acquired on task system account for differences in productivity levels with reference to the adoption of labour-intensive methods where beneficiaries from the community are engaged as construction workers.

Hence, their knowledge of what is expected of them and their skill is critical in achieving productivity. The aim of this research is to develop a work based conditions framework for estimating the optimal Construction labour Productivity for labour-intensive works in the Ghanaian construction industry. The objectives of the study are to identify the factors influencing work - based condition on labour productivity in Ghanaian construction firms; to determine the level of labour productivity on labour - intensive works in Ghanaian construction firms and to the examine the extent to which the construction labour productivity framework fits into the identified factors the Ghanaian construction firms.

Khosrowpour, et al. (2014) noted one efficient way to manage workers' performance is to monitor their activity on site, analyze the operation in real-time, and optimize the workflow dynamically. Recognition of worker behaviour can be performed at various levels of abstraction.

2 Theoretical Framework on Labour Productivity of Labour Intensive Works

This study is grounded on the works of Thomas and Sakarcan (1994) who used the factor model to develop task framework that predicted labour-productivity curve and Zayed and Halpin (2005), they concluded that personnel for pile construction is also a contributing component in ensuring productivity in the construction sites. The skill of the labourers was considered as paramount when it comes to this specialized form of construction.

Bernold and AbouRizk (2010) argued that workforce factor plays a significant role in the construction project implementation process since the construction industry is labour intensive nature. Jarkas and Bitar (2012) noted that workforce or labour cost accounts for 30–50% of the total project. Thus, considering the workforce plays a key role in achieving a higher level of productivity performance, construction professionals should pay more attention to the workforce dimension (Durdyev, et al. 2018). According to Abdel-Wahab (2008), the effective utilization of skills rather than a mere increase in the supply of skills is key to bringing about productivity improvements.

Sibande and Agumba (2018) reiterated that adherence to construction specifications, ensuring the quality of works delivered. Ugulu (2017) noted that the nature of the construction project might necessitate high-quality workmanship and meet the required construction method may affect the productivity of workers. Tabassi et al. (2012) argued that the application of new technology in the construction industry and effective construction techniques have a various influence on time, requirements of labour and costs.

Poor scheduling can result in unnecessary waste of time caused by delays as labourers wait for materials of equipment to become available or proceeding tasks to be completed (Chester and Hendrickson 2005). In order to successfully schedule a project, there must be some methodology for the process.

Work scheduled or reassigned during holidays such as independent day, founders' day and other statutory holidays often affected with stop-starts. Workers tend to discuss the time off and lose the previous momentum with a drop in productivity before they get back in the routine.

The work-based conditions focus on the work itself, which include the task to be carried out by the beneficiaries or workers. The various task systems are explained in the following paragraphs, which will form the basis of understanding the work-based conditions. The labour force is best utilized if it is divided into gangs. The intention is to ensure that the labour is used in the most efficient way and that each operation succeeds approximately at the same pace. Hence, the gang balancing is important because it also determines the length of the construction site.

In addressing the gap of understanding the work-based condition with specific attention on beneficiaries' knowledge task theory by Zayed and Halpin (2005) was employed to establish that as part of the conceptual framework of the labour productivity framework for labour-intensive works on road construction. The expectancy theory developed by Vroom (1964) and the theory was improved on by Maloney and McFillen (1987) relating it to the construction industry.

In the study of organizational behaviour, expectancy theory is a motivation theory first proposed by Victor Vroom in 1964.

3 Research Methodology

The study adopted a combination of survey research and experimental research designs. These designs are considered most appropriate due to the nature of the data required and study population.

Records available at the Ghana Social Opportunity Project (GSOP) indicated that there are 920 professionals involved in labour-intensive works comprises 200 Contractors; 200 Site Engineers; 200 Facilitators; 200 Time Keepers; 60 District Engineers and 60 Ghana Social Opportunity Project (GSOP) desk officers.

Ghana Social Opportunity Project is divided into five Zonal offices, namely Bolgatanga, Wa, Temale, Kumasi and Accra offices. There are 60 district offices for all the zonal offices, where Bolgatanga have 12 district offices, Wa has 10 district offices, Temale have 11 district offices, Kumasi has 14 district offices and Accra has 13 district offices. Since not all the district offices were handling road construction projects, purposive sampling technique was used to select 40 districts as they were into road construction projects. Of the 40 districts, one district engineer and one GSOP desk officer were selected from each district making 80 respondents. Again, 3 sites from each district were selected making a total of 120 districts. Of the 120 sites, one facilitator, one-time keeper, one site engineer and one contractor from each site were selected making a total of 480 respondents. In all, 560 respondents were considered for the study.

The questionnaire was used in gathering, the items in the questionnaire in the rest of the sections were based on a five-point Likert type scale. The scores were coded using a continuum of Excellent (E) to Very poor (VP). Respondents were instructed to either select by ticking (√) the appropriate number to indicate their level of Excellent, Good,

Average, poor and very poor to each of the statement about factors influencing productivity and measuring productivity of the companies (where; E = 5, G = 4, A = 3, P = 2 and VP = 1).

The validity and reliability of the instruments were then pre-tested at Ajumako Enyan Essiam, Assin South and Ati Morkwa districts all in the Central Region of Ghana and Accra Zonal office to help evaluate and refine the statements. Questionnaires were given to respondents who could read to be completed by them and where necessary, were given clarity and 543 out of 560 sets of questionnaire were collected and analyzed. Also, the actual task used for the various activities in the road construction was determined by measuring the works executed on sites through the use of work-study. The summary of the data consisted of means, standard deviations, and percentages, cross-tabulations, frequencies, figures and charts. Also, factor analysis and multiple regression model analysis were used.

4 Findings and Discussion

4.1 Results from Exploratory Factor Analysis

In Table 1, a Cronbach alpha of 0.817 was obtained for Work-Based Conditions. This satisfies the benchmark of Pallant (2013) and Fellows and Liu (2008), which stated that the Cronbach alpha coefficient of a scale should be above 0.7. The closer the alpha (α) is to 1, the greater the internal consistency of items in the instrument is assumed Table 2.

Table 1. Cronbach's alpha coefficient for work-based conditions

Reliability statistics		
Cronbach's alpha	Cronbach's alpha based on standardized items	N of items
0.817	0.835	13

There are four components identified Task system; Beneficiary knowledge of task; Work Expectation and Wage system.

Component 1: Task System

As presented in Table 3, the six (6) extracted Work based condition component (WBC), variables on component 1 were Crew size and composition of the labour force to carry out an activity is estimated (80.9%), The method of work to be carried out is determined/discussed (80.1%), Worker is free from the day's work on completion (79.8%), Supervisor approves completed task before releasing the worker (79.1%), In a piece work system workers are paid for the quantity of work produced with no reference to time taken for completion (65.7%) and Payment is made only upon production (52.8%).

Table 2. Total variance explained

Component	Initial eigenvalues			Extraction sums of squared loadings			Rotation sums of squared loadings[a]
	Total	% of Variance	Cumulative %	Total	% of Variance	Cumulative %	Total
1	4.204	32.342	32.342	4.204	32.342	32.342	3.607
2	2.569	19.763	52.105	2.569	19.763	52.105	2.664
3	1.553	11.949	64.053	1.553	11.949	64.053	1.584
4	1.245	9.575	73.628	1.245	9.575	73.628	2.569
5	.901	6.935	80.563				
6	.573	4.408	84.971				
7	.544	4.181	89.152				
8	.402	3.089	92.241				
9	.365	2.805	95.046				
10	.254	1.950	96.997				
11	.151	1.160	98.157				
12	.126	.966	99.123				
13	.114	.877	100.000				

Component 2: Beneficiary's Knowledge of Task

The two (2) extracted work based conditions component (WBC), variables for Component 2 were Worker understands daily task (88.6%) and Workers can earn more than the standard wage (77.7%).

Component 3: Work Expectation

Two (2) were extracted work based conditions component variables for component 3 were Limit/day is fixed (74.7%) and Expectations of worker performance change based on local conditions (e.g. poor weather) (46.8%).

Component 4: Wage System

Three (3) were extracted work based conditions component (WBC), variables for Component 4 were Daily wage rate (81.7%), Worker is released and paid after working effectively for the duration of normal working hours. (79.7%), and Task rate (56.4%). Fig. 1 also shows the work based conditions component construct based on the exploratory factor analysis.

These results confirm the findings of Sibande and Agumba (2018) they stressed that there is a need for the workers to comply with construction specifications, ensuring the quality of works delivered.

Table 3. Actual task output of the activities for road construction on sites in ghana Source: Fieldwork, 2018

No	Activity	Standard task rate (for 6 work hrs)	Actual task rate	Percentage coverage
1.0	Bush clearing			
1.01	Bush clearing including disposal of cuttings out of clearing width			
	In thick bush	170.00 m^2/md	70.00 m^2/md	41%
	In light bush	220.00 m^2/md	120.00 m^2/md	54%
	In savanna bush	270.00 m^2/md	190.00 m^2/md	70%
1.02	Grubbing including disposal of grubbed material out of clearing width			
	Depth not more than 250 mm thick	30.00 m^2/md	25.00 m^2/md	83%
	Depth more than 250 mm up to 500 mm thick	15.00 m^2/md	12.00 m^2/md	80%
1.03	Tree and stump removal including disposal of cuttings out of clearing width	2.00/md	1.00/md	50%
	Fell trees, girth 0.6–1 m and destump	3–4.00/md	2.00/md	50%
	Fell trees, girth 1–2.0 m and destump	1–2.00/md	1.00/md	50%
	Fell trees, girth 2.0–3.0 m and destump	0.5.00/md	0.3.00/md	60%
1.04	Boulder removal including disposal out of clearing width	1.50 m^3/md	1.00 m^3/md	66.7%
2.0	Earthwork			
2.01	Excavation only (excluding gravel excavation)	2.00 m^3/md	1.30 m^3/md	65%
	In soft/Loose soil	3.00 m^3/md	2.10 m^3/md	70%
	In hard soil	2.00 m^3/md	1.30 m^3/md	65%
	In very hard soil	1.50 m^3/md	1.00 m^3/md	67%

(continued)

Table 3. (*continued*)

No	Activity	Standard task rate (for 6 work hrs)	Actual task rate	Percentage coverage
2.02	Excavation including loading (excluding gravel excavation)			
	In soft/Loose soil	2.00 m^3/md	1.00 m^3/md	60%
	In hard soil	1.50 m^3/md	0.80 m^3/md	53%
	In very hard soil	1.20 m^3/md	0.60 m^3/md	50%
2.03	Loading of excavated soil (excluding gravel material)	5.00 m^3/md	2.50 m^3/md	50%
2.04	Off-loading of fill material by labor	7.50 m^3/md	5.00 m^3/md	67%
2.05	Spreading of fill material including mixing and watering	120 m^3/md	10.00 m^3/md	83%
2.06	Ditching and throwing suitable excavated material to the centre of road or throwing and spreading outside of drain if not suitable			
	In soft/Loose soil	2.50 m^3/md	1.60 m^3/md	72%
	In hard soil	1.70 m^3/md	1.10 m^3/md	64%
	In very hard soil	1.00 m^3/md	0.60 m^3/md	60%
2.07	Sloping and back sloping and throwing suitable excavated material to the centre of road or throwing and spreading outside of drain if not suitable			
	In soft/Loose soil	2.50 m^3/md	1.50 m^3/md	60%
	In hard soil	1.70 m^3/md	1.00 m^3/md	59%
	In very hard soil	1.00 m^3/md	0.50 m^3/md	50%
3.0	Camber formation/Base and Sub-base construction			
	Spreading and forming camber including mixing and watering	72.00 m^2/md	60.00 m^2/md	83%

(*continued*)

Table 3. (*continued*)

No	Activity	Standard task rate (for 6 work hrs)	Actual task rate	Percentage coverage
4.0	Gravelling			
4.01	Gravel excavation and stockpiling			
	In wet soil condition	3.00 m^3/md	2.00 m^3/md	67%
	In dry soil condition	2.00 m^3/md	1.20 m^3/md	60%
4.02	Gravel excavation including loading			
	In normal weathered rock/Lateritic gravel	2.00 m^3/md	1.10 m^3/md	55%
	In very hard material/With boulders	1.00 m^3/md	0.50 m^3/md	50%
4.03	Loading gravel by labour	5.00 m^3/md	2.00 m^3/md	40%
4.04	Off-loading gravel by labour	7.50 m^3/md	4.00 m^3/md	53%
4.05	Spreading of gravel including watering	90.00 m^2/md	70.00 m^2/md	78%
4.06	Reinstatement of borrow pit	3.00 m^3/md	2.00 m^3/md	67
5.0	Hauling of loose material			
5.01	Hauling material by head pan			
	0 to 50 m	3.00 m^3/md	2.50 m^3/md	83%
	50 to 100 m	2.50 m^3/md	2.00 m^3/md	80%
	100 to 200 m	1.50 m^3/md	1.00 m^3/md	67%
	200 to 250 m	0.70 m^3/md	0.40 m^3/md	57%
5.02	Hauling material by wheelbarrow			
	0 to 20 m	10.00 m^3/md	8.00 m^3/md	80%
	20 to 40 m	8.30 m^3/md	7.00 m^3/md	84%
	40 to 60 m	6.00 m^3/md	5.00 m^3/md	83%
	60 to 80 m	5.00 m^3/md	4.00 m^3/md	80%
	80 to 100 m	4.00 m^3/md	3.00 m^3/md	75%
	100 to 150 m	3.00 m^3/md	1.80 m^3/md	60%

(*continued*)

Table 3. (*continued*)

No	Activity	Standard task rate (for 6 work hrs)	Actual task rate	Percentage coverage
6.0	Equipment productivity			
6.01	Hauling material by a tractor with 2 trailers on average route condition			
	Hauling distance: 0–1 km	17 Trips/Day		
	Hauling distance: 1–2 km	13 Trips/Day		
	Hauling distance: 2–3 km	10 Trips/Day		
6.02	Compaction by pedestrian roller at maximum thickness layer <15 cm	375.00 m^2/day	300.00 m^2/day	80%

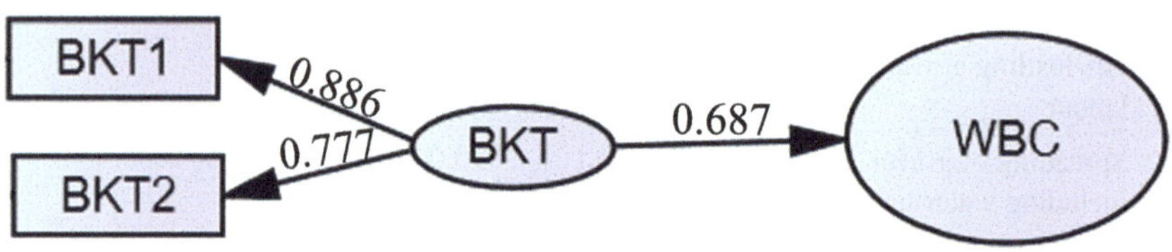

Fig. 1. Work-based conditions component construct based on regression analysis

As a result of the measured works of all the activities taken through the 120 sites under studied most of the activities had an average of 60% of task given completed. The reason for the low productivity included overcrowding of beneficiaries, since the programme is a social intervention programme to support the poor in the community government encouraged many beneficiaries to be recruited for the programme hence do not follow the work study schedule to determine the required number of beneficiaries for a given task.

Measurement Framework of Work-Based Conditions Component Construct
There is a need for participants to understand the daily task so as productivity can be achieved. The work-based condition had 0.687 as the regression correlation over labour productivity.

Work-based conditions factor 1 which is the Beneficiary's Knowledge of Task (BKT) system was significant. Indeed, construction methods are one among other constraints affecting construction productivity. Very often work that is not directly part of the construction of the structure is simply forgotten. Hence construction professionals need to subdivide the work into all working activities that have to be carried out on a step by step basis using the method statement. The number of workers inspected and the responsibility area of each supervisor should be at the optimum level. Meanwhile, it is also very advantageous and effective on labour that top managers audit the works on-site at intervals. When a task is risky they should be done by skilled paid workers (Table 4).

Table 4. Guide for the work–based conditions framework on labour intensive works

No	Component	
1	Work-based conditions	Beneficiary knowledge of task worker understands the daily task • Realistic task rate must be set • The local condition must be taken into consideration when setting out the task • The worker must understand the daily task. The unskilled workers need to be fully briefed on how tasks are carried out and how they will be assessed as satisfactory • The completed task needs approval from the supervisor before releasing the worker • A worker is free from the day's work on completion • Each worker is given a fixed quantity of work to do for the day and gets paid for the day • The supervisor should demonstrate how the work should be done by actually doing the work for a short period Workers can earn more than the standard wage • The remuneration system must be understandable and related to the way work is actually organised

5 Conclusion and Recommendation

The novelty of this study has developed a new metric measure which allows construction professionals to analyze effectively level of productivity. Based on the exploratory factor analysis Thirteen (13) factors were identified and were categorised into four components namely Task system; Beneficiary knowledge of task; Work Expectation and Wage system. It has been able to demonstrate that labour intensive method would be useful in reducing the duration of completing a project. Built environment professionals can use the labour productivity construct derived in this study in understanding whether or not their management techniques such as taking consideration of the work based conditions in achieving productivity at construction sites. There is the need to train students pursuing construction related programmes at the technical universities to be trained in understanding the task system that is used in measuring the work technique in achieving productivity on sites.

Further, the framework informs as to the components that determine labour productivity of labor-intensive works on road construction in the Ghanaian construction industry. Similarly, the latent variables which led to the labour productivity outcome variables could be used for firms' labour productivity measurement in the Ghanaian construction industry.

References

Abdel-Wahab, M.S.: An Examination of the Relationship Between Skills Development and Productivity in the Construction Industry. Loughborough University, Loughborough (2008)

Bernold, L.E., AbouRizk, S.M.: Managing Performance in Construction. John Wiley & Sons, New Jersey (2010)

Chester, M., Hendrickson, C.: Cost impacts, scheduling impacts, and the claims process during construction. J. Constr. Eng. Manag. **131**(1), 102–107 (2005)

Dixit, S., Pandey, A.K., Mandal, S.N., Bansal, S.: A study of enabling factors affecting construction productivity: indian scenario. Int. J. Civil Eng. Technol. **8**(6), 741–758 (2017)

Durdyev, S., Mbachu, J.: Key constraints to labour productivity in residential building projects: evidence from cambodia. Int. J. Constr. Manag. **18**(5), 385–393 (2018)

Han, S.H., Park, S.H., Jin, E.J., Kim, H., Seong, Y.K.: Critical issues and possible solutions for motivating foreign construction workers. J. Manag. Eng. **24**(4), 217–226 (2008)

Jang, H., Kim, K., Kim, J., Kim, J., Labour productivity model for reinforced concrete construction projects. Constr. Innov. **11**(1), 92–113 (2011). http://www.emeraldinsight.com/doi/abs/, https://doi.org/10.1108/14714171111104655

Jarkas, A., Bitar, C.: Factors affecting construction labor productivity in Kuwait. J. Constr. Eng. Manag. **138**(7), 811–820 (2012)

Khosrowpour, A., Niebles, J.C., Golparvar-Fard, M.: Vision-based workforce assessment using depth images for activity analysis of interior construction operations. Autom. Constr. **48**, 74–87 (2014)

Maloney, W.F., McFillen, J.M.: Motivational impact of work crews. J. Constr. Eng. Manag. **113**(2), 208–221 (1987)

Pallant, J.: SPSS Survival Manual. McGraw-Hill Education, UK (2013)

Rosenauer, D., Homan, A.C., Horstmeier, C.A., Voelpel, S.C.: Managing nationality diversity: the interactive effect of leaders' cultural intelligence and task interdependence. Br. J. Manag. **27**(3), 628–645 (2016)

Sambasivan, M., Deepak, T.J., Salim, A.N., Ponniah, V.: Analysis of delays in the tanzanian construction industry: transaction cost economics (TCE) and structural equation modelling (SEM) approach. Eng. Constr. Architectural Manag. **24**(2), 308–325 (2017)

Schwalbe, M.: In search of craft. Soc. Psychol. Q. **73**(2), 107–111 (2010)

Sibande, A.S., Agumba, N.J.: Construction work productivity in South Africa: a case of gauteng province construction industry. In: Proceedings of the 21st International Symposium on Advancement of Construction Management and Real Estate, pp. 523–533. Springer, Singapore (2018)

Tabassi, A.A., Ramli, M., Bakar, A.H.A.: Effects of training and motivation practices on teamwork improvement and task efficiency: the case of construction firms. Int. J. Project Manage. **30**(2), 213–224 (2012)

Thomas, H.R., Sakarcan, A.S.: Forecasting labour productivity using the factor model. J. Constr. Eng. Manag. **120**(1), 228–239 (1994)

Udris, I., Nibel, H.: Situational diagnosis vs. social construction of jobs a meta-analysis of the questionnaire "subjective job analysis". In: Recent Developments in Job Analysis, pp. 79–80. Routledge (2017)

Ugulu, R.A.: Investigating the role of on-site learning in the optimisation of craft gang's productivity in the construction industry (Doctoral dissertation) (2017)

Zayed, T.M., Halpin, D.W.: Productivity and cost regression models for pile construction. J. Constr. Eng. Manag. **131**(7), 779–789 (2005)

Developing Description Onion: A Tool for Improving Communication Effectiveness in Bills of Quantities for Construction Works

G. Nani(✉)

Department of Construction Technology and Management, Kwame Nkrumah University of Science and Technology, Kumasi, Ghana

Abstract. In measurement of construction work items, words are employed to describe the work, whose quantities are measured. These descriptions are used to communicate measured-quantities or measurement information to project stakeholders. The construction industry has experienced various kinds of such descriptions in various environments at various times. Though efforts were made to structure the description of measured work items, the strength of the various descriptors that culminate in these descriptions has not been identified. Consequently, content analysis of bill of quantities, questionnaire survey, and price-estimating analysis was used to determine and categorise the various descriptors relevant to the description of measured construction work items. The descriptors were grouped into primary, secondary, and tertiary descriptors. It was noted that primary descriptors were the ones required to provide fundamental information about measured work items and in many instances provides adequate information. Secondary and tertiary descriptors were noted to reinforce and improve the quality information in descriptions of measured work items. This categorisation therefore helps to understand how descriptionof work items in bills of quantities can be enriched to the benefit of project stakeholders. Strategic use of words from these categories of descriptors shall result in reduced verbosity; and improved quality of communication with project stakeholders.

Keywords: 'Bill of quantities' · 'Standard method of measurement' · SMM · Communication · Description · Construction work items

1 Introduction

Law (1994) described a bill of quantities as a document that lists every item of work (involved in a construction project) in a standardised format with quantities measured using strict measurement rules. Similarly, Uher (1996) and Cox (1994) portrayed a bill of quantities as a schedule of items giving brief identifying descriptions and quantities of work involved in the execution of building construction works. Uher (1996) and Cox (1994) definition matches the Institution of Civil Engineers' perception of bill of quantities (ICE 2012). Considering the above definitions, Law (1994) may be referring to the preparation of bills of quantities according to a stated measurement standard. The

J. N. Mojekwu et al. (Eds.): *Sustainable Education and Development*, pp. 131–143, 2021.
https://doi.org/10.1007/978-3-030-68836-3_13

similarity between all these definitions is that construction work items listed in bills of quantities must be given sufficient description, in order to provide adequate information to project stakeholders. The descriptions are usually intended to communicate measurement information about the relevant work item.

A cursory look at a typical bill of quantities indicates a document with six columns; of which the description column is one (Fig. 1). The content of the description provided is very relevant in decoding the information provided in the bill of quantities. Consequently, descriptions are composed mostly with the guidance of a Standard Method of Measurement (SMM), so as to enhance the effectiveness of the communication. Consequently, the SMM becomes the reference for encoding and decoding measurement information. Alternatively, descriptions are determined by the measurer, based on what he deemed relevant to the intended audience in decoding the measurement information presented in the bill of quantities. Even where SMMs were used, emphasis on aspects of descriptions depends on the discretion of the measurer. Consequently, knowledge about the relative relevance of the various descriptors involved in the composition of descriptions is important, in enhancing communication of bills of quantities.

ITEM	DESCRIPTION	QTY	UNIT	RATE	AMOUNT
				GHC	GHC
	SUBSTRUCTURE (ALL PROVISIONAL)				
	Excavation				
A	Excavate trenches to receive foundation starting from formation level not exceeding 1500mm deep	106	m^3	1.50	159.00
B	Excavate pits for column base starting from formation level not exceeding 150mm	14	m^3	1.60	22.40
	Disposal				
C	Back filling with selected excavated materials well ramming around foundation	72	m^3	1.45	104.40
	Hardcore				
D	Approved imported hardcore or laterite filling in making up level deposited and well compacted in 150mm layers and blinding with fine materials to receive concrete	220	m^3	8.00	1,760.00

Fig. 1. Typical bill of quantities format.

2 Position of Previous Research on Nature of Descriptions and Measurement

Several researches in the area of measurement of construction works noted the excessive nature of unnecessary details in measurement information, complexity of rules prescribed by standard methods of measurement, and inadequacy of measurement information provided in bills of quantities.

Morledge and King (2005) and Foster (2005) observed that the measurement information provided in a bill of quantities, was inadequate for specialist sub-contractors. The made reference to bills of quantities prepared in accordance with the seventh edition of the Standard Method of Measurement for Building Works (published in the United Kingdom). They indicated, it was difficult to estimate real cost of work items based on the bill of quantities information. Similarly, a survey by BCIS/RICS (2004) indicated estimators frequently amend SMM7 (UK) to suit their estimating practices, whenever they carry out measurement. In a recommendation to the Australian Institute of Quantity Surveyors (AIQS) and the Royal Institution of Surveyors (RICS), Mills et al. (2006) elaborated the relevance of simplified measurement information, which does not contain unnecessary detail. Similar recommendations were suggested by Davis and Baccarini (2004), Edwards and Edwards (1995). There were also similar indications in various countries, usually in the preface of existing SMMs. This suggests that measurement (including description) rules need review to streamline descriptions.

In response to the identified shortfalls of measurement information, researchers proposed and demonstrated the use of cost significant items in reducing the number of work items listed in bills of quantities (Edwards and Edwards 1995; Horner and Zakieh 1996). Jaggar et al. (2001) also suggested realignment of measurement to contribute effectively to information management. In studying measurement practices in Ghana, Nani et al. (2008) noted that the fifth edition of the standard method of measurement of building works (RICS and NFBTE 1964) was amended using principles that seek to simplify measurement information. These principles include the elimination of 'cost insignificant items'; streamlining of descriptions by eliminating information that were deemed to be insignificant to users.

While these principles simplify measurement to some extent, much attention was not paid to strategic use of descriptors, with the intent of promoting effective communication of bills of quantities information. It is noteworthy that to avoid communication failure, it is necessary to eliminate what is referred in communication science as noise, as much as possible (Saunders and Stewart 1990). One common noise, which had been responsible for most communication failures is verboseness, especially when several irrelevant words are used in a description. This communication problem may be minimised by employing carefully selected relevant descriptors in composing concise descriptions for measured construction work items. This has the tendency to reduce the volume of descriptions in bill of quantities, without compromising the quality of information required of such descriptions.

3 The Research Method

In this study a "Description Onion" was developed to aid description of measured construction work items. The purpose of the Description Onion is to improve the effectiveness of information transmitted in descriptions of measured construction work items. Relevant descriptors used in descriptions of measured construction work items were identified through literature review and content analysis of existing bill of quantities. Further, the relevance of descriptors were established through expert assessment of the various identified descriptors. The descriptor relevance assessment resulted in the ranking of the various descriptors.

Following this, a critical thinking process was adopted in categorising the various descriptors identified. This categorisation resulted in the development of the "Description

Onion". Additional content analysis of existing bill of quantities was conducted, followed by "pricing information analysis" to test the effectiveness of the "Description Onion". Details of these processes are provided in subsequent sections of this article.

4 Identification of Descriptors

Various descriptors were identified through a process of content analysis of descriptions of typical bills of quantities (prepared in Ghana). The descriptors were identified based on the type of information they provide to the users of bills of quantities. Five (5) Bill of Quantities prepared in Ghana were analysed for this purpose. The content of each

Table 1. Bill of quantities work item descriptors

Descriptors	Details
Identity	Identity of item (i.e. name) e.g. frame, foundation, lock, switch
Materials	Materials that constitute the components of the item; e.g. wood, steel, concrete (mix stated), plastic, aluminium, glass, etc.
Location	Part of the structure with which the item is identified; e.g. in substructure, in slabs, in walls, in roof, ceiling etc.
Level of workmanship	Workmanship required for the item; e.g. finish smooth, finish matt, pointed smooth, fair faced, etc.
Functions	Function of element produced by work item; e.g. construct window to exclude driving rain, etc.
Dimensions	Dimensions of major item components e.g. 300 mm thick, 750 mm wide, 6 m long, 50 × 100 mm, 3 × 150 × 900 mm, etc.
Treatment to items	Treatment to components (material) of item; e.g. kiln seasoned (wood), well vibrated (concrete), wrought (hardwood),
Handling of item	Handling of item (constituent materials); e.g. keep under shed (reinforcement), keep in enclosure above 28 °C (cement) etc.
Geometry	Geometry or shape of major component of item; e.g. circular, curved, rectangular, irregular, curvature (state), etc.
Discrete quantity	Number of discrete items in a lumped quantity; e.g. in 14Nr. (Columns), in 6Nr. (frames) etc.
Restrictions	Restrictions to work (if any); e.g. near busy traffic (excavation), noise limit, in habited structure etc.
Sundry components	Subsidiary items which were components (e.g. nails), water in concrete,
Unusual properties	Unusual properties of item; copper nails (to assemble wood), flexible (pipe), knots–free wood, etc.
Background	Background to which item (material) is applied; e.g. poured on earth (concrete), hacked concrete surface (plaster), etc.
Quantity	Quantity of item involved e.g. 6 m^3, 35 m^2, 11 m, 16 Nr. etc.

construction work item description was examined to identify the descriptors used. The descriptors were identified based on the type of information they provide to the users of the Bill of Quantities. The identification was carried out by examining descriptions in each Bill of Quantities one after the other, recording descriptors as they were found. The process was terminated when it was identified that subsequent Bill of Quantities and descriptions presented similar descriptors. Standard Methods of Measurements (SMMs) from various countries were also similarly examined to ensure the descriptors identified are exhaustive. The various SMMs consulted are listed in the appendix to this article. The descriptors obtained in the process together with details and examples are presented in Table 1.

During the content analysis of the documents mentioned above, it was noted that not all descriptors were found in all descriptions. Some were used much more frequently than others. This gives an indication that various descriptors provide varied levels of relevant information, when used in description of construction work items. This observation provided a hint for the need to conduct a relevance assessment of the various descriptors identified. The relevance assessment was conducted through questionnaire survey.

5 Relevance Assessment of Descriptors

In distinguishing the relevance of the descriptors identified in Table 1, an assessment (survey) was conducted, basically to exact the levels of relevance of the information provided by each descriptor. Respondents in this survey are certified members of the Ghana Institution of Surveyors (GhIS). All professional class members, who could be reached on the contacts provided at the GhIS secretariat were consulted. However, the questionnaires were administered to only those who were ready to partake in the survey. A five-point Likert Scale was used with a questionnaire instrument to measure the relevance of information each descriptor contributes to a description of a construction work item. Each respondent indicated their expert assessment on the Likert Scale. A rating of "1" on the scale indicates the information provided by the descriptor in a typical construction work item description is "highly relevant"; "2" indicates "very relevant", "3" indicates "moderately relevant", "4" indicates "rarely relevant", and "5" indicates "irrelevant". A descriptor is generally regarded a relevant if more than 50% of respondents rate it as "moderately relevant", "very relevant" or "highly relevant" (i.e. rating of "1", "2" or "3" on the Likert scale). In addition, a significant test was conducted at 5% level for each descriptor to determine the probability (p-value) that the descriptor could be rated by respondents as not significantly relevant (i.e. a rating scale of "4", or "5" on the Likert Scale). A summary of survey responses and analysis are shown in Table 2.

Descriptors that were rated as "highly relevant" (modal rating) are *identity*, *quantity*, *dimensions*, *location* and *constituent materials* of construction work items. At least 95% of respondents rated these descriptors as "relevant". All respondents rated '*identity*' of the construction work item as highly or very relevant, which is logical because this is the descriptor which identifies what is being measured. All respondents also considered the '*location*' of the work item as significantly relevant in a description, while 97%, 95% and 95% similarly rated '*quantity*, *dimensions*, and *materials* respectively. A significance test for these descriptors at 5% level yielded approximately zero "p-values".

Table 2. Analysis of survey results and relevance of descriptors

		Mode	Mean	% Rating ≤ moderate	p-value	Total responses	Mode and mean interpretation
Descriptors	Identity	1	1.3	100	0.00	111	High
	Quantity	1	1.6	97	0.00	108	High
	Dimensions	1	1.7	95	0.00	111	High
	Location	1	1.8	100	0.00	111	High
	Materials	1	1.9	95	0.00	111	High
	Treatment	2	1.9	97	0.00	111	Very
	Workmanship	2	2.2	89	0.00	111	Very
	Geometry	2	2.3	84	0.00	111	Very
	Background	3	2.3	92	0.00	111	Moderately
	Discrete quantity	2	2.5	81	0.00	111	Very
	Function of element	2	2.7	84	0.00	111	Very
	Restrictions	2	2.7	71	0.02	102	Very
	Handling	3	2.8	81	0.01	111	Moderate
	Unusual properties	3	2.8	75	0.05	108	Moderate
	Sundry components	4	3.4	49	1.00	111	Rare

Key to Likert scale ratings: 1 = highly relevant; 2 = very relevant; 3 = moderately relevant; 4 = rarely relevant; 5 = irrelevant.

This is an indication that there is nearly 100% certainty that the information contribution of these descriptors are significantly relevant to the quality of description for a typical construction work item. Consequently, it is deducible that these descriptors are fundamental to every work item description and their presence is relevant to all descriptions for construction work items.

The next set of descriptors, which were rated as "very relevant" (i.e. '2' on the Likert scale) by most respondents (modal rating) include: *treatments to materials*, *workmanship*, *geometry*, *discrete quantity*, *function of the element*, and *restrictions to work*. These descriptors attracted 97%–71% of respondents, who rated them as significantly relevant. Considering "*background*", the modal rating is 'moderate' (i.e. '3' on Likert scale), while the mean rating is skewed (can be approximated) towards 'very relevant' (i.e. '2' on Likert scale). In addition, 57% (simple majority) of the respondents indicated that this descriptor is either highly or very relevant. The descriptor is, therefore, considered as very relevant rather than moderately relevant. On the other hand, '*restrictions*' could be considered as moderately relevant rather than very relevant as the mean rating is highly skewed towards moderate. In addition, this descriptor yielded a p-value of 0.02 higher than zero compared to other descriptors in this group. Further, only 48%

(less than simple majority) of respondents indicated that this descriptor is either highly or very relevant. Consequently, the second group of descriptors, which are considered as "very relevant", include: *treatments to materials, workmanship, geometry, discrete quantity, function of the element*, and *background*. These descriptors provide information that may be required on a construction work item after the fundamental descriptors were considered. They present further clarification to the nature of construction work item under measurement. A significance test for these descriptors shows that respondents will almost always rate this group of descriptors as contributing very relevant information to descriptions. This is based on inference from p-values (p-values = 0) obtained at 5% significance level (Table 2).

The third group of descriptors includes *'restrictions, handling, and unusual properties of work'*, which were mostly rated as "moderately relevant" (modal rating). About 81% and 75% of the respondents hold the view that, *handling* and description of *unusual properties* respectively provide significantly relevant information to descriptions. A significant test on these descriptors indicates that they are "significantly" relevant at 5% level, though *'unusual properties'* would have been rejected at 1% significance level. These two descriptors together with "*restrictions*" are therefore regarded as a third group of descriptors which are "moderately relevant". This implies that mostly, while describing or decoding descriptions of measured construction work items, stakeholders may not always seek information carried by these descriptors.

The last descriptor is '*sundry components*' which achieved a modal rating of "rarely relevant". In fact, 49% of respondents rated this descriptor as significantly relevant while the rest 51% rated it as insignificant or irrelevant. A significant test for this descriptor indicates nearly 100% certainty (p-value = 1) that it would always be considered by stakeholders as irrelevant. The above inference on this descriptor is generally consistent with the practice of most SMMs. Most SMMs do not consider the inclusion of "*sundry components*" in descriptions as necessary. In effect this descriptor may be disregarded or treated as insignificant in the description of an item of building work. However, in exceptional instances, it may be included, where it assumes considerable information significance.

Though, the identified descriptors are grouped according to their relevance, some are individually more relevant than others within a group. This order of relevance was determined based on the calculation of the respective relative importance indexes. The descriptors were accordingly ranked in decreasing order of relevance as follows: *identity of the work item, quantity*, the *dimensions, location, materials, treatments, workmanship, geometry, background, functions of element, discrete quantity, restrictions, handling requirements, unusual properties of work item, and sundry components*. This provides further useful guide in the development of the Description Onion and subsequent composition of simple and concise descriptions of construction work items. The above inferences are organised and presented in a Description Onion in Fig. 2.

6 Description Onion

The various groups of descriptors are presented pictorially in an onion-like model (Fig. 2). Inferences from analysis of survey results suggested four groups of descriptors.

The relevant three groups (shown in Fig. 2) are referred to as Primary Descriptors, Secondary Descriptors, and Tertiary Descriptors. The fourth group of descriptors was found to be trivial for the purpose of composing descriptions for measured construction work items. These trivial descriptors include "sundry components of construction work items" such as nails in wood, etc. This group of items are often deemed to be included in the major items in which they occur. This group of descriptors is therefore excluded from the Description Onion on the grounds of their triviality. The Onion therefore has its core part and two skins, which denote the various groups of descriptors and the relevance of the information they provide in the description of an item of building construction work.

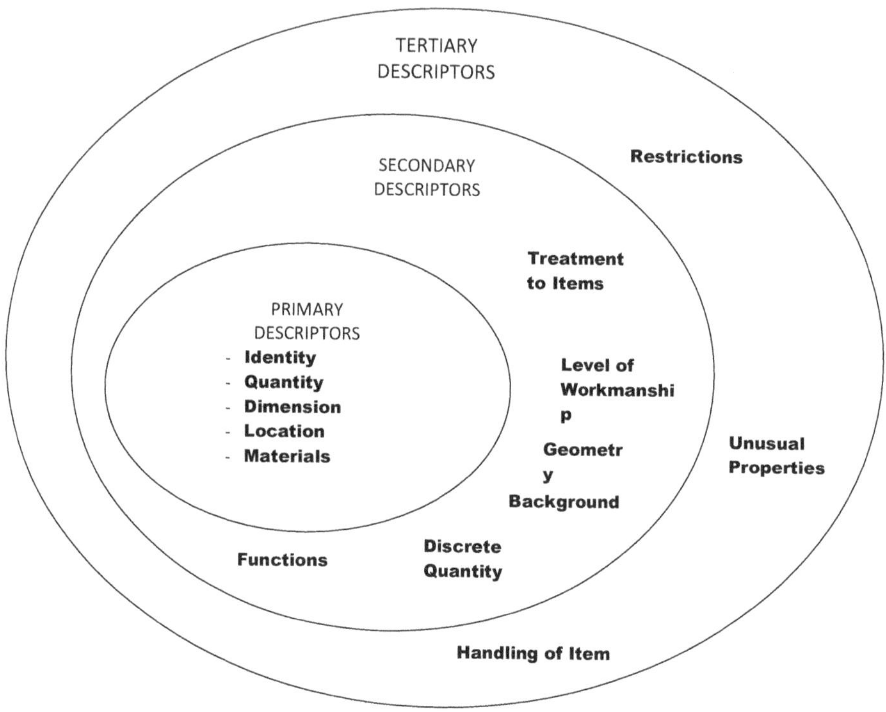

Fig. 2. Description onion

Primary Descriptors are at the core of the onion. They provide the core or basic information about a construction work item, which is highly relevant to the description of such work items. The other skins of the onion, which surround this core, represent the secondary and tertiary descriptors. They provide supplementary information to that of the Primary Descriptors. The relevance of the descriptors reduce towards the outer skin of the Onion.

The basic information provided by Primary Descriptors could be useful in a "shorthand-like" manner of descriptions. It is especially useful, where the description will be used by a smaller group of stakeholders, who are already familiar with the object of the description. In some instances, a description composed of only Primary Descriptors may be adequate. It is necessary that every SMM and bill of quantities descriptions cater for these basic descriptors. But generally, it is expected that SMMs would provide rules, based on the knowledge presented in the Onion, to support a strategic and a systematic approach to composing descriptions. This approach would simplify descriptions, and also aid software application to description of construction work items.

It is noteworthy that Primary Descriptors include the quantity of the construction work item, because it is considered as an integral part of the measurement information. Apart from the identity of the item the quantity is the most relevant descriptor of the item as far as measurement is concerned. However certain descriptor words may connote more than one descriptor, hence not all descriptors would be distinctly represented within a particular description for an item. In spite of the fact that "dimensions" and "materials" are Primary Descriptors, certain instances render their express inclusion in a description unnecessary.

Un-quantified dimensions of an item may not be stated, if the un-quantified dimension is negligible with regard to the quantified one (e.g. the thickness of paint on the wall, which was quantified in square meters); the un-quantified dimension is at the discretion of the contractor; (e.g. the thickness of formwork material), or the un-quantified dimension is standard, hence cannot be confused (e.g. 75 × 75 mm 'MEM" wall switch, etc.). Similarly, "materials" require no express mention if, they are specified at the discretion of the contractor (e.g. formwork). Again the mention of the materials is irrelevant if the item is proprietary; hence it is of a standard material which cannot be altered; e.g. ironmongery; or the material is intrinsically linked to the identity of the item (identification of the item implies knowledge of the material). This illustrates the instances that these descriptors may not be expressly found in a description.

In further analysis, the theory propounded in the Description Onion was validated through further content analysis of bill of quantities and pricing analysis. The pricing analysis was conducted on priced descriptions (descriptions that were formulated based on the Description Onion).

7 Test of Description Onion

Content analysis was conducted on the five sampled bills of quantities to identify the relative usage of the three groups of descriptors in the various item descriptions in the bill of quantities. This is intended to confirm the grouping of descriptors proposed in the Description Onion. A high usage in descriptions indicates high relevance, while low usage indicates irrelevance of descriptor. For each description in each bill of quantities, descriptors from each group were tallied as they were observed.

The findings indicate that descriptions in bill of quantities' construction work currently contain averagely 93% of the Primary Descriptors per item-description, 25% of Secondary Descriptors per item-description, and 3% of Tertiary Descriptors per item-description (Table 3). This confirms the assertion in the Description Onion that the most relevant descriptors, in in a typical description for a measured construction work item are the primary descriptors, followed by secondary descriptors, and then tertiary descriptors. This finding was further confirmed by a pricing analysis test.

Table 3. The rate of use of various descriptors in bill of quantities descriptions

Example BQ examined	Primary descriptors (%)	Secondary descriptors (%)	Tertiary descriptors (%)
1	94	24	2
2	92	23	4
3	96	28	3
4	93	25	3
5	90	23	2
Average	**93%**	**25%**	**3%**

Table 4. t-Test: paired two sample for means of two descriptions (first description used only primary descriptors, while second description used all groups of descriptors).

	Variable 1	*Variable 2*
Mean	0.984117647	0.994117647
Variance	0.000825735	0.000388235
Observations	17	17
Pearson correlation	−0.087009759	
Hypothesized mean difference	0	
Df	16	
t stat	−1.138085276	
P(T < = t) one-tail	0.135920177	
t Critical one-tail	1.745883669	
P(T < = t) two-tail	0.271840355	
t critical two-tail	2.119905285	

In the pricing analysis test, two sets of descriptions were formulated for each of 17 different work items selected from bill of quantities. The first description was formulated with only primary descriptors. The second description was formulated using primary, secondary and tertiary descriptors. The test-respondents, who were quantity surveyors sampled from among members of GhIS, priced the 2 sets of descriptions for each work item. The prices were standardised and a statistical t-test was conducted at 5% significance level to identify any significant difference between the prices of the two descriptions. The result of the test, shown in Table 4, indicates that there was no significant difference between the means of the prices for the two descriptions. This result also confirms the first validation test above, which was based on content analysis for bill of quantities. Consequently, it is therefore true that Primary Descriptors provide the basic information that is relevant construction work item descriptions. The primary

Descriptors are complemented by both secondary and tertiary descriptors. Generally, the information provided by the secondary and the tertiary descriptors enrich and reinforce effectiveness of communication emanating from a description. The grouping of descriptors as proposed in the Description Onion is therefore considered as useful.

8 Conclusion

Generally, descriptors that are relevant in describing measured construction work items could be categorised into primary, secondary and tertiary descriptors. Primary descriptors convey basic information about a work item, while secondary and tertiary descriptors usually enrich and reinforce it. A description containing only primary descriptors provide almost all the necessary information about the item under consideration, in which case the secondary and tertiary descriptors may not be necessary. The Description Onion is expected to promote a systematic approach and simplify description for the purpose of preparing bills of quantities for construction works. The concept could also be applied other forms of descriptions such as specification writing. This knowledge is useful in formulating the rules of measurement for standard methods of measurement (SMMs) and also aid description for measured construction work items.

Notably, the Description Onion has introduced the concept of significant descriptors (i.e. Primary Descriptors). This approach achieves simplicity of measurement through reduction of verboseness in descriptions, and numerousness of bill of quantities items. It was noted that items that were split as a result of inclusion of irrelevant descriptors would be combined, when the irrelevant descriptor is eliminated; this reduces the number of construction work items in bills of quantities. The theory propounded in the Description Onion is still in an early stage, and further research and tests must be conducted to fully establish the theory.

ANNEX

SMMs Used in Identification of Descriptors

1. Standard Method of Measurement of Building Works (7th edition), by Royal Institution of Chartered Surveyors (RICS and BEC 1998; RICS and BEC 1988)
2. Standard Method of Measurement of Building Works (6th edition), by Royal Institution of Chartered Surveyors (RICS and NFBTE 1978)
3. Standard Method of Measurement of Building Works (5th edition), by Royal Institution of Chartered Surveyors (RICS and NFBTE 1964)
4. Australian Standard Method of Measurement of Building Works by the Australian Institute of Quantity Surveyors (AIQS 2001a; AIQS and MBFA 1980)
5. Construction electronic measurement standards by (CEMS) by SPRING Singapore (SPRING 2002)
6. Building and Engineering Standard Method of Measurement (2nd edition) by Nigerian Institute of Quantity Surveyors (NIQS 2003)
7. Standard System of Measuring of Building Works by the Association of South African Quantity Surveyors (ASAQS 1999; ASAQS 1977)

8. Method of Measurement of Highway Works (Department of Transport, Scottish Development Department, Welsh Office and Department of the Environment for Northern Ireland 1987)
9. Standard Method of Measurement of civil Engineering Quantities (ICE 1968)
10. Australian Standard 1181-1982: Method of Measurement of Civil Engineering Works and Associated Building Works (Standards Association of Australia 1982)
11. South African Standard Method of Measurement of Civil Engineering Quantities (South African Institution of Engineers 1960)
12. Singapore Standard Method of Measurement of Building Works (Singapore Institute of Surveyors and Valuers 1986)
13. Kenyan Standard Method of Measurement of Building Works (Architectural Association of Kenya 1996)
14. Standard Method of Measurement for Industrial Engineering Construction (ACE and RICS 1984)
15. Irish Agreed Rules of Measurement (Society of Chartered Surveyors and Construction Industry Federation 2003)
16. CESMM3: Civil Engineering Standard Method of Measurement (ICE 1991)
17. Canadian Method of Measurement of Construction Works (Hadley 2000)
18. Measurement Rules for Contractors Quantities by Tweeds Quantity Surveyors, Cost Engineers and Construction Economists (Tweeds 1996)
19. Handbook of Measurement of Building Works by Bureau of Indian Standards (Bureau of Indian Standards 1987)
20. Standard Method of Measurement of Building Works by New Zealand Standards (New Zealand Standard 1995)
21. Rider Hunt System of Measurement for Construction Works (Rider Hunt 1988)

References

BCIS: Measurement based procurement of buildings: a survey of who measures buildings. In: Proceedings of RICS Measurement Conference, RICS, 30th September 2004

Cox, P.J.: Writing Specification for Construction. McGraw Hill, London (1994)

Davis, P., Baccarini, D.: The use of BoQ in construction projects - Australian survey, COBRA 2004. In: The International Construction Research Conference of the Royal Institution of Chartered Surveyors, RICS Foundation, Leeds, 7–8 September 2004

Edwards, P.J., Edwards, M.: A price - rationalized approach to item separation in the measurement of concrete work. Constr. Manage. Econ. **13**, 485–491 (1995)

Foster, C.: Mechanical an electrical measurement - do the rules need changing? Royal Institute of Chartered Surveyors. https://www.rics.org. 12 June 2005

Horner, M., Zakieh, R.: Characteristic items - a new approach to pricing and controlling construction projects. Constr. Manage. Econ. **14**, 241–252 (1996)

ICE: Civil Engineering Standard Method of Measurement, 4th edn. Thomas Telford, London (2012)

ICE: Civil Engineering Standard Method of Measurement, 3rd edn. Thomas Telford, London (1991)

Jaggar, D., Ross, A., Love, P.E.D., Smith, S.: Overcoming information opacity in construction: a commentary. Logistic Inf. Manage. **14**, 413–421 (2001)

Law, C.: Building contractor estimating: British style. Cost Eng. **36**, 23–28 (1994)
Mills, A., Lawther, P., Jones, D.: Standard methods of measurement – a comparative study of national and regional publications. In: Australian Institute of Quantity Surveyors and Royal Institution Chartered Surveyors (2006)
Morledge, R., King, S.: The effectiveness of current pricing documentation from the perspective of the contractor's estimator. In: CIB W92/ T23/W107 International Symposium on Procurement, NY USA, pp 609–616 (2005)
Nani, G., Edwards, P.J., Adjei-Kumi, T., Badu, E., Amoah, P.: Customisation and desirable characteristics of a standard method of measurement for building works in Ghana. Aust. J. Constr. Econ. Build. **8**(2), 30–40 (2008)
Saunders, R.G., Stewart, P.W.: Failure of communication in research and development. Proj. Manage. Res. Dev. **18**(2), 71–78 (1990)
Uher, T.E.: A probabilistic cost engineering model. Cost Eng. **38**, 33 (1996)

Theoretical Framework for Assessing Self-help Housing Projects Affordability

C. A. Dafeamekpor(✉), T. Adjei-Kumi, G. Nani, and E. Kissi

Department of Construction Technology and Management, Kwame Nkrumah University of Science and Technology, Kumasi, Ghana

Abstract. Extant studies on Self-Help Housing (SHH) approach focused substantially on the types, processes and the challenges, but very rare on the review of a set of criteria for its affordability measurement. However, every housing affordability measure requires a decision criterion for the measurement and subsequent judgement on affordability situations. This paper aims to address the gap by reviewing academic papers on the criteria for Self-Help Housing 'Projects' Affordability measurement. The study begun with a desktop search under the "T/A/K (title/abstract/keywords)" field of mainly of Scopus and with assistance of other search engines such Google scholar, Emerald and Taylor and Francis online data bases. A total of 113 papers were initially identified. The breakdown was as follows, 93 peer review and 20 no-peer review papers. But only peer review journals were selected for the study, thus a sample of 93 was used. However, after filtering, 21 of papers were found not to be relevant to the subject and thus the remaining 72 papers were finally subjected to critical content analysis. The study identified a total set of eight (8) criteria with thirty-one (31) associated determining factors for SHH affordability measurement. The criteria set were classified primarily into eight key categories; financing, access to land, building quality, development controls and planning regulations, building cost, locational effects, infrastructure and services and social issues. The outcome of this study broadens the understanding of housing policy formulators and researchers on Self-help housing affordability. By reviewing available existing literature on self-help housing, this study it provides the opportunity for further empirical studies on self-help housing affordability.

Keywords: Self-help housing · Self-help housing affordability criteria · Self-help housing Determinants · Self-help housing projects · Urban households · Developing countries

1 Introduction

Theoretically, it could be argued from a historical perspective that the human race has been fulfilling its shelter needs through self-construction, guided by different motivations for the adoption of the preferred housing delivery approach. To Murillo (2012), the motivation could be based on an individual or a collective decision. Perceptively, it could be argued that these housing decisions can be executed through formal or informal

J. N. Mojekwu et al. (Eds.): *Sustainable Education and Development*, pp. 144–163, 2021.
https://doi.org/10.1007/978-3-030-68836-3_14

means or both. Thus, Self-help housing (SHH) has its informal historical antecedent in developing countries largely in the global south. However, beyond the 1960s Turner (1976), internationalized its vital role in terms of the provision of shelter for the majority of urban households in developing countries.

Conceptually, SHH can be defined as a housing delivery approach predominately adopted by households in developing countries; where the houseowner buys a plot of land, self-manage the resources (labour, materials and funds) and construct a shelter/house formally or informally. It has been described it as a substitute solution to the conventional state-led housing delivery for most urban households, due to the failings of public housing policies in developing countries (Gilbert 2014; Arku 2009b). Similarly, the Centre for Affordable Housing Finance in Africa (CAHF), (CAHF 2019) asserted that conventional housing do not have capacity in Ghana and other countries in the sub-Sahara Africa to deliver adequately housing to the populace. Karley (2008), posited that public housing delivery is only for higher income earners in Ghana and those in the diaspora. In effect, this leaves the low to middle incomes households to construct their houses privately through self-help.

Ghana Statistical Service (2014), revealed that Ghana's current home ownership rates is mostly from the contribution of SHH. Impliedly, this housing delivery approach will continue to be the main source of supply of housing tenancy in Ghana, and the situation could be the same in many other developing countries. Some authors argued that it has been the main housing delivery approach among cultures of developing countries since time immemorial (Bangdome-Dery et al. 2014; Nnamdi 2011; Pugh 2001). Murillo (2012), claimed that urbanization in developing countries happens mostly through self-build practices. To (Bredenoord and Lindert 2010), cities in the developing countries are continuously been built mainly through SHH. According to Greene and Rojas (2008), self-help housing delivered incrementally has become the key strategy that facilitate access to housing for households in developing countries. Nonetheless to Smet (1999), most of these SHH households are trapped in housing affordability (HA) dilemmas due to financing and other peculiar socioeconomic challenges.

2 The Case For Self-help Housing Affordability Measurement

Several previous studies have identified that SHH contributes immensely both; to the upliftment of households' socioeconomic status, and the national economies of developing countries (CAHF 2019; Arku 2009). Despite its contribution, it is faced with serious socioeconomic problems of affordability (Afrane et al. 2016; Ahadzie and Badu 2011; Boamah 2010). Existing literature identified some of the affordability problems as; access to land and the lack of adequate financing (Nwuba et al. 2015). Longer construction period due to the incremental nature was observed to be a problem affected by exogenous economic factors; such as hikes in building materials prices (Bangdome-Dery et al. 2014) and land ligation problems (Owusu-Ansah et al. 2019). Consequently, studies claimed that SHH construction process takes between 5–15 years to complete (Arku 2009b; Greene and Rojas 2008). It presupposes that the overall cost of these housing projects at completion could be far beyond the initial cost estimates. This could be due to unstable inflationary tendencies and foreign exchange fluctuations situations in developing countries; thus affecting its affordability.

One would have expected that these SHH affordability problems could be addressed through the existing methodological approaches and researches on HA measurement, such as the price income ratios (PIR) and others. Therefore, a critical observation of these extant literature on its measurement was sourced from Scopus and other online data bases. The search had shown a clear paucity in literature on the precise metric classification that could promote an effective assessment of incremental SHH affordability measure for households in Ghana's housing market. More so, it revealed that much attention was rather focused more on the conventional HA measurement; which depends mostly on housing price and income as the main determinants. However, HA measure that depends exclusively on price and income have been debunked by the studies as not being effective in capturing all the affordability outcomes of the households (Nwuba et al. 2015; Mulliner and Maliene 2012; Gabriel 2005). This collective assertion is anchored theoretically on the premise that HA has economic, social and environmental dimensions. To Mulliner and Maliene (2012), these dimensions are also being influenced by factors that determines the outcomes of households seeking to meet their housing aspirations in their respective housing markets. This argument could justifiably be stretched for the case of measuring SHH affordability. That is to say, SHH households in a developing country like Ghana are also equally affected by affordability of same, but in strands of issues such as; financing problems (Karley 2008; Smet 2006), the difficulties in accessing land for SHH projects (Mselle and Sanga 2018; Afrane et al. 2016). A study has revealed that housing affordability is a problem, especially in Ghana's urban centres (Boamah 2010). This implied SHH affordability is a problem because, other researchers have discovered that it accounts for over 75% of Ghana's national housing stock annually (Arku 2009b). There is the need therefore, to develop a metric system that can enable SHH affordability measurement in Ghana's urban housing market.

In addition, Ezennia and Hoskara (2019), claimed that there no optimal metric for HA. Impliedly, the existing methodological approaches for HA could fail to reveal the optimal outcome if adopted for SHH affordability measurement, especially in a developing country's housing market like Ghana where self-built of housing is the predominant route to homeownership. Consequently, this study seeks to review literature to identify the criteria that will enable development of a metric for SHH affordability measurement. It is envisaged the identification of these criteria will broaden knowledge on SHH affordability. Furthermore, it seeks to provide empirical linkage connecting SHH affordability to the existing HA knowledge areas in literature.

Consequently, the focus of the study was to identify, organize and select the criteria through a comprehensive literature search, using Scopus and other credible search sources for criteria that influence SHH affordability. It is also envisaged that at the end, the outcome of this study will serve as a pedestal for further studies and broader understanding of self-help housing affordability. The identified affordability criteria have been subsequently categorized into the various classification to aid the selection of the appropriate measurement approach.

3 Research Methodology

This study adopted procedure for critical systematic review of literature to gain new knowledge construction management studies. The research method outlined below was used in similar built environment studies by Lam and Yu (2011); (Afshar et al. 2017); and Acheamfour, Kissi et al. (2019).Thus, the research framework (see Fig. 1) by Ke et al. (2009) was the guide for this study, on how the criteria for the SHH affordability metric could be selected. The previous studies that adopted Ke et al. (2009) research framework outlined four (4) process/phases for such studies. Namely: (i) selection of criteria; (ii) weighting of the criteria; (iii) scoring of SHH affordability' against individual criterion; and (iv) the selection of the ranking system. Thus, this study has been limited to the first phase of the selection process which is essentially the assessment and selection of criteria for SHH affordability measure. In this review, this paper seeks to present a complete examination of literature on SHH affordability criteria.

This study was primarily qualitative in nature. It comprehensively reviewed existing literature with the focus on only relevant past studies that are linked to SHH affordability criteria. Literature review is frequently been used for studies of this nature in housing research; through qualitative methodology for expanding knowledge on specific topic (Darko et al. 2017). Several housing literature review studies used data source from credible existing data bases to expand knowledge. For instance, Adabre and Chan (2019), used qualitative review of literature to identify success factors for sustainable affordable housing using Scopus data base. Li (2015), did a study on the trend on housing affordability research with same. It could be argued that the success of a qualitative research such as literature review is largely dependent on the credibility of the data source. In affirmation Adabre and Chan (2019), asserted that a qualitative literature review with the application of a structured literature search strategy provide important credible results. Therefore, Pollock et al. (2016), credible results are assured when qualitative studies adopted systematic research approach combine with multiples of related primary studies that provide answers to a specific gap in literature.

Accordingly, Ke et al. (2009) three-stage research approach framework has been adopted for this study. This same research framework also guided previous qualitative literature review studies by Acheamfour et al. (2019); Darko et al. (2017); and Hong and Chan (2014). Therefore, same research framework has been adopted for the study (see Fig. 1) below via title/abstract/keywords (T/A/Ks).

Consequently, these specific key terms; "Self-help housing", criteria influencing Self-help housing", and "Self-help housing affordability measurement criteria" were used in T/A/Ks of Scopus, Google scholar search engine fields, and other supplementary search databases (e.g. Taylor and Francis online, Science direct, Emerald insight, Sages and Research gate) in the first stage to identify the related peer review journal papers. Thereafter, the second stage begun by filtering further all the papers using the Scopus search engine and other the research databases to select the relevant papers. This is because same has been used in similar qualitative literature reviews in related studies as mentioned above. Two selection criteria were used to filter after the selected targeted journals were picked. These were; (i) the journal should have published a paper related to self-help housing (ii), the journal papers should also have touched on the criteria and determinants influencing self -help housing development. In the third or final stage, the contents of all the selected papers were critically examined and analysed as set out in Sect. 3.1 in order to classify them into various criteria as and in line with the research framework (see Fig. 1).

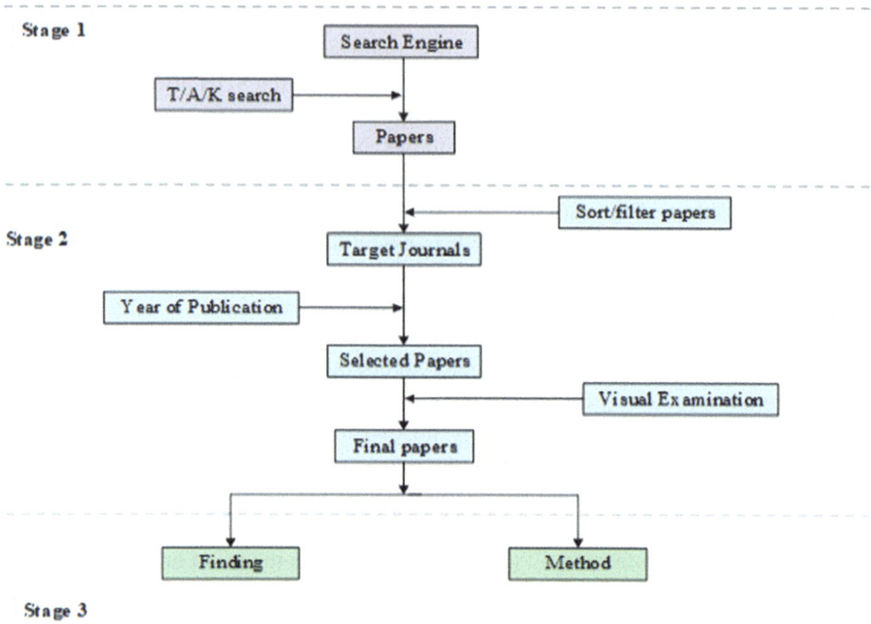

Fig. 1. Research Source: Ke et al. (2009), cited in Acheamfour et al. (2019)

3.1 Identification of Journal for the SHH Affordability Criteria

This study is conducted through a comprehensive review of literature, with much attention on relevant past empirical studies on the criteria for measuring self-help housing affordability. The journal paper identification process followed the commonly used methodology for epistemological advancement on specific topics in built environment studies by several authors such as Acheamfour et al. (2019); Darko, et al. (2017); Li et al. (2014). Thus, structured review of the literature using a three-stage refinement process by (Ke et al. (2009), was adopted for this study (see Fig. 1). The articles were sourced mostly through Scopus, with inputs from other online data bases such as Google scholar online databases under the "T/A/K (title/ abstract/keyword)" field of the search engines. This database was selected because of the following four reasons:

(a) It has been adopted extensively for literature review for studies in both built environment and housing domains (Adabre and Chan 2019; Serin 2018);
(b) Majority of research papers in the field of self-help housing and housing affordability were archived in Scopus (Li 2014);
(c) It is the best and most efficient search engine for conducting a literature review (Acheamfour et al. 2019);
(d) Scopus large data covers a wide range of literature in different areas in comparison with the Web of Science (wos), Google scholar, and Sociindex (Adabre and Chan 2019 and Serin, 2018).

3.2 Selecting Target Journal Papers Relevant to the Study

The search was limited to self-help housing affordability criteria and determinants its measurement. A total of 93 peer reviewed (see Table 1 in appendix) papers were initially identified (18 June, 2020) using "TITLE-ABS-KEY" at stage 1; in line with the research framework (Fig. 1). In the second stage, two criteria approaches were also adopted in order to select the 79 targeted journal papers because the large number of papers retrieved needed to be trimmed. These were;

i. First, all the papers relevant to self-help housing were selected,
ii. Second, papers with SHH affordability problems discussions that were relevant to the study were thereafter selected. Thus, a broad visual scrutiny has been done towards the selection of the target journal papers during the second stage as depicted in the search framework (Fig. 1).

Every paper that qualified in the selected journals were further subjected to the visual checks in terms of SHH, and including the year it was published. More so, only peer reviewed journals were selected at the end of the stage 2; therefore, a sample of 81 peer review publications were selected from 52 journals.

The papers were first purposively selected during the second stage by focusing on criteria that influences Self-help housing affordability that could provide a metric system. In addition and including discussion on the determining factors of SHH. A total of 81 papers relevant to the subject were selected out of the 132, with 53 rejected for their non-relevance. Thus, after the application of the second selection criteria, the number of final valid research papers was reduced from 132 to papers 81. Consequently, the 79-peer review papers were found in 46 different journals. These were finally identified according to the set selection criteria for further analysis in the third (final) stage. In effect, the 52 journals have qualified and were selected in this study had met the criterion set by Hong et al. (2012). That is; the journal contains a significant number of papers in the initial search. Hong et al. (2012), pegged the 'significant number' at a 'benchmark' of 1% of the total papers identified to be included in a review work. Thus, 81 out of 132 papers represented 61.36%, which far exceeded the 1% minimum benchmark.

The 79 sampled papers provide an in-depth perspective on the status of knowledge gap on SHH affordability measurement for further studies. Qualitative literature studies by Owusu et al. (Owusu-Ansah et al. 2019) and Acheamfour et al. (2019) used 46 and 37 peer reviewed journal papers respectively to present review. Consequently, the sample size of 81 was the maximum relevant saturation point per the Scopus search. In addition, it was considered acceptable, representative and realistic to enable meaningful conclusions to be drawn when compared with other related studies. Further, each of the criteria identifies from these 81 peer reviewed papers has some level influence on the affordability outcome of households, especially in the urban centres of a developing country like Ghana. Thus, using them to develop a metric for SHH affordability is novel.

3.3 Examination of Target Papers Related to Criteria for SHH Affordability

The research process adopted for this study centred on content analysis. As such, and as stated previously in Sect. 4.2, each of the 81 identified papers contents were subjected to critical content analysis in line with the position of Kolbe and Burnett (1991). Content analysis can be best explained as an observational research tool that greatly help to evaluate contents of all recorded forms of communication. Fellows and Liu (2008), posited that content analysis has been used often for the determination of the various aspects of a set of data by simply counting the number of times that an activity happens or a topic is depicted. According to Giannantonio (2010), the adoption of either qualitative or quantitative or both methods are allowed for doing content analysis in research. Therefore, this this study adopted qualitative method in order to place emphasis on understanding the meaning or influencers of the data (i.e. grouping the data into categories), as asserted Fellows and Liu (2008). Other forms content analysis-quantitively, concerns about the ability to generate numerical values for categorized data into; frequencies, ratings and rankings for statistical analysis. This analysis not only promotes easier comparison, but present better opportunity for examining the hierarchical order for categories within a data set. However, this study focused on the identification and classification of the criteria and their associated determinants; for developing a metric for SHH affordability SHH in a developing country from 91 eligible publications. Nonetheless, a quasi-quantitative content analysis was applied in this to statistically classify and enumerate the identified criteria against the associated determinants that can provide effective guide for assessing SHH affordability in Ghana.

4 Result and Discussion

This section provides a summary of how the results of the study were realized based on the research objectives and including the discussion on the results obtained.

4.1 List of Journal for the SHH Affordability Criteria

First of all, the research objective of identifying and organizing a set of criteria for SHH affordability measurement as set out in Sect. 3. In order to achieve this goal 81 publications that focused studies on self-help housing affordability measurement were selected through a methodical review.

4.2 Status and Credibility of Selected Papers

Though the primary focus of this study is to review literature from the 81 selected journal articles, in order to; broaden the discussion on the scope of literature on self-help housing. These includes; books, research reports and policy documents, and other published technical papers, written by institutions, organizations and agencies which were non-peer reviewed. The reason being that it promotes an all-inclusive and in-depth discussion (Darko et al. 2017). Out of a total of 132 papers presented, 81 were found to be relevant to the objective of the discussion. This represents 62.36% reviewed journals papers written by experts. Secondly, these papers were further reviewed by several other experts who published in their respective journals; which help to maintain the standard of quality, which also goes to ensure this article's quality.

4.3 Classification of SHH Affordability Measurement Criteria

Study by Acheamfour et al. (2019), revealed two clear basis for criteria classification in qualitative review studies. (i) suitable name description of a set of identified criteria, (ii) the quantitatively/qualitatively measure of the individual criterion. Thus, the classification of the criteria for this study was based on partly on (ii), but also on the works of Ezennia and Hoskara (2019) and Jewkes and Delgadillo (2010). As such, the literature review for this study have identified several SHH affordability determinants from the various papers published online. These identified determinants have been classified into 8 criteria groupings for easy understanding, and also to enable differentiation between them. The reasons for classifying these determinants into criteria set is as follows:

a) There is scanty literature on this form of classification for SHH affordability amongst the selected publications;
b) There was a lack of consensus on criteria for measuring housing affordability in general (Ezennia and Hoskara 2019; Jewkes and Delgadillo 2010), and particularly for SHH either quantitatively or qualitatively from the literature.

It should be noted that a full understanding of the importance of the determinants is very essential. Thus, even though this study is purely based on literature from published works in peer reviewed journal, relevant materials from non-peer review sources (e.g. books, reports, dissertations reports and articles) were also employed to lend support for an in-depth discussion on the subject matter. Accordingly, eight (8) criteria set, with a total of 31 associated determinants identified in literature are being considered. These are classified under the following considerations; Finance, Access to Land, building quality, Development controls and planning regulations, Building cost, Locational effect, Infrastructure and services and Social. The reasons for these criteria choices was due to fact that the definition and the assessment of housing affordability in literature by tradition, has mainly been confined largely to normative economic criteria (Ezennia and Hoskara 2019; Jewkes and Delgadillo 2010. Weaknesses of Housing Affordability Indices Used by Practioners. Journal of Financial Counseling and Planning, 21(1), pp. 43–52.," n.d.) which talk about the relationships between housing costs and incomes, particularly of the conventional housing delivery mode.

According to the various studies SHH is also guided by certain criteria set choices of the households that are influenced by array of key determinants. The process is largely dependent on the philosophy of self-governance in terms of the financial arrangement and the management of the process. From the review of 81 academic publications in 53 peer reviewed journals.

4.3.1 Financing

Most developing countries are having challenges with affordable housing financing, due to rapidly growing urban populations and fiscal constraints. In Ghana, the problem is not different. Addaney, et al. (2015) and CAHF (2019), have revealed that accessibility and availability of housing financing schemes have become affordability problems for the majority of the households developing countries. Collectively, these studies asserted that, inadequate housing financing for these self-home building households have become a big hurdle to affordable housing delivery rates in developing countries in Africa; because they supply most of the housing units. According to Ferguson and Smet (2010) and Teye et al. (2015), the housing financing challenges exist in these housing markets because lending policies were very unfavourable to self-home builders. Smet (1999), argued that the affordability criteria these institutions use to lend to self-builders are wrong. The reason attributed was self-builders adopt incremental approach to building their homes; and that lending affordability criteria should be linked with the financing sources for SHH developmental approach. Consequently, incremental housing funding schemes is the most appropriate in these housing markets.

Research has identified that generally, SHH construction process is largely financed incrementally. Several studies have identified the determinant influencing its financing. They were; savings, regular income earnings and loans/credit from families, friends and cooperative societies (Mselle and Sanga 2018; Chepeleva et al. 2018; Rameli et al. 2016; Adeyeni et al. 2016; Afram et al. 2015; Nwuba and Kalu 2015; Addaney et al. (2015); Bangdome-Dery et al. 2014; Decardi-Nelson et al. 2012; Henman and Jones 2012; Acioly 2011; Ahadzie and Badu 2011; Ferguson and Smets 2010; Gough ang Yankson 2010; Greene and Rojas 2008; Karley 2008: Sheuya 2007; Smets 2006; Stein and Castillo, 2005; Malhotra 2002; Pamuk 2000; Smets 1999). Financial windfall fall such as the sale of personal assets (CAHF 2019; Smets 2006) and the speculative sale of lands in the urban land markets in Ghana (Bangdome-Dery et al. 2014) have been identified as another common incremental financing pool for the self-builder.

It can be seen that financing self-help housing incrementally involves several stake holding factors as identified in previous studies, that determine its affordability. Thus, *financing* has been identified as a major criteria for SHH affordability measurement in this study; with focus on the funding mode adopted by self-home builder for the whole construction process. The determinants under this criteria were; regular income, savings, credit/loans/remittances from relatives and friends, and sale of personal assets.

4.3.2 Access to Land

Land is valuable commodity to the self-builder, as every developmental step taken is gauged by the availability of a parcel of land (Bangdome-Dery et al. 2014; Costello and Rowley 2010; Greene and Rojas 2008). Thus, the very first step that begins the SHH journey is by securing access to a land suitable for residential purpose. In this context, studies have cited land cost as a key determinant of access to SHH (Afrane et al. 2016; Nwuba et al. 2015). The cost of plot of lands in urban land market affect access to affordable SHH construction projects (Bangdome-Dery et al. 2014; Acioly, 2011; Ahadzie and Badu 2011; Greene and Rojas 2008; Mayer and Somerville 2000). To Makinde (2014), identified land cost as a major hindering factor for SHH delivery in developing countries. For Gough and Yankson (2000), high cost of land undermines its access affordability, prevailing in the urban land market in Ghana. Studies have indicated that prices of land for housing have risen sharply, affecting affordability of buildable lands in urban land market in developing countries (Kirst 2020; Agyemang and Morrison 2018; Afram et al. 2015).

Impliedly, it could be argued that the success of SHH affordability is hinged on households' access to plots of land for the building projects in developing countries; and thus, it is a key criteria for the success of SHH building projects in developing countries. Yet, in Ghana the allodial title/ownership of lands located at the various urban peripheries are vested in traditional authorities-chiefs and customary families (Kirst 2020; Gyamera et al. 2018). As a result, the allodial land tenure system is affecting land affordability, because there is lack of effective control (Agyemang and Morrison 2018). SHH could have been moderately affordable, but for the problematic land tenure systems in developing countries (Owusu-Ansah et al. 2019; Gyamera, et al. 2018; Mselle and Sanga 2018; Ferguson and Smets 2010; Smets 2006).

Similarly studies have identified that the high demand of land for housing in urban Ghana, has led to challenges of double sale and multiple ownership claims, which has resulted into many high land litigation costs (Brobbey 2019; Gyamera, et al. 2018; Mireku et al. 2016). To Afrane et al. (2016), revealed that numerous legal suits in Ghana's urban market have created unaffordability situations because, it delays individual's self-help building projects. Land acquisition processes, as well as title registration and pricing remain major problems to affordable SHH development in a developing country like Ghana (Brobbey 2019; Gyamera et al. 2018; Mireku et al. 2016; Bangdome-Dery et al. 2014).

In nut shell, land is a key criteria dimension of SHH affordability, because its easy access will determine the annual housing units' addition to national stocks in developing countries. As a result, the following determinants; land cost, land litigation cost, land title acquisition process and land tenure systems have been considered under *access to land* criteria.

4.3.3 Building Quality

Mulliner et al. (2013) asserted that quality of the building is an essential environmental criteria for assessing housing affordability because it provides better affordability outcomes in comparison to focusing solely on financial attributes such as income and housing price. Landman and Napier (2010), suggested that building quality can affect the affordability of housing within a community. They further asserted that owner-built housing is of the same quality as formal or conventional housing stock in most developing countries. However, it could said that self-building of one's own home could be a daunting the task. Ahadzie and Badu (2011), revealed that self-built owners may not have the skills set needed for effective management of the construction activities on site to achieve the optimum quality for housing project. Besides, the attainment of optimum building quality is costly (Cunningham 2013). Cunningham (2013), further identified factors such as; procurement choices for building materials, specifications, whole life costs, physical and environmental site conditions exert considerable pressure on the costs of attaining quality housing. In translation to SHH, ensuring that the best quality materials are incorporated into the building during construction can be stressful. Landman and Napier (2010), revealed that quality building materials coupled with good supervision are costly in housing construction, but can lead to better quality SHH. Studies by Ahadzie and Amoa-Mensah (2010) and Bangdome-Dery et al. (2014), also revealed that not all SHH developers have the requisite skills to self-manage their housing construction projects to achieve the needed quality. Listokin and Hattis (2005), identified that a quality SHH emanates from proper adherence to building codes and zoning regulations. They further articulated that these can enhance built environment for the self-built housing community, but its affordability may not be guaranteed because of the cost implication. Fiadzo et al. (2001), discovered that SHH affordability could be measured using quality indicators such as types of building materials procured and incorporated into building and good supervision of the works on site. Fiadzo, et al. (2001), again identified that conformance to design standards and specification enhanced SHH quality. This assertion was ably supported by Vaughan and Turner (2013) and Bangdome-Dery et al. (2014). The collective opinions from these authors indicated that self-builder's ability to adhere to the design standards, the specification, and the building codes could promote better living environment and housing quality.

Since studies have established that quality of the building is a vital environmental criteria for assessing housing affordability, the following determinants have been considered under this criteria for SHH affordability metric. These are; building materials quality, lack of specifications conformance and adherence to building code, lack of managerial skills and technical supervision.

4.3.4 Development Controls and Planning Regulations

Self-help housing provides the opportunity for most households in developing countries to meet their housing aspirations (Adegun and Olusoga 2019), and the development process are usually informally formal (Wibowo and Larasati 2018). For instance, in Ghana, they mostly formally obtain the construction permit from statutory bodies such as the metropolitan, municipal and district and Assembles (MMDAs), before embarking on informal site construction. However, a study by Asiedu-Danquah (2016), revealed that these self-builders in Ghana are constraint with costly numerous development controls and planning regulatory systems due to the inherent weakness and internal bureaucracy. Studies have asserted that though development control measures such as permission for construction and zoning have enhance envirnmental sustainability and promote effective land utilization policy in urban centres (Calder 2018; Glaeser and Gyourko 2003).

However, one could argue that these measures have also tend to hinder quick supply of the needed affordable housing in adeveloping countries, such as Ghana. Asiedu-Danquah (2016), has identified that the housing sector in Ghana is being saddled with high cost for the acquisition of building construction permits; including bureaucratic tendencies, which has posed daunting challenge for SHH. One could argue these group of households are already burdened with so many payments such as healthcare, children school fees and utility bills. To Boamah et al. (2012), construction permit acquisition cost and delays do not only greatly frustrate SHH in urban areas, but it has significantly impacted negatively on the development costs of self-builders in Ghana. Impliedly, this could be a hinder to SHH supply; thus, escalting the housing deficit problems with adverse effects on urban housing unaffordability situations. Again, construction permit acquisition fees payment have been identified in studies as major costs challenges affecting SHH in Ghana (Afram et al. 2015; Ahadzie and Badu 2011). According to Asiedu-Danduah (2016), the individual self-home builder goes through the same bureaucratic building permit acquisition process just like any established real estate firm that is into housing development, which invariably makes their housing projects more expensive. Thus, expensive building permit payment, coupled with bureaucratic bottlenecks become an impediment to realizing self-help affordable housing delivery in cities in Ghana.

In this regards, Development controls and Planning regulations has been identified as a good criteria for measuring SHH affordability in Ghana, and the determinants being considered under this criterion include; costly building permit and bureaucracy of the permit process.

4.3.5 Building Cost

The building cost in this study carries same meaning as the physical construction cost of the self-help housing project. In construction, the key cost constituents includes materials, labour and overheads. In effect, apart from paying for the cost of land and other statutory developmental costs, the self-builder also bears the overall cost of the actual physical construction cost of the building through the procurement of both materials and labour.

In Ghana the housing construction sector (like any other developing country) is noted to be heavily dependent on the importation of building materials, and they are subjected to rapid price increases due to the local currency depreciation (Owoo and Lambon-Quayefio 2020). This is because the local industry production do not have the capacity. The increasing the cost of this critical housing construction input (Afrane and Amoako 2011; Ahadzie and Badu 2011), affect the supply of SHH building materials import constitute 65–70% of the cost of construction in Ghana (Osei-Tutu and Adjei-Kumi 2009). Studies have revealed that building materials cost was about 70–71% of the total construction cost (Adjei et al. 2015; Odeyinka et al. 2006). Materials cost form a major component of the project cost in Ghana's housing construction industry (Owusu-Ansah et al. 2019; Danso and Obeng-Ahenkora 2018; Afram et al. 2015; Adinyira et al. 2012; Karley 2008). Thus, it could be argued also building material cost has become a severe constraints to the provision of self-help affordable housing; thus could affects the supply of SHH, which can lead to low housing affordability levels in Ghana.

Studies have also identified that the sustained increase in labour and transportation cost is affecting SHH supply in developing countries (Haas et al. 2016; Bangdome-Dery et al. 2014; Boyd et al. 2013; Adinyira et al. 2012). Several researchers have acknowledged that most self-builders have been unable to seek for adequate cost information on housing projects before initiation; which led to cost overruns and, thus its affordability (Afrane et al. 2016; Bangdome-Dery et al. 2014; Ahadzie and Badu 2011; Ahadzie and Amoa-Mensah 2010). Studies have also shown that the incremental approach to SHH projects increases the completion time longer than the conventional counterparts (Ward 2019; Ferguson and Smet 2010; Boamah 2010b; Arku 2009b). The reasons could be due to lack of financial capacity and the numerous land litigation challenges in Ghana's housing industry.

To this end, the *Building Cost* of SHH projects is being considered as key criterion for its affordability metric development. The identified corresponding determinants gleaned from authors include; building materials cost, labour and transportation costs, and inadequate cost information, and longer construction period being considered.

4.3.6 Location

Location criterion relates to specific issues of welfare and transport connections. It relates directly to land use and accessibility issues (Litman 2017). This is because it affects SHH households' transportation affordability, due to higher non-housing expenditures. Mulliner and Maliene (2013) asserted that location consideration such as transportation attributes provides better linkage in the livelihood and socioeconomic assessment in housing affordability measurement, especially for SHH affordability measure. It interplays with not only the easiness and the accessibility of transportation system, but also the economic opportunities that influences neighbourhood vitality (Hartell 2016; Mulliner and Maliene 2012). Similarly, location of a housing unit has been identified to have transportation affordability impact because it creates disparities in access to economic opportunities (Ganning 2017; Bieri and Dawkins 2016).

Impliedly, the peri-urban location SHH projects (Gillespie 2017), have effects on the households' access to transportation systems. However, to Bangdome-Dery et al. (2014), most self-builders do not give consideration to this issue. Researchers also identified that affordability measures that include the influence of location provides better housing affordability indicators on housing stress (Litman 2017; Saberi et al. 2017; Hartell 2016; Mattingly and Morrissey 2014). Payne (2004), asserted that the priority of the urban households in developing countries is to obtain a land where they can take full advantage of their livelihood opportunities. However, most of these lands are usually located in peri-urban fringes of cities in developing countries (Owusu-Ansah and O'Connor, 2009; Payne 2004). Lands for SHH housing in most cities of developing world are in urban peripheral locations (Ward 2019; Nuhu 2019; Sullivan and Olmedo 2015; Bangdome-Dery et al. 2014; Ahadzie and Badu 2011; Gough and Yankson 2010). Studies by Gillespie (2017) and Adedire, et al., (2017) in Ghana and Nigeria respectively, revealed that high patronage of peri-urban location for SHH projects because it offers relatively cheaper buildable lands.

Location factors such as transportation costs (i.e. fares, fuel and maintenance) and proximity to employment opportunities have been identified to affect housing affordability assessment because of the extra financial burdens place households (Fisher et al. (2009). Another location factor directly link to SHH affordability is the stress on self-built homeowners. Studies have identified that longer commuting distance between home and work and the vehicular traffic affect affordability due to higher fares and maintenance costs (Mattioli et al. 2018; Saberi et al. 2017; Litman 2017; Renne et al. 2016; Mattingly and Morrissey 2014). In addition, research has revealed that high vehicular traffics on the roads linking homes to places of works affect Self-home builders' employment, in terms of labour productivity and traffic stress (Agyapong and Ojo 2018. Acolin and Greene 2017; Oz et al. 2010; Graham 2007). A study by Wu and Zhao (2015), also identified that longer travel times between home and work have negative effects on the individual's housing affordability outcomes.

In summary, location considerations in housing affordability assessment provides deeper understanding on socio-economic issues. Under this criteria, the determinants in consideration are; urban peripheral location of land, accessible transportation services, housing stress and vehicular traffic effects due longer commuting distance commuting distance between home and work.

4.3.7 Infrastructure and Services

Infrastructure facilities such as roads and utilities services are very important to the development of functional housing system, as it provides the foundation for economic growth. However, in developing countries inadequate provision of infrastructure facilities and utilities services in urban centres have drew policy attention to issues of housing affordability (Gabriel and Painter 2018), which in effects has led to problems of widespread consequences slum development and urban sprawls.

Infrastructure and utility provision have always been state led in developing countries. However, Ezebilo (2020), asserted that governments in recent decades are unable to provide trunk infrastructure facilities in the cities of these countries. One can argued that, this development can have limiting effect on the individual household's capacity to participate in the provision of self-help affordable housing. Afrane et al. (2016), has identified that the state's inability to provide adequate infrastructure facilities has worsened the housing provision burden for the self-builder in Ghana and many other developing countries. Ibem (2009) and Dagdeviren (2011), asserted that governments are relegating urban infrastructure provision to community-led approach in most developing countries. This changing role of government has led to community-based approach; where the community by itself mobilise resources to construct roads and drains within their local community level, but these resources are not enough. For instance, UN-Habitat (2011) confirmed that infrastructure and sanitation facilities are lacking in the local communities of newly developing urban areas. Thus, to Afrane et al. (2016), many households are self-providing these facilities, but resources are limited; and it is affecting the individual's cost of housing production. UN-Habitat (2011), confirmed this claim and posited that the state do not readily provide water and sanitation facilities to urban households. Impliedly, self-home builders construct their own pipelines to connect to public water supply system and also construct cesspit within their premises for sanitation purposes; which the state should have provided. For Gillespie (2018), lack of access to basic infrastructure and services in the urban centres in Ghana is increasing the cost self-help housing development; thus a barrier to housing affordability.

Studies have reiterated that self-built homeowners in developing countries usually form themselves into groups for promoting the welfare of their communities (Bieri and Dawkins 2018; Boamah 2010b). These groups collaborate amongst themselves through mutual aid to construct roads and streets. The group also help members to connect their dwellings to electricity and water through lobbying state institutions. For instance, Gillespie (2018), also articulated that due to the peri-urban locations of SHH projects in Ghana, it become necessary that households most times construct access road to their building sites and pay state institutions for the provision of utility services such as water and electricity to the site. Rai (2018), did a study in Turkey which revealed that the cost of connecting roads and utility services to self-built homes have effects on non-housing expenses.

In summary, the availability of *Infrastructure and Services* have been identified in literature to have influence on SHH affordability because households are rather providing these facilities in a developing country like Ghana. Under this criterion therefore, the following determinants are considered towards SHH affordability assessment. These are; self-provision of community access roads, costs of connecting to water & electricity, and

Sanitation provision. This is, it believed that these determinants impact heavily on the access to self-built home ownership affordability.

5 Research Implication

A search through the plethora of literature on housing affordability, either on the concept or the measurement methods have been concentrated on the conventional housing approach in the developed and emerging economies (Li 2014). However, for Pugh (2001), Arnott (2008) and Murillo (2012), the non-conventional housing delivery approach (i.e. Self-help housing) is predominantly the best and the most credible route to meeting housing aspirations in the global south. In affirmation, Bang-dome Dery et al. (2014), asserted that self-help housing has been the commonest housing construction method in developing countries before the advent of conventional housing to developing countries. However, the rapid spike in urban population in these countries, especially in sub-Sahara Africa (Mahendra and Seto 2019), have resulted into a corresponding sharp increase in the demand for SHH by households particularly at the urban periphery of cities (Gillespie 2018; Kamua 2006). But it is faced with some affordability problems of inadequate infrastructure marred with land access problems. Studies have identified that self-builders faced development control challenges at the various MMDAs, and the lack of adequate housing financing schemes and the unstable prices of building inputs in a developing country such as Ghana; are signs of SHH affordability pressures.

Nevertheless, an examination of existing literature has showed paucity of research on metric system SHH affordability. However, studies have labelled this housing delivery approach as being incrementally based, and the most common route to meeting homeownership aspirations in most developing countries, especially those in sub-Sahara Africa (Mselle and Sanga 2018; Bang-Dome Dery et al. 2014). This study is an attempt to fill this gap; by identifying the criteria for SHH, so as provide the opportunity to measure its affordability in a developing country such as Ghana. This is because studies a by (Arku 2009b) affirmed that it contributes at least 75% of the nation's housing stock annual. Studies have indicated that adds at least \$300 million to Ghana's GDP annually (Bang-Dome Dery et al. 2014; Ahadzie and Badu 2011). In addition, studies on SHH have focused more on the definition, the approach, processes and the challenges, but attempt to measure its affordability is very scanty. Only one study by Nwuba et al. (2015) was identified in literature. It investigated the determinants of affordability of access to self-help homeownership in Nigeria, but this study focused on a broader issues of SHH affordability by developing a criteria set that can adequately measure its affordability in urban markets of developing countries. Also, many studies have focused on the measuring conventional HA through the development of various indices, but no known research on developing a criteria set for measuring SHH affordability through models or any form of algorithms has been identified.

The theoretical ideology underpinning housing affordability matters from socioeconomic point of view, is centrally welfare inclined. That is to say in the face of global rising housing costs against stagnant incomes, more housing burdens have been put on households' incomes (Gabriel and Painter 2018). Therefore, governments in the developed countries through welfare-targeted policy initiatives; have decided to assist households underserved by the housing markets through subsidies. But same cannot said of households in the developing countries, because they are overburdened with self-provision of shelter, but there are metric system measures this burden. Thus, there is need to measure the housing affordability burdens on these self-built households who might not only be devoting an excessive share of incomes on housing, but also self-financed and managed the whole housing provision process. This necessitate the identification of criteria set to ensure the affordability measurement of SHH in a developing country such as Ghana. Again, the outcome of this study should provide the basis for future studies on the development of indices for measuring SHH affordability. The outcome could also guide policy formulation on guidelines for governments assistance for an accelerate self-help housing provision; which could help to reduce the increasing housing deficits, because studies have shown it as the number one housing supplier in Ghana.

6 Conclusion

The concept of this study is that the issues of housing affordability for the self-builder is not only simply about income and housing costs; rather, it embodies how households in developing countries through self-help, are addressing one of the basic human needs-shelter in terms of; financing strategies, access to land, zoning and planning regulation, location related challenges; infrastructure provision and social related problems. Hence, the need has arisen for identification of a criteria set by which self-help housing affordability can be assessed; in this case through a model development. But, either the application of indices or models in the determination housing affordability have been conventionally based on a set of pre-determined factors such as income and housing costs in main stay housing affordability studies. Thus, if SHH affordability is to be measured, then there is need for a collection of well-defined decision criteria for it. As a result, this review sought to identify and classify the decision criteria provided the impetus and the ingredients for SHH affordability measurement.

In all, the study has shown eight (8) criteria set, and these were; Financing, Access to land, Building Quality, Development controls and planning regulations, Building Cost, Locational effects, Infrastructure and Services and Social issues.

The outcome of this study has not only contributed to greatly expanding the existing knowledge on housing, but also broaden the understanding on other possible forms of housing affordability measurement. Particularly, this study provides prospects for future research on self-help housing affordability measurement; which can guide the development of an inclusive housing policy development, especially in developing countries where SHH is the predominant housing delivery mode. Also, the lack of affordable housing delivery has led to mounting housing affordability challenges and sprawling urbanization in developing countries. Certainly, this study has provided a profound evidence that self-help housing affordability measurement criteria could be one major area that could attract attention for further studies in housing affordability studies.

In conclusion, this study may not be devoid of limitation by issues which affects the generalizability of the research findings just like any other category of review papers. The limitation is mainly seen in our overly dependence on Scopus and few search engines. Again, the number of papers used for the review could be another source of limitation, however the study covered all the relevant papers in achieving the aim of the study.

Future studies can aim at classifying the criteria set on quantitative or qualitative measurement approach that can be useful in developing an affordability index or model development for self-help housing for housing markets in developing markets.

Acknowledgements. This paper forms part of a PhD research project on Self -Help Housing Affordability measurement. The authors acknowledge that this paper shares a similar background and methodology with other related papers, but with different scopes and objectives. This study was taken on in the Department of Construction Technology and Management, at Kwame Nkrumah University of Science and Technology, Kumasi, Ghana. In conclusion, the authors are extremely grateful to the editors and all the invaluable contributions that will assist in enhancing the quality of this paper.

Disclosure Statement

The authors confirm no potential conflict of interest was reported by this paper.

References

Acheamfour, V.K., Kissi, E., Adjei-Kumi, T., Adinyira, E.: Review of empirical arguments on contractor pre-qualification criteria. J. Eng. Des. Technol. **18**, 70–83 (2019)

Acolin, A., Green, R.K.: Measuring housing affordability in São Paulo metropolitan region: Incorporating location. Cities **62**, 41–49 (2017)

Adabre, M.A., Chan, A.P.: Critical success factors (CSFs) for sustainable affordable housing. Build. Environ. **156**, 203–214 (2019)

Adedire, F.M., Adegbile, M.B.: Effects of urbanization on spatial demography change in Ibeju-Lekki. Lagos peri-urban settlement. Community Dev. **49**(3), 292–311 (2018)

Adegun, O.B., Olusoga, O.O.: Self-help housing: cooperative societies' contributions and professionals' views in akure. Nigeria. Built Environ. **45**(3), 332–345 (2019)

Adeyeni, G.O., Olayiwola, L.M., Oladehinde, G.J.: Challenges to incremental housing development in Ibadan Municipality, Nigeria. Asian Res. J. Arts Soc. Sci. **1**, 1–10 (2016)

Adinyira, E., Botchey, E.A., Kwofie, T.E.: Determining critical project success criteria for public housing building projects (PHBPS) in Ghana (2012)

Adjei, K. O., Fobiri, G., Owiredu, G.K.: Policies and barriers in the provision of affordable housing in Ghana. African Journal of Applied Research (AJAR), 1(1) (2015)

Afram, S.O., Bangdome-Dery, A., Eghan, G.E., Kwofie, T.E.: Analysis of causes of delay in middle and high income self-build housing projects (SBHPs) in Wa, Ghana. J. Building Constr. Plann. Res. **3**(04), 171 (2015)

Afrane, E., Ariffian, A., Bujang, B., Shuaibu, H., Kasim, I.: Major factors causing housing deficit in ghana. Dev. Country Stud. **6**(2), 139–147 (2016)

Afshar, M.R., Alipouri, Y., Sebt, M.H., Chan, W.T.: A type-2 fuzzy set model for contractor prequalification. Autom. Constr. **84**, 356–366 (2017)

Agyapong, F., Ojo, T.K.: Managing traffic congestion in the Accra central market. Ghana. J. Urban Manag. **7**(2), 85–96 (2018)

Agyemang, F.S., Morrison, N.: Recognising the barriers to securing affordable housing through the land use planning system in Sub-Saharan Africa: a perspective from Ghana. Urban Stud. **55**(12), 2640–2659 (2018)

Ahadzie, D.K., Badu, E.: Success indicators for selfbuild houses in two Ghanaian cities. J. Sci. Technol. (Ghana) **31**(3), 86–96 (2011)

Arku, G.: Housing policy changes in ghana in the 1990s. Hous. Stud. **24**(2), 261–272 (2009). https://doi.org/10.1080/02673030902719763

Arnott, R.: Housing policy in developing countries: The importance of the informal economy. Urbanization and growth, pp. 167–198 (2008). https://www.semanticscholar.org/paper/Housing-policy-in-developing-countries.-The-of-the-Arnott/a7d086fe76ba9082ee8b402c7b6ee57e183fc64f

Ashley, L.D., Mcloughlin, C., Aslam, M., Engel, J., Wales, J., Rawal, S., Nicolai, S.: The role and impact of private schools in developing countries–bibliography and literature reviews (2014)

Asiedu-Danquah, Y.A.: Building regulations and the development of unauthorized structures in urban Ghana: A case study of the Tema Metropolis (Doctoral dissertation, University of Ghana) (2016)

Bangdome-Dery, A., Eghan, G.E., Afram, S.O.: Overview of self-help (self-build) housing provision in Ghana: policies and challenges. Methodology **4**(6), 23–34 (2014)

Bieri, D.S., Dawkins, C.J.: Quality of life, transportation costs, and federal housing assistance: leveling the playing field. Hous. Policy Debate **26**(4–5), 646–669 (2016)

Bieri, D.S., Dawkins, C.J.: Amenities, affordability, and housing vouchers. J. Reg. Sci. **59**(1), 56–82 (2019)

Boamah, N.A.: Housing affordability in Ghana: a focus on Kumasi and Tamale. Ethiopian journal of environmental studies and management, 3(3) (2010)

Bogdon, A.S., Can, A.: Indicators of local housing affordability: Comparative and spatial approaches. Real Estate Econ. **25**(1), 43–80 (1997)

Bredenoord, J., van Lindert, P.: Affordable Housing in the Global south: Seeking sustainable Solution. In: Bredenoord, P., Lindert, V., Smets, P., (eds.)Backing the self-builders: Affordable Housing in the Urban Global South. Abingdon, Oxford, UK: Routldge, pp. 55–72 (2014)

Bredenoord, J., Van Lindert, P.: Pro-poor housing policies: rethinking the potential of assisted self-help housing. Habitat Int. **34**(3), 278–287 (2010)

CAHF, 2018. Urbanisation and housing challenges in Sub Saharan Africa. https://www.housingfinanceafrica.org/urbanisation-and-housing-challenges-is-sub-saharan-africa/. Accessed 23 April 2019

Danso, H., Obeng-Ahenkora, N.K.: Major determinants of prices increase of building materials on ghanaian construction. Open J. Civil Eng. **8**, 142–154 (2018). https://doi.org/10.4236/ojce.2018.82012

Darko, A., Chan, A., Zhang, C.: Drivers for green building: a review of empirical studies. Habitat Int. **60**, 34–49 (2017)

Ezebilo, E.E.: Evaluation of construction, marketing and management in housing delivery by a private developer: evidence from Papua New Guinea. J. Housing Built Environ. **35**, 1–25 (2020)

Ezennia, S.I., Hoskara, S.O.: Methodological weaknesses in the measurement approaches and concept of housing affordability used in housing research: a qualitative study. PloS one **14**(8) 2019

Fellows, R., Liu, A.: Impact of participants' values on construction sustainability. In: Proceedings of the Institution of Civil Engineers-Engineering Sustainability, vol. 161, (4), pp. 219–227. Thomas Telford Ltd. (2008)

Ferguson, B., Smets, P.: Finance for incremental housing; current status and prospects for expansion'. Habitat Int. **34**(3), 288–298 (2010)

Gabriel, M., Jacobs, K., Arthurson, K., Burke, T., Yates, J.: Conceptualising and measuring the housing affordability problem (2005)

Gabriel, S., Painter, G.: Why affordability matters. Regional Science and Urban Economics, Volume 80 (2020) 103378, pp. 1–6 (2018)

Ganning, J.P.: It's good but is it right? An under-the-hood view of the location affordability index. Hous. Policy Debate **27**(6), 807–824 (2017)

Ghana Statistical Service: 2010 Population and Housing Census: Housing in Ghana. Ghana Statistical Service, Accra (2014)

Giannantonio, C.M.: Book Review (2010). Krippendorff, K.(2004). Content Analysis: An Introduction to Its Methodology. Thousand Oaks, CA: Sage. Organizational Research Methods, 13(2), 392–394

Gillespie, T.: Collective Self-Help, Financial Inclusion, and the Commons: Searching for Solutions to Accra's Housing Crisis. Hous. Policy Debate **28**(1), 64–78 (2017)

Gough, K.V., Yankson, P.: A neglected Aspect of the housing Market. The caretakers of Peri-urban in Accra, Accra. Urban Studies **48**(4), 793–810 (2010)

Gough, K., Yankson, P.: Land markets in African cities: the case of peri-urban Accra. Ghana. Urban Stud. **37**(13), 2485–2500 (2000)

Greene, M., Rojas, E.: Incremental construction: A strategy to facilitate access to housing. Environ. Urbanization. Environ. Urbanization **20**(1), 89–108 (2008)

Hong, Y., Chan, D.: Research trend of joint ventures in construction: a two-decade taxonomic review. J. Facility Manage. **12**(2), 118–141 (2014)

Ibem, E.: Community-led infrastructure provision in low-income urban communities in developing countries: a study on Ohafia. Nigeria. Cities **26**(3), 125–132 (2009)

Jewkes, M.D., Delgadillo, L.M.: Weaknesses of housing affordability indices used by practioners. J. Financ. Couns. Plan. **21**(1), 43–52 (2010)

Karley, N.: Ghana residential property delivery constraints and affordability analysis. Housing Financ. Int. **22**(4), 22–29 (2008)

Ke, Y., Wang, S., Chan, A., Cheung, E.: Research trend of public-private partnership in construction journals. J. Constr. Eng. Manag. **135**(10), 1076–1086 (2009)

Kirst, S.: Chiefs do not talk law, most of them talk power: Traditional authorities in conflicts over land grabbing in Ghana. Canadian J. African Stud. **54**, 519–539 (2020)

Kolbe, R.H., Burnett, M.S.: Content-analysis research: An examination of applications with directives for improving research reliability and objectivity. J. Consum. Res. **18**(2), 243–250 (1991)

Li, J.: Recent trends on housing affordability research: where are we up to? Hong Kong, Urban Research Group Urban-City on Cities Working Paper Series, WP No. 5/2014 (2014)

Liu, Y., Li, Z.: Determinants of housing purchase decision: an empirical study of the high education cohort in Urban China. J. Asian Architecture Build. Eng. **17**(2), 299–305 (2018)

Mahendra, A., Seto, K.C.: Upward and outward growth: managing urban expansion for more equitable cities in the global south (2019)

Makinde, O.: Housing delivery system, need and demand. Environ. Dev. Sustain. **16**, 49–69 (2014)

Mselle, J.M., Sanga, S.A.: Constraints facing incremental housing construction in Dar es Salaam, Tanzania. J. Constr. Dev. Countries **23**(1), 1–20 (2018)

Mulliner, E., Maliene, V.: What attributes determine housing affordability? Int. J. Soc. Behav. Educ. Econ. Bus. Ind. Eng. **6**(7), 576–581 (2012)

Murillo, F.: Self-Build: Global South. International Encyclopedia of Housing and Home, pp. 265–277 (2012)

Nnamdi, E.: Perspectives on the architecture of Africa's underprivileged urban dwellers. Soc. Dyn. J. Afr. Stud. **37**(1), 43–77 (2011)

Nwuba, C.C., Kalu, I.U., Umeh, J.A.: Determinants of homeownership affordability in Nigeria's urban housing markets. Int. J. Housing Markets Anal. (2015)

Owusu-Ansah, A., Soyeh, K.W., Asabere, P.K.: Developer constraints on housing supply in urban Ghana. Int. J. Housing Markets Anal. (2019)

Owusu-Ansah, J.K., O'Connor, K.B.: Housing demand in the urban fringe around Kumasi, Ghana. J. Housing Built Environ. **25**(1), 1–17 (2010)

Pollock, M., Fernandes, R.M., Becker, L.A., Featherstone, R., Hartling, L.: What guidance is available for researchers conducting overviews of reviews of healthcare interventions? a scoping review and qualitative metasummary. Syst. Control Found. Appl. **5**(1), 190 (2016)

Pugh, C.: The theory and practice of housing sector development for developing countries, 1950–99. Hous. Stud. **16**(4), 399–423 (2001)

Rolleston, C., Adefeso-Olateju, M.: De facto privatisation of basic education in Africa: a market response to government failure? a comparative study of the cases of Ghana and Nigeria, pp. 25–44. Case Studies from Africa, South Asia and South East Asia, Education, Privatisation and Social Justice (2014)

Saidu, A.I., Yeom, C.: Success criteria evaluation for a sustainable and affordable housing model: a case for improving household welfare in Nigeria Cities. Sustainability **12**(2), 656 (2020)

Smets, P.: Small is beautiful, but big is often the practice: Housing microfinance in discussion. Habitat Int. **30**(3), 595–613 (2006)

Sullivan, E., Olmedo, C.: Informality on the urban periphery: housing conditions and self-help strategies in Texas informal. Urban Stud. **52**(6), 1037–1053 (2015)

Teye, J.K., Teye, I., Asiedu, M.O.: Financing housing in Ghana: challenges to the development of formal mortgage system. J. Housing Built Environ. **30**(1), 1–16 (2015)

UN-Habitat, : Ghana Housing Profile. Nairobi, UN-Habitat (2011)

Vaughan, E., Turner, J.: The value and impact of building codes (White Paper), Washington, D.C., United States: Environmental and Energy Study Institute (EESI) (2013)

Isohyperthermic Temperature Regime on Productivity of Labour Intensive Works on Construction in Ghana

E. Bamfo-Agyei[1](✉), C. Aigbavboa[2], and W. D. Thwala[2]

[1] Department of Building Technology, Cape Coast Technical University, Cape Coast, Ghana
emmanuel.bamfo-agyei@cctu.edu.gh

[2] Department of Construction Management and Quantity Surveying, University of Johannesburg, Johannesburg, South Africa
{caigbavboa,didibhukut}@uj.ac.za

Abstract. The aim of this paper is to investigate the principal components of temperature that affect productivity of labour intensive public works in the Ghana. The objectives are to identify the temperature components that affect labour productivity on the sites and develop a holistic construction labour productivity constructs on temperature component. Stratified method was used to select 560 respondents at the one hundred and twenty sites. Exploratory factor analysis was used to classify the factors into components. Regression analysis was carried out. Data was subjected to principal component analysis (PCA) with varimax rotation. The hourly Wet Bulb Globe Temperature indicates that from 5 am to 10 am there are no risk however from 1 pm to 3 pm there is extreme risk for the workers working out door due to the direct contact of the sun. Then the intensity of the temperature declines from 4 pm to 6 pm work session. Road contractors, especially in Ghana, have not realised the significance of temperature in relation to the labour productivity of their construction sites. However, the Exploratory factor analysis and regression analysis results have indicated that the temperature component significantly influence firms' labour productivity. The implication of the study to construction workers that the temperature construct emerged as the most influential construct that would aid firms in achieving productivity. Instead of conducting the construction activities at 8:00 to 15:00 it is recommended that the activities begin at 5:00–10:00 and resumes at 16:00 to 17:00 when the temperature is at an optimal level and the wet bulb globe temperature will not affect the productivity of the workers.

Keywords: Temperature · Productivity · Labour · Road · Ghana

1 Introduction

In the construction industry of developing countries, productivity loss is one of the greatest and most severe problems arising from lack of documented data for the estimating, scheduling and control of the project. Concerns over non-availability of accurate measures of labour productivity data for the industry and its sub-sectors have been constantly raised (Chapman and Butry 2008).

J. N. Mojekwu et al. (Eds.): *Sustainable Education and Development*, pp. 164–172, 2021.
https://doi.org/10.1007/978-3-030-68836-3_15

There has been limited research on frameworks reflecting the relationship between thermal environment and CLP in Ghana. However, these limited frameworks even failed to accurately demonstrate the productivity performance in hot and humid environments considering the human body heat tolerance limit.

Increases in temperature related to global climate change have continually drawn concerns regarding the occupational health of the public. In 2018, the Inter-Governmental Panel on Climate Change (IPCC) reported that the land and ocean surface temperature had increased by approximately 1 °C since 1880, and the number and length of heat waves are estimated to continue increasing during this century. An outdoor environment is considered a high temperature when the temperature exceeds 32 °C and the wet bulb globe temperature exceeds 26 °C (National Oceanic and Atmospheric Administration National Weather Service 2017). Thus, working environments and work activities that continuously expose people to high temperatures increase the risk of heat-related illness.

Labour-intensive public works on road construction of rural roads involving employees working in direct sunlight tend to be more vulnerable to high temperatures in outdoor working environments.

The productivity of workers in an outdoor high-temperature environment may decrease because of workers automatically decreasing their activity to prevent their bodies from generating heat excessive heat. Weather is to some extent unpredictable. When not scheduled adequately, weather can cause delays due to forced changes in the schedule as well as damages causing rework. Productivity decreases in poor weather conditions for many reasons.

Kissi (2015) cited Song and AbouRizk (2008) which argued that there is no systematic approach for measuring and estimating labour productivity, an assertion that implies that there are no standards to validate historical data as suitable for either estimating or evaluating productivity.

However most of the research works on productivity are yet to consider temperature and geographical location as some of the challenges affecting productivity on sites.

The aim of this paper is to investigate the principal components of temperature that affect productivity of labour intensive public works in the Ghana. The objectives are to identify the temperature components that affect labour productivity on the sites and develop a holistic construction labour productivity constructs on temperature component.

1.1 Theoretical Framework

Fugar and Agyakwah-Baah (2010) identified bad weather and unfavourable site conditions as some of the environmental challenges that affects productivity on most construction sites in the tropical regions. Fugar and Agyakwah-Baah (2010) noted that during the rainy season construction work may be disrupted especially outdoor activities. The rainy season temperatures range from 21 °C to 32 °C and the humidity is relatively high. The rest of the year is hot and dry with temperatures reaching 38 °C. Frimpong et al. (2003) confirms that high temperatures and high humidity certainly affect the productivity of construction workers as a result of dullness of their senses, poor coordination and discomfort from body heat.

Femia and Panfili (2005) asserted that the core stream of productivity enhancement is the one linked to labour productivity, and that test is on whether environmental efficiency is positively or negatively correlated to the primary technologically driven dynamics. Mazzanti and Zoboli (2009) argued that labour productivity dynamics seem to be complementary to a decreasing emission intensity of productive processes.

Soil temperature is often a significant factor, especially in agriculture and land treatment of organic wastes, because growth of biological systems is closely controlled by soil temperature. Soil temperature influences the physical, chemical, and microbiological processes that take place in soil (Yolcubal et al. (2004). These processes may control the transport and fate of contaminants in the subsurface environment. The practical aspect of this soil property is that seasonal soil temperatures seldom have to be considered when constructing roads.

Research Methodology

The research design is quantitative in nature and the population is made up of all 315 road construction projects that have a total workforce of 12,000.

Stratified method was used to select 560 respondents at the one hundred and twenty sites. Exploratory factor analysis was used to classify the factors into components. Regression analysis was carried out. Data was subjected to principal component analysis (PCA) with varimax rotation. To determine the number of factors to extract using Kaiser's criterion, the total number of components that have an eigenvalue of 1 or more are determined and adopted. The eigenvalue is described as a mathematical property of a matrix deployed both as a criterion of establishing the number of factors to extract and as a measure of variance.

Findings and Discussion

This section presents the results of the questionnaire which determines the temperature component that can promote labour Productivity in labour intensive works on road construction in Ghana. The mean item score (MIS) of the questions, skewness as well as the exploratory factor analysis (EFA) of the results are presented. The descriptive results reveal the ranking of all the factors from the highest to the lowest with the table also showing the individual mean and standard deviation of the factors.

Results from Descriptive Analysis

The results of the MIS of the questions and skewness of the data are presented and discussed in the following sessions (Table 1).

Table 1. Temperature component (TC)

Factor	VP	P	A	G	E	MEAN	SD	Rank
Quality of soil condition		5.0	8.5	42.0	44.6	4.26	0.814	**1**
Planning for inclement weather		6.1	29.3	11.6	53.0	4.12	1.027	**2**
Suitability of temperature for working	2.4	8.3	5.3	46.4	37.6	4.08	0.985	**3**
Quality of site conditions		5.0	7.0	69.2	18.8	4.02	0.676	**4**
Access to appropriate rain gear	.6	8.1	25.8	37.4	28.2	3.85	0.944	**5**

The temperature component that can promote labour productivity of labour intensive works on road construction. It shows that 'Quality of soil condition' was ranked first with a mean score of 4.26 and standard deviation (SD) of 0.814; 'Planning for inclement weather' was ranked second with a mean score of 4.12 and SD of 1.027; 'Suitability of temperature for working' was ranked third with a mean score of 4.08 and SD of 0.985; 'Quality of site conditions' was ranked fourth with a mean score of 4.02 and SD of 0.676; and 'Access to appropriate rain gear' was ranked fifth with a mean score of 3.85 and SD of 0.944.

Results from Exploratory Factor Analysis

The results from the EFA on the temperature component that can promote labour productivity of labour intensive works on road construction are presented in Tables 2, 3, 4, 5, 6 and 7 and Fig. 1. All five (5) variables listed temperature component were identified with the potential to promote labour productivity of labour intensive works on road construction in Ghana.

Table 2. Pattern matrix

Code		Component
		1
TC3	TC3 Planning for inclement weather	0.91
TC2	TC2 Access to appropriate rain gear	0.874
TC1	TC1 Suitability of temperature for working	0.856
TC4	TC4 Quality of site conditions	0.806
TC5	TC5 Quality of soil condition	0.616
	Extraction Method: Principal Component Analysis	

The data was subjected to PCA (with varimax rotation). The eigenvalue was set at conventional high values of 1.0. This is shown in Table 3.

Table 3. Matrix

	TC1	TC2	TC3	TC4	TC5
TC1	1	0.677	0.747	0.441	0.633
TC2	0.677	1	0.86	0.727	0.18
TC3	0.747	0.86	1	0.637	0.385
TC4	0.441	0.727	0.637	1	0.498
TC5	0.633	0.18	0.385	0.498	1

As shown in Table 4, the KMO measure of sampling was not adequate its value was 0.801, was high, the recommended minimum value of 0.6 and the Bartlett's test of sphericity was also statistically significant (less than 0.05), thus supporting the factorability of the correlation matrix.

Table 4. KMO and Bartlett's test

Kaiser-Meyer-Olkin measure of sampling adequacy		0.801
Bartlett's test of sphericity	Approx. Chi-Square	2803.103
	Df	10
	Sig	.000

Prior to performing the Principal Component Analysis (PCA), the suitability of the data for factor analysis was assessed. Inspection of the correlation matrix revealed the presence of coefficients of above 0.3 as presented in Table 5.

Table 5. Rotated factor matrix[a] for temperature component

		Component
		1
TC3	TC3 Planning for inclement weather	0.91
TC2	TC2 Access to appropriate rain gear	0.874
TC1	TC1 Suitability of temperature for working	0.856
TC4	TC4 Quality of site conditions	0.806
TC5	TC5 Quality of soil condition	0.616
	Extraction Method: Principal Component Analysis	

As shown in Table 3, one (1) factor with eigenvalues exceeding 1.0 were extracted. The total variance explained by each of the extracted factor is as follows: Factor 1 (67.10%).Thus, the final statistics of the PCA and the extracted factors accounted for approximately 67.10 percent of the total cumulative variance.

Component 1: Isohyperthermic Temperature Regime

As presented in Table 5, one (1) extracted Temperature component (TC), variables on component 1 were TC3 Planning for inclement weather is estimated (91%), Access to appropriate rain gear (87.4%), Suitability of temperature for working (85.6%), Quality of site conditions (80.6%) and Quality of soil condition (61.6%). The number in parenthesis indicates the respective factor loadings. This cluster accounted for 67.1percent of the variance. Figure 2 also shows the construct based on the exploratory factor analysis.

Table 6. Correlations

Item	Labprod_factor2	Temperature factor
labprod_factor2	1.000	0.564
Temperature _factor	0.564	1.000

Based on the correlation coefficient, the influence of temperature component to labour productivity was 0.564 that on the framework temperature need to be considered first in achieving the success of labour intensive works. This component comprises five variables which comprises access to appropriate rain gear; suitability of temperature for working; quality of site conditions and quality of soil condition which was renamed Isohyperthermic temperature regime.

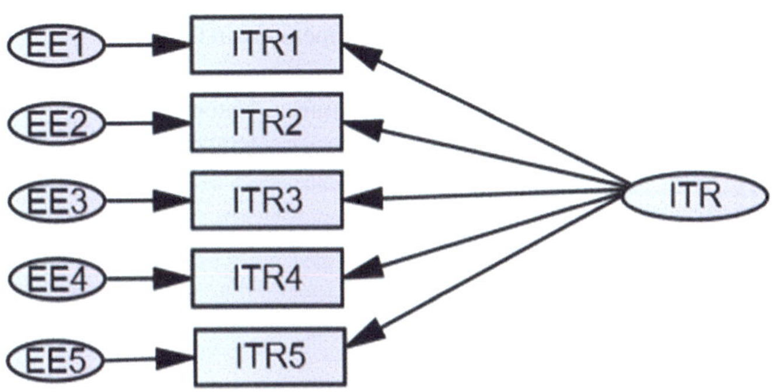

Fig. 1. Temperature component construct derived from the EFA

Isohyperthermic Temperature Regime

This is identified as factor 1 under the temperature component which comprises five (5) variables. This variables were extracted from temperature component they also influence labour productivity and company performance as shown in Table 4. The variables include: Planning for inclement weather is estimated; Access to appropriate rain gear; Suitability of temperature for working; Quality of site conditions; and Quality of soil condition, they had the following Cronbach's alpha 0.810; 0.830;0.823; 0.854 and 0.893 which had impact on productivity.

1.2 Findings on Climatic Heat Stress on Construction Sites

Further analysis on hourly Wet Bulb Globe Temperature indicates that from 5 am to 10 am there are no risk however from 1 pm to 3 pm there is extreme risk for the workers working out door due to the direct contact of the sun. Then the intensity of the temperature declines from 4 pm to 6 pm work session (Table 8).

Table 7. Welt bulb globe temperature in Ghana

Period	Dry bulb temperature (DB) (∘C)	Globe temperature (GT) (∘C)	Natural wet bulb temperature (WB) (∘C)	WBGT (∘C)
8:00–9:00	21	23	22	22.2
9:00–10:00	22	26	25	24.9
10:00–11:00	24	29	27	28.1
11:00–12:00	28	33	32	31.8
13:00–14:00	32	37	33	33.7
14:00–15:00	34	39	35	35.7
16:00–17:00	25	28	25	26.0

Source: field study 2019

Table 8. Welt bulb globe temperature in Ghana

Period	Ambient or dry bulb temperature (∘C)	Globe temperature (∘C)	Natural wet bulb temperature (∘C)	WBGT (∘C)
5:00–6:00	15	17	16	16.1
6:00- 7:00	16	18	17	17.1
7:00–8:00	20	22	20	20.4

Source: field study 2019

Usually the Isohyperthermic temperature regime has mean annual soil temperatures of 22 °C or more. The nature of the road being constructed falls in this category.

Based on the correlation coefficient, the influence of temperature component to labour productivity was 0.864 that on the framework temperature need to be considered first in achieving the success of labour intensive works. Temperature component had all the variables as contributing to productivity of labour intensive works on road construction and these variables are suitability of temperature for working, the quality of site condition and soil, planning for inclement weather and access to appropriate rain. The quality of soil which forms the primary construction material especially on road projects. It is therefore important for contractors to know how to recognize which soils are suitable for road works and which are not. Often simple field tests are necessary to make the required choice of suitable material.

That means contractors need to encourage workers to start their task in the early hours in the morning when the temperature is not very high to disrupt the activities of the workers for the given period in order to achieve high productivity. This component comprises five variables which comprises access to appropriate rain gear; suitability of temperature for working; quality of site conditions and quality of soil condition which was renamed Isohyperthermic temperature regime.

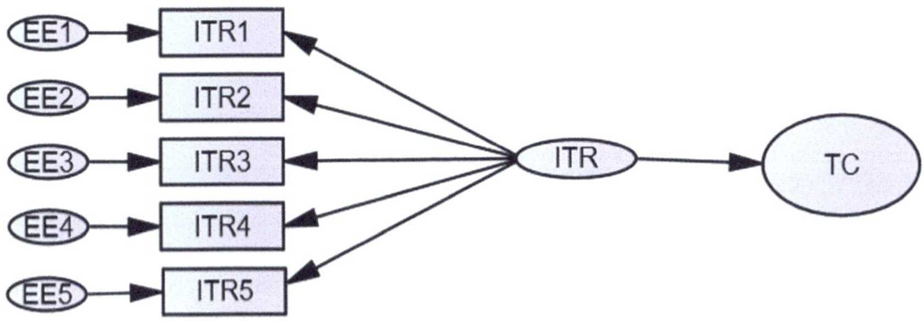

Fig. 2. Temperature component construct based on regression analysis

2 Conclusion

The results from the descriptive analysis, it was observed that five (5) variables listed of the work based conditions components were identified. The findings indicated that rankings of the temperature component that can promote labour productivity of labour intensive works on road construction. It shows that 'Quality of soil condition' was ranked first with a mean score of 4.26; 'Planning for inclement weather' was ranked second with a mean score of 4.12; 'Suitability of temperature for working' was ranked third with a mean score of 4.08; 'Quality of site conditions' was ranked fourth with a mean score of 4.02; and 'Access to appropriate rain gear' was ranked fifth with a mean score of 3.85.

The results from the exploratory factor analysis on the temperature component that can promote labour productivity of labour intensive works on road construction and this include temperature and soil characteristic.

There is the need for management to take the temperature component as part of their decision making when it comes to the start date or the timing of carrying out the project so as to improve labour productivity. The findings agree with the assertion of Mäki et al. (2001) that the workers would have to spend more time executing a task working on a poor quality of soil.

The knowledge advanced in this study will inform road contractors or owners of construction firms of the factors that significantly influence productivity on sites. It will guide them in taking decisions that impact on the labour productivity of their firms.

Nevertheless this research contributes to the development of an insight into the addition of temperature component and its influence on construction labour productivity. This will assist in improving the construction productivity by selecting the best project start time for an activity, since the beneficiaries are expected to work for eight hours in labour intensive works Ghana, from 8 am to 5 pm. Construction workers need to be encouraged to work at early hours in the morning from 5 am to 11 am before and resume at 4 pm to 6 pm, when both the temperature is at optimal level.

References

Al-Kaisi, M. M., Lal, R., Olson, K.R., Lowery, B.: Fundamentals and functions of soil environment. In: Soil Health and Intensification of Agroecosytems, pp. 1–23. Academic Press (2017)

Buol, S.W.: Tropical soils| humid tropical (2013)
Chapman, R.E., Butry, D.T.: Measuring and improving the productivity of the US construction industry: issues, challenges, and opportunities (2008)
Femia, A., Panfili, P.: Analytical applications of the NAMEA. In: Paper Presented at the Annual Meeting of the Italian Statistics society, Rome (2005)
Frimpong, Y., Oluwoye, J., Crawford, L.: Causes of delay and cost overruns in construction of ground water projects in developing countries: Ghana as a case study. Int. J. Project Manag. **21**, 321–326 (2003)
Fugar, F.D., Agyakwah-Baah, A.B.: Delays in building construction projects in Ghana. Constr. Econ. Build. **10**(1–2), 103–116 (2010)
Kisi, K.P.: Estimation of optimal productivity in labor-intensive construction operations. construction systems - dissertations & theses (2015). https://digitalcommons.unl.edu/constructiondiss/19, Accessed 14 Nov 2017
Kuykendall, C.J.: Key Factors Affecting Labour Productivity in the Construction Industry Master's Thesis, University of Florida (2007)
Mäki, S., Kalliola, R., Vuorinen: Road construction in the Peruvian Amazon: process, causes and consequences. Environ. Conserv. **28**(3), 199–214 (2001)
Marx, K.: Das Kapital: kritik der politischen ökonomie. Verlag von Otto Meisner, Germany1885, 1894 (1867)
Mazzanti, M., Zoboli, R.: Environmental efficiency and labour productivity Trade-off or joint dynamics? A theoretical investigation and empirical evidence from Italy using NAMEA. Ecol. Econ. **68**(4), 1182–1194 (2009)
Mincks, W.R., Johnston, H.: Construction jobsite management. Cengage Learning (2010)
National oceanic and atmospheric administration national weather service: a new high-resolution sea surface temperature blended analysis (2017)
Song, L., AbouRizk, S.M.: Measuring and modeling labor productivity using historical data. J. Constr. Eng. Manag. **134**(10), 786–794 (2008)
Thomas, H.R., Maloney, W.F., Horner, R.M.W., Smith, G.R., Handa, V.K., Sanders, S.R.: Modeling construction labor productivity. J. Constr. Eng. Manag. **116**(4), 705–726 (1990)
Vickers, M., Manicom, C., Schwarzkopf, L.: Extending the cost-benefit model of thermoregulation: high-temperature environments. Am. Nat. **177**(4), 452–461 (2011)
Yolcubal, I., Brusseau, M.L., Artiola, J.F., Wierenga, P.J., Wilson, L.G.: Environmental physical properties and processes. In: Environmental Monitoring and Characterization, pp. 207–239. Elsevier Inc. (2004)
Zhao, J., Zhu, N., Lu, S.L.: Productivity model in hot and humid environment based on heat tolerance time analysis. Build. Environ. **44**(11), 2202–2207 (2009)

Modeling Efficiency in the Presence of Volunteering Agency Hospitals and Council Designated Hospitals in Tanzania: An Application of Non Parametric Approach

K. M. Bwana(✉)

Department of Accountancy College of Business Education, P. O. Box 2077, Dodoma, Tanzania

Abstract. This study measures and compares efficiency of Council Designated Hospitals (CDHs) and Volunteering Agency Hospitals (VAHs) in Tanzania. The study employs 34 hospitals in Data Envelopment Analysis (DEA) from 2009 to 2013. Mann Whitney U was adopted to test the null hypothesis that means distribution is equal across the CDHs and VAHs. Output variables used were inpatients days, admissions, outpatients visit, total birth, and minor surgical operation, while the hospitals' beds and full-time equivalents (FTEs) were adopted as hospitals' inputs. Findings revealed that mean variable return to scale (VRTS) technical efficiency for CDHs was 0.744%, only 9 CDHs were found to be technically efficient and 6 were experiencing scale efficiency. However, most of CDHs hospitals were operating close to the scale efficiency as they have mean scale efficiency of 0.88823%. VAHs hospitals had mean VRTS technical efficiency of 0.702% and 7 hospitals were found to be scale efficient. Since the p-value is less than the 5% we rejected the null hypothesis that Mean distribution of technical efficiency score is equal across the CDHs and VAHs hospitals. The study recommends that hospitals experiencing a decreasing return to scale (DRS) or diseconomies of scale their size should be revisited to make them efficient. Hospitals sharing economies of scale should be equally supplied with health resources to increase their activities. This study suggests that the extension of this work should focus on how inefficient hospitals could improve their performance, given the available scarce resources.

Keywords: Modeling · Efficiency · Hospitals · Tanzania

1 Introduction

In health care systems, efficiency measurement is usually the first step in auditing the individual performance of health facility. Hospital's efficiency involves rational frameworks for the allocation of human and other resources between and within the health care facility (Kontodimopoulos et al. 2006). Other researchers have gone far and try to link the resource utilization and performance with Hospital's size (Bwana 2018a; 2018b; 2018c) or forms of ownership. An allocation is considered to be Pareto efficient if there is no room of making someone better off without making the other one worse off. Efficiency

J. N. Mojekwu et al. (Eds.): *Sustainable Education and Development*, pp. 173–182, 2021.
https://doi.org/10.1007/978-3-030-68836-3_16

is defined as the Pareto optimal allocation of resources (Aday 2004). Farrell (1957) introduced a simplified way to measure efficiency that could involve multiple inputs and outputs within the context of technical, allocation and productive efficiency. A firm is technically efficient when it produces the maximums outputs from a given amount of inputs or, produces the given output with the minimum inputs quantities (Hollingsworth 2008). There are two approaches to measure firm's efficiency: non-parametric and parametric approach. A non-parametric approach is the piecewise linear convex isoquant constructed such that no observed point should lie to the left or below it on the other hand parametric approach is econometric approach or trans log form, fitted to the data such that no observed point should lie to the left or below (Moshiri et al. 2011). Cummins and Zi (1998) pointed out that non-parametric approach estimates the best practice frontier with the efficiency of specific decision-making unit (DMUs) measured relative to the frontier. The frontier efficiency /production frontier measures how well the firm performs relative to the predicted performance of the best firm in the industry/market conditions.

Measuring of hospitals efficiency plays a significant role in the evaluation of health policy initiatives, and comparatives analysis of health systems (Biornet et al. 2003; Gerdtharn et al. 1999). Coyne et al. (2009) carried out a study to measure cost indicators about hospitals size and ownership, they revealed that small and large not for profit hospitals appear to achieve higher efficiency levels than the government-owned hospitals. Still, those larger hospitals of both ownership types report higher efficiency than that achieved by small hospitals. Other researchers have examined the relationship between different forms of ownership and hospitals performance. For example, Hu and Huang (2004) conducted a study on the hospitals' ownerships and efficiency performance. They found that public ownership significantly worsens hospitals efficiency while higher ward capacity utilization helps improve efficiency. In a similar study by Jehu-Appiah et al. (2014) ownership and hospitals efficiency was examined in Ghana. Their results showed that quasi-government hospitals and public hospitals were more efficient than the mission (religious-based) and private hospitals. Though there is an increasing trend in the assessment of hospitals performance in recent years, Ancarani et al. (2009) argued that hospital efficiency had been overlooked in the research literature. For example, modelling of efficiency in two categories of private not for profit (PNFP) hospitals has been given less attention by hospital researchers in Tanzania.

Different studies have been conducted on hospitals performance in Tanzania; however, most of the previous studies have dealt with measuring productivity, capacity utilization, financial performance, and other forms of performance. For example, Bwana (2014) evaluated productivity of faith-based hospitals in Tanzania; findings indicated that faith-based hospitals were experiencing deterioration in the productivity during the period under review (2001/2–2011/12), a decline which was mainly caused derived by worsening in technical progress. In another study Bwana (2018a) examined financial strength of council designated hospitals (CDHs) from 2009 to 2013 and findings revealed that CDHs were manifesting fair financial conditions with strong liquidity position and insignificant debt contained in the capital structure of the CDHs. Bwana (2018b) examined the Impact of public private partnerships (PPPs) on financial performance of hospitals in Tanzania using ratios analysis, the result indicated that hospitals under the

PPP arrangements were showing features of not being able to remain in business over a long period without government support. However, modeling of efficiency of VAHs and CDHs has been neglected in the previous hospitals studies, and therefore this study tries to cover the gap on the same. Generally, the study aims at modelling resources utilization in CDHs and VAHs, precisely the objectives of the study are:

i. To measure and compare the technical and scale efficiency of the VAHs and CDHs
ii. To examine the causes of the inefficiency in the VAHs and CDHs category

This study has been built on the Resource Dependency Theory (RDT) which argues that the firm operating in a resources endowed environment are more likely to excel and attain financial strength. RDT implications for hospitals planning signify that hospitals solvency depends upon its ability to participate in acquisitions, joint ventures and limited partnership with other organizations (Semritc 2009), in this case, CDHs are participating in partnerships with the government. Therefore, the study intends to explore the performance difference between CDHs and VAHs based on resources difference, as argued in the RTD. The study is significant since it involves the comparison of the performance in the two categories, which defines the private not for profit health facilities in Tanzania. The government of Tanzania through the Ministry Of Health something is missing here entered into a contract to support health service delivery in different parts of the country through CDHs. Therefore, this study is expected to uncover the extent of resources utilization between the two categories, because CDHs are endowed with support from the government. The study also contributes to the existing body of knowledge on the performance of private, not for profit hospitals in Tanzania. The remaining parts of this paper consists Sect. 2, which includes the methodology used in obtaining and analyzing data, Sect. 3 presents findings and discussions of results concerning previous similar studies. Conclusion and recommendations are presented in Sect. 4.

2 Methodology

Not for profit hospitals in Tanzania are mapped into five Zones, namely Lake Zone, Eastern Zone, Northern Zone, Western Zone and Southern Zone. There is a population of 90 private not for-profit hospitals in the country from which a sample size of 34 hospitals has been drawn to measure technical and scale efficiency, the sample comprises 17 council designated hospitals (CDHs) and 17 volunteering agency hospitals (VAHs). The sample was established using a stratified sampling technique where each zone was treated as a stratum.

2.1 Data Envelopment Model and Variables Specification

Data Envelopment Analysis (DEA) model is the piecewise linear convex hull methods to frontier estimation which was proposed by Farrell (1957), authors such as Boles (1966) and Afriat (1972) suggested mathematical programming methods which could achieve the task. Still, the technique failed to achieve wider attention until the paper by Charnes et al. (1978), which introduced the term Data Envelopment Analysis (DEA).

Charnes et al. (1978) proposed the model that assumes input-oriented and Constant Return to Scale (CRS), in subsequent article Banker et al. (1984) considered the alternative set of assumptions, such as variable returns to scale (VRS). DEA model was used in measuring economic efficiency, usually, DEA requires information on hospitals outputs and inputs. Inputs- are variables that define resources used to produce results, while hospitals' outputs are services provided to hospitals clients. In general inputs in health services/healthcare consist of variables representing labor, capital assets and/or other operational expenses (Ozcan 1992). Labor is the category of the main input, and is measured by the number of hours per patient per day by skill mix (this group include medical staff (such as doctors, nurses) and non-medical staff (such as administrators). Capital assets, mainly defined as plants, equipment and support technology, due to variations in the accounting practices of hospitals number of beds in the units are used as the proxy measure to capture a unit level of capital assets (Ozcan 2008; Rosko 1990). Outputs-the outputs included depending on the appropriateness to the evaluation of the hospital's efficiency and availability of data/information.

Five (5) outputs and two (2) input variables were involved. The output variables included were inpatients days, admissions, outpatients visit, total birth, and minor surgical operation, meanwhile the hospitals' beds and FTEs (full-time equivalents) were used as hospitals' inputs. As suggested by Parkin and Hollingsworth (1997), we perform series of DEAs analysis while gradually increasing the number of inputs and outputs used, this sensitivity analysis aims to examine consistency between different results as we conducted the study. The number of outpatients' visits has been consistently used as a measure of outpatient output. Similarly, the number of admissions and post admissions days (inpatients days-admissions) have been used as a measure of inpatient outputs (Rosko and Mutter 2010; Nedelea 2012). Due to the heterogeneity of the hospitals outputs different researchers usually include variables such as emergencies room visits, Outpatients' surgeries and births to control outputs heterogeneity. In this study the choice of outputs was based on previous studies by Rosko and Mutter (2010) and Nedelea (2012) - the outputs may also be selected based on easy or availability of data. Given the data constraints, inputs variables are assumed to be similar in hospitals efficiency studies (Rosko and Mutter 2010; Nedelea 2012). Farrell (1957) suggested that firms' efficiency should involve two components: technical and allocative efficiency whose combination signifies a measure of productive efficiency. This study employs the technical efficiency (TE) under the assumptions of input-oriented measured and variable return to scale (VRS); TE can be calculated by solving the following DEA LP problems.

Min λj, such that:

$$\sum_{j=1}^{n} \lambda j Yrj \geq Yro,\ _{(r=1.........5)}$$

$$\sum_{j=1}^{n} \lambda i Xij \geq \theta Xio,\ _{(i=1,2)}$$

$$\sum_{j=1}^{n} \lambda j = 1,\ _{\lambda j \geq 0 (j=1.....n)}$$

The objective of the Linear Programming problem is to find the Min Θ that particularly reduces inputs vector to ΘXio, while guaranteeing at least the output level of Yro. The inputs-oriented model was adopted based on the assumption that hospitals administrators have no control over the outputs, rather the inputs. The optimal solution to the Linear Programming problem is $TE = 0 \leq 1$ where $TE = 1$ indicates a point on the efficient frontier and hence technically efficient hospitals. $TE < 1$, meaning that it is possible to produce the observed level of outputs using less than all inputs.

2.2 Hypothesis Development and Testing

With the specific objective of measuring the efficiency of the two categories of hospitals (VAHs and CDHs), we developed the null hypothesis that mean distribution is equal across CDHs and VAHs against the alternative hypothesis that the mean distribution of efficiency is not equal across the two categories.

H 01: Mean distribution of the efficiency score is equal across CDHs and VAHs Hospitals.
H 02: Mean distribution is not equal across the CDHs and VAHs hospitals.

Non-parametric Mann-Whitney U test has been undertaken to perform the hypothesis test, with support of SPSS 21. The method suits the requirement of the study since it is useful in comparison of two unpaired (independent) groups when the assumption of normality of efficiency distribution is not met. Using Mann Whitney U Test brings sense when the scatter is random (implying that any factor affecting one value/making one value to be too low or too high should not affect other values. In other words, the error term should be independent. Using Mann Whitney U requires the two groups to have the same or similar shape.

Mann Whitney u test statistics is expressed by U, whereby;

$$\mathrm{U1} = \mathrm{n1} \cdot \mathrm{n2} + n_1(n_1 + 1)/2 - R_1 \ \mathit{and} \ \mathrm{U2} = \mathrm{n1} \cdot \mathrm{n2} + n_2(n_2 + 1)/2 - R_2$$

R1 and R2 are the sums of the two ranks in groups 1&2 respectively, n1 and n2 are total sample size in group one and two, respectively.

3 Findings and Discussion

Findings revealed that there were some variations in the mean inputs and outputs variables between hospitals category, for example, the mean number of beds was 183.871 in the Council Designated Hospitals (CDHs) and 184.671 in the Volunteering Agency Hospitals (VAHs). The mean number of staff was 198.92 in the CDHs and 115.7 in the VAHs. Further analysis revealed that mean a constant return to scale technical efficiency for CDHs was 0.663 (66.3%) and 6 hospitals were found to be Constant return scale technically efficient (CRSTE) during the period under the study 2009–2013.

On the other hand, the mean variable return to scale technical efficiency (VRSTE) was 74.3% over the same period. Six hospitals were also experiencing scale efficiency; the six hospitals were found to be efficient in all aspects. The remaining 11 CDHs were not operating at their optimal size which means they either experienced increasing returns to scale (IRS) or decreasing returns to scale (DRS). On the other hand, 9 (52.9%) hospitals were found to be a variable return to scale technically efficient (VRSTE). However, most of the CDHs hospitals were performing close to their optimal size as they have the mean scale efficiency score of 88.6%, which is relatively higher than 87.4% of the VAHs. The result also revealed that the performance of the CDHs was stable compared to that of VAHs, since CDHs and VAHs had standard deviation of efficiency scores of 24% and 27% respectively (Table 1). On the other hand, the results show that VAHs hospitals had mean constant return to scale technical efficiency of 0.611 (61.1%), and 7 (41%) hospitals (in this category) were found to be technically efficient during the period under the study 2009–2013 in all aspects of efficiency.

Table 1. VRS technical efficiency and scale efficiency of CDHs and VAHs (2009–2013)

Hospitals	Variables	Observation	Mean	Std. Deviation	Min	Max	Hospitals of frontier
Council designated hospitals (CDHs)	Technical efficiency (CRS)	85	.663215	.2434845	.151544	1	6(35%)
	Pure technical efficiency (VRS)	85	.743559	.2165882	.330762	1	9(52.9%)
	Scale efficiency (CRS)	85	.8860073	.1612484	.419204	1	6(35%)
Volunteering agency hospitals (VAHs)	Technical efficiency (CRS)	85	.6117538	.2698061	.190525	1	07(41%)
	Pure technical efficiency (VRS)	85	.7017015	.258126	.220332	1	08(47.1%)
	Scale efficiency (CRS)	85	.8748721	.1766214	.255404	1	07(41%)

Source: Research Findings 2019

The same hospitals were experiencing scale efficiency and manifested the constant returns to scale (CRS) which means 7 (41.1%) hospitals were operating at their optimal level of activities over the study period. The VAHs had mean scale efficiency of 87.5%. Hospital with CRS neither experience economy of scale nor diseconomy of scale. The remaining 10 (58.9%) hospitals were not operating at their optimal sizes, which means they had either increasing returns to scale (IRS) or decreasing returns to scale (DRS). The VAHs category had the mean variable return to scale technical efficiency (VRSTE) of 70.1% which is less than 74.3% of CDHs.

Generally, the comparison of the two periods (2009 and 2013) tells us whether this particular category of hospitals (VAHs) had been experiencing efficiency improvement or not. In the year 2009 there were 16(94.1%) hospitals exhibited the increasing returns to scale, meaning the hospitals were operating below their capacity, therefore if resources could have been equally added they would have realized more outputs since they have room to enjoy economies of scale, one Hospital under this category exhibited the decreasing returns to scale (DRS) in the same period 2009. Such Hospital (with DRS) need to scale-down its size of operation to become efficient, any attempt to increase the level of activities would push the facility into more diseconomies of scale. In 2013 it was found that 11 hospitals (64.7%) had increasing return to scale (IRS) while 2 hospitals had decreasing return to scale (DRS), the remaining 4 (23.5%) hospitals manifested constant return to scale (CRS), meaning they were operating at their optimal level. This implies that there was an improvement in terms of resources utilization in the CDHs category between the two periods. Generally, the mean constant return to scale technical efficiency of CDHs (66.3%) is higher than that of VAHs (61.3%). The CDHs category also had mean variable return to scale technical efficiency (VRSTE) of 74.3% which is higher than that of VAHs 70.1%. (Ref. Table 1). Findings revealed that the performance of CDHs was stable as compared to the implementation of VAHs and this is because CDHs has lower standard deviation as compared to that of VAHs. However, VAHs have potential to increase their ability to manage and use their resources. The result also revealed that when all (both CDHs and VAHs) hospitals are ranked with regards to technical efficiency (CRS) and pure efficiency (VRS), out of first ten, the first three are CDHs hospitals in the aspect of technical efficiency. On the other hand, CDHs rank number two to nine concerning pure efficiency. Generally, as far as ranking is concerned CDHs rank high than VAHs particularly in relation to technical efficiency.

4 Conclusion and Recommendations

The study measures the efficiency of CDHs and VAHs in Tanzania from 2009–2013 using Data Envelopment Analysis (DEA) approach, the study also engages Man Whitney U in testing if the mean distribution of efficiency score in CDHs and VAHs are equal or not. Findings from the hypothesis testing revealed that the mean distribution of efficiency score is not equal across the VAHs and CDHs. CDHs were better in resource utilization as compared to VAHs. However, VAHs have potential to increase their ability to manage and use their resources efficiently more than CDHs counterpart, this is because most of the hospitals were experiencing an increasing return to scale which also implies that average hospitals cost was decreasing over the period under review. Most of the CDHs are operating close to their optimal sizes compared to VAHs. This is evidenced by the mean scale efficiency, which was larger than that of VAHs. Over the study period performance of CDHs seems to be stable as compared to the performance of VAHs, this is evidenced by higher standard deviation of VAHs as compared to that of CDHs. We recommends that hospitals operating under the increasing return to scale (IRS) should be considered for expansions and enlarging their scale of activities since they still have room to enjoy economies of scale and produce more outputs if resources will be equally added. The study recommends that hospitals experiencing a decreasing return to scale

(DRS) or experiencing diseconomies to scale should be downsized into a manageable size to make them efficient. This is because it seems the hospitals are too small for their activities, and therefore to make them efficient restructuring is inevitable. The two categories of hospitals should also fully utilize the idle capacity since the study revealed that both CDHs and VAHs had the unutilized capacity of 21.4 and 22.6% respectively.

Appendix 1: Variables Used in the Previous Similar Studies

Previous authors	Country	Applicability in previous studies
NG (2008)	China	Measure of productive efficiency of health care sector in China (hospitals beds and number of staff were used as inputs variables)
Barbara et al. (2009)	USA	Measuring technical efficiency in acute care units (hospitals beds and number of staff were used as inputs variables)
Gannon (2005)	Ireland	Measuring technical efficiency of hospitals in Ireland (hospitals beds and number of staff were used as inputs variables)
Harris et al. (2000)	USA	Impact of mergers on the hospitals efficiency performance. (total number of staff was used as the inputs variables)
Nedelea (2012)	USA	Measuring the impact of hospitals status conversion on hospitals efficiency (hospitals beds and number of staff were used as inputs variables while outpatient surgery and total birth was used as output variables)
Barbara et al. (2009)	USA	Measuring technical efficiency in acute care units (hospitals beds was used as inputs variables)
Park et al. (2011)	USA	Measuring hospitals operating efficiency (total admission was used as outputs variables)
Moshiri et al. (2011)	Malaysia	Measuring efficiency of teaching hospitals (total admission was used as outputs variables)
Rosko and Mutter (2010)	USA	Inefficiency difference between two groups of of systems (CAH and PPS) (total admission and outpatient surgery were used as outputs variables)
Yawe (2006)	Uganda	Measuring productivity growth of district referral hospitals in Uganda (total birth was used as output variable)

References

Aday, L.A.: Evaluating the Healthcare System: Effectiveness, Efficiency, and Equity. Health Administration press, Chicago (2004)

Afriat, S.N.: Efficiency estimation of production functions. Int. Econ. Rev. **13**(3), 568 (1972)
Ancarani, A., Di Mauro, C., Giammanco, M.D.: The impact of managerial and organizational aspects on hospital wards' efficiency: Evidence from a case study. Eur. J. Oper. Res. **194**(1), 280–293 (2009)
Banker, R.D., Charnes, A., Cooper, W.W.: Some models for estimating technical and scale inefficiencies in data envelopment analysis. Manag. Sci. **30**(9), 1078–1092 (1984)
Biørn, E., Hagen, T.P., Iversen, T., Magnussen, J.: The effect of activity-based financing on hospital efficiency: a panel data analysis of DEA efficiency scores 1992–2000. Health Care Manag. Sci. **6**(4), 271–283 (2003)
Boles, J.N.: Efficiency squared--efficient computation of efficiency indexes. In: Proceedings of the Annual Meeting (Western Farm Economics Association), vol. 39, pp. 137–142. Western Agricultural Economics Association (1966)
Bwana, K.M.: Evaluating the productivity of faith based hospitals in tanzania: application of malmquist productivity index (MPI) approach. Int. J. Finan. Econ. **3**(4), 207–216 (2014)
Bwana, K.M.: Investigating efficiency based on the hospitals size: an application of a non-parametric approach to the private hospitals in Tanzania: African. J. Appl. Res. **4**(1), 106–119 (2018a)
Bwana, K.M.: Evaluating financial strength of council designated hospitals (CDHs) in Tanzania using financial strength index (FSI) model. Afr. J. Appl. Res. **4**(2), 32–44 (2018b)
Bwana, K.M.: Impact of Public Private Partnerships (PPPs) financial performance of Council Designated Hospitals (CDHs) in Tanzania. Afr. J. Appl. Res. **4**(1), 120–129 (2018c)
Charnes, A., Cooper, W., Rhodes, E.: Measuring the efficiency of decision making units. Eur. J. Oper. Res. **2**(6), 429–444 (1978)
Coyne, J.S., Richards, M.T., Short, R., Schultz, K., Singh, S.G.: Hospital cost and efficiency: do hospital size and ownership type really matter? J. Healthcare Manag. **54**(3), 163–176 (2009)
Cummins, J.D., Zi, H.: Comparison of frontier efficiency methods: an application to the US life insurance industry. J. Prod. Anal. **10**(2), 131–152 (1998)
Farrell, M.J.: The measurement of productive efficiency. J. Roy. Stat. Soc. Ser. Gen. **120**(3), 253–290 (1957)
Gerdtham, U.G., Rehberg, C., Tambour, M.: The impact of internal market on health care efficiency. evidence from the health care reforms in Sweden. Appl. Econ. **31**, 935–945 (1999)
Hollingsworth, B.: The measurement of efficiency and productivity of health care delivery. Health Econ. **17**(10), 1107–1128 (2008)
Hu, J.L., Huang, Y.F.: Technical efficiencies in large hospitals: a managerial perspective. Int. J. Manag. **21**(4), 506–513 (2004)
Jehu-Appiah, C., Sekidde, S., Adjuik, M., Akazili, J., Almeida, S., Nyonator, F., Baltussen, R., Asbu, E., Kirigia, J.: Ownership and technical efficiency of hospitals: evidence from Ghana using data envelopment analysis. Cost Effect. Resour. Allocation **12**(1), 9 (2014). https://doi.org/10.1186/1478-7547-12-9
Kontodimopontos, N., Nanos, P., Niakas, D.: Balancing efficiency of health services and equity of access in remote areas in Greece. Health Policy **76**, 49–57 (2006)
Moshiri, H., Aljunid, S., Amin, R.M., Dahlui, M., Ibrahim, W.N.: Measuring efficiency of teaching hospitals in Malaysia. Int. J. Bus. Manag. **6**(4), 207–213 (2011)
Nedelea, J.: Impact of Conversion to Critical Access Hospital Status on Hospital Efficiency: A PhD Thesis. Louisiana State University, USA (2012)
Ozcan, Y.A.: Sensitivity analysis of hospitals efficiency under alternative output/input and peer groups: a reviewer. Knowl. Politics **5**, 1–29 (1992)
Ozcan, Y.A.: Healthcare Benchmarking and Performance Evaluation: An Assessment of DEA. Springer, Norwell (2008)
Parking, D., Hollingsworth, B.: Measuring production efficiency of acute hospitals in Scotland, 1991–4: validity issues in data envelopment analysis. Appl. Econ. **29**, 1425–1433 (1997)

Rosko, M.: Measuring technical efficiency in health organization. J. Med. Syst. **14**(5), 307–322 (1990)

Rosko, M.D., Mutter, R.: Inefficiency Differences between the critical access hospitals and prospectively paid rural hospitals. J. Health Politics Policy Laws **35**(1), 95–126 (2010)

Semritc, A.V.: Indicators of Financial and Health Systems: A Systematic Review of the Literatures, Washington State University: Masters of Health Policy and Administration, Published Dissertation (2009)

Equality and Access to Urban Public Open Spaces by the Poor Urban Street Vendors in Dar Es Salaam

M. H. Kirumirah(✉)

Department of Business Administration, College of Business Education, P. O. Box 1968, Dar es Salaam, Tanzania
m.kirumirah@cbe.ac.tz

Abstract. This study aims at investigating the state of urban street vendors in in accessing open spaces Dar es Salaam. Specifically, the study explored factors influencing poor urban vendors in accessing public space and to examine the functionality and vendors' opinion on the sustainability of current state of affairs. The study was qualitative in nature with a case study design and was conducted in Dar es Salaam using street vendors and city authority officers sampled randomly and purposively. Data were collected by using interviews and focus group discussions and were analysed by the use of content analysis. Findings reveal that, while the government has taken initiatives to help the operations of street vending business, such initiatives have been successful. Pressing by-laws and actions have been enacted by local authorities influenced by big retail store owner. It is further revealed that due to contradictions among government actors, sustainability of government efforts to enhance the operations of street vending business is questionable. The study recommends the government to enact a national wide policy to govern the operations of street vending business.

Keywords: Street vending · Poverty · Equality · Access · Urban public open space

1 Introduction and Background to the Problem

The proliferation of street vending business in different countries across the world is a fact that urban authorities should not ignore (Nani 2016). Studies indicate that, the business is a great livelihood strategy and a weapon against poverty to the urban poor (Mahadevia and Vyas 2012; Mubarack 2018; Munishi and Casmir 2019). It has been reported that, street vending contributes in the provision of employment, for instance, in the New York City alone, it is said to provide more than 17960 jobs (Carpenter 2015), arrests the rate of crime in the city (Mramba 2015; Mutarubukwa 2015), becomes a shock absorber when the country is experiencing economic quagmires and extreme poverty among residents(Mubarack 2018) and a means for the livelihood to the disadvantaged poor and sidelined urban dwellers (Xue and Huang 2015).

J. N. Mojekwu et al. (Eds.): *Sustainable Education and Development*, pp. 183–193, 2021.
https://doi.org/10.1007/978-3-030-68836-3_17

Despite the fact that street vending is an integral part of the urban economy in most countries in the world, it is still considered illegal and its practitioners have been subjected to unequal treatment by authorities (Meneses 2013). They have been restricted to access and use urban spaces in conducting their businesses. Studies (Bhowmik 2010; Crossa 2013) indicate that, a great number of cities in the world are in the move to creating modern and smart cities free from street vendors, competitive in nature and attractive in the eyes of the tourists at the expense of urban poor who use them to earn a living. Thus, this move has led to suppressing vendors, closing their means of livelihood and incapacitating their means of fighting against poverty. In such a situation, authorities define street vending as an informal and unacceptable business in favour of their interest (Xue and Huang 2015), without thinking of the impact it has to people's economy and urban life in general.

With such motives, authorities have enacted exclusionary policies, laws and bylaws restricting vendors from accessing urban public open spaces (Reover and Skinner 2016). Such policies have led into uncountable evictions, harassment, and relocation which are accompanied with destruction of vendors' physical, economic and social assets. While the same situation has been reported in Ghana, (Muirui 2010), illegality has been ascribed to vendors in Uganda, and some moments dubbed criminals and a source of traffic congestion in Kampala (Nakibuuka 2016). In Tanzania the situation has been the same to that of Ghana and Uganda, with an exception of what is happening currently, when vendors are operating under the mercy of the current President. Although, apart from this political pronouncement no legal document has been prepared for the total legalization of vendors' operations.

Access to urban open spaces has been a contested issue especially when used by street vendors. Many city authorities have not been in favour of street vendors using these spaces and instead have been advocating for Public, Private Partnership (PPP). It is evident that most of vendors have been resettled, evicted and suppressed by different law enforcing bodies. While city authority official understand the importance of street vendors to peoples livelihood and a weapon against poverty, it is not known why they still suppress vendors and instead prefer allowing affluent people to use these spaces. Although authorities reiterate that they prefer giving these open spaces to affluent ones because they can pay more than street vendors, this is not a reason enough to explain double standards existing between the affluent and the poor urban street vendors who use these spaces for their livelihood and as a means of escaping from poverty. Despite the fact that a number of studies have been carried in Tanzania with regard to the street vending business, (Lyons and Brown 2009; Lyons et al. 2014; Mramba et al. 2014; Mramba 2015; Msoka and Ackson 2017; Mubarack 2018; Munishi and Casmir 2019) their central focus was on vendors' business reforms, street vending business for poverty reduction, street vending business and the use of ICTs, vendors' business challenges and resilience strategies and the training needs among street vendors and gave little attention on equality in accessing the available open spaces, what influences this uneven access, and the need for regulatory guidelines to safeguard such equality among city dweller. Based on the available gap in literature and practice, this study investigates inequalities with regard to accessing open spaces by the poor street vendors in Dar es Salaam and what influences this inequality.

1.1 Objectives of the Study

The study aims at exploring the state of urban street vendors in accessing open spaces in Dar es Salaam. Specifically, the study intends to identify factors influencing uneven access to public open spaces by the urban poor street vendors and explore usability and vendors' opinions on the sustainability of the president's currently enjoyed permission and freedom.

2 Theoretical Framework of the Study

The study used the theory of right to the city created by Lefebvre in 1968. The theory has become a widely used theory in urban studies (Marcuse 2009) rooted from Lefebvre (1996) [1968]. In his view, Lefebvre considers the concept to contain demands to be thought through. It is a cry and demand for more (Lefebvre 1996) from the oppressed, marginalized, underpaid and insecure members and groups of people in the city (Marcuse 2009). It is a cry for habitation, appropriation and participation in the city. However, in the current state, the concept means a lot basing from different angles considered by different authors (Brenner et al. 2012).

While other authors consider it as the right to urban life (Mitchell 2003), right to participate in urban issues, the struggle to solving urban problems (Brenner et al. 2012), the right to change cities to peoples heart's desire (Harvey 2003) and the right to access and occupy city facilities (Capron 2002; Lamb 2002); and more others, Lefebvre's meaning on the right to the city centres on the right to creating and using urban spaces freely with no restrictions by urban authorities through their created policies that impede urban dwellers from using these spaces in favour of profit making capitalist. The theory is in line with this study in the sense that the study agitates for equality in accessing urban open spaces by all. It further opposes the city authority actions of intending to create repressive policies that restrict street vendors to access urban spaces and bestow such rights to capitalists for profit making intentions at the expense of the majority poor. By using this theory, the study calls for collective actions by city stakeholders to collectively work for equality in accessing the available open spaces.

3 Methodology

A qualitative research approach with a case study design was employed in this study. The approach allowed the researcher to qualitatively study respondents' views and opinions on the topic under the study (Bryman 2003). The study was carried out in Dar es Salaam. The city was chosen because of being a business capital in the country and has attracted a number of street vendors of different characteristics in comparison to any other city in Tanzania, because of continuous contestations between street vendors and the middle class residents backed by the city authorities on access to the available open spaces, and because of a number of pressing bylaws against street vending enacted while a number Public Private Partnership projects on the available open spaces are underway. Convenient and purposive sampling techniques were used in data collection. Convenient sampling was used to sample 100 street vendors selected mainly in hotspots near open spaces. Purposive sampling was employed to sample city authority officials with vast knowledge regarding the operations of street vendors, rights over the use of available open spaces and investment projects that city authority wishes to take on the available open urban spaces.

In this study, data was collected by means of the interview, Focus Group Discussions (FGD) and documentary reviews. The interview and FGD guide involved a list of questions that were administered to respondents concerning the topic under the study. The questions were centred on the rights to use spaces, factors influencing uneven access to inequalities in accessing urban spaces among street vendors and their assessment on the prevailing situation and their future prospects. The interview and FGD guide were translated in Kiswahili the commonly spoken language in Tanzania by two independent professional translators to ensure translation equivalence.

With regards to FGDs, the discussions were moderated by the researcher in Kiswahili and voice recorded by an audio recorder. With regard to interviews, they were carried in two different scenarios. The first scenario included interviewing sampled street vendors and the second one involved interviewing city officials. While the former were interviewed on the spot as soon as they consented, the latter were interviewed based on their schedule and interviews were carried in their offices. In both cases proceedings were carried in Swahili. Data collected were transcribed verbatim in Kiswahili then text extracts to support findings were translated into English.

Data collected from different respondents through interviews and Focus Group discussion were summarized coded and grouped according to similarities in their contents. By employing content analysis data were analyzed according to Denscombe (2010) with the aid of MAXQDA 10 software.

4 Presentation of Findings and Discussion

4.1 Factors Influencing Uneven Access to Public Open Spaces by the Urban Poor Street Vendors

In this objective of the study. The researcher builds from the previous literature that the government had prohibited street vending and at times it was allowed to operate. In such lapses street vendors faced challenges when they wanted to access open spaces. City authorities used even security organs to ensure that vendors do not use open spaces for vending. Instead, such spaces were left for big business persons and at times through Public, Private Partnership, municipal authorities wanted to use these spaces for money generation projects supervised by big business persons. The objective intends to find out what influences such uneven access to open spaces in Dar es Salaam. Results are presented below;

The Need for Improving City and Municipal Revenues

It was revealed by data that, street vendors were restricted to use open spaces and there was a move of giving such spaces to big business owners because the authorities wanted to increase their monetary generations. It was revealed that big business owners have strong financial muscles, and can use the open spaces more productively than street vendors and through their activities they are able to pay a lot in form of rent, they are paying tax to the government among others. During an interview, one city official disclosed that,

These big business owners are more productive than vendors, imagine they would pay for the space, they would pay tax, provide employment and would have increased our collections. But to vendors you would end up getting just a little amount of money from them (City official, DCC).

Data indicate that it was based on monetary needs and financial muscles of big business owners and investors that city authority was influenced to grant the use right of public open spaces to them than allowing vendors to use them.

Political Influence

Politicians are among the policy makers at the national level and implementers of the same policies at their municipal levels as councillors. They were also part of teams that formulated street vendors' repressive laws and by laws. At the same time, their close ties with business persons and investors led to city authorities to ban vendors from using urban public spaces at the expense of street vendors. In their view, politicians preferred big business owners and investors to be in control of open space because some of the investors were representatives of politician while others cemented the idea that investors would have an extensive contribution to the city and municipal revenue. During a FGD, a vendor said, "*politicians had two faces, while they were part of investors aspiring to take the open spaces, but when they came to us they only showed that they are with us and fighting for our course*".

With their influence, the city authority had no objection rather than using whatever means possible to ensure that vendors are kept out of such spaces so that politicians and their allies could take control of the spaces.

The Need for Maintaining Environmental Health

While it is the fact that vendors were blamed of destructing the environment by littering garbage in areas where they worked from. Thus, the city authority would end up using its income to clean the environment and maintaining it for city beautification. Data indicate that city authorities embarked on beautifying the city by planting trees, flowers and ensuring that all the spaces are attractive. As a means of maintaining these, authorities banned vendors from accessing the spaces for their business giving a reason that they are not easily manageable. During an interview, a trade officer at Ilala MC said

> Considering what we had invested, it was not easy for us to allow them use those spaces. By allowing them means that you are putting the environment and all the structures we had put in place for beautifying the city. You cannot know who damaged the structures, because they are many. But still after doing their business they do not think of cleaning their surroundings (Trade officer, Ilala MC)

This means that allowing vendors to operate was considered a risk to the environment and the city beautification plan. However, vendors contested this and they said they used to pay 500Tshs on a daily basis for cleaning and garbage collection. One of them was quoted saying, "*we used to pay for garbage collection, we had our leaders they used to ensure that we do not destroy anything and at times we used to water trees and flowers they had planted. Unless they had other motives than considering us as a risk to the environment*".

Such contrasting statements mean that vendors and city authority were on different angles as to why one banned the other from using open spaces. While the reason was to maintain the beauty of the city, the city was ready to give it away to an investor giving a reason that the investor was controllable as compared to vendors.

The Need to Safeguard Interest of Big Retail Store Owners

The competition existing between formal and street vendors in one way or the other caused city authorities to bar street vendors from using open spaces available in the city. Data indicate that the general complaints tendered by big business owners about the parasitic nature id vendors led authorities to ban vending at different times. This was because their influence was big and they were the ones paying a huge sum of tax as compared to vendors who were paying nothing. During an interview, one city official said,

> We used to receive several complaints from business persons around the city that street vendors are benefiting at their expense. Their complaints were sometimes alarming. At times they were threatening to close their businesses if we had not banned street vendors. By considering that they are the major tax payers, we had to restrict vendors so that we avoid the worst from happening (City officer 3, DCC).

Such a quotation implies that vendors were zeroed because of the influence from the big business owners who at times though that the presence of these vendors would cause lowering their volumes of sales. It was also partly because of the influence from business owners in Kariakoo that the vendors' market in Lumumba was closed.

Data collected from this objective indicate that different reasons have been involved and have caused city and municipal authorities to bar street vendors from using urban open spaces for their business at the expense of big business owners. The need for collecting more taxes, political influence, the influence from big business owners and investors and environmental factors were cited. Data are in consistent with some of the existing literature which clearly indicate that city and municipal actions are normally influenced by politicians (Munoz 2018) who are in most cases are fighting to ensure that they maximize their revenues. Such stances are sometimes directed by the directions of the incumbent president (Msoka and Ackson 2017). Literature further indicate that the need for pleasing big business owners lead authorities into victimizing street vendors by denying them the right to use urban spaces. Such facts influence authorities to take sides by supporting big business owners at the expense of vendors. It was further articulated that vendors are dirty, destruct the environment and cause environmental pollution. The fact is supported by many authority officials who dreamt of creating smart cities which are attractive to visitors and tourists. This is similar to what (Bhowmik 2010; Crossa 2013) write that the need to create smart cities influence city authorities to prefer big business owner at the expense of vendors, claiming that vendors destroy the environment. However, the claim was totally contested by vendors and who clearly stated that to them cleanliness was key and they used to pay daily contribution for garbage collection and cleanliness. At Zanaki Street, vendors even showed the contract they had signed with

Green Waste Pro (a garbage collecting company) for cleaning their area as well as copies of receipts they used to pay to the same company. This indicates that, despite have such claims from officials, it was revealed that there might have been other reasons that led city officials from preferring big business owners than vendors who also had their right to use the city spaces for their livelihood. Such elements of inequalities may be associated with bribes from business owners to city authority officials.

4.2 Sustainability of the State of Vendors in the Country

This objective was created to tap vendors' views on the sustainability of the current state of vendors. This comes as a result of the presidents' pronunciation of allowing vendors to operate across the country. With such a pronunciation, it was wondered whether the state would be continuous or not. Findings of this study portray three sides. While the first one are sure that the state will continue to be the way it is, others think the state will not last for a long after 2020 and the last segment of vendors indicate that they do not know and cannot predict what will happen. All their vies are presented as follows.

The State Will Continue To Be Like The Way It Is Today

It was revealed by a group of vendors that following the state of affairs and the current state of street vendors, in which they are allowed to vend at anytime and anywhere, they claimed that since it is a presidential statement, the state will continue to be the way it is whether the incumbent president is in power or not. On vendor said, *"I am not even afraid that anyone will revoke the president's statement. We shall always be allowed to vend"*. Such a statement was also supported by another vendor who said, *"I don't think if there is anyone who can revoke the president's decree. Even another president will always respect the prior president's decree"*. Such statements indicate that vendors are sure that nobody will ever eject them from streets and it is their presidential given permission since he even gave them the opportunity of being registered and recognized through giving them special Identification Cards (vendors' IDs).

The Permission Will Not Las Longer After 2020

This was another segment of vendors who among others appreciated the president's given permission, but knew that the state of affairs would not go beyond 2020. To most of respondents in this segment believed that this was a political move that intended to win street vendors' votes in the forthcoming elections. During a FGD some vendors said, *"We have always been used as a political ladder, in the sense that politicians use us as their political agenda and after elections dump us"*. Another vendor put it clear that, "*What we are enjoying is out of presidential political motive of winning trust among vendors. I assure you, after 2020 we shall return to the previous state of being chased in town*". The discussion collected different views regarding the issue. One of them while connecting the permission given through IDs and the current practice he said they might be enjoying the last moments of the permission. He opined,

> The government provided us with IDs and said we shall have to renew them every year, but nothing has ever been done ever since we bought the IDs. To me it implies that it was a political statement and soon we are going back to our old times of fighting with militias and police (Vendor 33, Makumbusho).

Such statements indicate that because vendors have always been used as political agenda, they think that even this time after the 2020 elections, the permission they are enjoying will end. To some they think it may last up to the end of the fifth government reign but will never be enjoyed continuously.

Uncertain of Whether the State of Affairs Will Last or Change

The other segment of vendors indicate that they are not sure as to whether vendors will keep on enjoying the freedom they have today or not. It was captured from data that vendors were not sure of their tomorrow. Most of them kept reiterating that this is not the first moment when vendors were allowed. But in most cases after sometimes they used to be chased. In an interview session with a vendor who never knew of his tomorrow said, "*the problem is that we are here because of the president's pronunciation. And actually no one knows the intention of such a pronunciation. What it was for political popularity? In actual sense I don't know if this permission is going to last for a long time*". Supporting this another said, "*If you look closely, even the municipal officials do not want us here. They are only quiet because they can't go against the president. But the reality is that we might not be needed in town anytime sooner. We are not certain about our stay here*". Such quotations represent a group of vendors whose certainty on the continuous freedom enjoyed by vendors is at a very low stage.

Data from this objective are consistent with other literature which mostly show that, the absence of any regulatory framework that allows the operation of street vending business leads vendors' operations being at stake. Despite the fact that the government has taken a number of initiative to ensure that vendors are legalized and formalized, requirements for legalization have been a great burden to vendors (Lyon and Brown 2009) and the regulatory framework is full of contradictions (Recaud et al. 2018). With such contradictions and stumbling blocks, street vending has not achieved having a pronounced regulatory framework for vendors. This situation leaves them unaware of their tomorrow. It has also been identified that political motives are sometimes driving politicians to make statements that will ensure that they win popularity among vendors but after satisfying their motives they leave them without anyone to fight for them (Munoz 2018). A major fact that has been experienced in different countries show that politicians have been repeatedly calling for the halt of eviction and harassment of vendors towards elections and ordering for their serious eviction after elections (Etzold 2014). In a similar trend, the contrasting actions of different political figures including municipal and city directors to the current state of vendors (Kisembo 2017) is yet another reason leaving vendors unaware of the continuity of the freedom they are currently enjoying. The continuous contradiction in laws and contestation among authorities on the status of vendors has widely been reported by different authors (Msoka and Ackson 2017; Recaud et al. 2018). Of recent, city directors in Mwanza and Dodoma have been trying to evict vendors from their areas of operations, despite the presidential call for halting all actions against vendors in the country. Such situations suggest that may be the current freedom may continue in the presence of the current president or may be revoked at any time.

5 Conclusion and Recommendations

The study among other things has explained the need for vendors' access to city spaces as given by the right to the city theory. It discloses that vendors have the right to use the city, its opportunities and to participate in whatever takes place in the city. The study however shows city authorities deprive vendors' rights by favouring the affluent fellows when it comes to accessing urban spaces. Despite all these, some efforts were done by the government to save the business, however, efforts were half linked, top down and had no political intentions of solving the situation once and for all. As a result, vendors do not know their actual status as to whether they are legal or not. This study concludes that the city belongs to all and should be used by all sustainably, without considering ones economic standards. For economic and social harmony, formal and informal economic activities should be harnessed and allowed to operate by complementing one another.

6 Implication of the Study

The study informs policy makers that street vending is a viable economic opportunity for those who have missed to be absorbed in the formal system. It informs them that this opportunity serves to combat poverty among the urban poor who have been side-lined. Thus supportive policies to help vendors are of paramount importance than side-lining them and restricting them from using urban public open spaces. The study brings to city authority's attention that street vending is a reality that supports the life of many urban poor dwellers and is not going to vanish despite being treated with harsh and unequal policies and laws. The study further informs authorities that, because street vending is a viable economic activity, it should be legalized and national wide policy should be formulated to allow vending across the country. The study informs policy and decision makers that inclusive planning and decision making will help the city and the country at large to benefit from the street vending business other than treating the business with harsh and restrictive policies.

Area for Future Research
This study investigated general issues regarding to vendors' access to urban open spaces by the use of qualitative means. It recommends another qualitative study to be conducted to investigate the source of contradiction between municipal/city directors and the central government on the issue of street vendors in the country.

References

Bhowmik, S.: Street vendors in Asia: survey of research. In: Bhowmik, S. (ed.) Street Vendors in the Global Urban Economy, pp. 49–61. Routledge, New Delhi, India (2010)

Brenner, N., Marcuse, P., Mayer, M.: Cities for people, not for profit, city: analysis of urban trends, culture, theory, policy, action, **13**(2–3), 176–184 (2012)

Bryman, A.: Research Methods and Organization Studies, vol. 20. Routledge, New York, NY (2003)

Capron G.: Accessibility for'modern urban public spaces' in Latin- American cities: Physical appearances and socio-spatial pertinences. Paper presented at a conference on Rights to the city, Rome, May 2002

Crossa, V.: Play for protest, protest for play: artisan and vendors' resistance to displacement in Mexico city. Antipode **45**(4), 826–843 (2013)

Harvey, D.: The right to the city. Int. J. Urban Region. Res. **27**(4), 939–941 (2003)

Kirumirah, M.: The Role of Universities in Enhancing Community Outreach Services. A Case of street Vendors' Training in Dar es Salaam (Master's Thesis). University of Dar es Salaam September, 2018, Dar es Salaam (2018)

Kisembo, P.: Order not to evict hawkers, vendors confuses officials. The Citizen, 27 February (2017). http://www.thecitizen.co.tz/News/Order-not-to-evict-hawkers-vendorsconfuses-officials/1840340-3830627-c99fnlz/index.html. Accessed 3 May 2017

Lamb, M.: Vernacular Practice and the Emergence of Policy: An Analysis of Trespassing on a Brooklyn Golf Course. Paper presented at a conference on Rights to the city, Rome (2002)

Lefebvre, H.: The right to the city. Writings cities. 63181 (1996)

Lyons, M., Brown, A.: Legal pluralism and development: street-trade and regulatory reformin Tanzania. London South Bank University (2009)

Mahadevia, D., Vyas, S.: Law, regulations and rights of street vendors: Ahmedabad. Ahmedabad, India: Centre for Urban Equity (2012)

Marcuse, P.: From critical urban theory to the right to the city. City **13**(2–3), 185–197 (2009)

Meneses, R.: Out of place, still in motion: Shaping immobility/mobility through urban regulation. Soc. Leg. Stud. **22**(3), 335–356 (2013)

Mitchell, D.: The Right to the City: Social Justice and the Fight for Public Space. Guilford press, New York (2003)

Mramba, N.: The conception of street vending business (SVB) in income poverty reduction. Int. Bus. Res. **8**(5) (2015)

Mramba, N., Sutinen, E., Haule, M., Msami, P.: Survey of mobile phone usage patterns among street vendors in Dar es Salaam city- Tanzania: Int. J. Inf. Technol. Bus. Manage. JITBM. **28**(1) (2014)

Msoka, C., Ackson, T.: The politics and regulation of street trading in Dares Salaam. In: Rebel Streets and the Informal Economy, pp. 183–204. Routledge (2017)

Muiruri, P.: Women street vendors in Nairobi, Kenya: A Situational and policy analysis within a human rights framework. Organization for Social Science Research in Eastern and Southern Africa, pp. 1–23 (2010)

Munishi, E.J., Casmir, R.O.: Overcoming business capital inadequacy and resilience: implications for the urban street vendors' operations in Morogoro municipality. Bus. Educ. J. (BEJ), **1**(1), 1–18 (2019)

Mutarubukwa, P.: The role of entrepreneurship in combating youth unemployment and social crime in Tanzania. Bus. Educ. J. (BEJ), **1**(1), 1–18 (2015)

Nakibuuka, M.: The vulnerable livelihoods of street vendors in Uganda: A case of Kampala Central Division. (Unpublished masters' dissertation) Institute of social studies. The Hague, Netherlands (2016)

Nani, G.V.: A synthesis of changing patterns in the demographic profiles of urban street vendors in Botswana, South Africa and Zimbabwe. J. Prob. Perspect. Manage. **14**(3), 549–555 (2016)

Racaud, S., Kago, J., Owuor, S.: Introduction: Contested Street: Informal Street Vending and its Contradictions. Articulo-J. Urban Res. 17–18 (2018)

Roever, S., Skinner, C.: Street vendors and cities. Urbanization and environment, **28**(2), 1–28 (2016). https://journals.sagepub.com/doi/full/10.1177/0956247816653898

Xue, D., Huang, G.: Informality and the state's ambivalence in the regulation of street vending in transforming Guangzhou, China. Geoforum **62**, 156–165 (2015)

Yin, R.K.: Case study research: Design and methods. Sage publications, Thousand Oaks, CA (2013)

Customers' Satisfaction on Bus Rapid Transit Services in Tanzania: The Servqual Model Perspective

M. A. Mapunda(✉)

Department of Marketing, College of Business Education, P. O. Box 1968, Dar Es Salaam, Tanzania
m.mapunda@cbe.ac.tz

Abstract. As competition becomes intense worldwide, service providers, including Bus Rapid Transit (BRT) need to make service quality improvement as an endless process to satisfy their customers. This is because customers' satisfaction would encourage a modal shift from private motor vehicles to public transport. Currently, the BRT system operates in five African countries including Tanzania. Since it is a new form of mass transit, its ability to provide high-quality transport services remains largely unexplored. Therefore, this study aims at examining customers' satisfaction with Bus Rapid Transit services in Tanzania using the SERVQUAL Model. The study applied a quantitative method using a structured questionnaire. Data were collected from customers who use BRT services in Dar Es Salaam, Tanzania from five BRT's bus terminals. 200 respondents were randomly selected, and the data was analyzed using multiple linear regression models through SPSS version 25. The findings revealed that customers were somehow satisfied but some elements need to be improved. Responsiveness, reliability, and tangibility significantly influence customers' satisfaction while assurance and empathy were not. The value of $R^2 = 0.474$ was significant at $P < 0.001$, and all five service quality dimensions had positive beta coefficients with an overall dominance of the responsiveness dimension. This study is important as the results will provide insights into the customers' satisfaction in relation to the Bus Rapid Transit services. Besides, the study's findings will help the decision-makers and BRT's planners to focus on the service quality dimensions which are found to be significant in enhancing customers' satisfaction. This could improve public transport and reduce the use of private cars in the city.

Keywords: Customers' satisfaction · SERVQUAL · Bus Rapid Transit · Dar Es Salaam · BRT · UDART · Tanzania

1 Introduction

Customer satisfaction is one of the essential aspects of a business's success in the world. It is a person's feeling of pleasure or disappointment resulting from comparing the perceptions and expectations (Kotler 1997). Customers feel satisfied when a product or

J. N. Mojekwu et al. (Eds.): *Sustainable Education and Development*, pp. 194–208, 2021.
https://doi.org/10.1007/978-3-030-68836-3_18

service meets or goes beyond their expectations, otherwise, they are dissatisfied. There are some benefits related to customer satisfaction which include but are not limited to: customers' retention, customers' attraction, customers' trust-building as well as good corporate image portrayal (Mulatsih et al. 2017). From the benefits obtained, Chatzoglou et al. (2014) suggested that due to intense global competition, service providers need to make service quality improvement as an endless process to satisfy their customers. This is because customers' satisfaction would encourage a modal shift from private motor vehicles to public transport (Ojo 2017). In addition, the use of public transport would reduce wastage of time, air pollution, accidents, and increase economic health (Kumar et al. 2016). Therefore, there is a need to measure service quality for public transport to enhance customer satisfaction. Li (2016) advised that customer satisfaction is the mainly used approach for observing and measuring the quality of public transport services such as the Bus Rapid Transit (BRT).

According to the BRT Global Report, the BRT system operates in 172 cities worldwide, but only in five cities in Africa (BRT 2020) including Tanzania. In most countries, BRT was adopted as one of the public transportation developments to overcome traffic problems and congestion (Feye et al. 2014). Empirical evidence also shows that BRT is considered to be a high-capacity public means of transport that can operate within a short period and at low expenses (Velásquez et al. 2017; Cao et al. 2016). Despite the BRT being a modern form of public transport, Chandrakumara (2014) identified that bus transport remains extremely criticized by customers in terms of quality. Thus, the quality evaluation of the BRT services from customers' perception is very important since it gives direction on what needs to be rectified based on received criticisms (Aquino et al. 2018).

Customers' evaluation of service quality is based on various attributes as proposed by various scholars (Aquino et al. 2018; Iran-Nejad-Parizi and Khedmati 2016; Nelloh et al. 2019; Ugo 2014). For instance, Aquino et al. (2018) used fluency in the provision of services, staff training, physical conditions, convenience or accessibility, and integration between transport lines. In a study of Iran-Nejad-Parizi and Khedmati (2016) the attributes include physical, reliability, responsiveness, assurance, and empathy. Nelloh et al. (2019) mentioned the space of individual customer during the trip, vehicle conditions and maintenance, ticket line services, staffs' skills, information provision, social environment, safety, off-board services, and waiting time. In another study by Ugo (2014) the attributes include transport fare and accessibility of ticket sales outlets.

1.1 Problem Statement

Customer satisfaction is one of the essential aspects of any business success in the world including BRT. It could result in customers': retention, attraction, trust-building as well as good corporate image portrayal (Mulatsih et al. 2017). On the other hand, measuring service quality from the customer's perception is very important. As it is argued by Aquino et al. (2018) that the assessment of the BRT's services quality from customers' perception is very significant as it gives direction on what needs to be rectified based on received criticisms. Despite the importance of customers' satisfaction on the BRT services, there are few studies in the developing countries as identified by various scholars (Iran-Nejad-Parizi and Khedmati 2016; Cao et al. 2016). Similarly, Poku-Boansi et al. (2018) noted the slow adoption of BRT in African countries compared to South America and Southeast Asia. Besides, as the BRT being a new form of mass transit in Tanzania, its ability to provide quality transport services in the country remains largely unexplored. Therefore, this study aimed at examining customers' satisfaction on the Bus Rapid Transit services in Tanzania using the SERVQUAL model by (Parasuraman et al. 1988). The selection of this model has been justified by Izogo and Ogba (2015) that service quality dimensions are significant predictors of customers' satisfaction. Thus, the constructs from the SERVQUAL model are being used in this study to formulate objectives and hypotheses.

1.2 Aim

This study aimed at examining customers' satisfaction with Bus Rapid Transit services in Tanzania.

1.2.1 Specific Objectives

i. To find out the relationship between tangibility and customers' satisfaction on BRT services in Dar Es Salaam, Tanzania;
ii. To ascertain the relationship between reliability and customers' satisfaction on BRT services in Dar Es Salaam, Tanzania;
iii. To measure the relationship between responsiveness and customers' satisfaction on BRT services in Dar Es Salaam, Tanzania.
iv. To determine the relationship between assurance and customers' satisfaction on BRT services in Dar Es Salaam, Tanzania.
v. To test the relationship between *e*mpathy and customers' satisfaction on BRT services in Dar Es Salaam, Tanzania.

2 Theoretical Framework

2.1 Service Quality and Customer Satisfaction

Service quality is regarded as a key source of competitive advantage, as it helps in retaining and attracting new customers (Irfan et al. 2016). Similarly, customers' satisfaction is the outcome of an organization's service quality which either meets or goes beyond their expectations (Izogo and Ogba 2015). Terefe and Singh (2016) suggested that an increase in each service quality dimension is probably lead to an increase in customers' satisfaction.

Various studies have been done worldwide to show the importance of assessing service quality from customer's perception using service quality attributes. For instance, Aquino et al. (2018) did a study on factors influencing BRT service quality in Brazil. Their findings revealed that fluency in the provision of services, staff training, physical conditions in the provision of services, convenience or accessibility, and integration between transport lines significantly influenced customers' satisfaction. Similarly, Iran-Nejad-Parizi and Khedmati (2016) evaluated the BRT transport system among citizens of Tehran city in Iran. Their findings showed that physical, reliability, responsiveness, assurance, and empathy significantly influenced customers' satisfaction who use the BRT services in Tehran city.

Furthermore, Nelloh et al. (2019) researched factors that enhance travel satisfaction and loyalty among customers using BRT services in Indonesia. Their findings revealed that customers' were satisfied with the space of individual customers during a trip, vehicle conditions and maintenance, ticket line services, and staff skills. On the other hand, customers' were not satisfied with information provision, social environment, safety, off-board services, and waiting time. Moreover, Ugo (2014) did a survey study to assess service quality dimensions of the BTR on customers' satisfaction in South Africa in the city of Cape Town. The findings revealed that customers were not satisfied in the area of transport fare and accessibility of ticket sales outlets.

The empirical literature reveals that the service quality attributes which contribute to customers' satisfaction on BRT services vary across the countries. For instance, Nelloh et al. (2019) findings revealed that among other attributes customers' were satisfied with ticket line services, on BRT services in Indonesia. On the other hand, Ugo (2014) found that customers were not satisfied in the area of accessing ticket sales outlets on BRT services in South Africa in the city of Cape Town. Given this disparity, thus, there is a need for examining customers' satisfaction on the Bus Rapid Transit services in Tanzania.

2.2 The SERVQUAL Model

The study adopted a SERVQUAL model proposed by Parasuraman et al. (1988). This model has been widely used in assessing service quality. The original SERVQUAL had ten dimensions of service quality and were applied in the different service contexts (Parasuraman et al. 1985). Further, the ten dimensions were refined to produce a multi-item measurement scale which covers five dimensions of service quality which are: Tangibles, Reliability, Responsiveness, Assurance, and Empathy (Parasuraman et al. 1988).

2.2.1 Tangibility

Tangibles include physical facilities, equipment, and staff appearance (Parashurama et al. 1988). Previous studies reveal that tangibility significantly influences customers' satisfaction in using public transport services. For instance, the study by Bakti et al. (2018) revealed that there is a significant positive relationship between tangibility and customers' satisfaction in using public transport services. Scholars in different geographical locations considering different sectors found that tangibility is an important factor in influencing customers' satisfaction (Badarch and Zanabar, 2017; Shah et al. 2018). Thus, leading to the hypothesis.

H1: *Tangibility has a positive significant relationship with customers' satisfaction on BRT services in Dar Es Salaam, Tanzania.*

2.2.2 Reliability

Reliability is the ability of a service provider to maintain the operation schedule as promised and accurately (Kalokola 2019). Its attributes include the amount of public transport, waiting, and travel time, as well as the consistency of delivering public transport (Ojo 2017). The past studies by several scholars found that reliability significantly influences customers' satisfaction in using public service transport (Quddus et al. 2019; Aquino et al. 2018). For example, Quddus et al. (2019) findings revealed that reliability has a significant influence on customers' satisfaction in using public transport services. Researchers in different geographical locations and different sectors found that reliability is an important factor in influencing customers' satisfaction (Shah et al. 2018; Badarch and Zanabar 2017). Therefore, the following hypothesis was proposed.

H2: *Reliability has a positive significant relationship with customers' satisfaction on BRT services in Dar Es Salaam, Tanzania.*

2.2.3 Responsiveness

Responsiveness refers to the readiness of the service provider to assist customers in delivering prompt service (Ulkhaq et al. 2019). Previous studies reveal that responsiveness significantly influences customers' satisfaction in using public transport services. For instance, the study by Sam et al. (2018) found that there is a significant positive relationship between responsiveness and customers' satisfaction in using public transport services. Some scholars researched other than service sectors their findings showed that responsiveness is an important factor in influencing customers' satisfaction (Badarch and Zanabar 2017; Shah et al. 2018). Thus, leading to the hypothesis.

H3: *Responsiveness has a positive significant relationship with customers' satisfaction on BRT services in Dar Es Salaam, Tanzania.*

2.2.4 Assurance

Assurance refers to the knowledge, skills, courtesy, and trustworthiness of the service providers' employees and their ability to convey confidence (Sam et al. 2018). Previous studies reveal that assurance significantly influences customers' satisfaction in using public transport services (Nelloh et al. 2019; Aquino et al. 2018). For instance, the study by Nelloh et al. (2019) revealed that there is a significant positive relationship between assurance and customers' satisfaction on using public transport services. Scholars in different geographical locations researched on different sectors and their findings showed that assurance is an important factor in influencing customers' satisfaction (Hafiz and Alam 2016; Terefe and Singh 2016). Thus, leading to the hypothesis.

H4: *Assurance has a positive significant relationship with customers' satisfaction on BRT services in Dar Es Salaam, Tanzania.*

2.2.5 Empathy

Empathy means concern, ease of relationship, personal attention given to the passengers to understand their needs (Ulkhaq et al. 2019). Previous research reveals that empathy significantly influences customers' satisfaction in using public transport services (Mishra 2013; Sabir et al. 2014). For instance, the study by Mishra (2013) showed that there is a significant positive relationship between empathy and customers' satisfaction in using public transport services. Scholars in different geographical locations considering different sectors found that empathy is an important factor in influencing customers' satisfaction (Hafiz and Alam 2016; Shah et al. 2018). Thus, leading to the hypothesis.

H5: *Empathy has a positive significant relationship with customers' satisfaction on BRT services in Dar Es Salaam, Tanzania.*

2.3 The Conceptual Model

See Fig. 1.

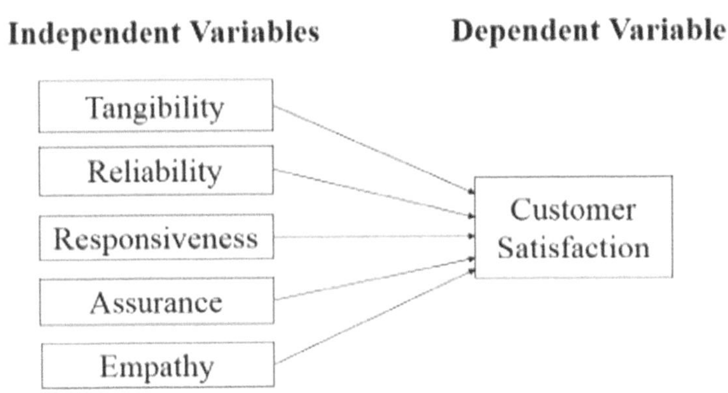

Fig. 1. Conceptual framework. Source: (Sabir et al. 2014; Yao et al. 2014; Minh et al. 2015)

3 Methodology

The study employed a quantitative design through a survey strategy using the SERVQUAL model to understand customer satisfaction in the process of using BRT services. A quantitative design was selected since the study objective was to examine the relationship among variables (Creswell 2014). Similarly, survey strategy was adopted since it is associated with quantitative methods and it is possible to generalize the findings from a sample to a population with minimum costs (Saunders et al. 2012).

The study was conducted in Dar Es Salaam city in Tanzania since it is the pioneer of the BRT service in the country. The target population was customers using BRT services which are operated by Usafiri Dar Es Salaam Rapid Transit (UDART). These were targeted because they are service recipients of the BRT services. According to Dar Es Salaam Transit (DART) passenger ridership data (2019), the population for the first eight months of 2019 was 37,435,866 with an average of 4,679,483 per month.

The simple random technique was used to select participants. The random sampling technique was preferred to reduce biases (Saunders et al. 2012). The study used a sample of 200 respondents who use BRT's services from the five bus terminals: Gerezani, Kimara, Kivukoni, Ubungo, and Morocco respectively.

Data for this study were collected using the questionnaire. The questionnaire was composed of five-point Likert scale items ranging from 1 = "*strongly disagree*" to 5 = "*strongly agree*" for six constructs that were adopted from (Randheer et al. 2011; Izogo and Ogba 2015). The six constructs together with their sample statements were: tangibility "*Inside environment of the bus is clean and hygienic*", reliability "*UDART services are punctual*", responsiveness "*Employees in UDART are always willing to help you*", assurance "*You feel safe in your transactions with UDART*", empathy "*UDART gives attention to pregnant women, children and handicapped*" (independent variables) and Customer satisfaction "*I encourage friends and relatives to use UDART*" (dependent variable). An English questionnaire's version was back-translated from English to Swahili the national language of Tanzania by three independent professional translators to ensure translation equivalence.

The questionnaires were administered by research assistants with the help of DART monitoring unit people who were found in the five listed BRT's terminals. The customers were briefed on the purpose of the study and those who were interested were asked questions and the research assistants were filling in the questionnaires. Data were collected from the first to the third week of August 2019, Monday to Friday during peak hours in the morning and afternoon. A total of 200 structured questionnaires were used, out of which 46 (23%) were incomplete, and 154 (77%) were complete. The incomplete questionnaires resulted because during the questionnaire administration some respondents just left and rushed for their buses.

3.1 Data Analysis

Data were analyzed using the multiple regression model through SPSS version 25 to predict customers' satisfaction based on their perceived service quality dimensions. All assumptions regarding the model were checked before the analysis. Descriptive statistics such as means, standard deviations, and percentages were used to analyze responses from respondents and respondents' demography respectively.

3.2 Ethical Consideration

The research clearance was sought from the relevant authorities including the BRT's management. The interviewers requested respondents' consent first before data collection, then explained the survey and its significance in improving BRT services. Confidentiality and anonymity were also ensured.

4 Results, and Discussions

4.1 Respondents' Demographic Characteristics

The demographic characteristics of the respondents were summarized based on their gender, age, education, and occupation. It revealed that a higher percentage were female (52.6%) compared to males (47.4%). Regarding the respondents' age, the survey revealed that (69.5%) of the BRT service users were between 20–50 years, which, belongs to the working-age group while the remained (30.5%) were above 50 years. In terms of occupation, the results found that (56.5%) of the BRT's service recipients were self- employed followed by (24. %) employed, (9.7%) of students, and others (9.7%) respectively. Concerning education, (18.9%) had primary education, (43.5%) had secondary education, (33.1%) had tertiary education, and (4.5%) informal education. In total (76.6%) of the respondents had formal education ranging from secondary to tertiary level, this could affect how they perceived BRT's service quality.

4.2 Descriptive Analysis

The results in Table 1 show the mean of customers' satisfaction is (M = 2.7549) and the standard deviation is (SD = .40268) which reveals that they are somehow satisfied with the service but some elements need to be improved. Their responses showed uniformity due to small dispersion in the standard deviation value. Tangibility was the highest with a mean score of (M = 3.8458) and a standard deviation of (SD = .57961). The last factor is reliability with a mean score of (M = 2.6607) and a standard deviation of (SD = .68818). Furthermore, Table 1 shows that standard deviation is very less signifying that values are not much dispersed around the mean and hence, the absence of outliers. Thus, the collected data are significant with small chances of errors.

Table 1. Descriptive statistics for service quality dimensions and customer satisfaction

	Mean	Std. Deviation	N
Customer satisfaction	2.7549	.40268	154
Tangibility	3.8458	.57961	154
Reliability	2.6607	.68818	154
Responsiveness	2.9188	.63199	154
Assurance	3.1905	.62953	154
Empathy	3.2955	.57484	154

4.3 Reliability and Validity

The reliability of data collection was computed using the Cronbach's alpha coefficient and the overall survey alpha value was 0.820. Besides, the individual alpha coefficient for each service quality dimension and dependent variable were: 0.717, 0.765, 0.756, 0.631, 0.705, and 0.697, for tangibility, reliability, responsiveness, assurance, empathy, and customer satisfaction respectively (see Table 2). Thus, the Cronbach's alpha value was in the acceptable range (Saunders et al. 2012).

The construct validity for all five service quality dimensions and customer satisfaction were assessed simultaneously using factor analysis in the form of principal component analysis (PCA) with direct rotation for scale items reduction to the cutoff point of 0.5 (Chawla and Sondhi 2016). The sampling adequacy was measured using the Kaiser-Meyer-Olkin (KMO) test and the overall value was 0.853 which is greater than the acceptable limit of 0.5 (Chawla and Sondhi 2016). Similarly, Bartlett's test of Sphericity indicated to be statistically significant with P-value < 0.001 (see Table 1) meaning that, the factor analysis was appropriate for this study. Through the PCA, six components with greater than or equal to one eigenvalue were extracted which fit into six variables (tangibility, reliability, responsiveness, assurance, empathy, and customer satisfaction) with 63.625% of the cumulative variance. The initial eigenvalues for the six components were 7.283, 2.263, 1.702, 1.229, 1.131, and 1.026 respectively (see Table 2).

4.4 Multiple Regression Analysis

The multiple regression model was conducted to predict customers' satisfaction with rapid bus transit using the SERVQUAL model's five service quality dimensions. The dependent variable was customers' satisfaction and the independent variables were: tangibility, reliability, responsiveness, assurance, and empathy (service quality dimensions). As shown in Table 3, the value of the coefficient of determination (R^2) = 0.474 which indicates that 47.4% of the variance in the dependent variable (customers' satisfaction) is explained by all five service quality dimensions (independent variables) at the 95% confidence level. Therefore, the five service quality dimensions can be manipulated to increase customer satisfaction.

From Table 4, the last column indicates that the overall regression model is statistically significant $F(5,148) = 26.713$, $P < 001$.

From Table 5, the second column shows regression coefficients of the independent variables which contribute to customers' satisfaction (dependent variable). The fourth column which has Beta coefficients shows the estimated increase or decrease in the independent variables given by the coefficient of the respective variable. Thus, the responsiveness is increased by 1, customers' satisfaction is estimated to rise by 0.338 (33.8%) if other variables remain constant. The sixth column shows a t-test for the significance of individual independent variables which indicates that tangibility, reliability, and responsiveness were statistically significant at $P < 0.05$. On the other hand, assurance and empathy were not significant. The last column shows the unique contribution of each predictor variable. From this study, the greatest unique contribution is for predictor reliability (0.215) (Table 5).

4.5 Hypotheses Results

H1: *Tangibility has a positive significant relationship with customers' satisfaction on BRT services in Dar Es Salaam, Tanzania.*

Table 2. Reliability and validity of research items

Items	1	2	3	4	5	6
T_1 T_2 T_3 T_4	0.762 0.632 0.773 0.779					
R_1 R_2 R_3 R_4		0.819 0.604 0.797 0.829				
RESP_1 RESP_2 RESP_3 RESP_4			0.787 0.784 0.802 0.670			
ASS_1 ASS_2 ASS_3				0.741 0.780 0.767		
EMP_1 EMP_3 EMP_4 EMP_5					0.713 0.784 0.777 0.633	
C_SAT1 C_SAT2 C_SAT3 C_SAT5						0.796 0.805 0.673 0.620
Eigen Values 1.131	 1.131	7.283	2.263	1.702	1.229	
Variance Explained 4.918	 4.462	31.663	9.840	7.399	5.343	
Total Variance				63.625		
Reliability of factors .705	 .697	.717	.765	.756	.631	
Reliability of the survey				.820		
KMO and Bartlett's Test .853 Kaiser-Meyer-Olkin Measure of Sampling Adequacy Approx. Chi-Square 1461.103 Bartlett's Test of Sphericity df 253 Sig. .000						

In hypothesis one, the study predicted that tangibility has a positive significant relationship with customers' satisfaction on BRT services in Dar Es Salaam, Tanzania. The results confirm the hypothesis by coefficients of Beta ($\beta = 0.166$) and significance level, ($P = 0.009$) which is significant. Also, a positive correlation scores of $r = 0.315$. This indicates that there is a mild positive relationship hence, the hypothesis is supported.

Table 3. Model summary results

Model summary									
Model	R	R square	Adjusted R square	Std. error of the estimate	Change statistics				
					R square change	F Change	df1	df2	Sig. F Change
1	.689[a]	.474	.457	.29683	.474	26.713	5	148	.000

a. Predictors: (Constant), Empathy Tangibility, Reliability, Assurance, Responsiveness
b. Dependent Variable: Customer Satisfaction

Table 4. ANOVA

ANOVA[a]						
Model		Sum of squares	df	Mean square	F	Sig
1	Regression	11.768	5	2.354	26.713	.000[b]
	Residual	13.040	148	.088		
	Total	24.809	153			

a. Dependent Variable: Customer Satisfaction
b. Predictors: (Constant), Empathy, Tangibility, Reliability, Assurance, Responsiveness

Table 5. Regression coefficients results

Coefficients									
Model		Unstandardized coefficients		Standardized coefficients	t	Sig.	Correlations		
		B	Std. Error	Beta			Zero-order	Partial	Part
1	(Constant)	.966	.196		4.939	.000			
	Tangibility	.115	.044	.166	2.645	.009	.315	.212	.158
	Reliability	.163	.045	.279	3.606	.000	.551	.284	.215
	Responsiveness	.215	.063	.338	3.439	.001	.618	.272	.205
	Assurance	.010	.056	.016	.186	.853	.503	.015	.011
	Empathy	.076	.054	.109	1.407	.161	.476	.115	.084

a. Dependent Variable: Customer Satisfaction

These findings corroborate other findings (Badarch and Zanabar 2017; Shah et al. 2018; Sabir et al. 2014) which indicated a positive and significant relationship between tangibility and customers' satisfaction.

H2: *Reliability has a positive significant relationship with customers' satisfaction on BRT services in Dar Es Salaam, Tanzania.*

Table 6. Pearson correlation analysis

		Customer sat	Tang	Reliab	Respo	Assur	Empat
Pearson correlations	Customer Sat	1.000	.315	.551	.618	.503	.476
	Tangibility	.315	1.000	.139	.225	.244	.277
	Reliability	.551	.139	1.000	.590	.583	.376
	Responsiveness	.618	.225	.590	1.000	.696	.619
	Assurance	.503	.244	.583	.696	1.000	.453
	Empathy	.476	.277	.376	.619	.453	1.000
Sig. (1-tailed)	Customer Sat		.000	.000	.000	.000	.000
	Tangibility	.000		.042	.002	.001	.000
	Reliability	.000	.042		.000	.000	.000
	Responsiveness	.000	.002	.000		.000	.000
	Assurance	.000	.001	.000	.000		.000
	Empathy	.000	.000	.000	.000	.000	
N	Customer Sat	154	154	154	154	154	154
	Tangibility	154	154	154	154	154	154
	Reliability	154	154	154	154	154	154
	Responsiveness	154	154	154	154	154	154
	Assurance	154	154	154	154	154	154
	Empathy	154	154	154	154	154	154

Hypothesis two predicts that reliability has a positive significant relationship with customers' satisfaction on BRT services in Dar Es Salaam Tanzania. The results show that reliability has a coefficient of Beta ($\beta = 0.279$) and significance level ($P = 0.000$) which is significant. Also, a positive correlation with scores of ($r = 0.551$). This indicates that there is a moderate positive relationship hence, the hypothesis is supported. These findings are similar to other findings (Shah et al. 2018; Badarch and Zanabar 2017; Yao et al. 2014), which revealed a positive and significant relationship between reliability and customer satisfaction.

H3: *Responsiveness has a positive significant relationship with customers' satisfaction on BRT services in Dar Es Salaam, Tanzania.*

In hypothesis three we predicted that responsiveness has a positive significant relationship with customers' satisfaction on BRT services in Dar Es Salaam, Tanzania. The results show that responsiveness has a coefficient of Beta ($\beta = 0.338$) and significance level ($P = 0.001$) which is significant. Also, a positive correlation with scores of ($r = 0.618$). This indicates that there is a strong positive relationship hence, the hypothesis is supported. These findings are similar to other findings (Badarch and Zanabar 2017; Shah et al. 2018; Sabir et al. 2014) which revealed a positive and significant relationship between responsiveness and customer satisfaction.

H4: *Assurance has a positive significant relationship with customers' satisfaction on BRT services in Dar Es Salaam, Tanzania.*

In hypothesis four we predicted that assurance has a positive significant relationship with customers' satisfaction on BRT services in Dar Es Salaam, Tanzania. The results show that assurance has a coefficient of Beta ($\beta = 0.016$) and significance level ($P = 0.853$) which is not significant. Also, a positive correlation with scores of ($r = 0.503$). This indicates that there is a moderate positive relationship but not significant. Hence, the hypothesis is not supported. The findings differ from that of (Terefe and Singh 2016), which showed a positive and significant relationship between assurance and customer satisfaction. However, the variation may be due to the context as the study was measuring Small and Medium Enterprises' satisfaction in using bank services.

H5: *Empathy has a positive significant relationship with customers' satisfaction on BRT services in Dar Es Salaam, Tanzania.*

In hypothesis three we predicted that empathy has a positive significant relationship with customers' satisfaction on BRT services in Dar Es Salaam, Tanzania. The results show that empathy has a coefficient of Beta ($\beta = 0.109$) and significance level ($P = 0.161$) which is not significant. Also, a positive correlation with scores of ($r = 0.476$). This indicates that there is a moderate positive relationship but not significant. Hence, the hypothesis is not supported. The findings differ from that of (Hafiz and Alam 2016), which revealed a positive and significant relationship between empathy and customer satisfaction. However, the difference may be due to the context since the study was assessing online customers' satisfaction in packaging and delivery services.

5 Conclusion, Implications, and Further Studies

The study assessed customers' satisfaction on Bus Rapid Transit Service in Tanzania using the SERVQUAL model perspective. It specifically used the SERVQUAL model's dimensions to formulate test the hypotheses. Tangibility, reliability, responsiveness, showed a positive and significant relationship with customers' satisfaction while assurance and empathy were not statistically significant.

This study implies that transport planners and decision-makers specifically those working with BRT services should focus on the service quality dimensions which were significant to enhance customers' satisfaction. This could improve public transport and reduce the use of private cars in the city.

The study is expected to make a contribution to the knowledge as little is known about service dimensions influencing customers' satisfaction in BRT services. This study will also add literature on customers' satisfaction on BRT services in general and developing countries' perspective.

The current study used a SERVQUAL model to assess the quality of BRT services based on customers' perception, the future research should consider both perception and expectation to measure the service quality gap using the same model.

References

Aquino, J.T., Souza, J.V., Silva, V.C., Jeronimo, T., Melo, F.: Factors that influence the quality of services provided by the bus rapid transit system: a look for user's perception. Benchmarking Int. J. **25**(6), 4035–4057 (2018)

Badarch, L., Zanabar, A.: Dimensions of hotel service quality in Mongolia. Jurnal Ilmiah Peuradeun **5**(2), 141–156 (2017)

Bakti, I.G., Rakhmawati, T., Damayanti, S., Sumaedi, S., Yarmen, M.: Testing and extending P-transqual public transport service quality model: a causal approach. In: IEEE International Conference on Industrial Engineering and Engineering Management (IEEM), Bangkok, Thailand, 16–19 December 2018. IEEE (2018). https://doi.org/10.1109/IEEM.2018.8607345

BRT: Global BRT Data, from BRT Global Report, 13 January 2020. https://www.brtdata.org/. Accessed 3rd Mar 2020

Cao, J., Cao, X., Zhang, C., Huang, X.: The gaps in satisfaction in transit services among BRT, metro, and bus riders: evidence from Guangzhou. J. Transp. Land Use **9**(3), 97–109 (2016)

Chandrakumara, D.P.: Urban dwellers satisfaction on public bus passengers transport in Sri Lanka. Asian J. Empirical Res. **4**(11), 514–525 (2014)

Chatzoglou, P., Chatzoudes, D., Vraimaki, E., Leivaditou, E.: Measuring citizen satisfaction using the SERQUAL approach: the case of the Hellenic Post. Procedia Econ. Financ. **9**, 349–360 (2014)

Chawla, D., Sondhi, N.: Research Methodology Concepts and Cases, 2nd edn. Vikas Publications, New Delhi (2016)

Creswell, J.W.: A Concise Introduction to Mixed Methods Research, 4th edn. Sage Publications, Calfornia (2014)

Feye, G.L., Evia, P., Benefoh, D.T.: Comparative assessment of success and failure factors for implementation of bus rapid transit system in Accra and Bogota. Term Paper - Doctral Studies, University of Bonn (2014)

Hafiz, N., Alam, A.F.: Applying SERVQUAL model to measure online customer satisfaction in package delivery services. J. Studia Universitatis Babes-Bolyai Negotia **LXI**(4), 121–136 (2016)

Iran-Nejad-Parizi, M., Khedmati, A.A.: Surveying satisfaction among Tehran citizens towars BRT transport system. Int. Bus. Manag. **10**(10), 1793–1798 (2016)

Irfan, M., Shamsudin, M.F., Hadi, N.U.: How important is customer satisfaction? Qualitative evidence from mobile telecommunication market. Int. J. Bus. Manag. **11**(6), 57–69 (2016)

Izogo, E.E., Ogba, I.E.: Service quality, customer satisfaction and loyalty in automobile repair service sector. J. Qual. Reliab. Manag. **32**(3), 250–269 (2015)

Kalokola, C.B.: Assessment of performance of BRT project in Tanzania: a case of Dar Es Salaam. Masters' dissertation, Mzumbe University, Dar Es Salaam (2019)

Kotler, P.: Marketing Management Analysis, Planning, Implementation, and Control, 9th edn. Prentice Hall International Inc., Upper Saddle River (1997)

Kumar, V., Kumar, V., Rao, M.: Preliminary assessment of bus rapid transit system for urban roads. Int. J. Technol. Res. Eng. **4**(3), 439–443 (2016)

Li, C.L.: Better, quicker, together enabling public transport service quality co-monitoring through a smartphone-based platform. Masters' thesis, Massachusetts Institute of Technology (2016)

Mishra, A.K.: Measuring commuters' perception on service quality using SERVQUAL in Delhi metro, pp. 1–30 (2013)

Minh, N.H., Ha, N.T., Anh, P.C., Matsui, Y.: Service quality and customer satisfaction: a case study of hotel industry in Vietnam. Asian Soc. Sci. **11**(10), 73–85 (2015)

Mulatsih, R., Andriyansah, Soesanto, H.: Corporate image of bus rapid transit antecedent customer repurchase. Int. J. Appl. Eng. Res. **12**(18), 7734–7740 (2017)

Nelloh, L.A., Handayani, S., Slamet, M.W., Santoso, A.S.: Travel experience on travel satisfaction and loyalty of BRT public transportation. Asian J. Technol. Manag. **12**(1), 15–30 (2019)

Ojo, T.K.: Quality of public transport service: an integrative review and research agenda. Transp. Lett. **11**(2), 104–116 (2017)

Parasuraman, A., Zeithaml, V.A., Berry, L.L.: A conceptual model of service quality and its implications for future research. J. Mark. **49**(4), 41–50 (1985)

Parasuraman, A., Zeithaml, V.A., Berry, L.L.: A multiple-item scale for measuring customer perception of service quality. J. Retail. **64**(1), 12–40 (1988)

Poku-Boansi, M., Marsden, G.: Bus rapid transit systems as a governance reform project. J. Transp. Geogr. **70**, 193–202 (2018)

Quddus, M.A., Rahman, F., Monsuur, F., de Ona, J., Enoch, M.P.: Analysing bus passengers' satisfaction in Dhaka using discrete choice models. Transp. Res. Rec. J. Transp. Res. Board **2673**, 758–768 (2019)

Randheer, K., Al-Motawa, A.A., Vijay, J.P.: Measuring commuters' perception on service quality using SERQUAL in public transportation. Int. J. Mark. Stud. **3**(1), 21–34 (2011)

Sabir, R.I., Javed, S., Ahmed, W., Noor, N., Munir, H.M.: Assessing customer satisfaction level of transport services using SERQUAL: a case of Daewoo Express, Pakistan. J. Basic Appl. Sci. Res. **4**(2), 207–213 (2014)

Sam, E.F., Hamidu, O., Daniels, S.: SERVQUAL analysis of public bus transport services in Kumasi metropolis, Ghana: core user perspectives. Case Stud. Transp. Policy **6**(1), 25–31 (2018)

Saunders, M.N., Lewis, P., Thornhill, A.: Business Research for Business Studies, 6th edn. Pearson Education Ltd., Harlow (2012)

Shah, S.N., Jan, S., Baloch, Q.B.: Role of service quality and customer satisfaction in firm's performance: evidence from Pakistan hotel industry. Pak. J. Commer. Soc. Sci. (PJCSS) **12**(1), 167–182 (2018)

Terefe, T., Singh, A.: The relationship between service quality and corporate customers' satisfaction with commercial banks working in Ethiopia. Int. J. Commer. Manag. Res. **2**(1), 8–13 (2016)

Ugo, P.D.: The bus rapid transit system: a service quality dimension of commuter uptake in Cape Town, South Africa. J. Transp. Supply Chain Manag. **8**(1), 1–10 (2014)

Ulkhaq, M.M., Ardiani, A.J., Farhan, M., Bagja, R.P., Hanif, R.Z.: Service quality analysis of bus rapid transit: a case in Semarang, Indonesia. In: 4th International Conference on Intelligent Transportation Engineering (ICITE) (2019)

Velásquez, J.M., Tun, T., Hidalgo, D., Ramos, C., Guarda, P., Guo, Z., Chen, X.: Bus rapid transit in China: a comparison of design features with international system. Working paper, World Resources Intitute, Washington DC (2017)

Yao, L., Siali, F., Bin Darun, M.R., Ismail, M.F.: Service quality and customer satisfaction: rapid Kuantan in Kuantan Route, Malaysia. In: SOCIOINT 14-International Conference on Social Science and Humanities, Istanbul, Turkey, 8th–10th September 2014 (2014)

Evaluating Customers' Satisfaction of Service Quality of State-Owned Transport Company: A Case of Kano State Transport Authority (Kano Line), Nigeria

J. A. Ojekunle(✉), S. D. Ibrahim, M. S. Oluwole, and A. S. Owoeye

Department of Transport Management Technology, School Entrepreneurship and Management Technology, Federal University of Technology, Minna, Niger, Nigeria

Abstract. Customers satisfaction and service quality are critical to the business survival of transport organisation. This is why this study attempts to examine the total customer satisfaction together with service quality of the inter-city transport service of Kano State Transport Authority, Nigeria. The data used for this study was obtained through the administration of 210 questionnaires to passengers at KSTA Loading Terminal using simple random sampling technique. The SERVQUAL model was adopted for measuring and management of service quality across different service contexts. Seven dimensions of service quality were used, these include; tangibility, reliability, Empathy, Responsiveness, Safety Comfortability and Assurance. After the analysis, the result shows that, the average mean score of 3.34 was calculated for customer level of satisfaction, which infers that users are fairly contented with the transport services rendered by KSTA. In terms of perception of quality of service of KSTA, the customer average mean score of 3.62 was calculated, implying that the customers perceptions of the quality of service of KSTA is moderately high. The findings also divulge that the satisfaction of Customer is meaningfully interrelated to all the dimensions of quality of service of satisfaction, reliability, responsiveness, assurance, empathy and tangible. Based on these findings, some specific measures that touch on improved vehicle maintenance management practices, passenger care, service reliability and effective service monitoring and regular feedback mechanism are recommended.

Keywords: Service quality · Customer satisfaction · Public transport

1 Introduction

Passenger transport service can be either intra-city or inter-city operations, inter-city bus carries travelers over lengthy distances between different metropolis, municipalities, or other populated locations. Conversely, intra-urban buses have regular stops throughout an urban or municipality. Whereas, inter-city buses commonly have only a stop at a Central Business District CBD) in the city, and covers long distances without stopover at all. Inter-city bus operations occur all over the globe and can be operated by public or private

J. N. Mojekwu et al. (Eds.): *Sustainable Education and Development*, pp. 209–223, 2021.
https://doi.org/10.1007/978-3-030-68836-3_19

establishments. Intra-city bus services frequently focus at densely populated urban zones, while inter-city inter-town bus facilities are of prominent values in lightly populated rural location that regularly have slight or no communal transportation. Although, there are other modes of moving people from cities to cities, bus operation remains the most common mean of transporting people between cities, as they can be found in both developed and developing countries (Ojekunle 2014).

One of the critical issues in public transport is service quality. The quality of service has implication on customer satisfaction as well as on the level of patronage. As customer satisfaction is low it also brings down patronage level which also adversely affects the revenue of public transport organization (Ojekunle 2014; Kostakis and Pandelis 2009). It is presently a verifiable truth that quality of service influences operational performance of transport organization and its economic fortune. The most unfavorable impact of poor service quality is lack of customer's satisfaction and therefore lack of patronage (Gabriella and Laura 2006).

The advent of globalization has brought about the breakdown of local and national exchange borders whereby markets that were up till now controlled by monopolists have brought competitors. In a new world of economic and business competition, transport organizations have come to understand that consumer loyalty is very important. Organizations that cannot devise means and management strategies that can consistently fulfill client's desire will not survive for a long time in a competitive business environment. The need to for business survival has therefore made many organizations to embrace service quality as a basic goal for survival. In recent times, studies have confirmed that quality of service has an encouraging connection with fulfillment of customer expectation and builds customer loyalty (Juan and Rocio 2014). Quality of service measurement is one of the most imperative real-world themes for service providers and regulatory bodies, but it also remains a formidable research subject. For these reasons, it is significant to recognize quality of service features and to certify their rank and impact on customer deeds (Gabriella and Laura 2006).

In a competitive business world, a large number of public transport operators attempt to enhance their service quality with aim of improving satisfaction of consumer to make them loyal and dedicated to the companies. Accordingly, communal transportation employs its peculiar strategies to improve its unique quality of service. These strategies are what differentiate one public transport organization from the others. Hence, transport operating company can survive compete favorably and remain in business for a wide range of time.

The search for explanation to quality of service rendered by public transport operators in the urban centres has long attracted the attention of researchers in the field of public transportation system. Since the early 1970's researchers have changed their focus away from the traditional studies of purpose and mode of intra-urban transport system to those that effectively capture the developments fundamental to service quality in the light of the existing technology and current planning procedures (Barabino et al. 2012). Moreover, competition among the transport operating organizations has become a kind of survival of the fittest, efforts to remain afloat in business must be vigorously pursued. Due to competition, the customers turn out to be further fastidious and anticipate improved services from service providing establishments. Therefore, the communal transportation company encounters the obstacle of rendering better and strong services to their customers. Therefore, failure to provide this key quality service may put the service provider at a disadvantage to those that can provide a superior service. This necessitates the research in order to provide explicit information that would unravel the main aspects of transport services that impact significantly on the customer satisfaction of public transport operating company.

This study therefore focuses on investigating overall customer satisfaction with service quality level of the inter-city transport service of Kano State Transport Authority (Kano Line). Nigeria.

2 Theoretical and Conceptual Framework

There are many underlying factors which can help our understanding of how to measure service quality. An appreciable list of researchers have produced lists of service quality factors; viz Armistead (1990); and Grönroos (1990) probably provided the best-known determinants emanate from Parasuraman et al. (1985). They provided a list of ten factors that determine service quality; which include communication, access, courtesy, competence, responsiveness, credibility, reliability, tangibles security and understanding. However, a high degree of correlation has been found to exist among courtesy, communication, credibility competence, and security, and between understanding and access (Robert 1997). Hence, they have been combined into two broad dimensions of assurance and empathy. Robert, then collapsed them into five scopes of tangibility, responsiveness, reliability, empathy and assurance as the indicators of measuring their quality of service.

SERVQUAL indicators as observed in Parasuraman et al. (1988) and Zeithaml et al. (1990), vary in their relative importance from a service company to anothers, but they have confidence in that the major factors of quality of service in many (if not all) consumer service company are encompassed in their list. However, in transport business, there other important factors of service quality which must he included these include safety and comfortability of the customers which were not explicitly captured in the Parasuraman et al. (1988) work.

3 Conceptual Issues

3.1 The MORI Model of Customer Satisfaction

Figure 1 depicts MORI Model of Customer Satisfaction, five major determinants of satisfaction in the public service have been identified, these are: 'Delivery', 'Timeliness', 'Information', 'Professionalism' and 'Staff Attitude'. Delivery infers that the service is rendered to customers while dealing with any down to earth issues that may emerge. Timeliness implies that the service is quickly given to the customers. Information implies that regardless of whether the data supplied to customers is accurate and far reaching. Professionalism discusses the capability and cleverness of worker in giving the service. Lastly, worker dispositions allude to the degree to which frontline staff are eager to offer approachable, obliging and empathetic service to customers.

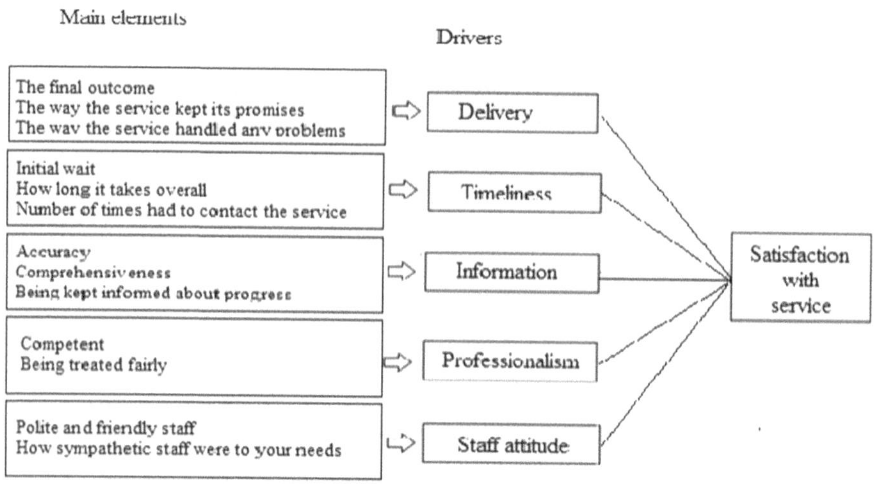

Fig. 1. Conceptual framework Source: MORI, (2004) and (2010)

However, beyond the variables identified by Mori's model of service quality, there are other factors that are key to measuring transport service; they include the comfort and safety of the customers. The level of passenger comfortability and safety are also considered important in evaluation transport service which are part of the consideration in this study. This is represented in Fig. 2 below.

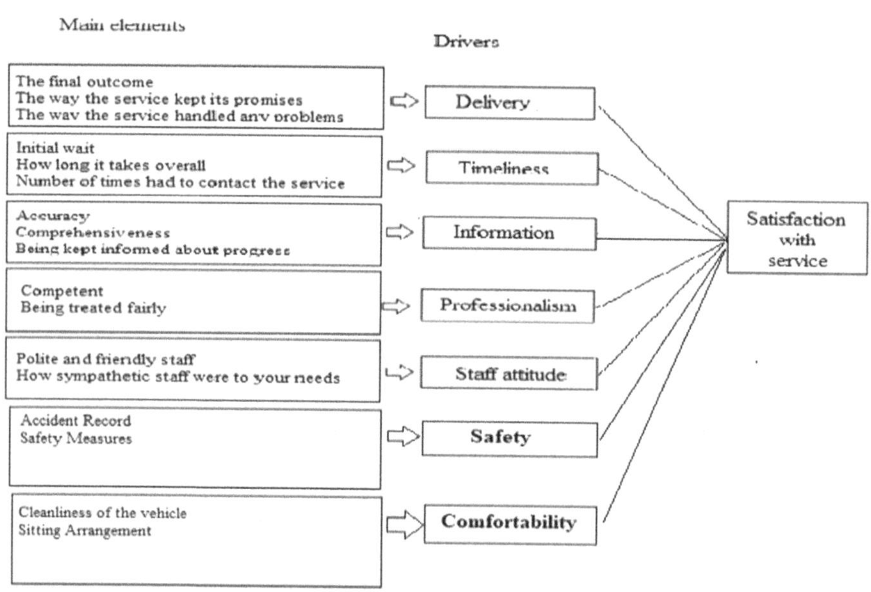

Fig. 2. Transport service quality measures. Source: Modified by the Author

4 Empirical Issues

Quality of service is considered as of the key factors of competitive benefit, as it assists to retain and charm customers. According to Shin and Kim (2008), and Cronin and Taylor (1992) quality of service is related with loyalty and satisfaction of customer. This correlation has been long-established, and researches have demonstrated the encouraging relationship between quality of service and satisfaction of customer, which ultimately result to loyalty of customer (Rashed and Abadi 2014; Santouridis and Trivellas 2010; Kim et al. 2004; Deng et al. 2009). Furthermore, quality of service is involved as an autonomous variable in forecasting loyalty of customer.

Generally, transport service organizations have focusing too much on profit gain and ignoring quality of service; they are basically cost efficient and cost effective oriented instead of service oriented. A degree of cost efficient is classically defined as rendered services (e.g. vehicle-kilometres), whereas, a degree of service effectiveness is defined as expended service (e.g. passenger-kilometres). Figure 3 illustrates the relationship between cost efficient and cost effectiveness. Nonetheless, transport operating bodies essentially do put concentration in obtaining a level quality of service that is high, considering travelers' primacies and necessities (El-Geneidy et al. 2007). For this reason, there is the need to use methods that can help to recognize the reputation of quality of service features on universal satisfaction clients as well as assessing quality of service.

From the reviewed publications, many methods that have been developed to quantify quality of service and satisfaction of customer of communal transport organizations just as in other service companies. These methods are grounded on patron evaluations. The appraisal of quality of service and satisfaction of customer can be gained in diverse means: by questioning customers of their observation or satisfaction on quality of service, by questioning the expectation or importance, or by questioning both observation and expectation. Furthermore, observation can be related with the zone of tolerance of expectations; this is defined as the range between the maximum desired level and minimum acceptable level of expectations (Figini 2003). A rating or ranking of each service features can be requested from patrons.

Govender and Qi (2011) observed that the inter-city bus service seems to offer safer, more cost effective and calm transport service than other alternative means of transportation in the cities. In spite of that they still observe there is great potential for improving service quality in order offer better service to its patrons. Therefore, giving consideration to quality of service could attest to make this approach of travel the ideal choice of travelling for local as well as international tourists. Litman (2015). Also, they discovered that luxury and suitability of travel environments has substantial straight and subsidiary influences on health, wealth and pleasure of customers.

The rapid urbanization and high rate of population growth with attendant traffic overcrowding and lessening regulation of communal transportation in many cities in developing countries compel majority of people in developing world to depend mainly on services giving by public transportation system for their movement wants. This further underscore the necessity for safer, more operative and more well-organized transport system, which is indispensable to ensuring satisfactory and reasonable approachability. Moreover, the enduring maintainable growth of livings in the rural and urban areas largely depends on the efficiency of public transport system (Rwebangira and Mounder 1999).

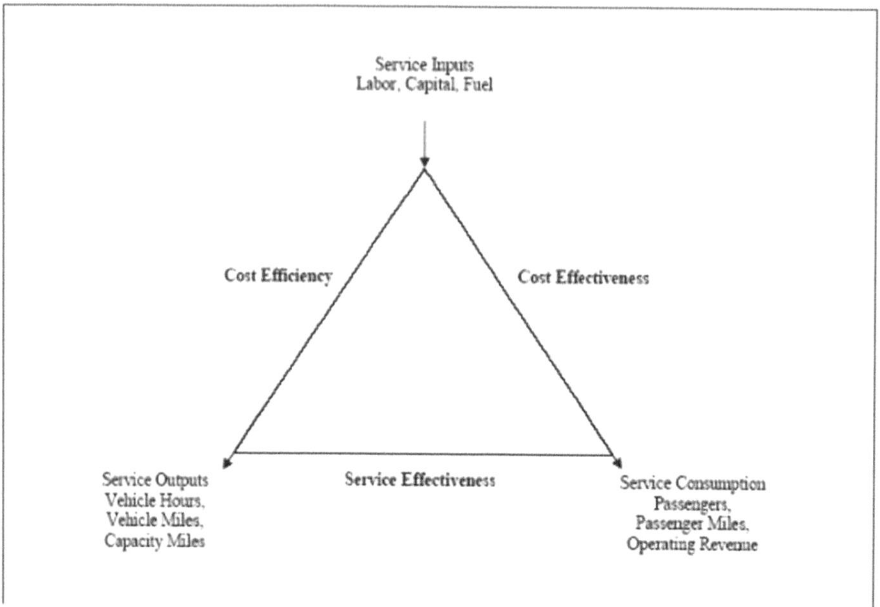

Fig. 3. Relationship between efficiency and effectiveness indicators. Source: Bertini R.L., El-Geneidy A., TRB, 2003.

The cost people are willing to pay for a transport service in order to travel from place to place differs dependent on the category of tour, travel period, traveler's choice and travel circumstances. Travelers always ready to reimburse additional cost or time for more suitability or luxury. For instance, travelers occasionally pay additional for advanced class facility, select slower styles such as trekking and biking since they appreciate the practice, or select a longer transportation path to circumvent transfers (Rwebangira and Mounder 1999).

It was further argued that an enhancement in the quality of service can further fascinate customers of users to the service provided. Base on this, the search to develop systems for measuring and identifying satisfaction of customer is still required. These systems permit the serious parts of the provided services to be acknowledged and satisfaction of customer to be improved (Nakanishi 1997). For transport operating companies for instance, service reliability is considered very vital since both the passengers and the transport service providers value consistent service. Moreover, a correct knowledge of performance evaluation of service can assist customers to be fully involve in the transportation policy and decision-making procedure and give transit operating companies helpful evidence to recognize and examine service difficulties (Nakanishi 1997).

Le-Klahn (2012) discovered that travelers were profoundly happy with Reliability Punctuality, Service Recurrence and Network Connection in the communal transportation while they were disappointed with the workers service, ease at bus stopovers, and the receipt cost. Antonucci et al. (2014) in Italy observed that Waiting Time, Punctuality, Reliability, Regularity, Security, Professionalism, Comfort, Neatness, and Courtesy of staff' were vital elements of passengers' gratification. Having explored a more extensive scope of elements of service in Italy. Barabino et al. (2012), discovered that 'neatness', 'bus reliability', 'recurrence' and 'on-board security', are more vital in deciding the service quality. Kostakis and Pandelis (2009) also uncovered that 'safety', 'service personnel', and 'service inside the bus', 'time', 'availability', 'route precise', and 'route recurrence' are as important service element or attributes that regulate the customer satisfaction of urban transportation in Greece.

Nwachukwu (2014) proved that, in Nigeria, 'comfort' assumed the highest consequence on inclusive satisfaction and seconded by accessibility. The features that followed were 'adequacy' and bus pack amenities'. It was revealed that 'comfort level' and 'waiting-time' as the primary features that move commuters from communal transport service to private automobiles in Dhaka. Kamaruddin et al. (2012) reveals that customer expectation on public transport services mostly depend on users' wellbeing in the Malaysian setting. Nonetheless, it was found that key quality of service fundamentals generally vary among different countries because of differences in social classes and quality of transport system. It was however observed that the priority of quality transportation not a particular transport mode but rather on providing effective transport system that will meet the need of the people. So, travel time, convenience, cost and flexibility are the crucial determinants of user-oriented transportation structure.

5 Methodology

A field survey approach was used to assess quality of service and satisfaction of customer in Kano State Transport Authority. From the operational records of KSTA, a total of 1050 passengers are carried daily. Out of these, 210 passengers were selected randomly from different bus terminals representing 20% of the total study population. The questionnaire survey was carried out at Kano State Transport Authority Loading Terminal. Passengers travelling to and from other cities in the country were the target population. After removing the defective ones, only 197 representing about 94% of the total questionnaire administered were eventually used for the analysis. The SERVQUAL model was chosen vis-à-vis the dimension and management of service quality across different service context. The SERVQUAL model was made up of ten dimensions of service quality these include; communication, tangibility, credibility, reliability, competence, responsiveness, courtesy, security, understanding the customer, and access. The SERVQUAL model is a good gauge for assessing quality of service of different specific industries. Nevertheless, it is appropriate to select the most vital dimension of this model which fit to that specific service being estimated with the goal of guaranteeing dependable and legitimate outcomes. Likewise, this model was utilized because it reflects customers expectation for service and in relation to perception of the service which is greatest ideal method to determine quality of service in the service segment (Shahin 2010). The research employed SERVQUAL to determine quality of service by means of the five paradigms of tangibles, empathy, assurance, responsiveness, and reliability to evaluate satisfaction of customer.

The Cronbach's alpha was adopted to evaluate whether the scale was reliable to measure the internal consistency because the higher the value the better the internal consistency level. Data analysis was carried out by descriptive statistics of Mean scale ranging from 5 (indicating highly satisfied) to 1 (indicting highly unsatisfied). The Product Moment Correlation Analysis was used to measure the type and strength of relationship between the dependent variable (customer satisfaction) and independent variable (service quality dimensions).

6 Findings and Discussion

Table 1. Customers perceptions on service quality

S/N	Factors of service quality	Mean	Std. Deviation	N
1	Comfortability	3.7326	0.87054	197
	Reliability	4.0241	0.92810	197
	Responsiveness	3.5685	0.91035	197
	Assurance	3.3553	0.79259	197
	Safety	3.2969	0.82949	197
	Empathy	3.6814	0.76518	197
	Tangibility	3.6954	0.82196	197
	Overall rating	**3.622**		

Source: Author's Computation (2018)

The mean in Table 1 is an excerpt of the scale of 5 = strongly agree to 1 = strongly disagree. Comfortability and Reliability were measured with three items. Also, Responsiveness, Assurance Dimension and Safety were measured by two items. Similarly, Empathy and Tangible dimension were also measured using four items. In terms of perception of quality of service of KSTA the customer average mean score of 3.622 was calculated from Table 1 which implies that customer perceived that the quality of service of KSTA is moderately high. In assessing customers' satisfaction from the services provided by KSTA, Table 2 depicts the passenger rate statement/items regarding satisfaction.

Six different statements of 5-point Likert scale was employed in the questionnaire to measure Satisfaction. The rating is how satisfied the respondent is with the price? The ratings are 5, 4, 3, 2, 1 which depicts Very Satisfied, Satisfied, Average Satisfied, Unsatisfied, Very Unsatisfied respectively. Also, if the respondent feels secured while traveling with Kano line, it is rated in these ratings 5, 4, 3, 2, 1 which depicts Very Secure, Secure, Average Secure, Insecure, and Very Insecure respectively. Conclusively, the customers were asked if they are happy with the transport service, if they will travel with Kano line again or will recommend Kano line to someone and if the service provided meets respondent satisfaction level.

Table 2 reveals the customers' level of satisfaction according to the adopted variables in relation to satisfaction of customer averagely with scores 3.42, 3.33, 3.43, 3.20, 3.17

Table 2. Customer satisfaction

S/N	Variables of customers satisfaction	Mean	Std. Deviation	N
1	Are you satisfied with the price?	3.4264	0.8695	197
2	Do you feel secured while traveling with Kano line	3.335	0.79504	197
3	Would you travel with Kano line again?	3.4315	0.80915	197
4	Would you recommend Kano line someone	3.2081	0.85853	197
5	Is the waiting time acceptable?	3.1777	0.81059	197
6	Does the service provided by Kano line meet your satisfaction level	3.6447	0.77961	197

Source: Author's Computation (2018)

and 3.64 respectively. Therefore, from the average mean score which is 3.37, by adhering to the scale, the result indicates that customers are generally satisfied with the transport services provided by Kano line.

6.1 Validity and Reliability of the Scale

To evaluate reliability and measure the internal consistency, Cronbach's alpha was employed Higher value of Cronbach's alpha implies that the internal consistency of items from the scale is higher (Nunnaly 1978). Cronbach's alpha is a function of the test items numbers and the average inter-correlation among the items. Conceptually, the formula for the Cronbach's alpha is shown:

$$\alpha = \frac{N \cdot \overline{c}}{\overline{v} + (N - 1) \cdot \overline{c}}$$

From the above equation, N represents equal to the number of items, c-bar represents the average inter-item covariance among the items and v-bar is the average variance.

From the equation, it implies that if you increase the number of items, you increase Cronbach's alpha. Additionally, if the average inter-item correlation is low, it implies alpha will be low. Cronbach's alpha increases as the average inter-item correlation increases as well (holding the number of items constant). From Table 3: Classification of the items based on reliability, responsiveness, assurance, empathy, tangibles and satisfaction was used to measure reliability.

As can be seen from Tables 3, 4, 5, 6 and 7, Cronbach's alphas for Tables 3 and 5 are very low, because they record alphas of less than 0.7 which is considered as the standard (UCLA, Statistical Consulting 2020). This implies service reliability and safety of Kano State Transport Authority are rated low, this is in line with earlier results in Table 1 above. However, Cronbach Alpha result for general customers' rating of staff's Responsiveness and Empathy as well as customers' satisfaction are relatively better as they record Cronbach's Alphas of 0.742, 0.708 and 0.85.

Table 3. Showing Cronbach's Alphaon reliability

Cronbach's Alpha	Items	No of items
0.582	* What is the waiting time of the bus? *Is the waiting time acceptable? * How convenient is the business time of the service? * What is your opinion on the on-time execution of services by Kano line?	**4**

Source: Author's Computation (2018)

Table 4. Showing Cronbach's Alphaon responsiveness

Cronbach's Alpha	Items	No of items
0.742	*Are employer willing to help/answer's customers questions? *Are employer willing to maintain error free records	**2**

Source: Author's Computation (2018)

Table 5. Showing Cronbach's Alpha on assurance

Cronbach's Alpha	Items	No of items
0.644	* How do you rate the safety of the transport service? * Drivers have sufficient driving skills * Personnel in bus station have knowledge and courtesy ascribed to employee's	**3**

Source: Author's Computation (2018)

Table 6. Showing Cronbach's Alphaon empathy

Cronbach's Alpha	Items	No of items
0.708	* How do you rate the handling of passenger's problems? * Do the give passengers personal attention? * Are drivers and conductors consistently polite?	**3**

Source: Author's Computation (2018)

6.2 Relationship Between Satisfaction of Customer and Service Quality Indicators

In this study, Table 8 shows a correlation matrix of both dependent and independent variables the findings of the study indicate that satisfaction of customer is meaningfully proportional to all quality of service scopes of satisfaction, assurance, responsiveness, reliability, empathy and tangible. Also, the result reveals that the relationship between satisfaction of customer and reliability, is high with two variables of $r = 0.704$ and p value

Table 7. Showing Cronbach's Alpha on customers' satisfaction

Cronbach's Alpha	Items	No of items
0.85	* Are you satisfied with the price? * Do you feel secure while travelling with Kano line? *Overall are you happy with the transport service? * would you travel with Kano line again? * Would you recommend Kano Line to someone? * Does the service provided by Kano Line meet your satisfaction level?	**6**

Source: Author's Computation (2018)

Table 8. Pearson correlation between dependent variable and independent variable

Variable	1	2	3	4	5	6
Combine variable for satisfaction	1					
Combine variable for reliability	0.704*					
Combine variable for responsiveness	0.755*	0.798*	1			
Combine variable for assurance	0.731*	0.678*	0.732*	1		
Combine variable for empathy	0.634*	0.632*	0.740*	0.716*	1	
Combine variable for tangible	0.678*	0.616*	0.568*	0.649*	0.599*	1

Correlation is significant at 0.01 level (2-tailed).
Source: Author's Computer Analysis (2018).

of <0.01. This implies that as more consistent services are provided, the more the patrons are satisfied with the services. The result in the Table 8 also indicates that there is a high encouraging correlation between satisfaction of customer and staff responsiveness with correlation coefficient of r = 0.755, at p value of <0.01. This implies that as the company has willingness to help and prompt service to passengers, improves its awareness, the more satisfied customers will be with the services. Consequently, there is a significant association between satisfaction of customer and assurance with correlation coefficient of r = 0.732 and p value of <0.01, which indicates that patron assurance has a profound influence on the satisfaction of customer.

Furthermore, from the Table 8 with correlation coefficient of 'r' = 0.634, with 'p' value <0.01 reveals equally a strong positive relationship between empathy and satisfaction of customer. This implies that the more compassionate the staff are to patrons the more pleased patrons are with the service provided. The result of the analysis also shows that the relationship between tangibility and satisfaction of customer is very significant with correlation coefficient r = 0.678 with p value of <0.01. This implies that the customers are satisfied with the service if the transportation service provider maintains and improves tangible things to be in good state and good-looking.

This study established that out of the five dimensions that were correlated with satisfaction of customer, three dimensions (i.e. Responsiveness, Reliability and Assurance) were very good satisfaction of customer predictors. McDougall and Levesque in 2000 earlier discussed that having knowledge of relative status of each dimension of quality of service can extremely support service contributors to rank their energies and properties and arrange them more successfully to enhance each dimension of quality of service. Consequently, this initial information helps transport operators to activate maximally on those dimensions that bid the extreme prospect to augment loyalty and satisfaction of customer. The outcomes of the research indicate that there is consistency with previous results. In 2011, Aldehayyat, conducted a research on Perception of Service Quality in Jordanian Hotels and evaluated the correlation amongst the quality of service dimensions and satisfaction of customer.

The findings illustrate that statistically the three dimensions of quality of service namely; Responsiveness, Reliability and Assurance have positive significant connection with satisfaction of customer; while the relationship between customers satisfaction on one hand and empathy and tangibility on the other is not very strong. This also was earlier confirmed by Akbaba (2006) who focused his studies on the hotel industry with different five-dimensional structure of quality of service. The findings support the claims that dissimilar procedures should be established for dissimilar service framework and the numbers of quality of service dimensions differ according to the specific package being rendered (Filipa et al. 2010; Thomas et al. 2014; Finn and Lamb 1991; Babakus and Boiler 1992; Bouman and Van der Wiele 1992).

7 Conclusion

One of the best ways of keeping customers' loyalty and patronage in a competitive business environment is having an effective and sustainable communication system amongst service providers and consumers. Now there is a significant indication that customers' perceptions of service quality performance of precise acts are very predictive over their overall satisfactions and readiness to patronize the service again, if desired. It is evident that customers are not satisfied with service frequency of the Kano Transport Authority because their rating of waiting time is very low. The safety and assurance of passenger aspects of the service are also considered below the passenger perception. The above findings will require some policy measures to improve the service quality.

8 Recommendations

The following recommendations were made from the research findings:

i. The Kano Line Transportation service reliability should be enhanced in three folds: Firstly, a constantly aligned set of features, procedures and standards that can define appropriately routing of KSTA vehicles should be established. Secondly, effort should be made to replace policy of equipment and spare parts and consistent maintenance of the KSTA buses. Thirdly, new and emerging technologies such as global positioning or tracking system should be introduced to monitor vehicles movement and drivers while on the roads.

ii. A healthier collaboration with current as well as probable travelers with a opinion to consider their needs more vibrantly should be put in place. Inspections should be carried out frequently and customer criticisms should be taken to cognizance and promptly attended to. Staff needs to be watchful of customer response as well as grievances so that the essential arrangements can be put in place.
iii. There is also need for Kano Line to consider changing their location of their loading points as customers complain a lot about it.
iv. Kano Line should implement an effective vehicle replacement policy by purchasing newer and better vehicles which guarantees good comfort for the passengers.

The study has so far helped our understanding of the way passenger perceive the service quality of state-owned transport operating companies in Nigeria and the aspects of their service that will require improvement from time to time.

References

Akbaba, A.: Measuring service quality in the hotel industry: a study in a business hotel in Turkey. Hospitality Manag. **25**, 170–192 (2006)

Aldehayyat, S.: Perception of service quality in Jordanian hotels. Int. J. Bus. Manag. **6**(7), 226 (2011)

Antonucci, L., Crocetta, C., d'Ovidio, F.D., Toma, E.: Passenger satisfaction: a multi-group analysis. Qual. Quant. **48**, 337–345 (2014)

Armistead, C.G.: Service operations strategy: framework for matching the service operations task and the service delivery system. Int. J. Serv. Ind. Manag. **1**(2), 6–17 (1990)

Babakus, E., Boller, G.W.: An empirical assessment of the SERVQUAL scale. J. Bus. Res. **24**(3), 253–268 (1992)

Barabino, B., Deiana, E., Tilocca, P.: Measuring service quality in urban bus transport: a modified SERVQUAL approach. Int. J. Qual. Serv. **4**(3), 238–252 (2012)

Bouman, M., Van der Wiele, T.: Measuring service quality in the car service industry: building and testing an instrument. Int. J. Serv. Ind. Manag. **3**(4), 4–16 (1992)

Carman, J.M.: Consumer perceptions of service quality: an assessment of the SERVQUAL dimensions. J. Retail. **66**(1), 33–55 (1990)

Cronin, J.J., Taylor, S.A.: Measuring service quality: a re-examination and extension. J. Mark. **56**, 55–68 (1992)

Finn, D.W., Lamb Jr, C.W.: An evaluation of the servqual scales retailing setting. In: NA - Advances in Consumer Research Volume 18, pp. 483–490 (1991)

Deng, Z., Lu, Y., Wei, K.K., Zhang, J.: Understanding customer satisfaction and loyalty: an empirical study of mobile instant messages in China. Int. J. Inf. Manag. **30**, 289–300 (2009)

Kim, M.K., Park, M.C., Jeong, D.H.: The effects of customer satisfaction and switching barrier on customer loyalty in Korean mobile telecommunication services. Telecommun. Policy **28**, 145–159 (2004)

Figini: Evaluating customer satisfaction and service quality. Fransco Milno (2003)

El-Geneidy, A., Horning, J., Krizek, K.J.: Using Archived ITS Data to Improve Transit Performance and Management. Minnesota Department of Transportation Research Services Section (2007)

Filipa, F., Sofia, P., Carlos, B.: Service quality and customer satisfaction in public transports. Int. J. Qual. Res. **4**(4), 125–130 (2010)

Gabriella, M., Laura, E.: A Service Quality experimental measure for public transport, pp. 42–53. University of Calabria – European Transport Faculty of Engineering Department of Territorial Planning (2006)
Grönroos, C.: Service Management and Marketing. Lexington Books, Lexington (1990)
Juan, D.O., Rocio, D.O.: Quality of service in public transport based on customer satisfaction surveys: a review and assessment of methodological approaches (2014). https://doi.org/10.1287/trsc.2014.0544
KajStorbacka, T.S., Christian, G.: Managing customer relationships for profit: the dynamics of relationship quality. Int. J. Serv. Ind. Manag. **5**(5), 21–38 (1994)
Kamaruddin, R., Osman, I., Pei, C.A.C.: Customer expectations and its relationship towards public transport in Klang valley: customer expectations and its relationship using SEM. Procedia-Soc. Behav. Sci. **36**, 431–438 (2012)
Rashed, A.F., Abadi, M.F.: Impact of service quality, trust and perceived value on customer loyalty in Malaysia services industries. Procedia Soc. Behav. Sci. **164**, 298–304 (2014)
Kostakis, A., Pandelis, I.: Measuring customer satisfaction in public transportation: an empirical study based in urban buses in the city of Larissa. The MUSA methodology. NIBES 260–275 (2009)
Le-Klahn, D.: Measuring tourists' satisfaction with public transport in Munich. Int. J. Bus. Tour. Appl. Sci. **1**(1), 74–83 (2012)
Litman, T.: Transportation Affordability, Evaluation and Improvement Strategies. Victoria Transport Policy institute (2015)
McDougall, G., Levesque, T.: Customer satisfaction with services: putting perceived value into the equation. J. Serv. Mark. **14**, 392–410 (2000)
Nakanishi, J.: Management of transport operations. Transp. Res. Rec. **1735**, 146–168 (1997)
Nunnaly, J.: Psychometric Theory. McGraw-Hill Inc, New York (1978)
Nwachukwu, A.A.: Assessment of passenger satisfaction with intra-city public bus. J. Public Transp. **17**, 99–119 (2014)
Ojekunle, J.A.: Analysis of fare structure and determination of bus operation in Nigerian cities. Int. J. Dev. Soc. **3**(2), 13–21 (2014)
Parasuraman, A., Zeithaml, V., Berry, L.L.: SERVQUAL: a multiple-item scale for measuring consumer perception of service quality. J. Retail. **69**(2 Summer), 193–215 (1988)
Parasuraman, A., Zeithaml, V.A., Berry, L.L.: A conceptual model of service quality and implications for future research. J. Mark. **49**(Autumn), 41–50 (1985)
Johnston, R.: Identifying the critical determinants of service quality in retail banking: importance and effect. Int. J. Bank Mark. **15**(4), 111–116 (1997)
Rwebangira, T., Mounder, D.: Investigating the impact of service quality and customer. Transportation Research Laboratory, Oxford University Press, UK (1999)
Santouridis, I., Trivellas, P.: Satisfaction on customer loyalty in mobile telephony in Greece. TQM J. **22**(3), 330–343 (2010)
Saravanan, R., Rao, K.S.P.: Measurement of service quality from the customer's perspective – an empirical study. Total Qual. Manag. **18**(4), 435–449 (2007)
Shahin, A.: SERVQUAL and Model of Service Quality Gaps: A Framework for Determining and Prioritizing Critical Factors in Delivering Quality Services (2010)
Shahin, A., Samea, M.: Developing the models of service quality gaps: a critical discussion. Bus. Manag. Strategy **1**(1), 1–11 (2010)
Shin, D.D.H., Kim, W.Y.: Forecasting customer switching intention in mobile service: an exploratory study of predictive factors in mobile number portability. Technol. Forecast. Soc. Change **75**(6), 854–874 (2008)
Thomas, K.O., Dauda, S., Rickey, Y.N., Dickson, O.M.: Service Quality and Customer Satisfaction of Public Transport on Cape Coast-Accra Route, Ghana (2014). https://www.researchgate.net/publication/266385664

Tran, T., Kleiner, B.H.: Managing for excellence in public transportation. Manag. Res. News **28**(11/12), 154–163 (2005)
UCLA, Statistical Consulting (2020). https://stats.idre.ucla.edu/spss/faq/what-does-cronbachs-alpha-mean/
Zeithaml, V.A., Parasuraman, A., Berry, L.L.: Delivering Service Quality. Free Press, New York (1990)

Effect of Service Quality of Weights and Measures Agency on Customer Satisfaction in Dodoma City, Tanzania

S. Ibrahim[1] and R. G. Mashenene[2](✉)

[1] Weights and Measures Agency, P. O. Box 266, Dodoma, Tanzania
[2] Department of Marketing, College of Business Education, Dodoma Campus, P. O. Box 2077, Dodoma, Tanzania
g.mashenene@cbe.ac.tz

Abstract. The study investigated the effect of service quality (SQ) on Weights and Measures Agency's customer satisfaction in Dodoma City of Tanzania. Specifically, the study (i) examined service quality gap between expectations and the performance of Weights and Measures Agency (WMA) and (ii) determined the influence of service quality on WMA customers' satisfaction. Across sectional research design was adopted. A sample of 91 respondents was included in a survey. Simple random sampling procedure was used to select WMA customers, and purposive sampling was used to select WMA Staff as key informants. A SERVQUAL Model with five SQ dimensions was adopted. Questionnaire, interview, observation and documentary review were used as data collection methods. Qualitative data were analyzed using content analysis. Descriptive statistics were used to assess SQ gap. The influence of quality of services on WMA customer satisfaction was determined using binary logistic regression model. Findings revealed tangibles, responsiveness and reliability were statistically significant dimensions to WMA customer satisfaction. The study recommends that WMA should strive to improve the aspects of SQ dimensions to enhance customer satisfaction.

Keywords: Service quality · Weights and Measures Agency · Customer satisfaction · SERVQUAL

1 Introduction

Worldwide, the concern of measuring quality of services provided by the Weights and Measures Agencies has become of great concern. For instance, USA established weights and measures departments as fully fledged legal metrology for the aim of tracing and monitoring quality of services provided (Racine 2011). This department was made responsible for ensuring that measurements operate reliably as well as to control quality of the service provided and shields consumers from dishonest operators (Racine 2011). From its conception, metrology was established to spearhead profitable trade and exchanges (Fanton 2019; Savio et al. 2016). In western countries, standardized weights

J. N. Mojekwu et al. (Eds.): *Sustainable Education and Development*, pp. 224–234, 2021.
https://doi.org/10.1007/978-3-030-68836-3_20

and measures, well established regulations and a well-developed set of laws and penalties for breaches have been developed accordingly (GAIN 2019). It has therefore been pointed that legal metrology has brought measurable societal and economic impact following its ability to regulate operating instruments to protect consumers and further it reduces chances for uncertainties of measuring instruments; as the result, it helps to enhanced customer satisfaction (Antwi and Matsui 2018; Filho and Gonçalves 2015).

In African countries, weights and measures as service delivery systems are underdeveloped compared to those in the western countries (Yiridoe 2005). Currently, a few existing studies in Africa have indicated a great concern on weights and measures which is directly connected to growth of profit margins and food security (Antwi and Matsui 2018). Most of the countries in the developing economies are constrained with inadequate government capacity to overcome technical barriers to trade and underdeveloped practices in standardization, weights and measures (RLDC 2014). It has been pointed out that the majority of farmers and marketers use standardized weighing instruments within the locally accessible markets with the aim of ensuring trade transactions are simple to execute whereas transparency, reliability, profits, and distinction of quality are well enhanced (Antwi and Matsui 2018).

In Tanzania, inadequate use of accurate measuring instruments results into a pronounced loss to smallholder farmers which is above 40% of sales per year and consequently consumers pay in excess of 25% to traders operating without standard weighing scales (Bengesi 2018; RLDC 2012). Weights and Measures has been one of government efforts in economic contribution through fair protection of trade in measurements among suppliers and consumers. Some of the measures the government has taken to improve WMA services include; strengthening workforce of the Weights and Measures Agency through recruiting temporally employees, allocating adequate budgets and rebuilding cooperation between the agency and other government machineries including the Tanzania Police Force (RLDC 2014). The Government also has prohibited the use of mechanical scales when buying produces instead digital scales have been prioritized to maximize accuracy. Despite the efforts taken by the government of Tanzania in improving and strengthening WMA, still the quality of services provided by WMA in Tanzania is not satisfactory as indicated by most of the previous studies which concentrated in measuring customer satisfaction and the use of weights and measures. For instance, Bengesi (2018) pointed out that customer dissatisfaction from services was one of the critical problems in a several agencies including Weights and Measures Agency in Tanzania. It has also been pointed out that there is slow improvement in performance of WMA through service delivery (RLDC 2014). The study of Kajungu (2014) when investigating the performance of the Kigoma Weights and Measures Agency on quality of customer service provision revealed unsatisfactory levels of customers resulting from poor customer care. The study of Mhoja (2017) on customer satisfaction of the Weights and Measures agency services in Mbeya city showed high level of customer dissatisfaction due to poor service delivery. The study of Bengesi (2018) pointed out that poor quality of service was one of the weak point of service delivery in the WMA systems. However, most of the current studies in Tanzania which have studied quality of service in WMA have not directly measured the effect of service quality on WMA customers' satisfaction (Bengesi 2018; Mhoja 2017; Kajungu 2014). Therefore, the current study investigated how service quality dimensions of Weight and Measure Agency affect customer satisfaction in Dodoma city in order to fill the knowledge gap that was left unfilled in the previous studies.

2 Theoretical Literature Review

This study was guided by SERVQUAL Model as Parasuraman et al. (1988) developed it. SERVQUAL model is a useful model in measuring quality of services and it has been applied in previous studies (Mashenene 2019). The SERVQUAL model is composed of five dimensions of service quality namely; empathy, assurance, reliability, tangible and responsiveness. The relevancy of SERQUAL model to this study is that both the researcher and the developer of the model intended to measure the service quality dimensions gaps. According to the model, customers before they are served with services, they build up expectations (E) in their minds and after they are served, they evaluate the service they have received and build up some perceptions (P). Therefore, the model suggests that, the difference between perceptions and expectations gives service quality (SQ) (i.e. $SQ = P - E$).

3 Empirical Literature Review

In Tanzania, information on service quality dimensions gaps between expectations and performance specifically for WMA is very limited. Few related studies have been conducted but still knowledge gap exist. For instance, Kajungu (2014) found that provision of customer service and levels of customer satisfaction are low and inadequate. Though the findings in this study depict improvement in revenue collection and financial matter but there was a huge gap between customer service provided and expectations and there were no specific dimensions of service quality which were measured in this study. Temba (2013) revealed that satisfaction of customers and service quality were related in the Tanzania Telecommunications Company Limited. The departure of this study from the current study is that the previous study was not carried to measure quality of services in WMAs. Mhoja (2017) adopted a case study design to investigate factors that influence customers' satisfaction on services provided by the Weights and Measures Agency. The study indicate that customer satisfaction and service quality are interlinked variables with a positive relationship between them. However, such a study did not employ SERQVUAL Model to establish service quality dimensions and measure quality of service using such dimensions and their effect on customer satisfaction.

4 Methodology

Cross-sectional research design was employed sine the researcher was constrained with time and financial resources (Yegidis et al. 2018). This study was carried out in Dodoma city which is the city that is growing quickly in Tanzania with exponential increasing need for WMA services to the customers due to increasing population in Dodoma city which has emanated from the government decision to shift its operations from Dar es

Salaam to Dodoma. The population of the study was staff and customers of WMA in Dodoma city. WMA Dodoma office has only nine (9) staff of which one of them is a regional Manager (WMA monthly reports 2018–2019). The target population in this study as stated herein, is WMA customers especially those who are doing business by using measuring instruments. According to WMA monthly reports (2018–2019), there are 2,248 WMA customers in Dodoma City. A multistage sampling was used in this study. Dodoma city as the study area was selected purposefully. Furthermore, wards and streets in which the study was conducted were also selected purposefully. The list of 2,248 WMA customers with weighing instruments for the period of one year and above was obtained from WMA office in Dodoma city. From WMA customers, an nth term (selection interval) was computed using the formula N/n (whereas N = population and n = sample size). Using systematic sampling final respondents were selected whereas the first respondent was randomly selected. To select key informants, purposive sampling was used because key informants were believed to be the WMA staff with a lot of information relevant to the study. The sample size used in this study was obtained by Slovin's formula (Muhoja 2017).

$$n = \frac{N}{\left(1 + Ne^2\right)} \tag{1}$$

$$= \frac{2248}{\left(1 + 2248 \times 0.1^2\right)} = 91$$

Where,
n = Sample size,
N = Total population and
e = Standard error (10%)

For this study, the desired margin of error (α) was 10%, and in our prior judgment it was hypothesized that majority (at least 50%) of customers that were satisfied with the service quality provided by the Weights and Measures Agency and the value of z = 1.966 (statistical tables at $\alpha = 0.1$ or 10%). Qquestionnaire, interview and observation methods were employed in collection of data from primary sources. Both closed and open-ended questions were used. 5-point likert-scale questions were used to capture customer's perceptions on quality of WMA services and customer satisfaction. Many previous related studies had used 5-point Likert scale questions to capture customer perceptions (Mashenene 2019). Before data collection, questionnaire was pre-tested in order to be able to omit questions which would not yield the required responses and which would be difficult to be comprehended by respondents. In addition, pre-test helped to add the missing questions, which were important to the study. Questionnaire for this study consisted of sections including demographic characteristics, a set of questions measuring customer perceptions and expectations. Also, the questionnaire consisted of questions in 5-point Likert scale measuring customer satisfaction. Interview method was used to capture detailed data from key informants. Every staff was interviewed separately by using the same questions in order to avoid undue influence. Each interview took 10 min in average, although the interview with Regional Manager took 22 min. Before interview session, consent to record was given from each interviewee. Data were recorded using notebook and some were recorded using mobile phone. In some special observable circumstances, observation method was used to collect the required data. Observation kit consisting of necessary data to be collected was prepared. Observation kit consisted issues of interest to be observed such as office space and working standards. Photos of different events were taken using mobile phones and events of interest were recorded using note books. In order to get some of the past useful information, some of the official documents were reviewed such as WMA strategic plan 2013–2018, 2018–2023, WMA monthly reports 2018–2019 and Weights and measures Act Cap 340 (RE: 2002).

Qualitative data were analysed using content analysis. During content analysis, recorded data in notebook and mobile phone were transcribed into text and later relevant themes were formulated. Thereafter, the qualitative findings were matched with the existing theory and literature elsewhere and were discussed intensively to bring the intended results. Quantitative data were analyzed using both descriptive and inferential statistics. To examine service quality dimensions' gap between customer expectation and performance of Weights and Measures Agency, the difference of means between customer perception (P) and expectation (E) for each dimension was computed. During the analysis, 5 – point Likert scale responses were computed into means. The difference of means between perceptions and expectations was computed as hereunder;

$$\mathrm{SQ} = \mathrm{P} - \mathrm{E} \tag{2}$$

Where by: SQ = Quality of services
P = Perceived value
E = Expected service

Then, the sum of P – E was divided by the number of items in each dimension in order to get the index score for each SQ dimension. Finally, the sum of all SQ index scores was computed and divided by the total number of SQ dimension (5 SQ dimensions). To determine the influence of service quality dimensions on WMA customer satisfaction, binary logistic regression model (BLRM) was employed. The reason for using BLRM was that the dependent variable (customer satisfaction) was treated as dummy variable. Dummy variable of customers' satisfaction was created using the criteria that the scores above the mean score were treated as 1 = dissatisfaction, 0 = satisfaction for scores below the mean. In treatment of independent variable, factor analysis was performed to establish index score for each service quality dimension. The 5 – point Likert scale responses of independent variables were subjected to factor analysis and the variable which had higher loading factor was considered for further analysis in the binary logistic regression model since each loading factor was treated as an index score. The BLRM was presented using the formula;

$$\mathrm{Y} = \frac{P_i}{1 - P_i} = \beta_0 + \beta_1 Ta + \beta_2 Re + \beta_3 Rs + \beta_4 Em + \beta_5 As + \varepsilon \tag{3}$$

Where;
Ta = Tangibles
Re = Reliability
Rs = Responsiveness
As = Assurance
Em = Empathy
ε = Error term and
Y = Service quality (SQ)

To assess the challenges facing WMA during service delivery, descriptive statistics through multiple responses were employed whereas per cent of cases for each challenge was established and presented in a table. Ranking of challenges using per cent cases was carried out in order to present severity of the challenges under the study.

5 Findings and Discussion

5.1 Service Quality Gap

The findings presented in Table 1 indicate that all service quality dimensions and their overall index for SERVQUAL model scored negative values, suggesting that WMA customers' perceptions on the quality of service provided was lower than their expectations.Generally, negative scores in all service quality dimensions and the index of the overall SERVQUAL model suggest that customers are dissatisfied with the service Quality offered by WMA. The ranking based on the magnitude of dissatisfaction revealed that responsiveness was ranked number 1 (−1.9228). This means that WMA customers had more expectations on responsiveness than the perceived response. That is, they expected that WMA officers are never too busy to save them, will give them prompt service and work on their complaints immediately. The findings of the current study are in harmony with (Akhlaghi et al. 2012) which pointed out that the most outstanding gap in service quality dimension was responsiveness but somehow different in the least one which was reliability while in this study the least was assurance. These results are almost the same as that of (Ibarra et al. 2017) which found that responsiveness was ranked number two; this was among the highly ranked dimension of service quality. These results are also supported by qualitative results from one of WMA customers who exhibited:

"*…I came in your office more than twice, I was first told that you are in Mpwapwa, when I came again, I was told that you left to Mrijo and today I am told you are here at Kikuyu verifying traders measuring instruments. It is now about two months I am not using my weighing scale*". Interview with WMA customer on 7th April, 2019.This qualitative finding reveals that WMA officers are too busy to give prompt service to their customers.

Empathy was ranked number 2 (−1.8821), implying that WMA customers had high expectations on empathy, especially on the affordability of the Government stamping fees. These results are different from that of (Mashenene 2019) which revealed that that empathy was ranked the fourth dimension in terms of service quality. These results are supported by the qualitative evidence from one of the WMA customers from Hombolo who exhibited:

"...I have brought this weighing scale, you said it is correct within the limits of error, why should I pay such big amount of money? Why don't you give discount...?" (WMA customer complained on 18 April 2019).

Reliability was ranked number 3 (−1.6768), which implies that customer expectation was not met by WMA officers in terms of reliability. These results are different from that of (Mbise 2015) which found that reliability was ranked number 1 (−1.404). The results are further supported by qualitative results from one of the customers who narrated;

"...they sometimes come to verify my scale once in a year, but last year they did not show up maybe they will come this year...." (claimed by the WMA customer at Ihumwa Ward on 19 April 2019.

Tangibles were ranked number 4 (−1.5772) which means that although the tangibles in WMA Dodoma office are not sufficient to impress the customers they are not as bad as like the first three service quality dimensions discussed above. These findings are quite different from that of Dehghan (2006) which found that all respondents were satisfied with the tangibles. The least service quality dimension was assurance, which was ranked number 5 (−1.2561). The negative value in assurance implies that WMA customers were not satisfied by the way they are handled by WMA staff in terms of knowledge, courtesy and confidence with the services they have been giving to the customers. These results were in harmony with that of Green (2014) which found that students had higher expectation in assurance than the perceived performance. Findings in general show that, the overall index score of service quality was −1.663, these results were consistent with those of Mashenene (2019) which indicated that customers were not satisfied with the quality of service provided by the College of Business Education with the overall index score of −0.634. Moreover, these results revealed that most of the customers had more expectations than what the service provider could offer. This was also revealed by (County 2016) who found that the overall index score was negative (−1.611), and all the individual scores of the five service quality dimensions were negative implying that customers had higher expectation than the perceived performance.

Table 1. Service quality dimensions gap score (n = 82)

Dimensions	Perceptions (P)	Expectations (E)	P – E	Rank
Responsiveness	1.9065	3.8293	−1.9228	1
Empathy	2.0244	3.5691	−1.8821	2
Reliability	1.9512	3.6280	−1.6768	3
Tangibles	1.9959	3.5732	−1.5772	4
Assurance	2.3130	3.9065	−1.2561	5
Overall gap score			**−1.6630**	

6 The Influence of Service Quality Dimensions on Customers Satisfaction

6.1 Findings from Binary Logistic Regression

At the beginning, some tests were performed to test if data fitted well into the binary regression model. These tests included Hosmer–Lemeshow (H–L) Test. The test for H–L was designed by their creators as a Goodness of Fit (GOF) test to assess the differences between the observed and expected or predicted probabilities as categorized across levels of predicted values (Hosmer and Lemeshow 2000). Since the p-value for Chi-square test is not significant (Chi-square = 3.667, p = 0.817), it is here by suggested that there is no enough evidence to support lack of fit of the suggested model in the results, hence, data fitted well in the model. In logistic regression, the lower the value of -2Log Likelihood implies the better fitting of the model (Hosmer and Lemeshow 2000). Also, higher values of Cox and Snell R square and Nagelkerke R square reveal greater model fit though such values are Pseudo values. The results in Table 2 show that the model used in this study contains variability between 44.9% and 59.9%, which is good enough for a model fit in logistic regression. Moreover, the results show -2Log Likelihood value of 64, which is small compared to the hundreds which are not wanted in logistic regression modeling.

Table 2. Findings from binary logistic regression (n = 82)

Service quality dimensions	B	S.E.	Sig.	Exp(β)
Tangibles	−1.618	0.701	0.021	1.198
Reliability	−1.461	0.698	0.036	1.232
Responsiveness	−1.303	0.688	0.058	1.272
Assurance	−0.403	0.672	0.549	1.668
Empathy	−0.725	0.656	0.269	1.484
Constant	2.786	0.742	0.000	16.219
Chi-square = 44.631, p = 0.000				
Hosmer and Lemeshow $-\chi 2 = 3.667$, p = 0.817				
Cox & Snell $R^2 = 0.449$				
Nagelkerke $R^2 = 0.599$				
-2 Log Likelihood = 64.437				

Generally, findings (Table 2) show that service quality dimensions; reliability, responsiveness and tangibles were significant predictors ($p < 0.05$) of customer satisfaction for WMA customers. The findings show that the coefficient of tangibles was negative (−1.618) related to customer satisfaction and significant (p = 0.021) suggesting a unit increase in unimproved tangibles will decrease customer satisfaction by 161.8%. The findings of the current study match Mashenene (2019) which found that tangibles were important attribute of service quality. The coefficient of reliability was negative (−1.461) related to customer satisfaction and significant at (p = 0.036) meaning that a unit increase in unimproved reliability will decrease customer satisfaction by 146.1%.

This further suggests that WMA should empower its staff through training in both professionalism and customer care. These results are similar to that of Nkyami (2016) which found that reliability had significant effect on customer satisfaction compared to tangibility and Empathy. In addition, responsiveness was another service quality dimension which had a negative coefficient of (−1.303) significant at ($p = 0.058$) meaning that a unit increase in unimproved responsiveness will decrease customer satisfaction by 130.3%. This suggests that WMA should improve in responding to customer request in order to improve customer satisfaction. These results were in harmony with those of Mwandosya (2013) which revealed that the overall expected services quality in regard to responsiveness as the predictor had high level. Further, the study showed that, customers are highly satisfied when they served quickly, likewise WMA customers would be satisfied if they get quick response from WMA staff. Assurance was found to be not significant at ($p = 0.549$) implying that assurance service quality dimension is not necessarily in making satisfaction to WMA customers. These findings were quite different from those of Janahi et al. (2017) which established strong and positive relationships between the service quality dimensions and customer satisfaction. Empathy was not significant at ($p = 0.269$) which means that empathy is not an important dimension of customer satisfaction in WMA. These findings are similar to that of Mhoja (2017) which found that empathy was not among the dimensions, which influence customer satisfaction.

7 Conclusion and Recommendations

The study concludes that wide service quality gaps between expected service quality and performance of the WMA. This means that in all SQ dimensions customer expectations were higher than the real services offered by WMA. With such existing gaps, the study further concludes that a quality of services and customer satisfaction were statistically related. The study recommends that the Ministry of Trade and Industry (MIT) should support WMA to improve infrastructures such as modern working standards, working spaces and equipment that will be adequately accommodate the available staff. MIT also should help the Agency to secure employment permits from the President's Office Public Service Management and Good Governance (PO – PSMGG) to fill staff shortage. Further, the PO – PSMGG should give priorities to expertise in metrology through giving employment permits to WMA when needed to increase the number of employees. WMA management should set budgets and conduct training to its inspectors of weights and measures in customer services including how to carry out regular surveys for the purpose of measuring levels of customer satisfaction. WMA management also should continue enforcing the law, rules and regulations that govern the day-to-day operations of WMA. The study further recommends to the public that every citizen should use verified instruments whenever they are making buying decisions. Based on the research findings, the following areas for future study are recommended; a similar study should be conducted with large sample size across regions so that findings can be generalized to a large population. Another study on legal framework should be conducted to measure its impact on customer satisfaction for WMA customers. Another study should be conducted in rural areas so that to be able to measure the difference in disposable income and its effect on WMA customer satisfaction.

References

Antwi, A.O., Matsui, K.: Price perception on weights and measures at the local markets of Ghana. Kasetsart J. Soc. Sci. **30**, 1–6 (2018). https://doi.org/10.1016/J.kjss.2018.01.011

Bengesi, K.M.K.: Factors hindering use of standard weights and measures along Irish potato supply chain in Njombe Region, Tanzania. Int. J. Bus. Manag. **13**(8), 196–206 (2018). https://doi.org/10.5539/ijbm.v13n8p196

County, N.: Original article gap analysis of educational services quality based on servqual model from Iranian medical students' Viewpoint (2014), **5**(2014), 87–96 (2016)

Dehghan, A.: Relationship between service quality and customer satisfaction: in the case of CCG (Customer Centric Group) CO. The Thesis for the Award of Master Degree in Continuation, Courses Marketing and e-commerce at the Tarbiat Modares University, Iran (2006)

Fanton, J.: A brief history of metrology: past, present, and future. Inter. J. Metrol. Qual. Eng. **10**(5), 1–8 (2019). https://doi.org/10.1051/Ijmqe/2019005

GAIN: USDA Foreign Agricultural Service. Global Agricultureal Information Network. GAIN Report Number: 1837 (2019). 7p.

Hosmer, D.W., Lemeshow, S.: Applied Logistic Regression, 2nd edn. Wiley, Hoboken (2000)

Janahi, A.M.A., Saeed, M.M., Mubarak, A.: The impact of customer service quality on customer satisfaction in Islamic banking. J. Islamic Mark. **8**(4), 595–604 (2017). https://doi.org/10.1108/JIMA-07-2015-0049

Kajungu, A.M.: Customer service provision performance in public organizations in Tanzania: the case of weights and measures agency in Kigoma Region. Mzumbe University, Morogoro, Tanzania (2014)

Mashenene, R.G.: Effect of service quality on students' satisfaction in Tanzania higher education. Bus. Educ. J. (BEJ) **2**(2), 1–8 (2019)

Mbise, E.R.: Students' perceived service quality of business schools in Tanzania?: a longitudinal study. Qual. Issues Insights 21st Century **4**(1), 28–44 (2015)

Mhoja, H.: Factors influencing customer satisfaction on the weights and measures agency services: a study of Mbeya City in Mbeya Region. Dissertation for Award of Master Degree in Business Studies at Mzumbe University, Morogoro, Tanzania (2017)

Mwandosya, J.: Assessment of customers' perception and expectations of service quality in Tanzania's commercial banks: the case of Azania Bank. Disseration for Award of Master Degree in Business Administration at Mzumbe University, Morogoro, Tanzania (2013)

Nkyami, R.T.: The influence of service quality on customer satisfaction in intercity public transportation: a case of alsaedy high class bus service. Thesis for the Award of Master Degree at the Open University of Tanzania (2016)

Racine, J.: Harnessing Quality for Global Competitiveness in Eastern Europe and Central Asia. Wold Bank Publications. The World Bank (2011).

Filho, B.A.R., Gonçalves, R.F.: Legal metrology, the economy and society: a systematic literature review. Measurement **69**, 155–163 (2015). https://doi.org/10.1016/j.measurement.2015.03.028

Rural Livelihood Development Company (RLDC): Assessment of Standardization, Weights and Measures and their Implication in Transaction Costs in the Agricultural Value Chains. Final Report, February 2014. https://agriknowledge.org/downloads/c821gj795

RLDC: Tanzania Markets Pan: Policies That Work 4 Markets: Assessment of Adherence to Recommended Weights and Measures in Grain Value Chain and Implication on Transaction Costs (2012)

Savio, E., Chiffre, L.D., Carmignato, S., Meinertz, J.: Economic benefits of metrology in manufacturing. Cirp Ann. **65**(1), 495–498 (2016). https://doi.org/10.1016/J.cirp.2016.04.020

Temba, M.L.: The Assessment of Service Quality and Customer (2013)

Yegidis, B.L., Weinbach, R.W., Myers, L.L.: Research Methods for Social Workers (Eight). Pearson, New York (2018)

Yiridoe, E.K.: A problem ignored: the role of a weights and measures system in food security in Africa. Outlook Agric. **34**(4), 233–241 (2005). https://doi.org/10.5367/000000005775454715

Determinants of Airline Selection at Nnamdi Azikwe International Airport, Abuja-Nigeria- A Researchers' Perspective

M. S. Oluwole[1], J. A. Ojekunle[1](✉), C. C. Adindu[2], R. O. Nwaogbe[3], and A. I. Muhammed[1]

[1] Department of Transport Management Technology, Federal University of Technology, PMB 65, Minna, Niger, Nigeria
[2] Department of Project Management Technology, Federal University of Technology, Minna, Nigeria
[3] Department of Maritime Logistics, Nigerian Maritime University, Okerenkoko, Delta State, Nigeria

Abstract. In 2016 the contribution of the air transport industry to the world economy is about USD $7.6 trillion, this accounts for over 10% of global gross domestic product. It is projected that the value of the overall travel industry will grow at an annual compound rate of 3.9% reaching USD $11.5 trillion between 2018–2017. This will represent more than 11% of global GDP. At the continental level, aviation sector contributes about USD $10 billion to the African economy. Furthermore, about 2000 airline operators with over 23,000 aircrafts are known to serve over 3,700 airports across the world. These developments continually stimulate airline operators towards increasing their market share on the global air transport landscape. Arising from these, the study examines the factors that determine passenger's airline selection decision taking at the Nnamdi Azikiwe International Airport, Abuja-Nigeria. The methodology of study involved structured questionnaire in which data was collected on passengers' attributes suggested by Ajzen theory of planned behavior and airline service qualities. Descriptive statistics, ANOVA and regression method were used in data analysis. Result shows that attitude, customer satisfaction scale and airline service reliability with mean score of: 4.42, 4.16, 4.13 respectively were the most significant variables influencing passengers' choice of airlines. The study recommends improvement of airline operation in the critical areas of service quality, reliability and strong public image to enhance current customer attraction and retention.

Keywords: Airline · Fare · Passengers · Ticketing and service qualities

1 Introduction

The Airline industry plays a major role in economic development of countries through its ability to open-up local and foreign investments. In 2016 the contribution of the air transport industry to the world economy is about USD $7.6 trillion, this accounts

J. N. Mojekwu et al. (Eds.): *Sustainable Education and Development*, pp. 235–244, 2021.
https://doi.org/10.1007/978-3-030-68836-3_21

for over 10% of global gross domestic product. It is projected that the value of the overall travel industry will grow at an annual compound rate of 3.9% reaching USD $11.5 trillion between 2018–2017. This will represent more than 11% of global GDP. At the continental level, aviation sector contributes about USD $10 billion to the African economy. Over 2000 airline operators with over 23,000 aircrafts are known to serve over 3,700 airports across the world. These developments continually stimulate airline operators towards increasing their market share on the global air transport landscape. In airline business, quality service determines the quantity of service demanded by air traveler. The demand of an airline service affects its revenue, through service patronage (Chikwendu et al. 2012). Passenger loyalty is best achieved when users are happy with the service offered by the airline. To this extent, airline service quality must be tailored towards better user satisfaction on the basis of service offered. Wanke et al. (2016), suggested that, identifying the gaps between service expectation and the actual service provided by any organization is what determines customer satisfaction is determined.

Nwaogbe et al. (2017) study on airline service quality at category 'one' airport in Kano, showed that based on comfort, affordability and service reliability indices, airline passengers are satisfied with the overall service provide by Arik Airline, Aero Contractors and Azman Air. Akpoyomare et al. (2016) study centered on domestic carriers service quality and passenger loyalty in Murtala Muhammed International Airport (MMIA), Lagos, the result shows a positive relationship between the service quality dimensions of customers' satisfaction and customer's loyalty. Okeudo and Chikwendu (2013) study also revealed that service attributes influence airlines corporate image and passenger loyalty in MMIA Lagos. The foregoing studies have shown the degree to which airline passengers' satisfaction relates to service attributes. As such, what is perhaps, lacking is how airline passengers can use each of the attributes in making choice of airline service for purposes of patronage. It is against this backdrop that this study seeks to assess the factors that determine choice of airlines by passengers at the Nnamdi Azikwe International Airport, Abuja. The study further investigated the influence of airline ticket pricing, safety, and service quality on airline choice in the study area. Three alternate hypotheses were formulated are, these are, there is no:

H1: Significant relationship between ticket price and airline selection
H1: Significant relationship between service quality and airline selection
H1: Significant relationship between safety and airline selection

2 Theoretical Framework

2.1 Theory of Planned Behaviour

Theory of planned behaviour states that intention toward attitude, subject norms, and perceived behavioural control, together shape an individual's behavioural intentions and behaviours. This theory links one's beliefs with behaviour, the theory which was proposed by Ajzen (1991) included perceived behavioural control to improve the predictive power of the theory of reasoned action that was earlier advanced by Ajzen and Fishbein (1975). The theory of planned behaviour suggests that people are much more likely to behave in certain way if they feel that they can exhibit them successfully. In other words, the more favourable the attitude toward behaviour and the subjective norm, the greater will be the perceived behavioural control and the stronger will be the person's intention to undertake the behaviour.

Put simply, behavioural intention as ensilaged by the theory of planned behaviour can be represented mathematically as:

$$BI = {}_{wA}A + {}_{wSN}SN + {}_{wPBC}PBC$$

The three factors being proportional to their underlying beliefs:

Where:
BI: Behavioural Intension
A: Attitude towards bahviour
b: The strength of each belief toward an outcome or an attribute
e: Evaluation of the outcome or attributes
SN: Subjective norm
n: The strength of each normative belief of each referent
m: The motivation to comply with the referent
PBC: Perceived Behaviour Control
c: The strength of each control belief
P: The perceived power of the control factor
$n =$ Empirically derived weight/co-efficient

To the extent that it is an accurate reflection of actual behavioural control, perceived behavioural control can together with intention be used to predict behaviour.

(https://en.wikipedia.org/wiki/Theory_of_planned_behavior).

$$B = {}_{wBI}BI + {}_{wPBC}PBC \quad \text{Where}$$

B: Behaviour
BI: Behavioural intention
PBC: Perceived Behavioural Control
c: the strength of each control belief
p: the perceived power of the control factor
w: empirically derived weight/coefficient.

3 Review on Airline Service Quality, Customer Behavior and Decision Criteria

Khan and Khan (2014), studied customer satisfaction in airline industry in Pakistan, the result shows that airlines offering better service to customers has higher patronage than carriers with less service satisfaction. Simsek and Demirbag (2017), airline modelled service quality, customer satisfaction and behavioural goals in Turkey, utilizing Structural Equation Model (SEM). The result indicates, dimension image has a strong significant perceived quality service by customer and in addition, staffs word of mouth was identified to have a positive importance on customer satisfaction, thereby enabling customers' loyalty.

Curtis et al. (2012) investigated Customer's satisfaction with airline service quality in US; aimed at examining the flight frequency issues and the difference in level of satisfaction between frequent and non-frequent flyers, their studies revealed that the more the level of service satisfaction with overall air carrier's quality and selected features decreased, the less air travelers flies. Adeola and Adebiyi (2014) study examined quality perceived value and customer loyalty as factors influencing the choice of airline in Nigeria, the result shows that airline passenger income, social state of road infrastructure and insecurity accounted for the sudden rise in air transport travelers. Rahim (2016) looked at customer loyalty and perceived service quality in Nigerian airline industry. The result indicates that perceived service quality is positively correlated to both customer's loyalty and satisfactions. Okeudo and Chikwendu (2013), studied the effects of service quality on airline image and passengers' loyalty using Arik airline as a case study, the result showed a positive association between airline service quality variables, image and customers repeated patronage.

4 Methodology

Descriptive survey research was used to investigate and report passengers and airline attributes determining the choice of airline. Parameters that control airline passengers buying behaviours as enunciated in the Adzen theory of planned behavior as well as other airline attributes which influences passengers buying decisions were used for the investigation. The study population consists of all passengers (domestic and international) of the selected airlines (Air Peace, Medview Airline, Aero Contractors, Max Air and Arik Air) which operate at the Nnamdi Azikiwe International Airport (NAIA), Abuja. The population of the study comprise of 200 airline passengers in the airport, each of the airlines was purposively administered with forty (40) sets of questionnaires. A combination of stratified and simple random techniques was used in drawing the target population from both domestic and international passengers of the airlines of interest. 176 questionnaires representing 88% of the sampled population was successfully filled, retrieved, and used for the analysis. Descriptive statistics combined with multiple regression in SPSS version 21 were used for data analysis. The three hypotheses were tested using ANOVA at the significant level of 0.05.

5 Results and Discussion of Findings

Majority of the airline passengers are male, this follows the norms in African society that male being mostly the bread winners of families is likely to be more mobile that female. The results show that respondents within the age bracket of 21–60 years are the most active users of the airline services and as such, accounts for about 86% of the airline passengers in the study area. This is expected as they constitute the most active ages and as such will be more mobile for business, education and leisure purposes. Majority (about 81%) of the passengers have first degree and above, implying that air transport being an elite means of transportation will consist mostly of educated class. High income

Table 1. Respondents socio-economic characteristics

S/N	Variables		Frequency	Percentage
1	**Gender**	**Male**	**99**	**56**
		Female	**77**	**44**
2	Age Groups	0- 20 Years	19	11
		21-30 Years	49	28
		31-40 Years	56	32
		41-50 Years	31	18
		51- 60 Years	15	08
		>60 Years	06	03
3	Educational Level	< Bachelor	33	19
		Bachelors	83	47
		Master	41	23
		> Masters	19	19
4	Income Brackets	<₦30,000	24	14
		₦30,001-₦50,000	19	11
		₦50,001-₦70,000	23	13
		₦70,001- ₦100,000	31	17
		₦100,001- ₦120,000	42	24
		>₦120,000	37	21
5	Occupation	Student	39	22
		Private Company	31	18
		Government Employees	58	33
		Entrepreneur	29	16
		Retiree	11	06
		Unemployed	08	05
6	Frequency of Travels	First time	26	15
		Once yearly	30	17
		Less than once a year	18	10
		2-3 time per year	50	28
		Above 3 times per year	52	30
7	Flight Destination	Within Nigeria	96	55
		Within Africa	55	31
		Outside Africa	25	14

(*continued*)

Table 1. (*continued*)

8	Airline Information Channel	Search Engines	15	9
		Social Media	26	15
		Airlines Websites	29	16
		Travel Agencies	55	31
		Family and Friends	37	21
		TV Adverts	09	5
		Travel Magazines	05	3
9	Ticket Purchasing Channel	At airport	58	33
		Airline website	48	26
		Airline offices	21	12
		Travel agencies	43	24
		Airline call centres	9	5
10	Purpose of travel	Business	59	34
		Leisure/vacation	29	16
		Seminar/meetings	32	18
		Education	16	9
		Visitation	14	8
		Others (Medicals)	26	15

earners (₦100, 001 above) accounted for 43% of the airline passengers, while 81% of airline passengers in NAIA, Abuja are educated above Bachelor's degree level, while majority (55%) undertake domestic flights, whose purpose is majorly for business. The travel agents, families and friends as well as airline websites remains the major channels of airline information in the study area as they accounted for 31%, 21%, and 16% respectively.. There are different avenues from which airlines tickets can be purchased in the study area, but the airline offices at the airport, airlines websites and travel agents are mostly used as they jointly accounted 83% of the distribution. The implication is that airline passengers at NAIA, Abuja are adopting virtual online approaches to access airline services because of the numerous advantages it offers (Table 1).

The mean score of airline choice determinants in the study area as presented in Table 2 shows that the Attitude scale has the highest mean score (M = 4.42), implying that attitude scale is the major factor which determines the selection of airline by passengers. This is followed by Airline reliability (M = 4.13), customer satisfaction (M = 4.16), airline convenient scale (M = 4.10), airline safety (M = 410) and airline reputation scale (M = 4.08) all have significant influence on airline selection in that order in the study area. The Perceived Behavioural scale with a mean score of 4.00, price scale and service quality scales with mean score of 3.68 and 3.84 respectively will also to a high degree influence airline selection in NAIA, Abuja.

Table 2. Determinants of airline choice

Factors	Average mean	Rank
Attitude scales	4.42	1
Subjective norm scale	3.41	10
Perceived behaviour control scale	4.00	7
Price scale	3.68	9
Airline reliability scale	4.13	2
Airline convenience scale	4.10	4
Airline service quality	3.84	8
Airline reputation scale	4.08	6
Airline safety scale	4.10	4
Frequent flier programme	3.23	11
Customer satisfaction scale	4.16	3
Buying intension scale	3.17	12
Buying behaviour	2.91	13

Source: Authors Computation (2019)

6 Test of Hypothesis

The ANOVA result was used to test the three hypotheses that were earlier formulated.

Hypotheses One: There is a significant statistical relationship between ticket price and airline selection.

Table 3. Airline ticket price analysis of variance

Model	Sum of squares	Df	Mean square	F	Sig.
Regression	6.793	3	2.264	5.664	.001[b]
Residual	66.363	166	.400		
Total	**73.156**	**169**			

a. Dependent Variable: Airline Selection
b. Predictors: (constant), purchasing ticket from this airline is easy for me, selection of a ticket type is my absolute decision and selection of airline is under my control.

Table 3 above, shows that the F-value is 5.664, degree of freedom is 169 and the calculated p-value is 0.001. The alternative hypothesis is therefore accepted since it is less than the tabulated p-value of 0.05. This finding aligns with the work of Nwaogbe et al. (2017) which posits that as the price of air tickets continues to drop, more passengers will be willing to travel by air.

Hypotheses Two: There is a significant statistical relationship between airline quality of service and airline choice.

Table 4. Airline quality of service variance

Model	Sum of squares	Df	Mean square	F	Sig.
Regression	90.121	3	30.040	566.465	.000[b]
Residual	8.379	158	.053		
Total	**98.500**	**161**			

a: Dependent Variable: Airline Choice and b: Predictors: (constant),

Table 4 above shows that the F-value is 566.465, degree of freedom is 161 and the calculated P-value is 0.00. Therefore H1 is accepted, since it is less than the tabulated p-value of 0.05, which means that there is a significant statistical relationship between quality of service and airline choice. Nwaogbe et al. (2013, 2017) states that, quality of service measurement regarding passengers perception of airline services (cleanliness, customer relation and reliability) has positive contribution towards the selection of airline.

Hypotheses Three: There is a significant statistical relationship between airline safety and airline selection.

Table 5. Airline safety analysis of variance

Model	Sum of squares	Df	Mean square	F	Sig.
Regression	77.381	3	−25.794	474.437	.000[b]
Residual	9.025	166	.054		
Total	86.406	169			

a. Dependent Variable: Airline Selection and b. Predictors (Constant).

From Table 5 above, it be seen that the F-calculated value is 474.437, degree of freedom = 169 and the calculated p-value is 0.00, therefore H1 is accepted since the calculated p-value is lower than the tabulated p-value of 0.05. The implication of the result is that, there is a significant relationship between safety and airline choice in the study area.

7 Recommendations and Conclusion

This study has examined the factors which determine airline selection at Nnamdi Azikwe International Airport, Abuja. The factors are: attitude scale, subjective norms and behavioral control parameters like- ticket price, service reliability, convenience, safety, customer satisfaction, buying intention and buying behaviour. In a bid to increase airline service patronage in the study area the following recommendations would suffice:

1. The pricing of Airline tickets should be reasonable and competitive.
2. The quality of service delivery should be improved upon on a sustainable basis based on the major parameters with highest mean score.
3. Airlines operations should strive to follow all laid-down safety procedures and protocols to ensure safety of customers life and properties all times.
4. The airline service offerings should be such that confers maximum value for money to passengers.

In conclusion, air transport industry is a key sector of Nigeria's national economy considering its high potentials for the development of trade, investment, culture and tourism within and among nations. The industry's capacity to facilitate global linkages among worlds' economies cannot be overemphasized especially at this period of recession, economic downturn and low pricing of Nigeria's oil resource.

References

Adeola, M.M., Adebiyi, S.O.: Service quality, perceived value and customer satisfaction as determinant of airline choice in Nigeria. Int. Lett. Soc. Humanistic Sci. **20**, 66–80 (2014). https://doi.org/10.18052/www.scipress.com/ILSHS.20.66. ISSN 2300-2697

Ajzen, I., Fishbein, M.: A Bayesian analysis of attribution processes. Psychol. Bull. **82**(2), 261 (1975). https://doi.org/10.1037/h0076477

Ajzen, I.: The theory of planned behavior. Organ. Behav. Hum. Decis. Process. **50**(2), 179–211 (1991). https://doi.org/10.1016/0749-5978(91)90020-T

Akpoyomare, O.B., KunleAdeosun, L.P., Ganiyu, R.A.: Airline service quality dimensions and customer loyalty: empirical evidence from air passengers' in Lagos State. Czech J. Tour. **5**(2), 155–171 (2016). https://doi.org/10.1515/cjot-2016-0009

Curtis, T., Rhoades, D.L., Waguespack, B.P.: Satisfaction with airline service quality: familiarity breeds contempt. Int. J. Aviat. Manag. **1**(4) (2012). https://doi.org/10.1504/IJAM.2012.050472

Chikwendu, D.U., Ejem, E., Ezenwa, A.: Evaluation of service quality of Nigerian airline using SERVQUAL model. J. Hospitality Manag. Tour. **3**(6), 117–125 (2012). https://doi.org/10.5897/JHMT12.019. http://academicjournals.org/JHMT. ISSN 2141-6575

Okeudo, G., Chikwendu, D.U.: Effects of airline service quality on airline image and passengers' loyalty: findings from Arik Air Nigeria Passengers. J. Hosp. Manag. Tour. **4**(2), 19–28 (2013). https://doi.org/10.5897/JHMT2013.0089. http://www.academicjournals.org/JHMT. ISSN 2141-6575

https://en.wikipedia.org/wiki/Theory_of_planned_behavior

Muhammed, A.I.: Assessment of factors that influence passengers' airline selection in Nigeria. Unpublished B.Tech thesis, Submitted to the Department of Transport Technology, School of Entreprenurship and Management Technology, Federal University of Technology Minna, Niger State-Nigeria (2017)

Nwaogbe, O.R., Abraham, P., Balogun, A.O., Ikeogu, C.C., Omoke, V.: Assessment of airline service quality in a category one nation: focus on MallamAminu Kano International Airport. Int. J. Aviat. Aeronaut. Aerosp. **4**(1) (2017). https://doi.org/10.15394/ijaaa.2017.1157

Rahim, A.G.: Perceived service quality and customer loyalty: the mediating effect of passenger satisfaction in the Nigerian Airline Industry. Int. J. Manag. Econ. **52**, 94–117 (2016). https://doi.org/10.1515/ijme-2016-0029

Simsek, K., Demirbag, O.: Modeling service quality, customer satisfaction and behavioral intentions in airline industry: a SEM approach. J. Int. Sci. Res. **2**(6), 11–29 (2017)

Khan, U., Khan, N.: Customer Satisfaction in Airline Industry. Department of Business Administration, Main Campus, Iqra University, Karachi – 75500, Pakistan (2014). https://doi.org/10.7763/IPEDR.2014.V76.12

Wanke, P., Barros, C.P., Nwaogbe, O.R.: Assessing productive efficiency in Nigerian airports using Fuzzy-DEA. Transp. Policy **49**, 9–19 (2016). https://doi.org/10.1016/j.tranpol.2016.03.012

Characterizing Street Vendors in the Urban Settings of Tanzania: Towards Sustainable Solutions to Vendors' Challenges

M. H. Kirumirah(✉) and E. J. Munishi

Department of Business Administration, College of Business Education, P. O. Box 1968, Dar es Salaam, Tanzania
{m.kirumirah,e.munishi}@cbe.ac.tz

Abstract. Despite the growth and expansion of street vending business along with its economic support to the poor urban dwellers, much facts regarding characteristics and general operations of each group is not known. Thus, this study intended to characterize street vendors in Dar es Salaam city, Tanzania, to unveil their characteristics, challenges and needs of each specific category. The study employed a mixed methods approach with a sample of 100 street vendors sampled conveniently. Findings indicate that, street vending business involves individuals of diverse characteristics in terms of gender, education, economic status, marital status, cultural practices among others. It was further revealed that, the operations of street vendors are different and the difference emanate from the nature of what one vends. Lack of training, lack of legal status, lack of recognition by different financial institutions are some of the general challenges however, each group had its pressing challenges. The study concludes that it is important to understand different characteristics of street vendors across the country so that measures taken to help them are relevant to their operations. Findings imply that, when dealing with street vendors, one should look at them differently because they possess different characteristics. Efforts to resolve their challenges thus, should be category specific.

Keywords: Street vending · Vendors · Characteristics · Tanzania

1 Introduction

Tanzania lies among the countries in the world whose economies are showing a growing pattern. According to the World Bank (2017), Tanzania economy is ranking the fifth among the developing economies, however, unemployment is cracking the heads of many in the country with unemployment rates standing at 13.7% (World Bank 2017). The country has over 800,000 graduates entering the labour market annually (ibid). The situation has been escalated by the increased enrollment of pupils as a result of fee free education in both Primary and secondary education in the country. Thus, a narrowing pattern in employment opportunity has been witnessed in the sense that the formal labour market cannot absorb all labour market entrants (ILO 2009).

J. N. Mojekwu et al. (Eds.): *Sustainable Education and Development*, pp. 245–261, 2021.
https://doi.org/10.1007/978-3-030-68836-3_22

Consequently, most of the young able bodied after failing to secure formal employment chances, as an alternative, have joined the informal sector. Statistics around the world confirm that, the sector contributes around two thirds of all the employed individuals, and its contribution to different countries' GDP is highly recognized (The World Bank 2019; Dell'Anno et al. 2018). Scholars attest that, the sector provides between 50–75% of employment and has attracted a wide range of individuals from different social background and most especially in the developing world (Sparks and Barnett 2010). In Tanzania the size of the informal economy has grown from 10% of GDP in 1960s, to 20% after the mid-1980s, 58.3% in 1999 and 2000, and around 52%–61% of GDP in 2013–2015 (Dell'Anno et al. 2018).The informal sector is a combination of different activities unregistered in the formal channel including urban farming, small manufacturing, software firms, and street vending to mention but a few (Oosthuizen 2008).

Despite the fact that street vending is considered illegal by the government and urban authorities since colonial times (Steiler 2018), circumstances of unemployment and unsupportive government economic stances from 1980s to present, have led to the development of this business. Literature reveal that, by 1993 when Dar es Salaam had a population of two million inhabitants, there were less than 10,000 vendors (May, 1993), however, the number has increased rapidly. By 2010 there were more than 700,000 street vendors around the city of Dar es Salaam (Lyon and Msoka 2007), and the number increased to more than one million by 2014 (Mramba et al. 2014). Such figures indicate that street vending has been growing widely in urban settings particularly in Dar es Salaam.

In Tanzania thus, street vending has attracted different people from different social background. It is an important survival strategy for many unemployed young and old, educated and uneducated, rich and the poor city dwellers in Tanzania and other developing countries (Mitullah 2003; Amis 2016. It has contributed widely to creating employment and economic development (Bhebhe 2012; IFRA 2016; Lyons and Msoka 2010; Mramba et al. 2014; Njaya 2014); helps in supplying limited products conveniently and at relatively cheap prices (Hassan and Alam 2015); minimizing the rate of crimes; improving people's standard of living most especially those involved in the business, and contributing to the country's economy at large (Suraiya and Noor 2012).

In spite of this variability, the actual nature of street vendors in Dar es Salaam city in terms of their activities, working environment, challenges, and their needs to curb their challenges are not well known. The available studies conducted in Tanzania provide shallow characterization (Muhanga 2017; Mramba et al. 2014), with others being done out of Tanzania (Adhikari 2017; Martínez et al. 2017; Mazhambe 2017; Beccles 2014; Tengeh and Lapa 2013; Martins 2006; Nirathron 2006; Manyanhaire et al. 2007) specifically in Nepal, Colombia, Zimbabwe, Ghana, South Africa, and Thailand respectively. This study intends to characterize street vending activities basing on their groups, challenges facing each specific group and needs of each specific group of vendors in Dar es Salaam city. The characterization will inform the general public, urban authorities and other policy makers the nature of street vendors there by enhancing them in creating supporting environment for each group of vendors based on their characteristics. It will also help in informing better policies in terms of financial enhancement, urban planning in general, and human capital development for improving small business in the country.

Specific Objectives

i. To survey on the main characteristics of street vendors operating in Dar es salaam;
ii. To categorize street vendors' operations and their main areas of comfort zone in Dar es salaam;
iii. To classify challenges facing each group of vendors in discharging its activities in Dar es salaam;

2 Theoretical Framework

2.1 The Structuralism and Neoliberal Theory

The study used both the structuralism and the neoliberal theories to complement each other's arguments. To structuralism theory street vending is a last resort survival strategy opted by urban dwellers who have failed to be employed in the formal employment. Street vending is a means from which they obtain economic needs (Williams and Gurtoo 2012) and a necessary means of survival in the absence of other livelihood strategy. The theory explains the Tanzanian urban street vending settings (Bhowmik 2007). The theory been used in India and China by Bhowmik (2007) and Xue and Huang (2015) respectively. The Neo liberal theory on its side considers street vending as a rational economic activity taken by many after the failure of the formal system and the state to provide citizens with friendly services and business frameworks leading them to poverty (Bhowmik 2012) and are further stifled by state imposed hurdles (Williams and Gurtoo 2012) and thus vendors are considered heroes. The theory has been used by different scholars (Mazhambe 2017; Bhowmik 2012; London and Hart 2004; Williams and Gurtoo 2012) in studying the street vending phenomena in urban settings in different parts of the world. Theories express the real life of vendors in Dar es salaam but fail to show what kind of individuals go for street vending. They have also failed to detail what faces street vendors after forcing to establish their businesses against the government wish. Thus hurdles street vendors face have not been given any focus.

2.2 The Relationship Between the Study and the Existing Studies

A number of studies have been conducted focusing on street vending subject across the world. These include (Bhowmik 2005; Williams and Gurtoo 2012; Vargas 2016; Mazhambe 2017) and many more. Such studies paid much of their focus on using street vending as a tool against poverty, causes of poverty, challenges facing poverty and a few studies focused on the components of street vendors. However, besides a number of studies conducted on street vendors, little have focused on vendors' characterisation, and those that tried, (Nirathron 2006; Adhikar 2017) were carried out of Tanzania. That being the fact, little is known on the real characteristics of street vending business in Tanzania.

2.3 Challenges Facing Street Vendors

Street vending has been a survival strategy to many especially the poor urban dwellers. However, street vendors have been facing a number of challenges on a daily basis. According to Mitullah (2003), there are common challenges facing vendors across the world. These include lack of legal status and right to vend, lack of space or poor location, restriction on licensing, cost of regulation, harassment, bribes, confiscation and evictions, lack of services and infrastructure and lack of representation or voice (Mitullah 2003: 2). It was reported by Beccle (2014) in Ghana that the heavy loads some vendors carry to sell, sometimes give them some form of body deformity. I is also evident that working in harsh conditions of the scorching sun expose them to lung associated diseases. Mramba et al. (2016) reports that poor business skills as result of low level of educataio among vendors. Lacking important skills like business management, communication skills, marketing skills and business record managing skills makes it difficult for vendors to excel (Kirumirah 2018, Marras 2018; Munishi and Casmir 2019).

It has been reported in several studies that street vending lacks legal recongintion in most of the African countries. This means that vendors are not recognized by the formal financial institutions and thus access to capital is limited (Otoo et al. 2012). In this regard, they cannot have a large stock of merchandise and neither can they achieve bigger profits. Bhowmik reports that they are exposed to accidents, arrests by urban military troops and harassment which leads them to lose their merchandise. Vendors also make losses twhen they fail to preserve their perishable products (Manyanhaire et al. 2007), face pricking ambiguous urban policies (Devlin 2010), arbitrary relocations from vending sites, anti-vending frameworks framed by urban authorities, and poor organization among street vendors (Mazhambe 2017).

Despite existing literatures in Tanzania and the rest of the world focus on challenges of street trade (Tonda and Thembela 2016; Beccles 2014; Lyons and Msoka 2007), little literature is available on the real characterization of street vendors in the city of Dar es Salaam. No study has so far focused on characterizing every group of vendors by

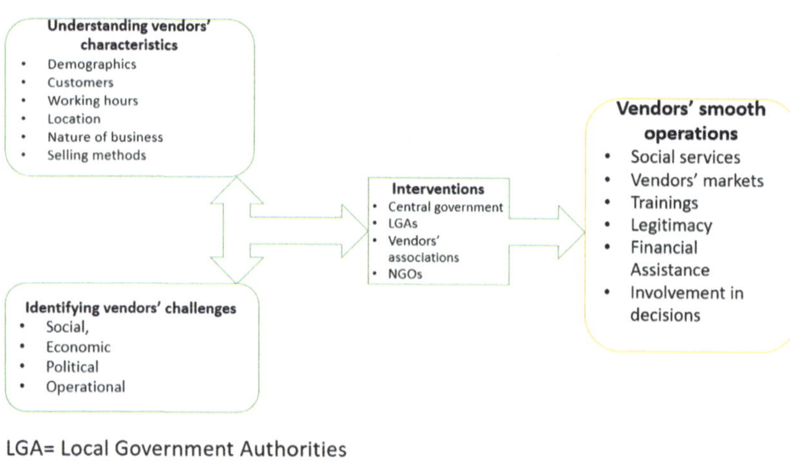

Fig. 1. The conceptual framework for vendors' characterization, challenges and intervention

showing their entire operations, challenges and special needs of every group. Thus with the existing gap in literature on the exact characteristics of street vendors, opened a chance for this study (Fig. 1).

3 Methodology

The study was carried out in Dar es Salaam city because of being a business hub with many street vendors from different parts of the country (Malefakis 2019). A mixed methods research approach was employed in which both qualitative and quantitative data were collected, analyzed and interpreted concurrently. It employed open and close ended interview guide, Focus Group Discussion and observation as the main tools for collecting data. From the intended population of street vendors, the sample size was determined based on Yamane's formula (1969) which states that at the significance level of 90%, the minimum sample size for the unknown population is 100 (Nirathron 2006). Thus the study involved 100 street vendors considering the fact that there is no exact number of street vendors in Dar es Salaam. Street vendors were obtained by convenient sampling technique because considering the nature of street vendors work, it was difficult to use other means. They were obtained from ten hot spots with a concentration of street vendors including Ferry-Kigamboni, Kivukoni, Bibi Titi Mohammed Street, Baridi to Mnazi mmoja, Kariakoo Msimbazi, Congo and Lindi streets, Biafra, Makumbusho, Mawasiliano, Kimara, and Mbezi Mwisho. At every spot, we sampled ten street vendors.

The qualitative data collected from different respondents through interviews and Focus Group discussion were summarized and grouped according to contents they possess. Important contents were coded and obtained from the texts. By the use of content analysis data were analyzed according to Denscombe (2010). As for quantitative data, cleaned, edited and coded data were entered in the Statistical Package for Social Sciences (SPSS) version 21 software which was used as a tool for quantitative data analysis. From this, descriptive statistics of frequencies, percentages, means and standard deviation were computed to determine the distribution of each group characteristics.

4 Findings and Discussion

4.1 The Main Characteristics of Street Vendors Operating in Dar es Salaam

The study intended to find out the main characteristics of street vendors in the urban settings, majorly Dar es Salaam. It was the researchers' intention to find out the major characteristics as the heart of the study is on characterizing street vendors. General characteristics determined here is of paramount importance as it informs of how street vendors look like in terms of their features. The subsequent sections presents main characteristics of street vendors in terms of gender, age, region of origin, education, marital status, distance to vending spot, size of the family, size of the capital, source of the capital, daily income, expenditure, and experience among others.

Age of respondents.

As highlighted earlier in this study, street vending combines a variety of different people from different social background. These include the young and the elder generation, the educated, immigrants, the single and married and much more. Table 1 presents data that indicate respondents, marital status, age, region they are coming from, education background, size of the family among others.

Table 1. Vendors' characteristics in terms of gender, age, marital status and family size

Characteristics	Description	Male	Female	Total
Age	Under 18	0	0	
	18–36 years	29	32	61
	37 + years	19	20	39
Total		48	52	100
Marital status	Single	25	14	39
	Married	17	24	41
	Divorced	5	12	17
	Widow(er)	1	12	13
Total		48	52	100
Place of origin	Dar es salaam	4	6	10
	Other regions	44	46	90
Total		48	52	100
Education	None	2	9	11
	Primary	19	21	40
	Secondary	18	16	34
	Cert/Dip	4	4	8
	Bachelor +	5	2	7
Total		48	52	100
Size of the family	1–2 members	21	15	37
	4 members	13	25	43
	More than 6	14	12	20
Total		48	52	100

Data from Table 1 indicate that, in terms of gender, currently, the number of female street vendors is almost equal or slightly surpassing that of male. Data in every segment indicate that, there were 52 female respondents as compared to that of 48 respondents among males. This indicates that, currently the city has more female street vendors than male street vendors. The study concurs with findings presented by different scholars (Martins 2006; Chen et al. 2005) that there are more female street vendors as compared to men. This is attributed to the changing nature of affairs in which women currently are more into entrepreneurship and are the most bread earners of different families in the African context. However, findings from other studies (Manyanhaire et al. 2007;

Muhanga 2017) showed that there were many male street vendors in Zimbabwe and Tanzania respectively. This could be attributed to different contexts in which the study was conducted.

With regards to age, data from Table 1 indicate that there are no street vendors who is under the age of 18 years of age because due to fee free education most of them are still in school. It is reported that there are very many street vendors at the age between 18 and 36 years. A group comprising of energetic and able bodied youth, who are in dire need for a livelihood strategy. Similarly, it is in this age group that most graduates from different education levels have completed their education, thus, while waiting for chances of employment they engage themselves in street vending. Data also indicate that there are people beyond the age of 36 who engage in street vending and most of them are women who are searching for their family survival. Findings are in line with other scholars (Manyanhaire et al. 2007; Muhanga 2017) who noted that there are very many street vendors at the age of 19–40 years and a few beyond the age of 40. Similar findings were reiterated by who found that the age of 20–40 years attract many street vendors.

Concerning marital status, the study reported both single and married respondents at an almost equal number (39 singles and 41 married ones) Most of the single respondents are male. It was also revealed that the divorced and the widow were among the group of street vendors. Being left with kids to feed and other responsibilities, the divorced and widow opt to become street vendors as a means of their survival. Findings are similar to those of Manyanhaire et al. (2007) and Adhikar (2017) who found that, there were more married individuals among street vendors than the unmarried and widowed ones. It was revealed further that most vendors come from the periphery to the Dar es Salaam metropolitan to search for their fortune. Scholars (Nirathron, 2006; Tengeh and Lapah 2013; Malefakis 2019) inform that, most street vendors come from different parts of a respective country with some being foreigners. For instance, many of street vendors in South Africa are from other countries apart for South Africa itself (Tengeh and Lapah 2013).

Education status was among the important aspect that was researched in this study. The study found with many vendors being primary and secondary school leavers, it was surprising that there were college graduates with certificate, diploma and bachelor's degree in different fields. Such findings imply that there is a serious problem of unemployment in the country that needs to be addressed so quickly. (World Bank Group 2017). Such findings are in line with those of Martins (2006) who among others revealed around 6.5% of his respondents holding certificate, diploma and degree levels of education.

The study further investigated other characteristics of street vendors in the urban settings of Dar es Salaam. In this regard, the size of the capital, source of capital, daily income and the working experience were probed. Data are presented in Table 2 above and are described as follows.

With regard to capital size, data express that most of the respondents had their capital ranging from 30,000 Tshs ($14) to more than one million Tshs ($450)with many (69) between 100,000–500,000 Tshs. Gender wise, there are few women with a capital size of more than 500,000 Tshs except those dealing in electronic money transfers bigger capital size than the rest. It was revealed that some vendors especially women do not

Table 2. Vendors' size and source of capital, daily income, expenditure and working experience

Characteristics	Description (Shs)	Response		Total
		Male	Female	
Size of capital	<100,000	4	13	17
	100,000–300,000	21	22	43
	310,000–500,000	15	11	26
	>500,000	8	6	14
Source of capital	Personal savings	12	10	22
	Previous work	22	11	33
	Relatives	6	8	14
	Borrowing/loans	0	9	9
	Hire purchase/Malikauli	8	10	18
	Merry go round	0	4	4
Daily income	<10000	30	35	65
	10000–30000	11	9	20
	31000–50000	3	4	7
	>50000	4	4	8
Working experience	<1 year	21	19	40
	1–2 years	10	18	28
	3–4 years	12	7	19
	>5 years	5	8	13

need capital rather start their business through hire purchase (Mali kauli). This could be associated to the fact that women are more trustworthy than men. Generally, findings are in line with Munishi and Casmir (2019) who reveal the same data that, street vendors have their capital between 30,000–1,000,000/ =. It was revealed that most vendors secured their capital form, personal savings (34%), family support, exploitative loans and *mali kauli*. The need for creating their own ventures drove them to save with an intention of establishing their business. With women, obtain their capital through merry go round in order to initiate their ventures. Due to the fact that most of street vendors have a small capital base, their daily income is also small. It was revealed that most of vendors (92%) earn between 10000–50000 Tshs. An earlier study by Nirathron (2006) identified that in Thailand food vendors earn little amount daily and it cannot suffice all their needs.

Regarding working experience, it was revealed that 40% of respondents were new in the street vending business as they had less than a year. This might be attributed to the permission given by the president of Tanzania that all street vendors should be allowed to vend but be given special IDs. Data further indicate that there are many women street vendors who have been in the business for a long time as compared to men. Out of 13% of vendors who have more than 5 years in the business, 8% are women. Similar data were found in the study conducted by Manyanhaire et al. (2007) who confirmed that more women began street vending activities earlier than men as there were 30% of women who had more than 6 years in vending as compared to only 10% of men.

4.2 Categories of Street Vendors' Operations and Their Salient Features

The second objective of the study intended to categorize street vendors basing on their operations, salient features. It was the researchers' argument that street vendors in their totality, have their own categories, sub categories as well as salient features. In this study a summary of their categories is presented in the following table and discussed in the subsequent sections (Table 3).

Table 3. Categories of street vendors.

Sn	Category	Frequency	
		Male	Female
1	Food	12	21
2	Electronic accessories	4	2
3	Mobile money	2	12
4	Kitchen ware	0	2
5	Outfit	4	3
6	Handicraft	2	1
7	Beverages	8	7
8	Shoes making and shining	2	0
9	Herbs	2	2
10	Fashion	4	1
11	Mixed products/kiosks	8	1
Total		48	52

4.2.1 Food and Beverages

This is the biggest category that includes a greatest segment of street vendors in Dar es salaam. This category includes sub categories like cooked food, fast food (fries), vegetables and fruits, condiments and spices, processed foods, fried seeds among others. As for beverages, soda, water, processed and natural juice, and confectionery. This category employs a greatest segment of street vendors. Data indicate that 48% of respondents are from this category. There are special features of this category. These are explained as follows.

Gender

In terms of gender, the category is dominated by more women as compared to men as

21% of women are involved in this category as compared to 12% of the men counterparts. The study, attributes this trend to the fact that women are used to the cooking sector and are willing to involve themselves in this business. It was observed that women are more into cooked food, vegetables and processed foods as men are involved in the fast foods (French fries/chips). However, it was observed that the number of men and women in the beverage category is almost the same. Men constitute 8% as women make 7% of respondent in the beverage category.

Location
In terms of location, the study has found out that, natural markets (bus stands, railway stations, ferry stations and nearby academic institutions. This is because street vendors and especially those dealing in the food category need a concentration of people. To them this concentration means readymade customers. Thus, such food vendors prefer staging their business in such areas to maximize their earnings by selling from the available people or people passing by going to board other means of transport.

Nature of the Business
It was observed from collected data that, most of the food vendors are stationed in places where there is a concentration of people. In this case therefore, some of food vendors and beverage sellers have built some temporary canvas thatched structures which they use to protect themselves and their customers in abnormal weather conditions. It was revealed that, food vendors steak in those areas because moving away from those areas means moving away from customers.

Customers
It has been observed that food vendors and beverage sellers serve a wide range of individuals. However, low income earners and students were associated to consuming food vendors' products. This is because they are sold at a cheaper price due to the fact that vendors do not pay tax and neither do they pay any kind of rent. It was also observed that, customers served by these vendors also include travelers.

Method of Selling
Food vendors and beverage sellers normally have their means of selling their products in their customers' acceptable standards. For instance, food vendors normally use hotpots to store the cooked food, have tables and chairs on which customers sit and sometimes they supply food to other vendors around. As for vegetable and fruit sellers, they normally sell their products in heaps displayed for customers' easy observation. Beverage sellers use destroyed refrigerators, put ice blocks in them and cover the refrigerators so that they keep the products cold.

Working Hours
Vendors selling cooked foods normally work from morning to evening as long as their customers are present. These vendors start by preparing breakfast, then lunch and supper at last. However, those selling fries/chips work from 10 morning to mid night because their customers are available most of the time. As for beverage sellers, they work for the entire day with oy = others extending to mid night especially those working near

academic institutions. This explains why there are more men dealing with fires and beverages as compared to women.

4.2.2 Electronic Accessories and Mobile Money Services

This another category of street vendors available in the city of Dar es salaam. The category involves a total of 20% of respondent and making it the second according to collected data. It can be observed that, while women dominate the mobile money section by 12% to 2% of men, men dominate that of accessories by 4% to 2% of women. As far as mobile money, vendors proved services for all the mobile money companies available in Tanzania (M-pes, TigoPesa, Airtel Money, Halopesa and TTCL money). As for accessories, these include phones, chargers, pouch, and home appliances among others. Features of this categories are revealed hereunder.

Gender
This is among the categories dominated by women. This is because it does not involve hard working. In the same manner, women are normally trustworthy and would like working where no hard work is involved. Men dominate selling electric accessories because they are in the position of fixing them in case they misbehave. Thus while women dominate the mobile money services, men dominate in selling electric accessories.

Location
It has been observed that most of these services are located where there is a collection of people. For example, Mobile money services are located in areas where there many people with many economic activities taking place or even there is a concentration of students from Colleges and Universities. As for those selling electronic accessories, they would prefer locating their places near bus stops and stations on street pavements, near government offices as well as nearby academic institutions.

Nature of Business
It has been observed in the field that while mobile money vendors are static and have built some temporary but movable structure to safeguard themselves or using umbrellas donated by cellular phone companies, those selling accessories are sometimes mobile. They normally change their location depending on where they anticipate customers to be located.

Customers
Students, workers, travelers, business persons form a great portion of this group of vendors. Unlike electronic accessory sellers, mobile money vendors serve customers of all types and caliber and financial muscles.

Method of Selling
It has been revealed that while mobile money vendors provide their services under the shade of their umbrella or the built structures from where their customers find them and seek their services right from there. As for sellers of electronic accessories, it has been

revealed that they display materials down, put them on temporary tables or hold them in their hands as they display them before their potential customers.

Working Hours
Mobile vendors normally work from morning to 6:00 in the evening. This is because most of these are women who are married and have some other family responsibilities to take at home. It was also revealed that for security purposes they prefer leaving early so as they get home safe and avoid any potential risks. It was also revealed that those selling electronic accessories close at 7:00 because no more potential customers are available and due to lack of light customers cannot see their products effectively.

4.2.3 Kiosks and Herb Vendors

This another category of vendors that also has many street vendors. The category is practices by both men and women with many men 8% holding kiosks than women. These are normally located near academic institutions and bus or ferry stations. The category involves selling mixed items including toiletry, beverages, electronic appliances, mobile money services, selling of processed foods as well as other medicinal herbs. These vendors depend on customer including students and street passers. By creating wooden drafted racks vendors display their commodities there. As for those selling herbs, temporary tables are used to display their products. Although running these kiosks illegitimately, vendors work almost for 24 h. This explains why vendors in this category are men as compared to the women counterparts.

4.2.4 Outfit, Fashion, Handcraft and Shoe Making

This is a category of street vendors with related materials. In total, they constitute 15% of the respondents in this study. This includes all vendors selling clothes, shoes, cosmetics and other household decorations. This category includes both men and women who display their commodities on the street or building walls. These vendor prefer displaying their materials near academic institutions and both public and private offices. While most of these vendors are stationed in one area, a few of them selling women clothes are mobile in nature moving from one location to the other looking for customers. Women and girls form a great segment of their customers' pool as most of these items are meant for girls. In most cases these vendors work from noon with those selling clothes beginning from 14:00 to 21:00 when students complete their daily routine.

Despite the fact that these characteristics were not known wholly, a number of earlier studies (Muhanga 2017; Beccles 2014; Mramba et al. 2014; William and Gurtoo 2012; Manyanhaire et al. 2007; Nirathron 2006) had tried to mention some of categories of street vendors existing in their study context. Different categories represent a number of activities carried by street vendors in Dar es Salaam city. It has been observed that dominance of women in food related category and mobile money services depict that women have become more active in earning bread for the family and contributing to family well-being. The existence of street pavements, offices, institutions, and ferry, railway and bus station serve street vendors need of customers. Customers coming to get services in these areas end up becoming potential customers of street vendors. The art of positioning where customers are available is a success factor among street vendors. Where vendors position themselves becomes a strategy for them to maximize their sales. Martins (2006) express that street vendors position themselves in offices, near the hospitals, transport parks, industrial areas among other areas.

4.3 Classifying Challenges Facing Each Group of Vendors in Discharging Its Activities in Dar Es Salaam

The third objective in this study wanted to identify and classify challenges facing street vendors while executing their tasks. It was the researchers' intention to reveal challenges facing each category of street vendors. This intended to fill the gap existing in literature in the sense that challenges facing street vendors are grouped and are considered whole and not divided according to each category of street vendors. Data collected indicate that there are general challenges facing street vendors while other challenges are category specific. These challenges are presented and grouped in the subsequent figure.

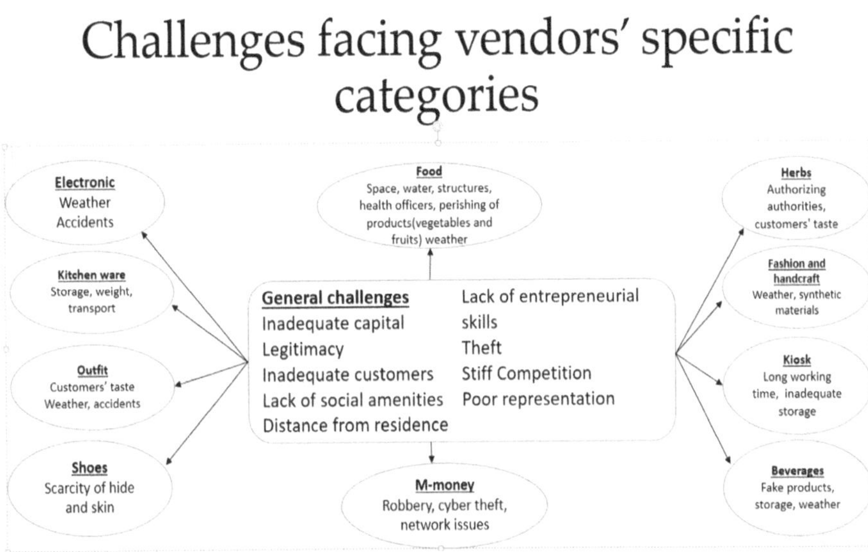

Fig. 2. Challenges facing vendors' specific categories

Data from Fig. 2 above indicate that, street vendors are faced with various challenges. These are political, social, technological and economic in nature. Some challenges are shared by all street vendors in the sense that they face these challenges equally while some others are category specific.

Regarding general challenges facing all street vendors, inadequacy of capital in the sense that they have limited capital and are not accepted to take loans from financial institutions because they do not meet all terms and conditions. Further, vendors are regarded illegal and this challenge deprives them of all other services they would acquire from city authorities. One among them was quoted saying, *"though we have IDs but we are not recognized as other business person. We cannot even register for youth and women funds given by every municipal, town or district council across the country".*

Inadequacy of customers was yet another challenge facing all vendors. It should be understood that the study was conducted after the outbreak of COVID 19 disaster and all schools and universities whose students are vendors' potential customers were closed. Social amenities like water and toilet, the distance vendors travel from their residence to the vending places, hostile weather, inadequate entrepreneurial skills, theft, stiff competition among themselves and poor representation in decision making bodies constitute their pressing challenges.

However, every category was observed to have its own challenges. Among others, the food and mobile money had serious challenges. The food category was hampered by inadequate space from where they can put their tables, chairs and other utensils, due to limited space, even stalls for those selling fruits cannot fit. And hence vendors and customers receive services in a non-conducive environment in which some fruits and vegetables are piled down on the floor. Further, water and other important structures like toilets and selling stalls. This means that such vendors cannot provide 100% hygienic services. As for Mobile money vendors, armed robbery, network problems as well as cyber theft were serious challenges.

Findings are in line with a number of different scholars who tried to discuss challenges hindering street vendors (Munishi and Casmir 2019; Kirumirah 2018; Marras 2018; Mazhambe 2017; Tonda and Thembela 2016; Mramba et al. 2016; Beccles 2014; Otoo et al. 2012; Devlin 2010; Lyons and Msoka 2007; Manyanhaire et al. 2007; Bhowmik 2005; Mitullah 2003). All these scholar agree to the reality that street vendors face a number of challenges that hinder vendors' prosperity in Tanzania.

5 Conclusion and Recommendations

According to this study, street vending is a viable economic opportunity that employs a great segment of young people in urban settings in the country. It shows that the number of street vendors has been increasing a day after the other. It has provided employment, improved people's stands of life, and has made it easy to get a variety of commodities at a reasonable price. While the available studies, indicated that street vending was of the poor, uneducated young men and a few women, the study has revealed a completely different picture. It shows that the venture involves more women than men and involves people of different characteristics including university graduates. Differences in social background and employment structures have been associated to the available trend. Unlike previous studies that considered street vending as a single category, this study has unveiled categories of street vendors and their salient features in terms of sex, location, method of selling, nature of customers among others. It has also been revealed that because vendors are of different categories in the city of Dar es salaam, thus they face different challenges. Each group has its challenges and thus have to be solved differently. Provision of social amenities, legitimizing of all street vendors in the country, provision of low interest rate loans, improving security in general, improving storage facilities and providing entrepreneurship training, and minimizing harsh regulations will relive vendors of their challenges.

Therefore, this study recommends that because street vending acts as a sponge to the available trend of unemployment, responsible authorities need to ensure that it is fully legitimized and vendors get recognized by financial institutions. The study recommends the Ministry of Labour, Employment and Youth Development should ensure that street vending is registered among viable and decent employment opportunities.

It is further recommended that, since every category of street vendors has its challenges, responsible authorities (City, Municipal and Ministries) should ensure that if vending is legal thus all vendors' challenges are solved not in a holistic manner but according to each category.

References

Adhikari, D.B.: Informal street food trade: a source of income generation in urban Nepal. Econ. J. Dev. **23 & 24**(1–2), 1–7 (2017)

Amis, P.: Symbolic politics, legalism and implementation: the case of street vendors in India. Commonwealth J. Local Gov. (18), 36–47 (2016). https://doi.org/10.5130/cjlg.v0i18.4841

Beccles, R.: Street Vending in Ghana, A solution or a Problem for development. Global Political Economy (2014)

Bhebhe, N.: Bulawayo's dying industry: is there hope for revival? News Day, November 2012, online. https://www.newsday.co.zw/bulawayo's-dying-industry-is-there-hope-for-revival. Accessed 08 Jan 2016

Bhowmik, S.: Street vendors in Asia: a review. Econ. Polit. Weekly **40**(22), 2256–2264 (2005)

Bhowmik, S.K.: Street vending in urban India: the struggle for recognition. In: Cross, J., Morales, A. (eds.) Street Entrepreneurs: People, Place and Politics in Local and Global Perspective, pp. 89–123. Routledge, London (2007)

Dell'Anno, R., AnaMaria, A., Balele, N.P.: Estimating shadow economy in Tanzania: an analysis with the MIMIC approach. J. Econ. Stud. **45**(1), 100–113 (2018)

Denscombe, M.: The Good Research Guide: For Small-Scale Social Research Projects (Open UP Study Skills). McGraw-Hill, New York (2010)

Devlin, R.T.: Informal urbanism: legal ambiguity, uncertainty, and the management of street vending in New York City (Doctoral dissertation). University of California, Berkeley (2010)

IFRA: Urbanization and Street Vending: How Street Vending an Individual and Collective Resource can be integrated into Urban Governance? IFRA. Nairobi (2016)

ILO: Supporting entrepreneurship education: a report on the global outreach of the ILO's Know about Business programme (No. 446902). International Labour Organization (2009)

Kirumirah, M.: The role of universities in enhancing community outreach services. a case of street vendors' training in Dar es Salaam. Master's thesis, University of Dar es Salaam, Dar es Salaam, September 2018

London, T., Hart, S.L.: Reinventing strategies for emerging markets: beyond the transnational model. J. Int. Bus. Stud. **35**(5), 350–370 (2004)

Lyons, M., Msoka, C.: Micro-trading in urban mainland Tanzania: The way forward. Final Report. Dar es Salaam, Development Partners Group on Private Sector (DPG-PSD/Trade), Development Consulting Services. Dar es Salaam: Development Consulting Services (2007)

Lyons, M., Msoka, C.: The world bank and the African street: doing business reforms in Tanzania. Urban Stud. **47**(5), 1079–1097 (2010)

Malefakis, A.: Creating a market where there is none: spatial practices of street vendors in Dar es Salaam, Tanzania. City Soc. **31**(1), 119–136 (2019)

Manyanhaire, O.I., Murenje, T., Chibisa, P., Munasirei, D., Svotwa, E.: Investigating gender dimensions in vending activities in the city of Mutare, Zimbabwe. J. Sustain. Dev. Africa **9**(4), 169–186 (2007)

Marras, S.: Street Food in Tanzania: A literature review: Food and Agriculture Organization of the United Nations (2018)

Martínez, L., Short, J.R., Estrada, D.: The urban informal economy: street vendors in Cali, Colombia. Cities **66**, 34–43 (2017)

Martins, J.H.: Socio-economic and hygiene features of street food vending in Gauteng. South Afr. J. Clin. Nutr. **19**(1), 18–25 (2006)

Mazhambe, A.: Assessment of the contribution of street vending to the Zimbabwe economy. A case of street vendors in Harare CBD. IOSR J. Bus. Manag. IOSR–JBM **19**(9), 91–100 (2017)

Mitullah, W.V.: Street Vending in African Cities: A Synthesis of Empirical findings From Kenya, Cote D'ivoire, Ghana, Zimbabwe, Uganda And South Africa, Background paper for the 2005 World Development Report (2003)

Mramba, N.R., Appiola, M., Kolog, A.E., Sutinen, E.: Technology for street traders in Tanzania: a design science research approach. Afr. J. Sci. Technol. Innov. Dev. **8**(1), 121–133 (2016)

Mramba, N.R.: The conception of street vending business (SVB) in income poverty reduction in Tanzania. Int. Bus. Res. **8**(5), 120–129 (2015)

Mramba, N., Sutinen, E., Haule, M., Msami, P.: Survey of mobile phone usage patterns among street vendors in Dar es Salaam city- Tanzania. Int. J. Inf. Technol. Bus. Manag. JITBM **28**(1), 1–10 (2014)

Muhanga, M.: Informal sector in urban areas in Tanzania: some socio-demographic, economic and legal aspects. Int. J. Account. Econ. Stud. **5**(2), 163–168 (2017)

Munishi, E.J., Casmir, R.O.: Overcoming business capital inadequacy and resilience implications for the urban street vendors' operations in Morogoro municipality. Bus. Educ. J. (BEJ) **1**(1), 1–8 (2019)

Nirathron, N.: Fighting poverty from the street. A Survey of Street Food Vendors in Bangkok. International Labour Organization (2006)

Njaya, T.: Nature, operations and socio-economic features of street food entrepreneurs of Harare, Zimbabwe. IOSR J. Humanit. Soc. Sci. **19**(4), 49–58 (2014)

Oosthuizen, C.L.: Skills needed to move from the street vendor to the shop owner. Masters dissertation, North-West University, South Africa (2008)

Otoo, M., Ibro, G., Fulton, J., Lowenberg-Deboer, J.: Micro-entrepreneurship in Niger: factors affecting the success of women street food vendors. J. Afr. Bus. **13**(1), 16–28 (2012)

Sparks, D., Barnett, S.: The informal sector in Sub-Saharan Africa: out of the Shadows to foster sustainable employment and equity. Int. Bus. Econ. Res. J. **9**(5) (2010). https://doi.org/10.19030/iber.v9i5.563

Steiler, I.: What's in a Word? The conceptual politics of 'informal' street trade in Dar es Salaam. Articulo-J. Urban Res. (17–18) (2018). https://doi.org/10.4000/articulo.3376

Suraiya, S., Noor, F.: An analysis of socioeconomic conditions of street vendors: a study on Dhaka city. Daffodil Int. Univ. J. Bus. Econ. **6**(1–2), 93–102 (2012)

Tengeh, R., Lapah, C.Y.: The socio-economic trajectories of migrant street vendors in urban South Africa. Mediterr. J. Soc. Sci. **4**(2), 109–127 (2013)

Tonda, N., Thembela, K.: Spaces of contention: tension around street vendors' struggle for livelihoods and spatial justice in Lilongwe, Malawi. Urban Forum **1–13**, (2016). https://doi.org/10.1007/s12132-016-9291-y

Vargas, A.: Outside the law: an ethnographic study of street vendors in Bogota. Lund Stud. Sociol. Law **45** (2016). https://ssrn.com/abstract=2837686

Verick, S.: The Impact of Globalization on the Informal Sector in Africa. Economic and Social Policy Division. United Nations Economic Cat Commission for Africa (2006)

Williams, C.C., Gurtoo, A.: Evaluating competing theories of street entrepreneurship: some lessons from a study of street vendors in Bangalore. India. Int. Entrep. Manag. J. **8**(4), 391–409 (2012)
World Bank: Tanzania: An Overview (2017). www.worldbank.org. Accessed 20 May 2017
Xue, D., Huang, G.: Informality and the state's ambivalence in the regulation of street vending in transforming Guangzhou, China. Geoforum **62**, 156–165 (2015)

Cluster Development Initiatives in Promoting Small and Medium Enterprises in Tanzania

B. S. Francis[1(✉)], A. Mwakalobo[2], and A. M. Nguyahambi[1]

[1] Department of Political Science and Public Administration, The University of Dodoma, P.O. Box 259, Dodoma, Tanzania

[2] Department of Economics, The University of Dodoma, P.O. Box 259, Dodoma, Tanzania

Abstract. This paper examined the implementation status of Cluster Development Initiatives (CDIs) in promoting Small and Medium Enterprises (SMEs) in Singida, Mbeya and Morogoro regions of Tanzania. Although much has been written on the contribution of CDIs in promoting SMEs, little attention has been given by scholars on the implementation status of CDIs particularly in Tanzania. In filling this knowledge gap, this paper focused on examining the implementation of technology, training, networking and capital supports. A cross-sectional research design with simple random sampling techniques were employed where by 150 SMEs owners in clusters were surveyed and key informants were interviewed for primary data. Both quantitative and qualitative data were analyzed by One Way ANOVA and thematic analysis respectively. The findings revealed that Implementation of CDIs supports in the study area was high on training and inadequate on capital with mean scores of .4819 and .2478 across both regions and clusters with statistically no significant difference at P Value = 0.18 and significant at P Value = 0.000 respectively in promoting SMEs. However, small loan sizes, long processes in loan processing and high reliance on donor funded projects were the major challenges on CDIs. It was concluded that CDIs have great potential towards promoting SMEs yet; it has not been explored and utilized to the maximum. It was therefore recommended that, policy makers via the responsible ministry should device a national strategy to provide clear guidance to all stakeholders as well as mainstreaming CDIs implementation in Local Government Authorities (LGAs) and special government budgets.

Keywords: Small and Medium Enterprises · Cluster Development Initiatives · Implementation

1 Introduction

Globally, Cluster Development Initiatives has been the promising mechanism that can expedite the promotion of Small and Medium Enterprises (SMEs) (UNIDO 2009; WorldBank 2017). This is premised from the fact that, clusters are associated with dynamism, innovation, competitiveness, joint actions, cooperation and externalities that enable enterprises to overcome many constraints including capital, skills and technology (Andersson et al. 2004; UNIDO 2009; Economic Development and in Africa Report

J. N. Mojekwu et al. (Eds.): *Sustainable Education and Development*, pp. 262–272, 2021.
https://doi.org/10.1007/978-3-030-68836-3_23

2011)). Recognizing the potentials of clusters, a number of public schemes for cluster based development initiatives have become functional in various parts of the world such as India, Canada and Italy to mention a few (UNIDO 2006). In India for instance, around 72% of employment, 59% output and 76% exports of the small scale industry sector exist in clusters (UNIDO 2015). Cluster achievements in these countries have been mainly due to comprehensive policy and promotional support from the government in terms of credit, technology and skill formation (UNIDO 2009; UNIDO 2015).

In most of Sub-Saharan African countries with exception of few countries like Ethiopia, SMEs are reported not to be well promoted such that they are locked in low-quality, low-income, poor information and technical knowhow and markets (Bigsten and Gebreeyesus 2007;Oyelaran-Oyeyinka & McCormick, 2007; Kenya's Industrial Transformation Programme, 2015; Iddrisu, Mano & Sonobe, 2012). However, in 2006 the Tanzania government adopted and started to implement CDIs as a strategy for promoting SMEs focusing on technology, training, capital support and networking (Diyamett and Komba 2008; Mwamila and Temu 2006). These components of CDIs were regarded as the major priority to cope with the main SMEs challenges in Tanzania (Kazimoto 2014; Mutalemwa 2009; Ministry of Trade and Industry 2012). Since its adoption in Tanzania, CDIs has been in operation but little is known on its implementation status. Some scholars, Musonda, (2007); Musonda, Adeya, & Abiola, (2008), Omolo, (2015) and Msuya, (2011) focused on knowledge, technology, cluster based growth, industrial dynamism as well as adoption and progress of CDIs in Tanzania. However, these studies shed little light on the status of implementation of CDIs for promoting SMEs. This paper therefore, aimed at examining the implementation status of CDIs in Tanzania focusing on the implementation of technology, training, networking and capital supports.

2 Theoretical Framework

This paper is underpinned by Resource Based Theory (RBT) and Institutional Economic theory (IET). RBT explains how various resources such as physical, financial, human and technological are essential for SMEs (Westhead, Wright, & Ucbasaran, 2001). CDIs, through its supports on capital, technology and training enhance SMEs resource acquisition. In order to capacitate SMEs resources, IET, insists on synergy through networking and linkages (Porter and Emmons 2003; Wares & Hadley, 2008). The question to be answered by this paper under the guidance of these theories is how resources like technology, training and capital (RBT) are linked with networking with various institutions (IET) under CDIs to meet diverse needs of SMEs business operations so as to promote SMEs in Tanzania.

3 Research Methodology

The research design for the study was cross sectional exploratory design which involved data collection at one point in time. The choice of this design based on the fact that it provided a very quick, efficient, accurate and economical means of accessing information about the population (Saunders 2011). This study was carried out in Singida, Morogoro and Mbeya regions, due to the fact that, Small Industries Development Organization

(SIDO) Cluster Development Initiatives were based in those regions and had been in operation for a significant period of time (Diyamett and Komba 2008; Msuya 2011). The population was owners of clustered SMEs under CDIs in Singida, Morogoro and Mbeya regions. The sample size was 150 SMEs owners. These respondents were proportionately sampled randomly from each SME in clusters in the respective regions. Key informants were sampled purposefully as follows; 1 MIT official, 8 SIDO officials, 2 COSTECH officials, 7 SMEs cluster chair persons. These made a total of 18 key informants. Data were collected from both primary and secondary sources. Primary data were collected through survey method in which questionnaire tool was used to collect quantitative data to 150 SMEs owners.

Also interview guide as a tool for qualitative data collection was used to interview the key informants. Observation method through the use of observation guide was also used to collect primary data. Secondary data were collected in which various reports related to SMEs cluster were used. Quantitative data were sorted, coded and then entered into Statistical Packages for Social Sciences (SPSS) for analysis. For each CDIs support respondents scored 1 in each element of the support if they received and 0 if they did not receive. Then the scores were summed up into and index score of each support relative to the number of elements in each support. Then the mean of an index score of each support were compared by One way ANOVA across regions and clusters so as to examine the implementation status of CDIs. Qualitative data were mainly analyzed by thematic analysis in which the recurring themes and subthemes were typed and presented in line with the paper objective.

4 Results and Discussion

The main objective of the paper was to examine the implementation status of Cluster Development Initiatives in promoting SMEs in Singida, Mbeya and Morogoro regions of Tanzania focusing on the implementation of technology, training, networking and capital supports as presented in Tables 1 and 2.

Table 1. Mean of CDIs supports implementation across Regions

Region	Kinds of support				
	n	Technological	Training	Networking	Capital
Singida	33	.3864	.5498	.4697	.4596
Mbeya	35	.3071	.4490	.5238	.1810
Morogoro	82	.3506	.4686	.4533	.1911
μ	150	.3483	.4819	.4733	.2478
Sign. level		.418	.182	.261	.000

Source: Survey Data, 2019

Table 2. Mean of CDIs supports implementation across clusters

Cluster	Kinds of support				
	n	Technological	Training	Networking	Capital
Mtinko sunflower oil processing	21	.4167	.5986	.5159	.4603
SIMUSOP	12	.3333	.4643	.3889	.4583
Mbeya rice group	12	.2917	.4881	.6667	.1806
Mbeya sunflower oil processing	23	.3152	.4286	.4493	.1812
Morogoro engineering	44	.2784	.3669	.3864	.1326
Morogoro food processing	11	.3182	.4675	.4545	.2121
Morogoro grain milling	27	.4815	.6349	.5617	.2778
μ	150	.3483	.4819	.4733	.2478
Sign. level		.024	.000	.000	.000

Source: Survey Data, 2019

5 Technological Support

Tanzania SME Development Policy of 2003 emphasizes on technology upgrading and transfers as significant aspects for SMEs development (URT 2003). Technological support under CDIs was implemented to clusters for enhancing technology upgrading and innovation on production process to enlarge production and improve the quality of the products. It was mainly in the form of operating machines, technological expertise, study tour to learn new technologies and inter firm technological learning and adoption.

Results in Table 1 indicate that, the overall average mean score of technological support implementation across regions was .3483 in which Singida region had mean implementation score of .3864 and Morogoro had mean implementation score of .3506 while Mbeya had mean implementation score of .3071. The differences in implementation of technological support across region was not statistically significant P value = 0 .418. On the other hand, results on Table 2 indicate that, the overall average mean score on implementation of technological support across clusters was .3483 with mean implementation score of .4167 at Mtinko sunflower oil processing cluster, .3333 in SIMUSOP sunflower oil processing cluster, .2917 in Mbeya rice group cluster, .3152 in Mbeya sunflower oil processing cluster, .2784 in Morogoro Engineering cluster, .3182 in Morogoro food processing cluster and .4815 in Morogoro grain milling cluster in which there was statistically significant differences in implementation of technological support at P value = 0 .024.

The findings implied that, the implementation of technological support across regions was almost the same. Notably, there was relatively higher implementation in Singida and Morogoro regions. This was supported by SIDO report which indicated that, most of the technological supports were implemented in Mtinko sunflower processing cluster, SIMUSOP in Singida region and Morogoro grain milling cluster in Morogoro region. Mtinko cluster received sunflower oil refinery machine from Market Infrastructure, Value Addition and Rural Finance (MIVARF) at a cost of TZS.71, 240,000 million and fortification machine from MEDA. They also received laboratory equipments and reagents from JICA for the refinery plant at a cost of about TZS. 20 million. Also in SIMUSOP cluster two SMEs were installed with fortification machines from MEDA while about 70% of SMEs in Morogoro milling cluster were installed with fortification machines from SANKU (SIDO, 2018). The findings conquer with the claim that, CDIs creates a competitive advantage that leads to absorb and create new technologies (Ali et al. 2016; Birhanu 2009). Moreover, during interview with SIDO and COSTECH officials it was reported that, COSTECH and SIDO in collaboration with JICA in the year 2018 organized one study tour to visit clusters in Davao city Philippines whereby some SMEs owners' representatives attended. From the findings, few abroad study tours implied that, most of technological knowledge used in the clusters especially in processing activities and engineering were learnt and adopted from within the country. In the same way, Zhihua Zeng, (2008) reported that, in most of SMEs clusters in Africa, knowledge and technology is acquired domestically; there are a few cases where the technology are adopted from abroad.

6 Training Support

Training support was implemented in the study area as part of CDIs to build capacity for SMEs in clusters to carry out various business activities in an effective and efficient manner. Training support under CDIs was provided in the form of business record keeping, marketing strategies; inter firm collaboration and networking, product value addition, product branding and promotion and bankable strategic business plan preparation.

The Results in Table 1 indicate that, the overall average mean score of training support implementation across regions was .4819 in which Singida region had mean implementation score of .5498 and Morogoro had mean implementation score of .4686 while Mbeya had mean implementation score of .4490. The differences in implementation of training support across regions was not statistically significant P value = 0.182. However, results on Table 2 indicate that, the overall average mean score on implementation of training support across clusters was .4819 with mean implementation score of .5986 at Mtinko sunflower oil processing cluster, .4643 in SIMUSOP sunflower oil processing cluster, .4881 in Mbeya rice group cluster, .4286 in Mbeya sunflower oil processing cluster, .3669 in Morogoro Engineering cluster, .4675 in Morogoro food processing cluster and .6349 in Morogoro grain milling cluster in which there was statistically significant differences in implementation of training support at P value = 0.000.

The findings implied that, though implementation of training support was the same across the regions, it was relatively high with mean implementation score of .4819 across clusters. This implied that there was high implementation of training support across regions and clusters in the study area. This signified that, training support implemented under CDIs in the study area provided broadly required skills and knowledge to SMEs in clusters. These findings align with Iddrisu, Mano, & Sonobe, (2012) that; training programs offered in the clusters are very important opportunities to acquire useful knowledge and skills. However, there were significant differences across clusters at P value = 0.000 in which Morogoro grain milling, Mtinko sunflower oil processing and Mbeya rice group clusters had mean score of 0.6349, 0.5986 and 0.4881 respectively on implementation of training support which was above the overall average mean score for training. This implied that training was highly implemented in these clusters compared to other clusters in the study area. COSTECH and SIDO officials during interviews affirmed;

> *"We organize several training for capacity building to cluster members depending on the needs and availability of funds. For instance, in Morogoro Municipality by the year 2015 TZS. 30 million was spent for training cluster facilitators in which Morogoro grain milling benefited much on training for preserving grains from poisonous fungus. Also JICA supported about TZS. 2,812,000 in July 2018 to hire experts for coaching machines operators and laboratory workers on sunflower oil refining process, hygiene and laboratory material preparation at Mtinko cluster in Singida region. Training on common product brands were also implemented at Mbeya rice and Mtinko sunflower oil processing clusters."*

The findings implied that, training support in the study area was implemented depending on the required knowledge and skills for cluster members. The results are in line with the resource based theory that; training should comprise human knowledge and innovative skills essential for SMEs business operations (Camelo-Ordaz et al. 2003).

7 Networking Support

Cluster Development Initiatives ensures SMEs form a complementary network or synergy (Cortright 2006; Gudda et al. 2013). In the study area networking support comprised of networking with raw material suppliers, academic/research institutions, donors/sponsors, financial institutions and Local Government Authorities (LGAs).

Results in Table 1 show that, the overall average mean score of networking support implementation across regions was .4733 in which Singida region had mean implementation score of .4697 and Morogoro had mean implementation score of .4533 while Mbeya had mean implementation score of .5238. The differences in implementation of networking support across regions was not statistically significant P value = 0.261. However, results on Table 2 indicate that, the overall average mean score on implementation of networking support across clusters was .4733 with mean implementation score of .5159 at Mtinko sunflower oil processing cluster, .3889 in SIMUSOP sunflower oil processing cluster, .6667 in Mbeya rice group cluster, .4493 in Mbeya sunflower oil processing cluster, .3864 in Morogoro Engineering cluster, .4545 in Morogoro food processing cluster and .5617 in Morogoro grain milling cluster in which there was statistically significant differences in implementation of networking support at p value = 0.000.

From the findings, the difference in implementation of networking support across regions was not statistically significant. This implied that, the number of networks established for clusters across regions were more less the same. A report by SIDO, (2017) indicated that, all SMEs under CDIs in Singida, Mbeya and Morogoro were linked to Local Government Authorities like district, municipal and city councils as well as financial institutions like banks and SACCOSS (SIDO 2018). During interview with clusster chairpersons it was revealed that, Mtinko and SIMUSOP sunflower oil processing cluster in Singida region and Sunflower oil processing cluster in Mbeya region were not directly linked to any academic/research institutions unlike other clusters in the study area. The findings implied that, though some important linkages like R&D institutions and raw material suppliers lacked in some clusters, CDIs formed both horizontal and vertical networks especially with a range of institutions depending on the need and type of SMEs business activities in the respective clusters in the study area.

The findings are supported by the argument that, creating a network with academic and research institutions, government authorities and private institutions, suppliers, retailers, wholesalers, banks and other service providers has proved to be success factor for SMEs in clusters due to minimizing the risk of failure (Alex 2014; Anwar et al. 2018). Similarly, institutional economic theory testifies that, an enterprise will enormously improve its performance in a specialized and networked environment (Gudda et al. 2013; Stamp 2013). In interview with SIDO and COSTECH officials it was also revealed that, CDIs created a network between clusters with various donors/sponsors in which most of the support programs implemented in the study area were funded by SIDA, JICA, MEDA and MIVARF. This implied that, CDIs attracted a network of sponsors/donors to SMEs in clusters whereby most of the supports implemented were donor funded.

However, there was statistically significant difference on implementation of networking support across clusters at P value = 0.000 in which Mbeya rice group, Mtinko sunflower oil processing and Morogoro grain milling clusters had higher mean score of networking support implementation which was 0.6667, 0.5159 and 0.5617 respectively. The means scores for these clusters were above the overall average mean score (0.4733) for networking support. This was due to the fact that, Mtinko and Mbeya rice group clusters were observed to be directly linked to suppliers of raw materials and output dealers in which Mbeya rice group cluster was linked to 2000 rice business dealers and over 1500 contracted small holder farmers in Momba, Mbarali, Kyela and Sumbawanga district for supplying raw materials (Mbeya Rice Group 2019). Also Mtinko Cluster leader in interview reported that, Mtinko sunflower oil processing cluster was linked to 52 farmers, 7 sunflower oil seeds businessmen, 5 transporters and 3 farmers groups. Likewise Morogoro grain milling cluster was observed to be linked to farmers, transporters and maize flour entrepreneurs (SIDO 2017). Evidently, networking in these clusters created both forward and backward linkages as well as taking into account the issue of combining cluster and value chain approach which is mostly appreciated for solving several constraints confronted by the entire sector, while rigorously emphasizing networks creation and interlinkages throughout every segment of the value chain (Ali et al. 2016).

8 Capital Support

Capital support was the form of support which was provided through CDIs to enable SMEs clusters to access fund for improving capital, purchase raw materials, machines, spare parts, equipment and meet the costs of other business operations. Capital support in CDIs was provided in the form of government funds directly to SMEs in clusters, loan from financial institutions linked to SMEs in clusters, SIDO loan to SMEs in clusters, fund from linked institutions interested with SMEs activities in clusters, subsidizing some clusters operational costs and special grants for supporting SMEs in clusters.

Results in Table 1 indicate that, the overall average mean score of capital support implementation across regions was .2478 in which Singida region had mean implementation score of .4596 and Morogoro had mean implementation level of .1911 while Mbeya had mean implementation score of .1810. The differences in implementation of capital support across regions was statistically significant P value = 0.000. However, results on Table 2 indicate that, the overall average mean score on implementation of capital support across clusters was .2478 with mean implementation level of .4603 at Mtinko sunflower oil processing cluster, .4583 in SIMUSOP sunflower oil processing cluster, .1808 in Mbeya rice group cluster, .1812 in Mbeya sunflower oil processing cluster, .1326 in Morogoro Engineering cluster, .2121 in Morogoro food processing cluster and .2778 in Morogoro grain milling cluster in which there was statistically significant differences in implementation of capital support at P value = 0.000.

Relatively low overall average mean score of .2478 in implementation of capital support with statistically significant difference at P value = 0.000 across regions and clusters implied that, capital support under CDIs was not sufficiently implemented in the study area. However, Mtinko sunflower cluster had high mean score on implementation of capital support compared to all other clusters in the study area. This was testified in a report by SIDO, (2018) which indicated that JICA covered the costs for business and preliminary processes for Tanzania Bureau of Standards (TBS) product permit and provided TZS.5, 841, 500 million to Mtinko cluster in Singida region to subsidize costs for official launching and promotion of the cluster. Moreover, some other linked institutions to the cluster like MIVARF provided TZS.342, 787,250 million for building a sunflower oil seeds storage facility with capacity of about 1000 tones. Furthermore, Singida Rural District Council provided directly TZS.45, 000,000 million to Mtinko cluster as contribution for construction of sunflower oil refinery plant. Findings are supported by the resource based theory which underlines that, CDIs should ensure availability of various resources including financial and physical resources to facilitate various business activities for SMEs in the clusters (Kozlenkova, Samaha, & Palmatier, 2014; Westhead, Wright, & Ucbasaran, 2001).

On the other hand, Ariksson, (2015); Hasan and Jamil 2014) reported that, in most developing countries loan has been the main source of capital for majorities of SMEs. Interviews with cluster chairpersons in the study area revealed;

> *"A few number of SMEs owners in clusters access loan from SIDO but majorities opt for loan using their collaterals from other linked financial institutions like NMB, CRDB, EQUIT, FINCA banks and SACCOSS simply because the loan size provided at SIDO is too small (NEDF/RRF TZS.6/6.5million maximum) to enable*

significant improvement of our SMEs business activities. Also the new Credit Guarantee Scheme (TZS.50million maximum) has long processes which lead to delays in securing loan. This sometimes culminated to some of us securing loan while the high season for business has already passed."

Findings further implied that, the main capital support to SMEs through loan in the study area was financial institutions like banks and SACCOSS linked to SMEs in clusters than SIDO loan. This could have been contributed by inadequate knowledge on SIDO loan schemes, small loan size and long processes leading to loan delay in some cases. All these jeopardized the implementation of capital support under CDIs. The findings tally with studies conducted in Ethiopia, Nigeria and Bangladesh which found that, some SMEs owners had to wait several months to secure fund they needed from the banks. Often, it was difficult to secure fund from the banks due to long assessment processes, these delays hindered a lot of business activities that could be carried out within the planned time (Ericksson 2015; Hasan and Jamil 2014).

Moreover, lowest mean score in Mbeya region for implementation of capital support implied that, SMEs in clusters in the region were not well supported on capital through CDIs. A financial report by SIDO, (2018) indicated that, between the year 2015 to 2018 a total loan amount of TZS.169 million was disbursed to 13 SMEs owners through NEDF and CGS loan schemes and none SME owner from Mbeya region received capital support through SIDO loan.

9 Conclusion and Recommendations

This paper contributes on understanding how resources (technology, training and capital) are linked with the aspects of networking with various institutions and stakeholders in the practice of promoting SMEs through CDIs. From the above results it is concluded that, Cluster Development Initiatives have great potential towards promoting SMEs yet; it has not been explored and utilized to the maximum in Tanzania since technological support base mostly on technological expertise rather than provision of modern machines, networking of SMEs in clusters do not adequately involve research/ academic institutions while capital support is mostly on loan by linked financial institutions due to small loan size and long processes of SIDO loan schemes and generally implementation of CDIs support highly depend on donor funded projects which make it to be unsustainable in most cases. It is therefore, recommended that, Policy makers especially on SME policies review the issues of sustainability on implementation of CDIs supports, device a national strategy for CDIs to provide clear implementation guidance to all stakeholders as well as mainstreaming CDIs implementation programs in Local Government Authorities (LGAs) and special government budgets.

References

Ali, M.,Godart,O., Görg, H., Seric, A.: Cluster Development Programs in Ethiopia: Evidence and Policy Implications. Kiel Institute for the World Economy, Kiel (2016)

Alex, A.N.: Industrial cluster-aboom for micro, small and medium enterprises. Int. J. Human. Arts Med. Sci. **2**(9), 61–66 (2014)

Andersson, T., Serger, S.S., Sörvik, J., Hansson, E.W.: The Cluster Policies Whitebook, vol. 49. Princeton, Citeseer (2004)

Anwar, M., Rehman, A.U., Shah, S.Z.A.: Networking and new venture's performance: mediating role of competitive advantage. Int. J. Emerg. Mark. **13**(5), 998–1025 (2018). https://doi.org/10.1108/IJoEM-07-2017-0263

Bigsten, A., Gebreeyesus, M.: The small, the young, and the productive: determinants of manufacturing firm growth in Ethiopia. Econ. Dev. Cult. Change **55**(4), 813–840 (2007)

Birhanu, D.: Small Scale Metalworking Industries Cluster (Case Study on Towns of Oromia Special Zone) The Thesis Submitted to School of Graduate Studies of Addis Ababa University in Partial Fulfillment of the Requirement for the Degree of Masters of Science in Mechani. Addis Ababa University (2009)

Camelo-Ordaz, C., Martín-Alcázar, F., Valle-Cabrera, R.: Intangible resources and strategic orientation of companies: an analysis in the Spanish context. J. Bus. Res. **56**(2), 95–103 (2003)

Cortright, J.: Making sense of clusters: regional competitiveness and economic development: Brookings Institution, Metropolitan Policy Program (2006)

Diyamett, B.D., Komba, A.A.: Tanzania Cluster Initiative Project: An Evaluation Report from the Eight Cluster Initiatives (2008)

Economic Development in Africa Report: Towards a new industrial policy in Africa: The why and the how of policy making. New York (2011)

Ericksson, E.: Demand of External finance by Manufacturing SMEs in Addis Ababa Ethiopia: Master thesis in Finance Gothernburg School of Business, Economics and Law (2015)

Gudda, P., M. Bwisa, H., M. Kihoro, J.: Effect of Clustering and Collaboration on Product Innovativeness: The Case of Manufacturing Small and Medium Enterprises (SMEs) in Kenya (2013)

Hasan, F., Jamil, G.M.H.: Financing small and medium enterprises in Bangladesh-issues and challenges. Asian J. Technol. Manag. **7**, 45–54 (2014). https://doi.org/10.12695/ajtm.2014.7.1.5

Iddrisu, A., Mano, Y., Sonobe, T.: Entrepreneurial skills and industrial development: the case of a car repair and metalworking cluster in Ghana. J. Knowl. Econ. **3**(3), 302–326 (2012)

Ivory, P.R.: Clusters and cluster initiatives: The role of collaboration and social capital in building a system of innovation in Ireland. Dublin City University (2012)

Kazimoto, P.: Assessment of challenges facing small and medium enterprises towards international marketing standards: a case study of Arusha Region Tanzania (2014)

Kenya's Industrial Transformation Programme: Ministration of Industrialization and enterprise development. Nairobi, Kenya (2015). http://www.industrialization.go.ke

Mbeya Rice Group: Five Years Strategic Plan (Jan 2019 - Dec 2024). Unpublished Report. Mwanjelwa SIDO Industrial Area, Mbeya (2019)

Ministry of Trade and Industry: Micro, Small and Medium Enterprises in Tanzania, National Baseline Survey Report. Government Printer, Dar es salaam (2012)

Ministry of Industry and Trade: Small and Medium Enterprise Development Policy. Government Printer, Dar es salaam (2003)

Msuya, F.E.: Status Report of Cluster Initiatives in Tanzania. Institute of Marine Sciences, Zanzibar (2011)

Musonda, F.M.: Small and micro enterprise clusters in Tanzania: can they generate industrial dynamism? In: Oyelaran-Oyeyinka, B., McCormick, D. (eds.) Industrial Clusters and Innovation Systems in Africa: Institutions, Markets and Policy, pp. 81–99. United Nations University Press, Hong Kong (2007)

Musonda, F.M., Adeya, C.N., Abiola, B.O.: Handicraft and Furniture Clusters in Tanzania. In: Rodrik, D. (ed.) Comments on Trade, Growth and Poverty, by D. Dollar and A. Kraay (2000). Retrieved from https://www.hks.harvard.edu/fs/drodrik/Researchpapers/ (2008)

Mutalemwa, D.K.: Barriers to SMEs development in the manufacturing sector: evidence from Tanzania. Afr. J. Bus. Econ. Res. **4**(23), 93–111 (2009)

Mwamila, B.L.M., Temu, A.K.E.: Innovation systems and clusters programme in Eastern Africa (ISCP-EA). In: 3rd Regional Conference on Innovation Systems and Innovative Clusters in Africa. Stimulating Competitiveness for Sustainable Economic Development 3–7 Sept 2006. Dar es salaam, Tanzania (2006)

Omolo, R.D.J.W.: Training and development on performance of small and medium enterprises in Kisumu County, Kenya. Int. J. Res. **26** (2015)

Oyelaran-Oyeyinka, B., McCormick, D.: Industrial Clusters and Innovation Systems in Africa. United Nations University Press (2007)

Porter, M.E., Emmons, W.: Institutions for collaboration: overview. HBS Case, 9–703 (2003)

Saunders, M.N.: Research Methods for Business Students, 5th edn. Pearson Education India, Chennai (2011)

Organization, S.I.D.: Promoting Industrialization in Tanzania Using Cluster Development Approach. Government Printers, Dar Es Salaam (2017)

SID Organization: A financial Report on the Disbursement of Loan to SMEs in clusters through NEDF and CGS Loan Schemes Unpublished Report, Dar Es Salaam (2018)

Stamp, M.: Guideline for Cluster Development, A Handbook for Practitioners. PLC, Croatia (2013)

UNIDO: Making Cluster Work, UNIDO Methodology. Foundation for MSME Clusters, New Delhi (2006)

UNIDO: Cluster DEVELOPMENT for Pro-poor Growth: The UNIDO Approach. United Nations Industrial Development Organization, Vienna (2009)

UNIDO: Changing Paradigms of Cluster Development. The global practitioners network for competitiveness clusters and Innovation (2015)

United Republic of Tanzania: Small and Medium Enterprise Development Policy. Government Printer, Dar es salaam, Tanzania (2003)

Wares, A.C., Hadley, S.J.: The cluster approach to economic development. Tech. Brief (7), 1–2 (2008)

Westhead, P., Wright, M., Ucbasaran, D.: The internationalization of new and small firms: a resource-based view. J. Bus. Ventur. **16**(4), 333–358 (2001)

WorldBank: Piecing together poverty puzzle. International Bank for Reconstruction and Development. World Bank, Washington, DC (2017)

The Influence of Firm Leverage on Performance Among Listed Firms in Dar es Salaam Stock Exchange

B. Mwenda[1(✉)], B. O. Ndiege[2], and D. Pastory[3]

[1] Department of Accountancy, College of Business Education, Mbeya, Tanzania
[2] Tanzania Co-operative Development Commission, Dodoma, Tanzania
[3] Department of Accountancy, College of Business Education, Dar es Salaam, Tanzania

Abstract. Many studies have looked at how firms make capital structure decisions. One important reasoning for capital structure decision is the consideration of agency costs and information asymmetry effects between the owners of the companies and the agents (managers of the companies). This study looked at the relationship between firm leverage and firm performance through the eyes of agency cost theory in the Tanzanian listed companies and thus expecting a positive relationship between the two. Panel data of 10 listed companies for 6 years was obtained for the fixed effect regression analysis of firm performance on firm leverage and other control variables. Results show that there is a negative relationship between firm leverage and firm performance in Dar es Salaam Stock Exchange (DSE) contrary to agency costs theory. Some studies have seen a similar trend in some countries, in Tanzania, the negative relationship can be explained by the underdeveloped and inefficient banking and corporate sector. Companies with low leverage have witnessed better financial performances.

Keywords: Firm performance · Capital structure · Agency cost · Fixed effect

1 Introduction

The primary goal of any business is profit maximization. In pursuit of this goal, managers may not necessarily seek to maximize utility of the shareholders. There is a conflict of interest which arises here. This conflict leads to the agency costs, the agents (managers) not being able to completely work in the interest of their principles (owners) (Jensen and Meckling 1976).

Information asymmetry theory argues that uncertainty can only lead to market inefficiency if one part has better information than the other. Parties will always have 'inside information' that concerns themselves that the other side does not have. The side with better information is said to have private information, equivalently, asymmetric information. One form of asymmetric information arises when an agent's service is being bought. The buyer may not always be able to monitor how hard and well the agent is working (Nicholson and Snyder 1972). Because of the information asymmetry problem, shareholders employ directors to monitor managers and run businesses on their behalf

J. N. Mojekwu et al. (Eds.): *Sustainable Education and Development*, pp. 273–283, 2021.
https://doi.org/10.1007/978-3-030-68836-3_24

and seek periodic feedback and reports in terms of financial statements. (Shiri et al. 2016; Kubota and Takehara 2016). Shiri et al. (2016) showed that firms with more disclosure practices were less prone to information asymmetry problem.

Agency costs arise as a consequence of information asymmetry between the owners and managers. Under imperfect markets, information asymmetry has a positive relationship with the cost of capital (Armstrong et al. 2011). These agency costs for a firm may come in many forms. In monetary terms, these consists of costs such as the incentives to the directors and remuneration packages as a means to make managers concentrate on maximizing utility of the owners of the business. Once satisfied with the remuneration, these directors are more likely to act properly on behalf of the principles to monitor the operations of the firms. Agency costs are also driven by the resources consumed by directors in the process of exercising their duties, example is the usage of company assets by directors.

The principles are also occasionally required to take part directly in meetings about the affairs of the firms. This is another agency cost, the time taken by the principles themselves in monitoring operations. When all these costs are exercised, total agency costs are likely to be minimized but not entirely wiped off. The remaining costs to the firm add up to residual losses which will always result as long as principles make use of agents (Jensen and Meckling 1976). Jensen and Meckling argues that, given agency costs, debt financing may help managers concentrate on profit maximization rather than individual utility maximization. Therefore, a more leveraged firm should result in a better financial performance.

Many studies have looked at the impact of capital structure decisions on firm performance. Modigliani and Miller, in their 1958 paper, assumed perfect market conditions to study the relationship between the choice of capital structure and firm performance. Perfect market conditions are those which are free of taxes, costs of transactions and other forms of friction such as agency costs. Market imperfections were later identified for the first time by Jensen and Meckling (1976). Many other studies were done building on the Jensen and Meckling paper. All the studies have had varying results on the relationship of capital structure on firm performance.

Capital of the firm, being made up of equity and debt has various costs involved with it. Equity shareholders expect to get returns based on their investment in the company, thus making the dividends the main costs associated with this source of capital. Firms acquire debts as well to finance both its short term and long term engagements. The cost of debt for a firm is the interest paid to the debtholders.

Trade-off theory and Pecking order theories have only suggested considerations before deciding on the nature of capital structure to adopt. The former argues that firms should look at the trade-off between tax benefits and bankruptcy when deciding on the level of debt while the later gives a hierarchy of considerations before going for external financing (Myers 1984). Under the assumptions of agency theory and the information asymmetry theories, it is expected that when a firm is less leveraged, agency costs will arise despite of the already present cost of capital. In this study, we look at the evidence from the Tanzanian listed companies to understand whether more leverage has helped managers concentrate more on profit maximization in order to be able to better service debts and hence reducing agency costs.

2 Leverage and Firm Performance

With the presence of agency costs, it is expected that firms will opt for more leverage to counter the increased costs of capital arising from the use of equity capital. Dawar (2014) found that in contrast to the assumptions of agency theory, leverage had a negative influence on financial performance of Indian firms. Many similar studies have also demonstrated this negative relationship including the study by Simerly and Li (2000) who found that debt had a negative impact on competitiveness of the firm as the imposition of covenants limits firm's ability to make decisions. Other studies, Majumdar and Chhibber (1999), Chiang et al. (2002), Abor (2007), Zeitun and Tian (2007), Onaolapo and Kajola (2010), Sadeghian et al. (2012), etc. have also reported similar results. Dawar (2014) argues that, the findings in his study may not be very surprising given the fact that most Indian firms obtain debt financing from the underdeveloped bond markets of India and the dominantly state-owned banks in India.

In conformity with the assumptions of agency theory, many studies have shown that the relationship between leverage and firm performance is not monotonic. In their 2010 paper, Margarities and Psillaki argues that at higher leverage a negative relationship can be expected but mostly there is a positive relationship between leverage and firm performance. Studies that have shown this relationship includes Hadlock and James (2002), Roden and Lewellen (1995), Williams (1987), Grossman and Hart (1982), Taub (1975), Lara et al. (2003) in case of the Brazilian companies, etc. In This study we look at the agency theory assumptions as observed in Tanzanian listed companies using panel data of 10 Tanzanian companies for a period from 2011 to 2016.

2.1 The Tanzanian Context

Most studies on capital structure and its impact on firm performance have been based on the more developed markets such as the USA, UK and Canada. (Dawar 2014). In Tanzania, some studies have been performed on this relationship. Kipesha and Moshi (2014) used 5 years panel data to look at the impact of capital structure on performance of 38 banks in Tanzania. Their study reveals a negative relationship between firm performance and firm leverage when firm performance is measured in terms of Return on Assets (ROA). This finding is contradicted by another result in their study which shows a positive relationship when firm performance is measured in terms of Return on Equity (ROE).

The study by Kipesha and Moshi did not control for other firm related or industry related variables. It also used only five years' data for the years from 2007 to 2011. Okiro, Aduda & Omoro in their 2015 paper, used data combined from the four stock exchanges in the East African Community, the Nairobi Stock Exchange (NSE), Dar es Salaam Stock Exchange (DSE), Uganda Stock Exchange (USE) and the Rwanda Stock Exchange (RSE). Their study only looked at the intervening effect of leverage on firm performance which was positive but they did not show separate trends within the individual stock exchanges. Lack of enough studies on firm leverage in Tanzania may be due to data availability problem. In this study, we have successfully obtained data for all the 10 listed companies that have been listed at DSE for at least 6 years and also at the same time controlling for other variables, firm size, sales growth and liquidity.

Other African studies on firm leverage and firm performance includes the study by Abor (2005), who studied the effect of capital structure on profitability of the listed companies in Ghana, David and Olorunfemi (2010) who studied the impact of capital structure on firm performance in the petroleum industry of Nigeria. This study on Tanzanian firms will be an important addition to the literature on firm leverage and firm performance in Africa.

3 Methodology

This study uses data on 10 listed firms in Dar es Salaam Stock Exchange (DSE). The focus of the study is to measure the influence of firm's leverage on DSE listed firms' performance, to do this, we have pooled data only for the Tanzanian firms listed at DSE for a period of at least 6 years. Only 10 firms qualified under these criteria due to the fact that DSE is still a young stock exchange and many firms in the country are not yet motivated to list in the stock exchange. Six years' panel data on these 10 firms was obtained from the DSE website.

The study uses two dependent variables, Return on Assets (ROA) and Return on Equity (ROE) to measure firm's performance. These variable (the ratios) are widely believed to be good measures of the firm's financial performance in an accounting period. Many similar studies have used the same variables in other countries including Kipesha et al. (2014), Dawar (2014), Okiro et al. (2015), etc.

Leverage of the firms is measured using the Short-term Debt Ratio (STDRATIO) and the Long-term Debt Ratio (LTDRATIO). Both of these ratios together represent the two possible leverage options that the firm can choose from. Mostly firms will have both types of leverage on their statements of financial position. Similar studies that have used same ratios to measure firm performance include Kipesha et al. (2014), Dawar (2014), Margaritis and Psillaki (2010), Nunes et al. (2009), Zeitun and Tian (2007). According to agency cost theory, firms with higher leverage are expected to perform better than those with less leverage (as argued in the above section). Managers of the more leveraged firms will focus more on the profitability of the businesses in order to be able to better service the acquired debts. Drawing from this theory and previous studies, we can state our two hypotheses as follows:

Ha0: Short-term debt has no relationship with firm's performance.

Ha1: Short-term debt has a positive relationship with firm's performance.

Hb0: Long-term debt has no relationship with firm's performance.

Hb1: Long-term debt has a positive relationship with firm's performance.

The study also controlled for other variables which are firm characteristics of size, sales growth and liquidity. Performance may be affected by firm size in the sense that it will make firms operate at different environments and hence getting different trading results. In this study, natural logarithm of the total assets has been used as the proxy for the firm size. Sales growth is another important variable since with increase in sales, profitability may also increase if firms manage their costs properly and consistently, liquidity on the other hand helps firms capitalize on short term financial deals and hence likely boosting their profitability. Similar studies that have controlled for some variables

Table 1. The explanatory variables and the expected impacts

Variable	Description	Expected sign
stdratio	This is the ratio of total short-term debts to the total assets of the firms for the years 2011 to 2016	+
ltdratio	This is the ratio of total long-term debts to the total assets of the firms for the years 2011 to 2016	+
sgrowth	This variable was measured by taking current year's sales minus previous year's sales dividing the result by the previous year's sales	+
liqd	Current ratio was chosen as the measure of the firm's liquidity. For each firm, this ratio was obtained from the year 2011 to 2016	+
lsize	Firm's size was measured by taking the natural logarithm of the total assets for the years 2011 to 2016	+

including the three variables in this study. (Dawar 2014: Margaritis and Psillaki 2010; Nunes et al. 2009; Zeitun and Tian 2007) (Table 1).

We can now write our two research models as;

$ROA_{i,t} = \beta_0 + \beta_1 STDRATIO_{i,t} + \beta_2 LTDRATIO_{i,t} + \beta_3 SGROWTH_{i,t} + \beta_4 LIQD_{i,t} + \beta_5 LSIZE_{i,t} + \mu.$

$ROE_{i,t} = \beta_0 + \beta_1 STDRATIO_{i,t} + \beta_2 LTDRATIO_{i,t} + \beta_3 SGROWTH_{i,t} + \beta_4 LIQD_{i,t} + \beta_5 LSIZE_{i,t} + \mu.$

4 Results

Table 2 shows the descriptive statistics of the secondary data obtained from listed companies at DSE. The total number of observations is 60, 2 observations have been removed by Eviews software for data missing reasons. Table 3 presents correlation analysis results of the independent variables. Only short term debt ratio has been seen to highly correlate with the liquidity (current ratio) of the firms.

Table 4 shows the results of the Hausman test on the choice of a regression method to use for the panel data. The results show that fixed effect method is more appropriate for the data on the listed Tanzanian firms. The chi-square statistic shows that we should reject the null hypothesis which is the use of the random effect method.

Tables 5 and 6 show the results of fixed effect regression analysis of ROA and ROE on short-term debt ratio, long-term debt ratio, sales growth, liquidity and natural logarithm of the total assets. Table 5 shows that only three variables are significant, short term debt ratio, long term debt ratio and sales growth while liquidity and size of the firms have an insignificant effect on firm's profitability in Tanzanian listed firms. Table 6 has only two variables significant, short term debt ratio and firm's size. Both tables have shown a negative relationship between firm's performance (as measured by both ROA and ROE) and firm's leverage (as measured by both STDRATIO and LTDRATIO).

Table 2. Descriptive statistics

	ROA	ROE	LIQD	LSIZE	LTDRATIO	SGROWTH	STDRATIO
Mean	19.71759	35.36879	7.174310	19.27890	0.129043	0.118460	0.418122
Median	10.17500	33.52000	2.735000	19.32895	0.089230	0.108299	0.279208
Maximum	69.26000	99.57000	29.55000	22.41257	0.457439	0.458423	0.888687
Minimum	−20.11000	−84.14000	0.460000	15.98759	3.25E−11	−0.242192	0.091906
Std. Dev.	21.06457	30.69328	8.236700	1.872308	0.125763	0.144984	0.278946
Skewness	0.587890	−0.665037	1.086903	0.052863	1.379993	0.019444	0.532889
Kurtosis	2.457624	5.839077	2.690922	2.012469	3.896517	3.241021	1.594586
Sum	1143.620	2051.390	416.1100	1118.176	7.484491	6.870682	24.25109
Observations	58	58	58	58	58	58	58

Table 3. Correlation aanalysis: independent variables

	LIQUIDITY	LSIZE	SGROWTH	STDRATIO	LTDRATIO
LIQUIDITY	1	0.5314	0.1887	0.7353	−0.5461
LSIZE	0.5314	1	0.1207	0.3476	−0.5986
SGROWTH	0.1887	0.1207	1	0.2637	−0.2448
STDRATIO	0.7353	0.3476	0.2637	1	−0.2682
LTDRATIO	−0.5461	−0.5986	−0.2448	−0.2682	1

Table 4. Hausman Test on the preferred effect (random or fixed effect panel data regression)

Correlated Random Effects - Hausman Test			
Test cross-section random effects			
Test Summary	Chi-Sq. Statistic	Chi-Sq. d.f	Prob.
Cross-section random	20.006671	5	0.0012

4.1 Discussion of the Findings

Contrary to agency theory, the results of this study indicates a negative relationship between firm performance and leverage (Tables 5 and 6). The more firms use leverage has been seen to cause less firm performance. Agency cost theory argues that more leverage should incline managers to focus on better performance so as to generate enough funds to repay the debts. This case of the Tanzanian firms is an indication of inefficiencies. These results are similar to the conclusion by Brewer and Featherstone (2016) who found that managers might improperly manage their affairs in order to get debt financing and hence end up with more inefficiencies.

Table 5. Results of regression analysis: ROA as dependent variable

Variable	Constant	stdratio	ltdratio	sgrowth	liqd	Lsize
Coefficient	94.3439	−16.8942	−42.7334	16.9972	0.3206	−3.4793
Std. Error	49.8728	7.4933	9.1860	5.8725	0.3674	2.5719
t-Statistic	1.8917	−2.2546	−4.6520	2.8944	0.8725	−1.3528
Prob.	0.0650**	0.0291*	0.0000*	0.0058*	0.3875	0.1829

Dependent Variable: ROA.
*significant at 5% level of significance.
**significant at 10% level of significance.

Table 6. Results of Regression Analysis: ROE as dependent variable

Variable	Constant	stdratio	ltdratio	sgrowth	liqd	lsize
Coefficient	336.1736	−69.3687	−7.28983	21.28418	−0.6592	−13.935
Std. Error	119.3536	30.76276	22.60405	13.8395	0.85863	5.985712
t-Statistic	2.816618	−2.25496	−0.3225	1.53793	−0.76773	−2.32804
Prob.	0.0073*	0.0293*	0.7486	0.1314	0.4468	0.0247*

*significant at 5% level of significance

Other reason could be the underdeveloped nature of the Tanzanian corporate sector, both financiers and the financed firms may participate in the poor management of the debt. The negative relationship between firm size and return on equity (Table 6) is another evidence of inefficiencies in the Tanzanian listed companies. More assets owned by companies should generate better financial returns. We can therefore say that the inefficiencies may come from generous terms from the debt providers and sluggish management of debt and assets by debt receivers can be a reason for the negative relationship. Similar results and conclusion were reached by Dawar (2014) for the case of Indian firms and Kipesha and Moshi (2014) for the case of Tanzanian commercial banks.

Similar to Dawar's (2014) argument, a prior paper by Bradford et al. (2011) argues that owner's private equity and private contribution to firm's debt has been seen to have a negative relationship with firm performance. In Tanzania, most big banks have some government share of ownership as well as most of the listed companies at DSE have government ownership. This can be related to this study's findings and Bradford et al. (2011) findings that such inefficiencies may be a result of the presence of government share of ownership on both listed companies and the providers of debt financing (the banks).

5 Conclusion

This study concludes that given the underdeveloped corporate sector in Tanzania, a negative relationship between firm leverage and firm performance can be expected. More leveraged firms perform poorer than the less leveraged firms due to inefficiencies. A further evidence for inefficiencies has been given by the observed negative relationship between firm size and firm performance. Further studies may look at the reason for the inefficiencies and where they result from and specifically pinpointing the reason for the negative relationship in Tanzania.

6 Appendices

Appendix 1: Eviews Output of the Regression of ROA on STDRATIO, LTDRATIO, SGROWTH, LIQD and LSIZE

Dependent Variable: ROA
Method: Panel Least Squares
Date: 01/03/18 Time: 09:54
Sample: 2011 2016
Periods included: 6
Cross-sections included: 10
Total panel (balanced) observations: 60

Variable	Coefficient	Std. Error	t-Statistic	Prob.
C	94.34391	49.87281	1.891690	0.0650
STDRATIO	−16.89415	7.493320	−2.254561	0.0291
LTDRATIO	−42.73341	9.185953	−4.652039	0.0000
SGROWTH	16.99716	5.872486	2.894373	0.0058
LIQD	0.320550	0.367373	0.872547	0.3875
LSIZE	−3.479313	2.571859	−1.352840	0.1829
Effects Specification				
Cross-section fixed (dummy variables)				
R-squared	0.957807	Mean dependent var		18.57317
Adjusted R-squared	0.944681	S.D. dependent var		21.78646
S.E. of regression	5.124177	Akaike info criterion		6.318135
Sum squared resid	1181.573	Schwarz criterion		6.841721
Log likelihood	−174.5440	Hannan-Quinn criter		6.522938
F-statistic	72.96712	Durbin-Watson stat		2.152846
Prob(F-statistic)	0.000000			

Appendix 2: Eviews Output of the Regression of ROE on STDRATIO, LTDRATIO, SGROWTH, LIQD and LSIZE

Dependent Variable: ROE
Method: Panel Least Squares
Date: 01/03/18 Time: 09:55
Sample: 2011 2016
Cross-sections included: 10
Total panel (unbalanced) observations: 58

Variable	Coefficient	Std. Error	t-Statistic	Prob.
C	336.1736	119.3536	2.816618	0.0073
STDRATIO	−69.36872	30.76276	−2.254958	0.0293
LTDRATIO	−7.289832	22.60405	−0.322501	0.7486
SALESGROWTH	21.28418	13.83950	1.537930	0.1314
LIQUIDITY	−0.659196	0.858630	−0.767731	0.4468
LSIZE	−13.93500	5.985712	−2.328044	0.0247
Effects Specification				
Cross-section fixed (dummy variables)				
R-squared	0.889524	Mean dependent var		35.36879
Adjusted R-squared	0.853555	S.D. dependent var		30.69328
S.E. of regression	11.74574	Akaike info criterion		7.982857
Sum squared resid	5932.386	Schwarz criterion		8.515730
Log likelihood	−216.5029	Hannan-Quinn criter		8.190422
F-statistic	24.73034	Durbin-Watson stat		2.999260
Prob(F-statistic)	0.000000			

Appendix 3: Eviews Output of the Hausman Test on the Choice of Random or Fixed Effect Regression Analysis for the Panel Data on 10 listed Firms at DSE

Correlated Random Effects - Hausman Test
Equation: EQ01
Test cross-section random effects

Test Summary		Chi-Sq. Statistic	Chi-Sq. d.f	Prob.
Cross-section random		20.006671	5	0.0012
Cross-section random effects test comparisons:				
Variable	Fixed	Random	Var (Diff.)	Prob.
STDRATIO	− 16.894149	− 30.232293	16.725785	0.0011
LTDRATIO	− 42.733411	− 51.128858	5.919813	0.0006
SALESGROWTH	16.997165	16.550202	3.548791	0.8125
LIQUIDITY	0.320550	− 0.131386	0.057294	0.0590
LSIZE	− 3.479313	− 2.050578	4.495612	0.5004

Cross-section random effects test equation:
Dependent Variable: ROA
Method: Panel Least Squares
Date: 01/03/18 Time: 11:30
Sample: 2011 2016
Periods included: 6
Cross-sections included: 10
Total panel (balanced) observations: 60

Variable	Coefficient	Std. Error	t-Statistic	Prob.
C	94.34391	49.87281	1.891690	0.0650
STDRATIO	− 16.89415	7.493320	− 2.254561	0.0291
LTDRATIO	− 42.73341	9.185953	− 4.652039	0.0000
SALESGROWTH	16.99716	5.872486	2.894373	0.0058
LIQUIDITY	0.320550	0.367373	0.872547	0.3875
LSIZE	− 3.479313	2.571859	− 1.352840	0.1829
Effects Specification				
Cross-section fixed (dummy variables)				
R-squared	0.957807	Mean dependent var		18.57317
Adjusted R-squared	0.944681	S.D. dependent var		21.78646
S.E. of regression	5.124177	Akaike info criterion		6.318135
Sum squared resid	1181.573	Schwarz criterion		6.841721
Log likelihood	− 174.5440	Hannan-Quinn criter		6.522938
F-statistic	72.96712	Durbin-Watson stat		2.152846
Prob (F-statistic)	0.000000			

References

Abor, J.: Effect of capital structure on profitability: empirical analysis of the listed firms in Ghana. J. Risk Financ. **6**(5), 438–447 (2005)

Armstrong, C.S., Core, E., Taylor, D.J., Verrecchia, R.E.: When does information asymmetry affect the cost of capital? J. Account. Res. **49**(1), March 2011. https://doi.org/10.1111/j.1475-679X.2010.00391.x

Bradford, W., Du, Q., Sokolyk, T.: Firm ownership, agency costs and firm performance. Researchgate, (a published paper, journal tittle and publisher not obtained yet) (2011)

Brewer, B., Featherstone, A.M.: Agency cost of debt: evidence from Kansas farm operations, Agricultural Finance Review, 77(1), 2017. Emerald Publishing Limited **111–124**, 0002–1466 (2016). https://doi.org/10.1108/AFR-03-2016-0023

David, D.F., Olorunfemi, S.: Capital structure & corporate performance in Nigerian petroleum industry: Panel data analysis. J. Math. Stat. **6**(2), 168 (2010)

Dawar, V.: Agency theory, capital structure and firm performance: some Indian evidence. Manag. Financ. **40**(12), 1190–1206 (2014). https://doi.org/10.1108/MF-10-2013-0275

Jensen, M.C., Meckling, W.H.: Theory of the firm: managerial behaviour, agency costs and ownership structure. J. Financ. Econ. **3**(4), 305–360 (1976)

Kipesha, E.F., Moshi, J.J.: Capital structure and firm performance: evidences from commercial banks in Tanzania. Res. J. Financ. Account. **5**(14), 168–178 (2014)

Kubota, K., Takehara, H.: (2016), Information asymmetry and quarterly disclosure decisions by firms: evidence from the Tokyo Stock Exchange. Int. Rev. Financ. **16**(1), 127–159 (2016). https://doi.org/10.1111/irfi.12068

Lara, J.E., Marcos, J., Mesquita, J.M.C.: Capital structure and profitability: the Brazillian case. *Researchgate*, (a published paper, journal tittle and publisher not obtained yet) (2003)

Margaritis, D., Psillaki, M.: Capital structure and firm efficiency. J. Bus. Financ. Acc. **34**(9–10), 1447–1469 (2007)

Modigliani, F., Miller, M.: The cost of capital, corporate finance and the theory of investment. Am. Econ. Rev. **48**(3), 261–297 (1958)

Myers, S.: The capital structure puzzle. Financ. **39**(3), 575–592 (1984)

Nicholson, W., Snyder, C.: Microeconomic theory: basic principles and extensions. South-western Cengage Learning, 3rd Edition (1972)

Okiro, K., Aduda, J., Omoro, N.: The effect of corporate governance and capital structure on performance of firms listed at the East African Community Securities Exchange. Eur. Sci. J. **11**(7) (2015)

Shiri, M.M., Salehi, M., Radbon, A.: A study of impact of ownership structure and disclosure quality on information asymmetry in Iran. VIKALPA J. Decision Mak. **41**(1), 51–60 (2016), Indian Institute of Management, Ahmedabad SAGE Publications sagepub.in/home.nav https://doi.org/10.1177/0256090915620876, https://vik.sagepub.com

Zeitun, R., Tian, G.: Capital structure and corporate performance: Evidence from Jordan. Australasian Account. Bus. Financ. J. **1**(4), 40–53 (2007)

External Factors Influencing Performance of Listed Firms on Dar es Salaam Stock Exchange

B. Mwenda[1(✉)], B. O. Ndiege[2], and D. Pastory[3]

[1] Department of Accountancy, College of Business Education, Mbeya, Tanzania
[2] Tanzania Co-operative Development Commission, Dodoma, Tanzania
[3] Department of Accountancy, College of Business Education, Dar es Salaam, Tanzania

Abstract. The prosperity of firm performance depends on external surrounding environment. However, in Tanzania, little is known about external factors influencing firm performance. The aim of this study was to determine the external factors influencing the performance of listed firms on Dar es Salaam Stock Exchange. The Study employed ex post facto research design as a guide. The sample size for this study consisted of 14 listed firms from 2011 to 2018. The study employed panel data, where secondary data for dependent variables were obtained from firms audited annual reports while independent variable data were obtained from National Bureau of Statistics, and Bank of Tanzania. The dependent variable (firm performance) was measured by Return on asset (ROA), while independent variables measured where; Exchange Rate, Gross domestic product, Lending Interest Rate, Inflation Rate, and Corporate tax rate with firm size and firm age as control variables. The study used two models (Model 1 and 2) during analysis. Model 1, the study included all variables, while model 2 dropped control variables (firm size and age) during analysis. Generalized Least Square method was used for analysis and testing the hypotheses. The findings indicated that inflation rate was positively significant to ROA at $p < 0.05$ and $p < 0.1$ in Model 1 and 2 respectively, while corporate tax rate was positively significant at $p < 0.01$ for Model 1 and 2. Exchange rate was negatively significant at $p < 0.01$ for model 1 and 2, while firm age had a positive significant influence on ROA at $p < 0.01$ in model 1. Such results have implications on firms since their survival, growth and performance highly depend on their interactions with the surrounding environment. The study recommends regulatory bodies and Bank of Tanzania to formulate policy frameworks to regulate and control effects of external factors in order to improve firm performance.

Keywords: Firm performance · External factors · Listed firms · Dar es Salaam Stock Exchange · Return on Assets

1 Introduction

Challenges of competition have led firms to realize the importance of good performance which would ensure firm sustainability. Firm performance is a general measure of firm's

J. N. Mojekwu et al. (Eds.): *Sustainable Education and Development*, pp. 284–296, 2021.
https://doi.org/10.1007/978-3-030-68836-3_25

overall financial health over a given period of time and how firms use their resources to generate profit (Obeng-Krampah 2018). The performance of a firm is affected by both internal and external factors. Internal factors exist within firm and under management control. These factors are capital turnover, leadership, organizational culture, sales growth, debt ratio and inventory level (Broadstock et al. 2011). External factors exist outside the firm and are out of management control. They include environmental and political condition, suppliers, government regulations, and competitors (Adidu and Olanye 2006). According to World Bank Group Report (2019) on economic monitoring, the main external factors include exchange rate, government expenditure, interest rate, inflation rate, corporate tax and gross domestic product. These main external factors can either give a threat to firm performance (Issah and Antwi 2017).

Before the 2008 global financial crisis, most of the business analysts paid more attention on firms' internal factors on business performance (Khan et al. 2018). It was until after the financial crisis of 2008, finance experts turned their focus on macroeconomic (external) factors which are out of management control to understand and predict future business performance (Issah and Antwi 2017). During the same financial crisis, Tanzania's Gross Domestic Product (GDP) was projected to be 8% and after the crisis the GDP was 5% for 2009/10. Also exchange rate depreciated by 13.2% from 2008 to 2009, whereby exchange rate in 2008 was about 1 USD to 1,162.9 Tshs and in 2009 it increased to about 1 USD to above 1,340 Tshs and ultimately affecting firms' performance (Ngowi 2015; Lunogelo et al. 2010).

Empirical evidence from both developed and developing countries depict the reality of the impact of macroeconomic (external) factors on firms' performance. For instance, a study by Zeitun et al. (2007) on macroeconomic determinants, conducted in Jordan documented that macroeconomic factor such as exchange rate of the country affect other sectors through cost of debt, as high exchange rate result into increase in interest rate. Supplementing this, another study by Rehman (2016) on the impact of macroeconomic variables on capital structure in textile industry of Pakistan revealed that out seven macroeconomic variables studied, corporate income tax variable was found to have a positive impact on firms' performance.

Similarly, a study by Dewi et al. (2019) on the impact of macroeconomic factors on firms' profitability in Indonesia, reported that inflation rate has a negative effect on profitability of listed firms in the same country. The experience form Turkey as depicted by Tuncay and Cengiz (2017) whose study focused on relationship between Corporate Profitability and Macroeconomic Indicators, shows that, there is a positive relationship between profitability (firms' performance) and GDP. Likewise, Ismail et al. (2018) examined how macroeconomic factors affect the performance of Insurance Companies in Malaysia Stock Exchange. Using Return on Asset (ROA) as a measure of performance of insurance companies, it was revealed that GDP and Interest rate have a positive effect on firm performance while Consumer Price Index (inflation rate) affected it negatively. A further study by Alibabaee and Khanmohammadi (2016) assessed economic variables and financial performance of listed companies in Iran Stock Exchange. Findings revealed that exchange rate had a positive influence on the performance of companies, while inflation and interest rate were insignificant.

In the African context, the influence of macroeconomic (external) factors on firms' performance has not been neglected. A study by Gatsi et al. (2013) which examined about corporate income tax and financial performance in Ghana listed firms found that, corporate income tax had a negative significant influence on financial performance while firm size and age were used as control variables had a positive significant influence on financial performance. However, Simiyu and Ngile (2015) found a negative relationship between GDP and firm performance in Kenya listed firms.

The reviewed studies have used different macroeconomic variables which have given both positive and negative implications to firm performance hence being inconclusive. In the same vein, some studies (Tuncay and Cengiz 2017; Ismail et al. 2018) were conducted from economies whose stock market exchange are powerful (save for those from the African context) and cannot be equated to that of Tanzania. Therefore, this study used the similar variables from previous studies and tested them using data from Tanzania.

In the Tanzanian context, little is documented on external factors influencing firm performance save for a few that have focused on internal factors. Naila (2013) and Norman (2012) examined internal factors such as environmental compliance on financial performance and usefulness of Financial Information in Capital Markets Investment Decision Making respectively. The scanty existing studies did not focus on external factors such as GDP, exchange rate, inflation, interest rate, and corporate tax rate. Yet it is an obvious fact that, the survival and growth of firm depends highly on the surrounding environment and their interactions (World Bank Group 2019).

Despite contradicting views from studies (Dewi et al. 2019; Tuncay and Cengiz 2017; Zetuin et al. 2007), on the relationship between external factors and firms' performance globally, insufficient empirical evidence exists in Tanzania and even those that exist are limited to internal factors (Naila 2013; Norman 2012). This gave a room for conducting further study and fill the notable knowledge gap in Tanzania by assessing the influence of external factors on firm performance. Therefore, the main objective of this study was to determine external factors influencing performance of listed firms on Dar es Salaam Stock Exchange. Specifically, the study sought to; (i) examine the influence of interest rate on performance of listed firms (ii) ascertain the influence of exchange rate on performance of listed firms (iii) examine the influence of corporate tax on performance of listed firms (iv) determine the influence of inflation rate on performance of listed firms (v) examine the influence of gross domestic product on performance of listed firms.

The study hypotheses was:

H_0 : External factors does not influence performance of listed firms on Dar es Salaam Stock Exchange.

2 Theoretical Framework

The study was guided by Open Systems Theory (Bertalanffy 1969), cited by Owolabi (2017) with an assumption that, Organizations exist in an open setting where their activities are highly influenced by the surrounding environment (external factors). The external factors are out of the organisation control. The factors include interest rate, exchange rate, corporate tax, inflation rate and gross domestic product among others.

The theory assumes that the organization cannot exist alone and must depend on external factors for survival. Thus, organizations should adopt from their environment and also gain advantage from risks posed by interactions (Owolabi 2017; Laszlo and Krippner 1998; Buckley 1967). Thus Owolabi (2017) argues firm managers should know there surrounding environment and the influence they pose on firm performance. The theory implication to this study is that firms will attain competitive advantage once having a properly structured and coordinated functioning with their external environment since external factors are a huge determinant of firm performance.

3 Methodology

This Study employed ex post facto research design. According to Kothari and Garg (2014) and Kerlinger and Rint (1986) ex post facto research design aims to investigate possible relationships between two or more observing variables (cause-effect relationship). Ex post facto design is considered to be suitable for this study because, the study is non-experimental, it only seeks to examine causal relationship between the dependent and independent variables of the study (Owolabi 2017).

The Targeted population of this study was 28 listed firms in DSE. Census approach was used to obtain 14 listed firms operating domestically and with an experience of 8 years of operation from 2011 to 2018. The remaining 14 firms were dropped since, 7 were inactive foreign firms and the other 7 are domestic but had less than 3 years of operation. According to Tekatel (2019) for a sound performance analysis, it is best to have data of more than three years of observation. Hence, this study observed data from 2011 to 2018 by taking firms with a minimum of 8 years of operation as a benchmark. The study employed panel data where, secondary data for dependent variable (ROA) were obtained from listed firms' audited annual reports such as income statement and statement of financial position. Panel data for external factors (independent variables) were obtained from National Bureau of Statistics (NBS), and Bank of Tanzania (BOT).

3.1 Operationalization of the Variables

Financial ratios, such as Return on Assets (ROA), Return on Equity (ROE), Return on Sales (ROS), Sales Growth (SG), and Operating Margin (OM) are used to measure firm performance. According to Gilchris (2013) ratios offer a wider understanding of a firm's performance by using information extracted from firms' annual reports. In this study, ROA was used to measure firm performance as a dependent variable since it shows how firm managers use their assets to generate profit. Other researchers such as Issah and Antwi (2017) as well as Kanwal and Nadeem (2013) used ROA in their studies to measure firm performance. ROA was calculated as;

$$ROA = \frac{profit\ before\ tax}{Total\ Assets} \tag{1}$$

The independent variables analyzed in this study were Exchange Rate, GDP, Lending Interest Rate, Inflation Rate, and Corporate tax rate while control variables where Firm size and age. The description of each variable and their expected sign are given in Table 1.

Table 1. Description of variables and their expected signs.

Variables	Formula	Type of variable	Expected sign
Return on Asset (ROA)	Profit before tax/Total assets	Dependent	
Natural Log of exchange rate	Exchange rate during a year between USD and TSh	Independent	(±)
Gross Domestic Product (GDP)	Final output of goods and services	Independent	(±)
Lending Interest Rate (LIR)	Lending rate during the year computed by Bank of Tanzania (BOT)	Independent	(±)
Inflation Rate (IR)	Consumer Price Index (CPI) annual percentage changes	Independent	(±)
Corporate Tax Rate (CTR)	Income tax/operating income × 100	Independent	(±)
Firm Size (FS)	Natural logarithm of total assets in the period	Control	(±)
Firm Age (FA)	Number of years since incorporated till the period of study	Control	(±)

3.2 Model Specification

This study used Multiple Regression Model for analysis. A number of studies (Dewi et al. 2019; Issah and Antwi 2017; Alibabaee and Khanmohammadi 2016) analyzing the influence of external factors on firm performance used panel data and multiple regression model for analysis. With this regard, Multiple Regression Model was suitable for analysing the objectives due to the nature of the dependent variable which was numerical (continuous) variable. The Model used in this study is stated below;

$$Y_{it} = \beta_0 + \beta_1 X_{it} + \beta_2 Z_{it} + \mu_i + \alpha_t + \varepsilon_{it} \tag{2}$$

where; Y is return on asset (ROA), β_0 is constant, β_1 and β_2 are coefficients to be estimated, X is set of treatment variables (GDP, LnExchange Rate, Lending Interest Rate, Inflation Rate and Corporate tax rate), Z is a vector of control variables (firm size and firm age), μ is firm dummy capturing time invariant firm's specific effect, α_t is time dummy capturing time variant specific effect, ε is error term assumed to be white noise, i and t are firm and time units respectively.

3.3 Diagnostic Tests

Before the regression analysis was conducted, important diagnostic tests were carried to ensure the assumptions such as multicollinearity, heteroskedasticity, autocorrelation and stationarity. These were checked to ascertain whether they satisfy data requirements (Kennedy 2008; Bryman and Cramer 2001).

3.3.1 Multicollinearity Test

Pearson Correlation matrix was used to test for the assumption of multicollinearity in this study. The assumption of multicollinearity is met when correlation coefficients are $\leq+0.9$ or ≥-0.9 between variables (Field 2013). When two variables are highly correlated, they violate multicollinearity assumptions; hence one variable is dropped because both variables measure the same effect. Table 2 summarizes the Pearson correlation matrix of variables.

Table 2. Pearson correlation matrix

Variable	ROA	Gross domestic product	Lending interest rate	Inflation rate	Lnexchange rate	Corporate tax rate	Firm size	Firm age
ROA	1							
Gross domestic product	−0.0375	1						
Lending interest rate	−0.1755	0.0033	1					
Inflation rate	0.1587	−0.3443	−0.715	1				
Lnexchange rate	−0.2309	0.1237	0.7779	−0.7726	1			
Corporate tax rate	0.2531	0.0456	0.0163	0.0482	0.0002	1		
Firm size	0.1142	−0.0793	−0.2619	0.0915	−0.1814	0.0967	1	
Firm age	0.3101	0.0092	0.1119	−0.1064	0.1185	0.1528	0.062	1

From Table 2, variables were retained for further analysis since there was no problem of multicollinearity among variables and the correlation coefficients were between the accepted range ($\leq+0.9$ or ≥-0.9). Also, the study tested multicollinearity using Variance Inflation Factor (VIF), where VIF results were less than 5 hence, there was no problem of multicollinearity (Table 3). These results are supported by Gikombo AND Mbugua (2018) who argued that for multicollinearity problem, the value of VIF should be greater than 5.

3.3.2 Heteroscedasticity Test

This study also tested for heteroskedasticity assumption to check the presence of constant variance within residuals. Breusch-Pagan/Cook-Weisberg was used to test the validity for this assumption. According to Biorn (2017) the assumption of heteroskedasticity is met when the ***p***-value is greater than 0.05. It was found that ***p*** value of chi^2-statistic (17.80) being 0.0000 which was below the significant level 0.05 for ROA. Hence, the study

Table 3. Variance Inflation Factor (VIF)

Variables	Inflation rate	Lnexchange rate	Lending interest rate	Gross domestic product	Firm size	Corporate tax rate	Firm age
VIF	3.67	3.38	3.31	1.39	1.16	1.06	1.05
1/VIF	0.272156	0.296273	0.302142	0.721904	0.860709	0.941381	0.955568

rejected the null hypotheses and concluded that there was heteroskedasticity problem in ROA.

3.3.3 Autocorrelation Test

Furthermore, autocorrelation was also tested in this study. The assumption of autocorrelation is met when values of the same variables have no similarities among them over consecutive period of time (Pallant 2010). This means that, past values cannot be used to predict future values. The Wooldridge (2002) test was used to check the validity of this assumption. The assumption is met when the p – value is greater than 0.05. For this study the p-value of F-statistic (0.247) was 0.6276 and greater than the significant level of 0.05 for ROA. Hence, the study failed to reject null hypotheses. Therefore, there is no first order autocorrelation problem in ROA.

3.3.4 Stationarity

Levin-Lin & Chu test was used to test the assumption of stationarity in this study. The assumption of stationarity is met when the p - value are less than 0.05 (Biorn 2017). The findings in Table 4 indicate that stationarity assumption was met since the p values were less than 0.05 hence all variables were retained for analysis.

Table 4. Levin-Lin-Chu unit-root test

Variables	Unadjusted t	Adjusted t*	p-value
Return on asset(ROA)	−8.9819	−6.5107	0.0000
Gross domestic product	−11.9118	−10.6533	0.0002
Lending interest rate	−15.8378	−16.9053	0.0000
Inflation rate	−37.8777	−36.5923	0.0000
Exchange rate	−4.1861	−3.1093	0.0009
Corporate tax	−51.8976	−48.5654	0.0000
Firm size	−7.7498	−4.4507	0.0000
Firm age	−4.0044	−3.9404	0.0001

The diagnostic tests conducted revealed that there was no problem with diagnostic assumptions with an exception of heteroskedasticity whose values (***p*** value of chi^2-statistic (17.80) being 0.0000) were less than the accepted value of 0.05 hence violating the assumption. In order to overcome this problem, the study adopted the Generalized Least Square (GLS) as a remedy to the problem as recommended by Gujarati (2004) and Ongore and Kusa (2013) that in order to overcome the problem of heteroscedasticity in the study data, Generalized Least Square (GLS) method is used for analysis to provide best estimates.

4 Findings and Discussion

4.1 Descriptive Statistics

The study intended to examine the external factors influencing the performance of listed firms. Both dependent and independent variables were measured in this study. To provide the overview of these variables, descriptive statistics were conducted. These involved Mean, Standard deviation, Minimum and maximum values. Table 5 presents a summary of dependent variable (ROA), independent variables (GDP, lending interest rate, inflation rate, Lnexchange rate, and corporate tax) and control variables (firm size and age).

Table 5. Descriptive statistics

Variable	Obs	Mean	Std. Dev.	Min	Max
ROA	112	9.169588	28.29236	−163.77	84.42
Gross domestic product	112	6.675	0.74453	5.1	7.9
Lending interest rate	112	16.22125	0.843393	14.96	17.62
Inflation rate	112	7.781387	4.051663	3.5	16.00054
Lnexchange rate	112	7.526726	0.157889	7.350773	7.7248
Corporate tax rate	112	0.2240657	0.202414	−0.3	1.133787
Firm size	112	7.826251	1.143296	4.678573	9.733656
Firm age	112	26.14286	18.4649	1	68

Results from Table 5 showed that the mean values of dependent variable was 9.17% for ROA which is less than its standard deviation of 28.29% indicating the presence of high variation in ROA while minimum and maximum were −163.77% and 84.42% respectively. The independent variables results showed that the mean value of GDP was 6.68% greater than its standard deviation of 0.74% and with a minimum value of 5.1% and maximum value of 7.9%. The mean value of Lending Interest Rate (LIR) was 16.22%, greater than its standard deviation of 0.84% with 14.96% and 17.62% for Minimum and Maximum respectively. Also the Inflation Rate (IR) was 7.78% which was greater than its standard deviation of 4.05% with 3.5% and 16% for minimum and maximum respectively. Natural log of Exchange Rate (LnEXR) had a mean value of

7.53% greater than its standard deviation of 0.16% and with the minimum value of 7.35% and maximum value of 7.72%. Corporate Tax Rate (CTR) had a mean value of 22.4% which was higher than standard deviation of 20.2% with the minimum value of 30% and maximum value of 113.3%. For control variables, mean values of Firm Size (FS) and Firm Age (FA) were 8 and 26 years of operation respectively.

4.2 Regression Results

Generalized Least Square method was used to analyze the influence of external factors on the performance of listed firms on DSE. This study used two models (model 1 and 2) during analysis. In model 1, the study included all variables; while model 2, dropped control variables (firm size and age) during analysis in order to check robustness (consistence) of the results. The coefficient of variables were considered to have either positive or negative statistically significant influence on firm performance at **p values** were less than 0.01, 0.05, or 0.1 (Field 2013). Results of panel regression model (GLS) are presented in Table 6.

From Table 6, the inflation rate had a positive statistical significance at $p < 0.05$ and $p < 0.1$ with coefficients of 8.3158 and 7.8163 for model 1 and 2 respectively. These findings imply that an increase in inflation improves performance of the listed firms due to positive coefficients on both models. Such results echo those of Hooshyari and Moghanloo (2015) whose study revealed that inflation has a positive correlation with profitability of firms in Iran. However, Dewi et al. (2019) reported contradicting results in which inflation had a negative effect on performance of firms in Indonesia. The difference in the above results could be attributed to environmental variations, economic policies in the two different countries and cultural practices. These results are in line with the Open System Theory since inflation had a positive influence on firm performance because organization activities are highly influenced by the surrounding environment.

The Coefficient of exchange rate showed a negative significant relationship with ROA at $p < 0.01$with a coefficient of −0.0203 for model 1 and −0.0317 for model 2. Equated to these findings, Alibabaee and Khanmohammadi, (2016) noted that, exchange rate has influence on firm performance only when economy of the country is exposed to international markets and its effect may be directed differently. Open System Theory supports this study results as exchange rate was found to influence firm performance.

Coefficient of Corporate Tax Rate (CTR) had a positive statistical significance correlation with ROA at $p < 0.01$ with coefficients of 30.7153 and 37.3576 for model 1 and 2 respectively. With the reality that the tax structure of listed firms are based on firm performance, thus there are expectations of having positive relationship between tax rate and firm performance. The results are in line with the findings of Rehman (2016), but contrasting with results of Gatsi et al. (2013). The articulated contradiction in findings above could be as a result of differenced in monetary policies, environmental and political conditions, government regulations, and competitors. These findings support Open System Theory which contend that, the increase in firm performance leads to increase in corporate tax rate which is an external environment.

The coefficient of firm age showed positive significant relationship between firm age and ROA at $p < 0.01$ with a coefficient of 0.9922 for model 1 only. This implies that more experienced firms have the advantage of increased customer base hence improving

Table 6. Panel regression results of generalized least square run against ROA

Variables	Model 1	Model 2
Gross domestic product	−10.7412	−9.6356
	(7.530)	(10.232)
Lending interest rate	−4.4944	−5.5882
	(4.569)	(6.205)
Inflation rate	8.3158**	7.8163*
	(4.006)	(4.002)
Lnexchange rate	−0.0203***	−0.0317***
	(0.007)	(0.011)
Corporate tax rate	30.7153***	37.3576***
	(11.913)	(12.346)
Firm size	−0.3087	
	(2.225)	
Firm age	0.9922***	
	(0.289)	
Time dummy	Yes	Yes
Firm dummy	Yes	Yes
Constant	−954.0989	410.6483***
	(645.069)	(154.902)
Observations	112	112
Number of firms	14	14

Standard errors in parentheses *** $p < 0.01$, ** $p < 0.05$, * $p < 0.1$

their operations as well as sales for better firm performance. These results are in line with Becker et al. (2006); Noor and Fadzillah (2010) who reported that firm age had a positive significant effect with the firm performance.

5 Conclusion and Recommendations

5.1 Conclusion

This study sought to examine external factors influencing firm performance in Tanzania. For the purpose of analysis, this study selected 14 listed firms in DSE having 8 years of operations from 2011 to 2018 as a benchmark. Multiple Panel Regression (Generalized Least Square) was used for analyzing variables in this study and found inflation rate, Corporate Tax Rate and firm age to have positive significant influence on ROA while exchange rate had a negative significant influence. The survival of firms depends on external factors for its growth and performance. This is because these influence the firm performance both positively and negatively. It is high time for firms to focus their attention on the external environment since they survive in an open surrounding environment that allows give and take. Once the external environment is neglected, the firm performance might be threatened.

5.2 Recommendations

Based on research findings, the study recommends the Bank of Tanzania (BOT) and other regulatory bodies to stabilize exchange rate by using foreign reserve available so as secure resources from foreign countries. When foreign currency appreciates, the central bank should increase supply of foreign currency in the economy. On the other hand, when it depreciates, the central bank should collect excess supply of foreign currency in the economy to maintain a constant exchange rate. Also the government should maintain reasonable range of interest and inflation rate in order to achieve higher corporate tax as a result of good firms' performance.

References

Adidu, F.A., Olanye, P.A.: Basic Small Business Entrepreneurship: A Modern Approach. Royal Pace Publishers, Agbor (2006)

Alibabaee, G., Khanmohammadi, H.M.: Economic variables and financial performance of company listed Stock Exchange. IRAN Int. Bus. Manag. **19**(10), 4561–4566 (2016)

Becker, J., Fuest, C., Hemmelgarn, T.: Corporate tax reform and foreign direct investment in Germany-evidence from firm-level data (2006)

Bertalanffy, L.V.: General Systems Theory. Braziller, New York (1969)

Bryman, A., Cramer, D.: Quantitative Data Analysis with SPSS Release 10 for Windows: A Guide for Social Scientists. Psychology Press, London (2001)

Broadstock, D.C., Shu, Y., Xu, B.: The heterogeneous impact of macroeconomic conditions on firms' earnings forecast. In: Macao, Macao International Symposium on Accounting and Finance (2011)

Buckley, W.: Sociology and Modern Systems Theory. Prentice- Hall, Englewood Cliffs (1967)

Biorn, E.: Economics of Panel Data: Methods and Applications. Oxford University Press, Oxford (2017)

Chaudhry, I.S., Ayyoub, M., Imran, F.: Does inflation matter for sectoral growth in Pakistan? an empirical analysis. Pak. Econ. Soc. Rev. **51**, 71–92 (2013)

Dewi, V.I., Soei, C.T.L., Surjoko, F.O.: The impact of macroeconomic factors on firms' profitability (evidence from fast moving consumer good firms listed on indonesian stock exchange). Acad. Account. Finan. Stud. J. **23**(1), 1–6 (2019)

DSE: Capital Market Product and Services Development, p. 45. Dar es Salaam, Tanzania (2017)

Field, A.: Discovering Statistics using IBM SPSS, 4th edn. SAGE publications Ltd., London (2013)

Gatsi, J.G., Gadzo, S.G., Kportorgbi, H.K.: The effect of corporate income tax on financial performance of listed manufacturing firms in Ghana. Res. J. Finan. Account. **4**(15), 118–124 (2013)

Gikombo, E.M., Mbugua, D.: Effect of select macro-economic variables on performance of listed commercial banks in Kenya. Int. Acad. J. Econ. Finan. **3**(1), 80–109 (2018)

Gilchris, M.: Influence of bank specific and macroeconomic factors on the profitability of 25 commercial banks in Pakistan during the time period 2007–2011. Am. J. Bus. Finan. **3**(2), 117–127 (2013)
Gujarati, D.N.: Basic Econometrics, 4th edn. McGraw-Hill, New York (2004)
Haider, S., Anjum, N., Sufyan, M., Khan, F., Ullah, A.: Impact of macroeconomic variables on financial performance: evidence of automobile assembling sector of Pakistan stock exchange. Sarhad J. Manag. Sci. **4**(2), 202–213 (2018)
Hooshyari, N., Moghanloo, A.P.: Evaluating the impact of inflation on profitability of banks. Arab. J. Bus. Manag. Rev. **9**(4), 19 (2015)
Ismail, N., Ishak, I., Manaf, N.A., Husin, M.M., Hasim, A.: Macroeconomic factors affecting performance of insurance companies in Malaysia. Acad. Account. Finan. Stud. J. **22**, 1–5 (2018)
Issah, M., Antwi, S.: Role of macroeconomic variables on firms' performance: Evidence from the UK. Cogent Econ. Finan. **5**(1), 1405581 (2017). https://doi.org/10.1080/23322039.2017.1405581
Kanwal, S., Nadeem, M.: The impact of macroeconomic variables on the profitability of listed commercial banks in Pakistan. Eur. J. Bus. Soc. Sci. **2**(9), 186–201 (2013)
Kennedy, P.: A Guide to Econometrics, 6th edn. Blackwell Publication, Oxford (2008)
Kerlinger, F.N., Rint, N.: Foundations of Behaviour Research. Winston, London (1986)
Khan, F., Ullah, A., Ali, M.A., Khan, M.I.: The relationship between macroeconomic variables and the dividend payout ratio of the textile sector listed on Pakistan stock market. Sarhad J. Manag. Sci. **4**(1), 111–121 (2018)
Kothari, C.R., Garg, G.: Research Methodology: Methods and Techniques. New Age International Limited, New Delhi (2014)
Lunogelo, H.B., Mbilinyi, A., Hangi, M.: Global financial crisis discussion series paper 20: Tanzania phase 2. Overseas Dev. Inst. **111**, 01–07 (2010)
Mwangi, E.N., Wekesa, S.: Influence of economic factors on organizational performance of airlines: a case study of Kenya Airways Ltd. J. Hum. Soc. Sci. **22**(5), 8–14 (2017)
Naila, D.L.: The effect of environmental regulations on financial performance in Tanzania: a survey of manufacturing companies quoted on the Dar Es Salaam Stock Exchange. Int. J. Econ. Finan. Issues **3**(1), 99–112 (2013)
Ngowi, P.H.: Economic crisis: implications and responses in the banking sector. Afr. J. Econ. Rev. **3**(1), 100–115 (2015)
Noor, R.M., Fadzillah, N.S.M.: Corporate tax planning: a study on corporate effective tax rates of Malaysian listed companies. Int. J. Trade Econ. Finan. **2**(1), 189–193 (2010)
Norman, A.S.: The usefulness of financial information in capital markets investment decision making In Tanzania: a case of Iringa Region. Int. J. Mark. Technol. **8**(2), 50–65 (2012)
Pallant, J.: SPSS Survival Manual: A Step by Step Guide to Data Analysis Using SPSS. Allen and Unwin (2010)
Omodero, C.O., Mlanga, S.: Evaluation of the impact of macroeconomic variables on stock market performance in Nigeria. Bus. Manag. Stud. **5**(2), 34–44 (2019)
Ongore, V.O., Kusa, G.B.: Determinants of financial performance of commercial banks in Kenya. Int. J. Econ. Finan. Issues **3**(1), 237 (2013)
Owolabi, B.A.: Economic characteristics and financial performance of selected manufacturing companies in Nigeria: Masters Dissertation, University of Babcock: Nigeria, p. 112 (2017)
Obeng-Krampah, K.D.: The Impact of Macroeconomic Factors on Firm Performance: Masters Dissertation, University of Ghana, p. 132 (2018)
Rehman, Z.U.: Impact of macroeconomic variables on capital structure choice: a case of textile industry of Pakistan. Pak. Dev. Rev. **55**(3), 227–239 (2016)
Simiyu, C.N., Ngile, L.: Effect of macroeconomic variables on profitability of commercial banks listed in the Nairobi securities exchange. Int. J. Econ. Commer. Manag. **4**(3), 1–6 (2015)

Singh, T., Mehta, S., Varsha, M.S.: Macroeconomic factors and stock returns: evidence from Taiwan. J. Econ. Int. Finan. **4**(3), 217–227 (2011)

Tekatel, L.W.: Financial Performance Analysis: A study on Selected Private Banks in Ethiopia: Masters Dissertation, University of Andhra, p. 55 (2019)

Tuncay, F., Cengiz, H.: The relationship between corporate profitability and macroeconomic indicators: evidence from 500 largest industrial organizations in Turkey. Int. Bus. Res. **10**(9), 87 (2017). https://doi.org/10.5539/ibr.v10n9p87

Usman, O.A., Adejare, A.T.: Inflation and capital market performance: the Nigerian outlook. J. Emerg. Trends Econ. Manag. Sci. (JETEMS) **5**(1), 93–99 (2013)

Wooldridge, J.: Econometric Analysis of Cross Section and Panel Data. MIT Press, Cambridge (2002)

World Bank Group (2019). https://www.worldbank.org/en/research/brief/economic-monitoring, Accessed 6 Sept 2019

Laszlo, A., Krippner, S.: Systems theories: their origins, foundations, and development. Adv. Psychol. Amsterdam **126**, 47–76 (1998)

Zeitun, R., Tian, G., Keen, S.: Macroeconomic determinants of corporate performance and failure: evidence from an emerging market the case of Jordan. Corp. Ownersh. Control. **5**(1), 179–194 (2007)

Zulfiqar, Z., Din, N.U.: Inflation, interest rate and firms' performance: the evidence from textile industry of Pakistan. Int. J. Arts Commer. **4**(2), 111–115 (2015)

Online Marketing Strategies in Creating Loyalty Among ALAF LTD Customers in Tanzania

Z. T. Lweno[1] and R. G. Mashenene[2(✉)]

[1] ALAF LTD., P.O. Box 169, Dodoma, Tanzania
zuberi.lweno@safalgroup.com

[2] Dodoma Campus, Department of Marketing, College of Business Education, P.O. Box 2077, Dodoma, Tanzania
g.mashenene@cbe.ac.tz

Abstract. This study examined the influence of online marketing strategies on creating loyalty to ALAF LTD customers in Tanzania. Specifically, the study dealt with (i) to identify online marketing strategies applied by ALAF Ltd, (ii) to assess customers' perception toward online marketing strategies adopted by ALAF Ltd, (iii) to determine the relationship between online marketing strategies and customer loyalty. The study adopted cross-sectional research design. The study involved Dodoma City ALAF Ltd customers and the sample size was 78 ALAF customers who were randomly selected. Data were collected using questionnaire, interview, and documentary review. To analyze qualitative data, the study adopted content analysis. To assess customers' perception toward online marketing strategies descriptive statistics were used whereas means and standard deviations were computed. To determine the relationship between online marketing strategies and customer loyalty, binary logistic regression model was performed. The findings revealed that Facebook, Instagram and website were highly used as online marketing strategies whereas Facebook, Instagram and WhatsApp were highly perceived by customer to be greatly used online market strategies. The binary logistic regression results indicated a positive relationship exist between online marketing strategies and customer loyalty. The study concludes that online marketing strategies are important ingredients to enhance customer loyalty. The study recommends that ALAF Ltd should improve usage of online marketing strategies.

Keywords: Online marketing strategies · Customer loyalty · ALAF LTD · Tanzania

1 Introduction

Online marketing strategies elsewhere globally have been crucial in creating customer loyalty. For instance, in Kenya, companies dealing with tour businesses such as travel agencies and those engaging with specialty tour businesses; have also managed to solicit a big number of new businesses via online platforms, mostly through electronic mail (Wanjau, Macharia and Ayodo 2012). Generically, the most successful websites are those which are easy to find names and they are registered with various search engines (WTO

J. N. Mojekwu et al. (Eds.): *Sustainable Education and Development*, pp. 297–309, 2021.
https://doi.org/10.1007/978-3-030-68836-3_26

2011). Similarly, in recent years e-retailing has become an alternative shopping channel (Brown et al. 2003); previous studies globally on e-shopping experiences revealed that a positive relationship between frequency of e-purchases and e-shopping tendency and negatively related to the probability to terminate an e-transaction (Brown et al. 2003). The study further revealed positive feelings of online shoppers towards online shopping compared to non-shoppers. A comparative study on on-line marketing usage between US and Irish students showed the US students were more exposed to online marketing than those in Irish (Mikalef et al. 2013), this implies that online marketing strategies have spread globally.

In Kenya, the success story about the development of tourism industry has been great and the contribution of the industry to the growth of the country's Gross Domestic Product (GDP) has also been significant, has created employment opportunities and it has raised the foreign exchange earning capacity. In Tanzania, internet users were approximately 20 million and the internet had penetrated at 20 percent number of 19,862,525 populations (Tanzania Communication Regulatory Authority (TCRA) 2016). In this view, digital marketing in the country is now at the elementary stage in a sense that there is a small number of online users and still there is a minimum usage of digital marketing visa vis the country population estimation of 50 million (National Bureau of Statistics (NBS) 2016). The number of internet users in Tanzania indicates government initiatives and efforts in developing communication and internet facilities. For instance, in 2009 Tanzania established the project known as the National Information and Communication Technology Broadband Backbone (NICTBB) as one of the initiatives (Kowero 2017). Also, in 2015 the government amended the National Act and established the Electronic Regulation with aim to protect operators and consumers on electronic transaction (BOT 2016) and in 2016 the ICT policy was enacted. Together, such efforts have fueled the use of on-line marketing as promotional strategy.

ALAF was established in October 1960 as a Tanzania's pioneer roofing solution manufacturer with its head office in Dar es Salaam region and strategic branches being located in Dodoma, Mwanza, Arusha and Mbeya. Adoption of online marketing strategies by ALAF has been one of the factors for its growth whereby customers are being frequently updated with new information. As the result, this strategy has been found to be cost effective and time saving, in addition, the company receives feedback from customers which remarks as one of the indicators of customer loyalty. As it is in the global perspective that online marketing is increasing with increase in the communication technology, likewise in Tanzania, currently number of firms and business agencies have started blending the traditional marketing strategies with the online marketing strategies as a way to reach several prospects and making their services well known to the customers. A number of initiatives to improve online marketing have been made by ALAF Management in support of the Government initiatives. Such initiatives include usage of social media such as Instagram, Facebook, WhatsApp, search engine, websites and e-Books. Despite these efforts, no any empirical study has been conducted by ALAF Company to establish online marketing strategies and their influence on customer loyalty. Therefore, this study aims at examining how online marketing strategies influence creation of loyalty among ALAF customers in Tanzania.

2 Methodology

2.1 Data

This study was conducted in Dodoma City whereas ALAF Ltd was purposefully selected due to being the producer of building and construction materials with the largest market share in Dodoma city and the use social media to communicate with its customers as one of its marketing strategies. The selection of Dodoma city was based on its current status of being the pronounced the quickest growing city in the country. The growth of Dodoma city has been accelerated by the government decision to shift its operations from Dar es Salaam city to Dodoma city. Following this shift, a lot of building and construction activities in Dodoma city are taking place which require ALAF LTD products. This study employed cross-sectional research design due to the fact that the design allows the researcher to collect data at one point and it is appropriate when the researcher is constrained with time and financial resources.

The population of ALAF was composed of three hundred and forty (340) permanent customers that was obtained from the company data base. It is from this study population a sample of seventy-eight (78) permanent customers was drawn. Determination of the sample size was performed using the formula by Yamane (1967) as follows;

$$n = \frac{N}{1 + N\,(e)^2} \tag{1}$$

Where by; -
n = Sample size
N = Population size
e = Precision level at 10%
$n = 340/$
$1 + 340\,(0.1)^2$
$n = 77.977 = 78$

To select final respondents from the population, the list of ALAF Ltd customers was obtained from the Dodoma ALAF Ltd office since the customer database was accessible to all ALAF Ltd staffs. It was from this list the researcher randomly selected the sample using lottery. The study used secondary and primary data. Data from primary sources were captured by the use of survey in which questionnaire and interview with key informants were used. The questionnaire included several closed ended and few open-ended questions. Mostly, questionnaire had 5-points Likert scale questions. Previous studies such as Mashenene (2020) and Mashenene and Kumburu (2020) argued that 5 – points Likert scale questions are suitable in studies that intend to generate index scores. Before data collection, the questionnaire was pre-tested in order to omit unsuitable questions and add important missing questions. To supplement quantitative data, interviews using interview guide were conducted for the purpose of collecting the firsthand information from the key informants who were the ALAF employees. Key informants were purposefully selected based on their knowledge and experience on issues related to online marketing. During the interview, data was recorded using note books and mobile phones. Secondary data were obtained from ALAF Ltd offices and various government reports through documentary review.

3 Analytical Model

Content analysis was employed in the analysis of qualitative data collected through interviews. Transcription of recorded data into text was first carried out which followed by categorizing them into relevant themes and sub-themes. Qualitative findings obtained from the analysis were interpreted and presented in the form of quotations and they were matched with the relevant theory and existing literature (Kumburu and Kessy 2018).

Microsoft Excel and version 23 of the Statistical Package for Social Sciences (SPSS) were employed as analytical tools for the analysis of quantitative. Before data analysis was carried out, data were edited and validated to omit unsuitable and irrelevant data. Thereafter, data were coded and entered into the SPSS for analysis.

To identify online marketing strategies, descriptive statistics were used whereas means and standard deviations were computed from the 5-points Likert scale responses. Interpretation of results was based on means generated. To determine customers' perceptions, data collected using 5-point Likert scale were subjected to descriptive statistics whereas means and standard deviations were computed. Interpretation of the results was based on means obtained. To determine the relationship between online marketing strategies and customers' loyalty among the ALAF Ltd customers, binary logistic regression model was employed as an econometric model. Customer loyalty which was measured using 5-points Likert scale, its responses were factored using factor analysis. Further, the factor scores were segregated using mean score into binary response (0,1). During analysis, ten identified online marketing strategies used by ALAL Ltd as independent variables namely; email marketing, search engine, Facebook, Instagram and WhatsApp, website, viral marketing, e-books, banner advertisement and online public relations were reduced into seven online marketing strategies after dropping e-book, banner advertisement and online public relations. The criterion for dropping e-book, banner advertisement and online public relations was based on the fact that these variables were perceived with customers with a mean score below 3.0. The online marketing strategies as independent variables were captured using 5-points Likert scale questions which during analysis were transformed into index scores. The binary logistic regression equation was presented as follows;

$$\Pr(Y = 1/x) = \beta_0 + \beta_1 x_1 + \beta_2 x_2 + \beta_3 x_3 + \beta_4 x_4 + \varepsilon \quad (2)$$

Whereby; -
Pr = the Probability function
Y = Customer loyalty
X = the linear predictor (independent variables to be predicted)
β_0 = Constant
X_1 = Email marketing
X_2 = Search engine optimization
X_3 = Social media and viral marketing
X_4 = e-Book, website and banner advertisement

To examine the challenges facing ALAF Ltd in the adoption of online marketing, descriptive statistics through multiple responses were performed in order to establish cases of occurrences for the respective challenges. During the analysis, the responses on the challenges which were summarized in "Yes" and "No" categories were subjected to multiple responses to determine cases of occurrence.

To ensure validity of data, triangulation approach was adopted whereas several data collection and analysis methods were used. Prior to the main survey, a pilot study was carried out from which questions in the questionnaire were validated and the questionnaire was improved based on what was observed during the pilot study. Reliability in this study was established using Cronbach's Alpha test. Cronbach (1951) pointed out that this test measures the overall consistency of the research instrument. The coefficient of Cronbach's alpha when is equal to 0.7 or above it is interpreted that data are reliable (Pallant 2011). Cronbach's alpha test for reliability has been widely used in several recent previous studies (Mashenene and Kumburu 2020; Mashenene 2016).

4 Findings and Discussion

4.1 Online Marketing Strategies Used by ALAF Ltd

The findings (Table 1) shows the mean score and standard deviations which were computed in the course of identifying online marketing strategies used by ALAF Ltd. The findings indicate that the mostly used online marketing strategies by ALAF Ltd are Website (mean = 4.12), Facebook (mean = 4.14) and Instagram (4.14).These findings imply that ALAF Ltd uses websites, Facebook, and Instagram as its popular marketing strategies since they were ranked with the highest mean score which was greater than the mean score of 3.0. Additionally, the findings (Table 1) show that e-books (mean 3.8718), search engine (mean = 3.3462) and viral marketing (mean = 3.2564) are popular online marketing strategies used by ALAF Ltd since they had mean scores greater than 3.0. Other findings (Table 3) show that email marketing (mean = 2.6923), WhatsApp (mean = 2.7821), banner advertisement (mean = 2.5385) and online public relations (mean

Table 1. Online marketing strategies applied by ALAF Ltd (n = 78)

Online marketing strategies	Min.	Max.	Mean	Std. Dev.
Email marketing	1.00	2.00	2.6923	1.46453
Search engine	1.00	2.00	3.3462	1.47882
Facebook	1.00	2.00	4.1410	.95030
Instagram	1.00	2.00	4.1410	.95030
E-books	1.00	2.00	3.8718	1.33648
Website	1.00	2.00	4.1538	.97314
WhatsApp	1.00	2.00	2.7821	1.41552
Viral marketing	1.00	2.00	3.2564	1.43948
Banner advertisement	1.00	2.00	2.5385	1.50175
Online public advertisement	1.00	2.00	2.7692	1.42405

Source: Field work, 2019

= 2.7692) were online marketing strategies moderately by ALAF Ltd since their mean scores were greater than 2.5. These findings are supported by those of Timilsina (2017) which indicated that Website, Facebook and Instagram were widely used online marketing strategies by companies in Finland. The findings also indicated that the online marketing strategies have created easily accessible and affordable marketing atmosphere in reaching several customers within a short period of time. These findings also are in line with those of Mashenene et al. (2019) which revealed that online marketing strategies are very powerful tools for enhancing customer loyalty in Tanzanian higher education.

5 Customer's Perception Toward ALAF Online Marketing Strategies

Generally, the findings (Table 2) indicate that the overall mean score of customers' perceptions was 3.59, implying that the customers' perception was high since it was above the mean score of 2.5. Specifically, the findings (Table 2) indicate that the highly perceived online marketing strategies used by ALAF Ltd are Facebook (Mean = 4.6923), Instagram (Mean = 4.7436) and WhatsApp (Mean = 4.4615), email marketing (Mean = 3.8718), search engine (Mean = 3.4487), Website (Mean = 3.6154) and Viral Marketing (Mean = 3.8974) which were above the average mean score of 3.0. These results imply that Facebook, Instagram and WhatsApp were important online marketing strategies and were perceived useful by ALAF customers. These findings match with those of Wanaque, Zeeshan and Imam (2016) which revealed that online marketing strategies were useful in creating customers' awareness, increase attractions and provide customers with search box and product categories to make products easily accessible to customers. Nevertheless, e-books scored mean of 2.423, banner advertisement scored a mean of 2.7821, and finally, online public relations had a mean of 2.0256. From these results, the

Table 2. Customer' perception on ALAF online marketing strategies (n = 78)

Online marketing strategies	Min.	Max.	Mean	Std. Dev.
Email marketing	1.00	5.00	3.8718	1.45369
Search engine	1.00	5.00	3.4487	1.01479
Facebook	2.00	5.00	4.6923	.79459
Instagram	3.00	5.00	4.7436	.56834
E-books	1.00	5.00	2.4231	1.08734
Website	2.00	5.00	3.6154	1.03486
WhatsApp	2.00	5.00	4.4615	.93548
Viral marketing	2.00	5.00	3.8974	1.08819
Banner advertisement	1.00	5.00	2.7821	1.27562
Online public relations	1.00	5.00	2.0256	1.25847
Overall Mean			**3.59**	

Source: Field work, 2019

variables had low customers' perceptions which imply that they were unfriendly applied by the ALAF Ltd customer.

6 Findings from Binary Logistic Regression

The coefficient of email marketing (Table 3) was 0.24 implying that a unit increase in the use of email marketing will result into 2.4% increase in customer loyalty. The results further indicate that email marketing was statistically significant and the odds ratio was 1.1, implying that the contribution of email marketing to customer loyalty was high. These findings are supported by those of Dilham et al. (2018) in Indonesia which revealed that internet marketing had a significant influence on customer loyalty. These findings were also supported by those of Lemmenett (2014) which entailed that email marketing strategy was a good strategy to reach customers directly and it was a famous strategy in cost saving.

Table 3. Findings from binary logistic regression

Predictors	B	S.E.	Exp (B)
Email marketing	0.024***	0.012	1.126
Search Engine	0.046***	0.068	1.347
Social media and viral marketing	0.037***	0.011	1.259
E-books, website, banner advertisement	0.012**	0.007	1.013
Constant	0.419	1.303	1.521

Source: Field work, 2019

Notes: ** and *** represent significance levels at 5% and 1% respectively.

The binary logistic regression results were supported by the qualitative findings which exhibited;

"*...our company use email at great extent in sharing information about our products and giving feedbacks to our customers on their customers. Basically, email marketing as one among our online marketing strategies helps us much in meeting customer demand and loyalty..." (The interview conducted with ALAF Ltd Branch manager on 12thApril 2019) ...*".

The coefficient of search engine (Table 3) was 0.046 implying that a unit increase used in search engine results into 4.6%. The results further indicate that search engine was statistically significant and the odd ratio was 1.4, implying that the contribution of search to customer loyalty was high. These findings are supported by those of Hidayanto et al. (2012) which indicated that search engine marketing was aimed at increasing company's visibility. As the implication, customers get a chance to access company's information via search engines. These findings were supported by the qualitative findings which entailed that;

"...Search Engine Marketing (SEM), support us through allowing our company to post adverts on search engines like Google, which stands as proven and an effective audience acquisition strategy. Our company search engine marketing strategy helps us to reach several customers and reasonably period realize return on investment..." (Interview conducted with ALAF Ltd Sales Manager on 15th May2019).

The findings (Table 3) indicate that the coefficient of social media and viral marketing was 0.037 implying that an increase in using social media and viral marketing results into 3.7% increase in customer loyalty. The results further indicate that social media and viral marketing were statistically significant and the odd ratio was 1.3, implying that the contribution of social media and viral marketing to customer loyalty was high. These results are in relation with those of Khan (2018) which found that social media and viral marketing had significant impact on brand equity.

The findings are in relation with those of interview as it was detailed by one of the key informants that;

"...Social media and viral marketing are among the important online marketing strategy in our company which support much in increasing the number of customers resulting into good sales returns. But as sales management team, we all know that, social media are not for everyone and social media should not be used just for the sake of technology but its potentiality on interaction, taking part in the discussion, and sharing knowledge..." (Interview held with ALAF Ltd Sales Manager on 27th May 2019) ...."

The findings (Table 3) indicate that the coefficient of e-books, website, and banner advertisement was 0.012 implying that an increase in the use of e-books, website, and banner advertisement results into 1.2% increase in customer loyalty. The results further indicate that e-books, website and banner advertisement were statistically significant and the odd ratio was 1.0, implying that the contribution of e-books, website and banner advertisement to customer loyalty was high. These findings were in harmony with those of Cyr et al. (2008) which showed that company websites enhance customer trust, satisfaction and loyalty.

7 Rating of the Online Marketing Strategies According to Loyalty

Basing on the issue of email marketing, the findings (Table 4) indicate that customers were served well and promised not to look for other suppliers as it was depicted mean score of 3.2179 which was above the average mean of 3.0 and taking arising issues easy and give them time and trust to fix them scored a mean of 3.2821. This means that customers were satisfied with the services offered by the ALAF Ltd. However, in case of making several repeat purchases via email scored mean of 2.5897 which was below the average mean of 3.0 actually indicate that there was moderate use of email for product purchases by the customers.

Additionally, based on search engine findings indicate that, it was good, and increased visiting frequently scored mean of 3.5769, not wasting of time to look for other sources scored mean of 3.5641, and finally referring to friends and contacts scored mean of 3.9872 which all variables were above the average mean. These results indicate that, in the concern of search engine customers had higher trustworthiness with the ALAF Ltd through the use of online marketing strategy.

Moreover, in case of social media and viral marketing results denote that, customer's advocacy for ALAF social media platforms scored a mean of 4.4103, customer frequently purchased through ALAF social media scored mean of 3.1538, and giving feedback to ALAF so that they can improve their products and services scored mean of 4.0000 which were all above the average mean of 3.0. This means that, social media and viral marketing with concentration of the above variables had higher support on the customer's loyalty in the ALAF Ltd. However, in case of daily visit ALAF Facebook, Instagram, WhatsApp pages to look for some new things scored mean of 2.7564 which was below the average mean of 3.0. This means that the variables had moderate support on the concern. These findings are supported by those of Salvador (2014) which indicated that viral marketing strategy is crucial to every company.

Furthermore, in case of e-books, website, banner advertisement results validate that, opening to other products and services offered by ALAF scored mean score of 3.9359, purchases volume have increased scored mean of 3.5769, being happy, and never look for other suppliers scored mean of 3.8205, and customer willing to buy variety of ALAF products scored mean of 3.6538 which are above the mean average of 3.0. These results

Table 4. Rating ALAF online marketing strategies according to loyalty (n = 78)

Online marketing strategies	Mean	Std. Dev
Email marketing		
I am served well; I will not look for other suppliers	3.2179	1.18044
I made several repeat purchases via email	2.5897	1.21073
I consider emerging issues easy and try to fix them	3.2821	1.12697
Search engine		
It's so good, increased my visiting frequently	3.5769	1.06319
I don't waste time to look for other sources	3.5641	1.25450
I always refer to friends the products	3.9872	.98684
Social media and viral marketing		
I do advocacy for social media platforms	4.4103	0.78021
I frequently purchase through social media	3.1538	1.20687
I always visit social media to look for new things	2.7564	1.17535
I give feedback for improvement of products	4.0000	1.03196
E-books, website, banner advertisement		
I am open to other products offered by ALAF	3.9359	1.17705
My purchase volume has increased	3.5769	0.91905
I am happy, I will never look for other suppliers	3.8205	1.10187
I am willing to buy variety of products	3.6538	1.33705

Source: Field work, 2019

imply that there was higher customer's satisfaction on the services offered by ALAF Ltd in the case of products and information services which results into customer loyalty.

8 Challenges Facing ALAF Customers in Adoption of Online Marketing Strategies

Findings (Table 5) indicate the cases for the challenges facing ALAF customers in the adoption of online marketing strategies. The findings (Table 5) show that customers had inadequate knowledge (68.7% cases) on how to use online frameworks and platforms implying that such a challenge has been a stumbling block to ALAF customers to fully use online marketing platforms. These findings are in harmony with those of United Nations (2017) and Ndlodo and Dhurup (2010) which found that lack of knowledge by customers inhibited the use of e-commerce in businesses. These findings were supported by qualitative findings which exhibited;

"*...our customers enjoy much the use of online marketing strategies like use of Website, Facebook, Instagram, and search engine as most of them declared that, such strategies help them to save time, cost and timely information sharing. Despite this potentiality, at large our customers face challenges to effectively make use of such online strategies due to inadequate knowledge on the use of social media ....*" (Interview conducted with ALAF Ltd Branch Manager on 23rd April 2019)".

The findings (Table 5) also indicated minimum security (34.3% cases of occurrence) was another challenge facing ALAF customers in the adoption of online marketing strategies. Implication of these findings is that if customers fear about security of online platforms, they will hardly use them. These findings are similar to these of Bostanshirin (2014) which revealed that security issues were among critical challenges facing online marketing users. These findings were supported by qualitative findings which exhibited;

"*...Despite the importance of online marketing strategies to our company, most of our customers perceive low security in using these online marketing such Website, Facebook, Instagram, and search engine. Therefore, this is an obstacle for ALAF Ltd in the adoption of e-marketing strategies and low security of e-platforms have resulted into several reported online theft cases on customers' transactions...*" (Interview conducted with ALAF Ltd Branch Manager on 23rd April 2019).

Limited privacy was a third challenge facing ALAF customers in the adoption of online marketing strategies mentioned by respondents with 20.9% cases of the multiple responses. The findings from this study are in harmony with Bostanshirin (2014) which pointed out that among challenges facing online marketing include privacy in the implementation of virtual space. These findings are supported by qualitative findings which exhibited.

"*...ALAF customers' personal information experience limited privacy. The majority of customers tend to avoid using which could make their personal information to be publicly known.....*" (Interview conducted with ALAF Ltd Branch Manager on 23rd April 2019) ....".

Table 5. Challenges facing ALAF Ltd in adoption of online marketing strategies (n = 78)

Challenges facing ALAF Ltd.	Responses		Percent of cases
	N	Percent	
Inadequate privacy	14	13.9	20.9
Time wasting on information search	7	6.9	10.4
High cost	6	5.9	9.0
They are not user friendly	5	5.0	7.5
Inadequate knowledge of how to use	46	45.5	68.7
Minimum security	23	22.8	34.3

Source: Authors

9 Conclusion and Recommendations

9.1 Conclusion

The conclusion for this study is presented according to the objectives. Regarding, online marketing strategies applied by the ALAF, it is concluded that the company has consider high application of websites, Facebook, search engine, Instagram, e-book as well viral marketing which were found to play great roles on creating platforms for customers to share information about the products which results into increased sales return and customer loyalty. Customers' perception towards online marketing strategies adopted by ALAF, the study concludes that overall mean perception of customers was 3.59 which imply that the customers' perception was high. In this regard, Facebook, Instagram, WhatsApp, e-mail marketing, search engine, website and viral marketing were highly perceived to be used by ALAF customers Moreover, the study findings conclude that relationship between online marketing strategies and customer loyalty. This implies that online marketing strategies were statistically significant to customer loyalty. i.e. (Email marketing $p = 0.006$, search engine $p = 0.002$, social media and viral marketing $p = 0.001$ and e-books, website, banner advertisement $p = 0.034$). Therefore, the contribution of email marketing, search engine, social media and viral marketing, e-books, website and banner advertisement to customer loyalty was high and important. Finally, pertaining the challenges facing ALAF Ltd in adoption of online marketing, there is a knowledge gap among ALAF Ltd customers on the uses of the online marketing strategies as it revealed by 68.7% cases of the multiple responses. Therefore, the company has to work on it effectively so that to increase the number of users with the focus of increasing sales rate and meet customer loyalty.

9.2 Recommendations

The following recommendations are presented based on the study findings;

i. The ALAF Ltd should improve the use of online marketing strategies for easy and time saving in accessing information and service. This can be done through promotional campaign to sensitize customers on the use of online service to access ALAF product information. Have ICT policy that directs customers to should use online service when making orders, payments, lodging complaints. This will help the company to improve customer loyalty through customer empowerment. Further, ALAF Ltd should build capacity to its employees through training on the use of online marketing strategies.

ii. The Telecommunication Regulatory Communication Authority (TCRA) has to work closely with internet providers and companies using online marketing strategies so as to strengthen internet connectivity and bandwidth and protect privacy and confidentiality of customers. Further, TCRA should ensure that the Cybercrime Act of 2015, is enforced accordingly to help operators and users of the ICT to reduce hesitations on the use of online marketing strategies due to the fear of security and privacy.

iii. ALAF Ltd customers should use online marketing platforms whenever they want to preview ALAF products, make order effect payment or lodge complains so as to save time, money and maximize their loyalty to the company.

9.3 Recommendation for Further Study

i. There is a need to conduct another study by involving customers from more than one organization other than ALAF Ltd for generalization.

ii. There is a need to conduct another study to measure the effect of online strategies on organizational performance by using performance indicator such as profitability.

iii. There is a need to conduct another study that will result into a technological solution application that will be used by ALAF Company to give feedback on customer loyalty.

References

Bostanshirin, S.: Online marketing: challenges and opportunities. In: International Conference on Social Sciences and Humanities, 8–10 Sept 2014. Istanbul, Turkey (2014)

BOT: Bank of Tanzania Annual Report 2016/2017 (2016). Retrieved 10 Aug 2020. https://www.bot.go.tz/

Brown, M., Pope, N.K.L., Voges, K.: Buying or browsing? An exploration of shopping orientations and online purchase intention. Eur. J. Mark. **37**(11–12), 1666–1684 (2003). https://doi.org/10.1108/03090560310495401

Cronbach, J.L.: Coefficient alpha and the internal structure of tests. Psychometrika **16**, 297–334 (1951)

Dilham, A., Sofiyah, R., Muda, I.: The internet marketing effect on the customer loyalty level with brand awareness as intervening variables. Int. J. Civil Eng. Technol. **9**(9), 681–695 (2018)

Hidayanto, A., Adha, M.S., Jiwanggi, M.A., Melia, T.: A study of impact of search engine optimisation to internet marketing strategy. Int. J. Serv. Econ. Manag. **4**(4), 298–316 (2012)

Khan, S.: Instagram as a marketing tool for luxury brands. Int. J. Manag. Bus. Res. **8**(2), 120–126 (2018)

Kowero, A.B.: Report: Exploiting the Potentials of the National Information and Communication Technology Broadband Backbone (NICTBB) in Tanzania. Tanzania Country Level Knowledge Network (2012)

Kumburu, N., Kessy, J.: Consumers' preference on imported and locally made furniture in Dar es Salaam and Arusha. Tanzania. Glob. Bus. Rev. **22**(2), 1–13 (2018). https://doi.org/10.1177/0972150918811519

Lammenett, E.: Praxiswissen Online-Marketing. Springer Gabler, Wiesbaden (2014)

Mashenene, R.G.: Performance of rural and urban women owned small and medium enterprises in Tanzania: do socio-cultural factors matter? J. Coop. Bus. Stud. **5**(1), 73–84 (2020)

Mashenene, R.G., Msendo, A., Msese, L.R.L.: The influence of customer retention strategies on customer loyalty in higher education in Tanzania. Afr. J. Appl. Res. **5**(1), 85–97 (2019). https://doi.org/10.26437/ajar.05.01.2019.07

Mashenene, R.G.: Socio-cultural Determinants of Entrepreneurial Capabilities among the Chagga and Sukuma Owned Small and Medium Enterprises in Tanzania. Thesis for Award of PhD Degree at Sokoine University of Agriculture, Morogoro, Tanzania, p. 274 (2016)

Mashenene, R.G., Kumburu, N.P.: Performance of small businesses in Tanzania: human resources. Based view global customer services. J. Retail. Consu. Serv. **21**(5), 773–779 (2020)

Pallant, J.: SPSS Survival Manual: A Step by Step Guide to Data Analysis Using SPSS for Windows, 4th edn., p. 335. Open University Press, McGraw Hill (2011)

Salvador, M.S.: The new on-line marketing medium: Viral Marketing. Analysis of the field through two case studies. Master's Thesis on Business Administration, Marketing. Unpublished (2014)

Timilsina, M.: Impacts of social media in restaurant businesses-A case study of restaurant based on Oulu region. Thesis for the Award of Bachelor Degree in Business and Information Technology of the Oulu University of Applied Sciences, Finland (2017)

Tonnesen, A.: Barriers and opportunities to car-use reduction. A study of land-use and transport policy in four Norwegian cities. Dissertation for the Award of PhD of University of Oslo (2015)

Wanjau, K., Macharia, N.R., Ayodo, E.M.A.: Factors affecting adoption of electronic commerce among small medium enterprises in Kenya: survey of tour and travel firms in Nairobi. Inter. J. Bus. Humanit. Technol. **2**(4), 76–91 (2012)

World Trade Organization Annual Report (2011)

United Nations: Consumers protection in electronic commerce. United Nations Conference on Trade and Development. Geneva, 3–4 July 2017 (2017)

Assessment of the Effects of ICT on Supply Chain Management Practices in Public Institutions in Tanzania – A Case Study at a Utility Company in Tanzania

A. P. Matay and E. A. Mjema(✉)

College of Business Education, P.O. Box 1968, Dar es Salaam, Tanzania
e.mjema@cbe.ac.tz

Abstract. Supply Chain Management (SCM) has been noted as an increasingly important management field to help enterprises improve supply chain operations. In recent years, the development of the applications of ICT in SCM has been seen by many parties and it is observed that innovations enabled by ICT are creating new ways for firms to manage supply chain relationships. The use of ICT has received significant attention in the supply chain context, which involves the flows of material, information, and finance in a network consisting of customers, suppliers, manufacturers, and distributors. However, the relationship between the two notions in term of the roles of ICT in SCM remains still as an area that requires more researches. Therefore, this study assessed the effects of ICT on the SCM practices at the Company that was taken as a Case Study. A case study approach shows the intensity of how the variables provided by the adaptation of ICT bring an effect in the SCM practices. The sampling frame of the study consisted of 100 workers from the ICT and Procurement departments at the ompany headquarters. The findings of the study show that ICT affects the SCM practices by increasing the financial performance of the Company. It was also found that there is also an increased customer service and satisfaction of the customer through the improvement of information availability and visibility. The increased effectiveness of operation was also highly rated effects of an integration of ICT into SCM practices of the Company.

Keywords: Information and Communication Technology (ICT) · Supply Chain Management (SCM)

1 Introduction

The increase in requirements to offer global supply chain service packages to better satisfy customer needs the ICT play a key role in this process, assuring the linkage between chain participants as well as a more effective control of time, cost and quality of the services for the flow of the material. The questions on how ICT can be used to enhance SCM operations in companies and organizations are also included by among

J. N. Mojekwu et al. (Eds.): *Sustainable Education and Development*, pp. 310–320, 2021.
https://doi.org/10.1007/978-3-030-68836-3_27

these researchers (Waters 2009). The SCM encompasses the management of all logistics process of a business, which include activities such as procurement, warehousing, inventory control, manufacturing, distribution and sales order of a business (Graham 2013).

As companies seek to improve supply chain efficiency through increased integration, ICT is considered as a useful aid for SCM in supporting information-sharing. SCM works simultaneous along with ICT and it is included in the supply chain information flow. Innovations enabled by ICT are creating new ways for firms to manage supply chain relationships (Sambamurthy et al. 2013).

In fact, both the academic literature and the practitioner literature have noted that business competitions in a number of industries are no longer between individual firms, but rather between supply chains (Lambert and Cooper 2010; Oh and Rhee 2008). One of the fundamental reasons that cause the paradigm shift in supply chain relationships is the advent of a knowledge-intensive economy. The value of most products and services in a knowledge-intensive economy depends primarily on the development of knowledge-based intangibles, like technological knowhow, product design, marketing, preferences of customers, and understanding of value-added networks. As new product development becomes more complex and market environments become more dynamic and competitive, it is likely that the knowledge and information needed to deliver value to the end customers are no longer confined in a single firm.

Despite the researches and surveys done by the aforementioned researchers, of which they expounded the importance and modalities of ICT in supply chain, there is no clear study which focused on the effects of ICT in supply chain. Previous studies have struggled to pinpoint important things regarding the emerging of ICT use in the Supply chain activities. Most of reviewed studies have strived to show the way ICT and related software and tools have been working as catalyst tools through which supply chain activities are transformed and improved. Altogether had similar focus but the failed to achieve the clearest intervention about the exact effects of ICT on SCM practices.

The main objective of this research was to measure the effects of ICT on SCM practices. The main objective was operationalized through the following specific objectives: a) to identify the challenges encountered when adapting ICT in their SCM practices; b) to examine the extent of usage of ICT in the Supply Chain; and c) to assess the effect of the usage of ICT on SCM at the Company.

2 Theoretical Framework

SCM is the integrated planning, co-ordination and control of all business processes and activities in the supply chain to deliver superior consumer value at less cost to the supply chain as a whole whilst satisfying requirements of other stakeholders in the supply chain (e.g. government and NGO's)[1]. SCM is a systemic, strategic coordination of the traditional business functions within a particular company and across businesses within the supply chain, for the purposes of improving the long-term performance of the individual companies and the supply chain as a whole.

[1] https://www.researchgate.net/publication/40122004_Supply_Chain_Management_theory_and_practices [accessed Sep 13 2018].

The Resource-Based View (RBV), developed by Wernerfelt (1984), is a managerial framework used to determine the strategic resources with the potential to deliver comparative advantage to a firm. These resources can be exploited by the firm in order to achieve sustainable competitive advantage. RBV proposes that firms are heterogeneous because they possess heterogeneous resources, meaning firms can have different strategies because they have different resource mixes[2]. The RBV focuses managerial attention on the firm's internal resources in an effort to identify those assets, capabilities and competencies with the potential to deliver superior competitive advantages. As we seek to study ICT value in digitally enabled supply chains, we draw primarily on the RBV on how technology creates value (Zhu and Kraemer 2012; 2015). The RBV attributes improvement in firm performance to valuable resources or resource bundles (Barney 1991; Peteraf 2013). From the RBV, one lens through which to look at ICT value creation is an indirect role for ICT in firm performance.

Revenue generation and cost reduction are the two major dimensions of process performance improvements through supply chain integration (Mukhopadhyay and Kekre 2012). Such improvements, seen from the RBV, stem from resource synergy along the supply chain. Effective SCM aims to synchronize supply, production, and delivery (Lee et al. 2010). For this to happen, firms needs to leverage the connectivity of the Internet to create an inter-firm digital platform, enabling real-time information sharing, and improving coordination of allocated resources across the supply chain (Lee 2014). The digital platform helps establish connections among separate resources owned by supply chain partners, thus translating them into bundles of coexisting resources responsive to each other (Zhu and Kraemer 2012). This is consistent with the notion of creating resource synergy as advocated by the RBV (Conner 2011). More broadly, integration across separate stages of a supply chain allows each supply chain partner to focus on the operation at its own stage. This may eliminate the burden of acquiring duplicate resources thus increasing resource utilization and decreasing operational costs. Cost reduction can be further achieved through resource synergy among horizontal partners (Lee 2012).

The Transaction Cost Economics (TCE), developed by Coase (1937), is a theory of organizational efficiency: how should a complex transaction be structured and governed so as to minimize waste? This can be understood through the lens of TCE. Explicitly recognizing the costs of coordination among economic entities in markets, TCE stresses that a firm's central task is to coordinate transactions efficiently (Williamson 2015). ICT can lower coordination costs, and in supply chain contexts, digitally enabled integration capability can substantially improve transactional efficiencies through increased information sharing and communications capabilities, resulting in improved supply chain performance (Zhu and Kraemer 2015).

The use of ICT in supply chain and logistics management has attracted increasing attention of the business and academic world. Lee and Wang (2011) addressed the possibilities of reducing the bullwhip effect in supply chains through Internet based collaboration. Technology application in supply chain context may provide benefits in the following areas: improve supply chain agility, reduce cycle time, achieve higher efficiency, and deliver products to customers in a timely manner (ibid).

[2] https://www.researchgate.net/publication/45072518/download accessed on 12th September 2018.

The most cited theory explaining about the adoption of ICT is the **Technology Acceptance Model (TAM)** developed by Davis (1989). TAM presented a theoretical model aiming to predict and explain ICT usage behaviour, that is, what causes potential adopters to accept or reject the use of information technology. Theoretically, TAM is based on the **Theory of Reasoned Action (TRA).** In TAM, two theoretical constructs, perceived usefulness and perceived ease of use, are the fundamental determinants of system use, and predict attitudes toward the use of the system, that is, the user's willingness to use the system. Perceived usefulness refers to "the degree to which a person believes that using a particular system would enhance his or her job performance", and perceived ease of use refers to "the degree to which a person believes that using a particular system would be free of effort" (Davis 1989).

Security and reliability issues significantly inhibit ICT adoption in an organization. The perceived potential of hackers gaining access to people's information and the level of fraud is one of the major barriers to ICT adoption. The majority of people do not believe that their information is safe online. For this reason, individuals and companies might be reluctant to perform transactions online that require the exchange of personal information (Olusegun et al. 2016). The lack of trust in supply chains can be argued not to be the fault of the company. This can be for reasons that include the potential for data or money theft (ibid). Such developments may also require a restructuring of the entire logistics and supply chain system to better serve and retain the customers and this may be the reason for a company to shun the idea of implementing ICT solutions.

Successful companies have developed focused e-business solutions for improving customer service elements that are success factors in their business operations. Electronic Data Interchange (EDI) for example contributes positively to order cycle time, product availability, distribution malfunctions, product availability, and distribution flexibility among other things (Lim and Palvia 2011). Information Technology has enabled companies to streamline logistics flows, reduce inventory and improving customer service thus improving efficiency in information transfer. The use of internet has made it easier to share information along the supply chain. This has led to improved operational performance, good customer service and solution development (Graham et al. 2013).

ICT in SCM also provides a reduction in cycle time, reduction in inventories, minimization of bullwhip effect and improvements in the effectiveness of distribution channels (Levary 2010). Vendor-Managed Inventory has enabled sharing of information between buyer and seller. Buyers are able to share their information on demand to their supplier. The supplier in turn manages this information and can be able to do forecasting based on the data received.

3 Methodology

The Case Study methodology was used in this research. Sampling frame of the study consisted of 100 workers from ICT and Procurement departments at the Company headquarters. The study used Yamane's formula to determine its sample size. But, since the level of precision or sampling error was $\pm 10\%$, 1 respondent was added to make a total of 51 respondents. The study used correlation to find the t-values and validate the predictions of the variables, the researchers considered and drew conclusion basing on the set base value of t-value among the variables of the study at hand. Stata was used to manipulate and analyze the quantitative data with the codes and label shown in Table 1 as they were used in the software.

3.1 Modeling

The study assumes and explains that the effects of ICT on SCM is basically attributed with the inclusion of the Extent to which ICT is being used, its effects when well adopted and integrated into the systems and operations, a set of well-played society and government roles, and, lastly a well address to the challenges that ICT encounters when adopted and integrated into the SCM practices. The relationship of the stated variables can be formulated as follows;

$$\mathbf{E_{IS}}_{\rightarrow}(\mathbf{E_u} \wedge \mathbf{E_{us}} \wedge \mathbf{G_r} \wedge \mathbf{S_r} \wedge \mathbf{S_c})$$

Whereas;
$\boldsymbol{E_{IS}}$ = effects of ICT on SCM practices, $\boldsymbol{E_u}$ = effect of the usage of ICT on SCM, $\boldsymbol{E_{us}}$ = extent of usage of ICT in the Supply Chain, $\boldsymbol{S_c}$ = challenges encountered by the Company when adapting Information Technology in their SCM practices, $\boldsymbol{G_r}$ = the role played by the Government; and $\boldsymbol{S_r}$ = the role played by the society.

4 Findings and Discussion

This study intended to seek opinions from respondents of supplies and transport department of the Company. Basically, 19.4% of the respondents held a diploma level of education while 80.6% of respondents held undergraduate level of education and above. The questionnaires grouped the working experience into below 2 years who comprised 27.8% of respondents, 2–5 years of experience who comprised 33.3% of all respondents, 6–10 years of experience who covered 22.2% of respondents and, lastly, 10 and above years of experience who also comprised 16.65% of all respondents. The large number of respondents which is 33.3% of all respondents implies the existence of mid-experienced workers with 2 to 5 years of experience.

Table 1. Codes and label of variables

Code	Label	Code	Label
I41	Improved product design	E61	Decision support
I42	Improved marketing strategies	E62	Transaction Execution
I43	Advanced production/power generation	E63	Collaboration and Coordination
I44	Increased financial performance	E64	Record tracking and keeping
I45	Increased customer service	E65	Resources Planning and Management
I46	Increased customer satisfaction	E71	Improving of information availability and visibility
C51	Lack of committed management	E72	Enabling single point of data
C52	Resistance of people/workers towards change	E73	Improve decision making (i.e. informed decision)
C53	Lack of skilled employees	E74	Improved supply chain agility
C54	Relatively high running cost	E75	Reduced inventory levels of spare parts
C55	Security and reliability perception	E76	Improved distribution systems
		E77	Reduction of cost of operation
		E78	Increased efficiency of operation
		E79	Increased effectiveness of operation

5 Effects of ICT in SCM Practices of the Company

In a scale of 0 to 10, the following was the average of each variable against the level of education and experience of the respondents as follows: the study found out that improved financial performance is the leading effect as it was nominated with an average of 5.54 of all respondents from all/ various working experiences. That was followed by increased customers' service with an average of 4.32 of all respondents and increased customer satisfaction with an average of 4.24 of all the respondents.

6 Challenges Encountered by the Company When Integrating ICT into SCM Practices

The study found that security and reliability perception is the biggest challenges that encounter the Company while integrating ICT into their SCM practices that has been weighted by an average of 3.46 of all respondents. That was followed by an average of 3.31 of all respondents who considered that the lack of committed management as a challenge. However, high running costs of the ICT related systems has been mentioned by an average 3.29 by all respondents while resistance of people /workers towards change lack of skilled employees to run and operate the systems shared the averages of 3.12 and 2.98 respectively.

7 Extent of Usage of ICT in Supply Chain Management Practices of the Company

Regarding the extent of usage of ICT in SCM it was found that ICT is highly used in record tracking and keeping. That was selected and highly weighed by an average of 4.12 of all respondent. Moreover, the usage of ICT in resources planning and management has been mentioned by an average of 4.09 of all respondents who termed transaction execution as another area of Supply Chain Management practices that ICT. Collaboration and coordination and decision support has respectively viewed as other areas integrate ICT to some extent. Table 6 shows the results of the means of the extent to which ICT has been used in SCM practices of the Company.

8 Regression Analysis of the Effect of ICT on SCM

In order to validate the research findings, the researcher run and conducted a linear regression analysis using Stata. The t-values tested the prior-mentioned responses that the coefficient is different from 0. The study rejected and considered all t-value greater than 1.96 (for 95% confidence) to have no statistical significance on explaining the effects of ICT in SCM practices of the Company. The results were categorized basing into two: level of education and job experience of the respondents for each of the objective. Table 2 summarizes the relationship and validity of each of the categorical response by looking at the t-values;

Table 2. Regression analysis on effects basing on level of education.

Source	SS	df	MS			
				Number of obs	=	137
				F(6, 131)	=	797.71
Model	1990.5195	6	331.75325	Prob > F	=	0.0000
Residual	54.4805013	131	.415881689	R-squared	=	0.9734
				Adj R-squared	=	0.9721
Total	2045	137	14.9270073	Root MSE	=	.64489

Educationa~l	Coef.	Std. Err.	t	P>|t|	[95% Conf.	Interval]
I41	-.0335604	.0873318	-0.38	0.701	-.2063234	.1392026
I42	.2147461	.0994149	2.16	0.033	.0180797	.4114125
I43	-.1064319	.088934	-1.20	0.234	-.2823646	.0695008
I44	-.0040443	.0069194	-0.58	0.560	-.0177325	.0096438
I45	.689403	.0977623	7.05	0.000	.4960058	.8828002
I46	.120204	.0584934	2.06	0.042	.0044901	.2359178

The results as shown in Table 2 shows that increased customer service and increased customer satisfactions coded as I45 and I46 to have no significance on explaining the effect of ICT in SCM practices of the Company with the t-value of 7.05 and 2.06 respectively, which were, basically larger than 1.96 for the 95% of confidence level. Furthermore, when a researcher drew an attention of the data basing on the job experience of the respondents, the following results as summarized in Table 3 were found;

Table 3. Regression analysis on effects basing on job experience.

Source	SS	df	MS			
				Number of obs	=	81
				F(6, 75)	=	108.67
Model	632.272356	6	105.378726	Prob > F	=	0.0000
Residual	72.7276443	75	.969701923	R-squared	=	0.8968
				Adj R-squared	=	0.8886
Total	705	81	8.7037037	Root MSE	=	.98473

Job_experi~e	Coef.	Std. Err.	t	P>|t|	[95% Conf.	Interval]
I41	-.5123204	.1577689	-3.25	0.002	-.8266122	-.1980286
I42	-.1203812	.2166115	-0.56	0.580	-.5518933	.311131
I43	.7375848	.1795815	4.11	0.000	.3798402	1.095329
I44	-.0143324	.0123434	-1.16	0.249	-.0389217	.0102569
I45	.5266995	.1955376	2.69	0.009	.1371686	.9162303
I46	-.0096454	.1182335	-0.08	0.935	-.2451787	.2258878

Table 3 provided the study with the fact that, by looking at the p-values, which was supposed to be not more than 0.05, improved product design (141) and increased customer satisfaction (146), had no significance on explaining on the effects that ICT has on SCM practices of the Company.

9 Challenges Encountered by the Company When Integrating ICT into SCM Practices

Table 4 summarizes the regression analysis results for the challenges that the Company encounter when integrating ICT into its SCM practices.

Table 4. Regression analysis on challenges basing on level of education.

Source	SS	df	MS			
				Number of obs	=	131
				F(5, 125)	=	1.37
Model	.691506792	5	.138301358	Prob > F	=	0.2389
Residual	12.590936	125	.100727488	R-squared	=	0.0521
				Adj R-squared	=	0.0141
Total	13.2824427	130	.102172637	Root MSE	=	.31738

Educationa~l	Coef.	Std. Err.	t	P>|t|	[95% Conf.	Interval]
C51	-.054477	.028487	-1.91	0.058	-.1108563	.0019024
C52	-.0050745	.0246795	-0.21	0.837	-.0539183	.0437694
C53	.0348176	.0364749	0.95	0.342	-.0373708	.107006
C54	-.0058808	.0288873	-0.20	0.839	-.0630524	.0512908
C55	.0372088	.0333637	1.12	0.267	-.0288221	.1032397
_cons	3.868579	.1048695	36.89	0.000	3.661029	4.076129

Table 4 depicted the fact that all responses had significance on explaining the challenges that the Company encounter when integrating ICT into their SCM practices. On the contrary, job experience of the respondents had a slight difference as shown on Table 5.

Table 5 stipulates unexpected result that security and reliability perception (C55) had no significance on explaining about the challenges that the Company encounter when integrating ICT in its SCM practices with the t-value of 3.59 which is, basically, large that the limit of 1.96. That information contradicts with the majority when descriptive analysis was considered.

10 Effects of the Usage of ICT on SCM at the Company

The results of the regression analysis on the extent of usage of ICT in SCM practices of the Company as shown on Table 6 contradicts with previous analysis made basing on the averages of the responses. The t-value of 2.21 for the response Resource Planning and Management (E65) means that there was no significance on explaining the areas that ICT is widely used at the Company.

Table 5. Regression analysis on challenges basing on level of education.

Source	SS	df	MS			
				Number of obs	=	75
				F(5, 69)	=	6.36
Model	22.9235181	5	4.58470362	Prob > F	=	0.0001
Residual	49.7431486	69	.720915197	R-squared	=	0.3155
				Adj R-squared	=	0.2659
Total	72.6666667	74	.981981982	Root MSE	=	.84907

Job_experi~e	Coef.	Std. Err.	t	P>|t|	[95% Conf.	Interval]
C51	-.4251824	.0955014	-4.45	0.000	-.6157025	-.2346622
C52	.0479651	.0947987	0.51	0.614	-.1411532	.2370834
C53	-.0340835	.1250867	-0.27	0.786	-.2836247	.2154577
C54	-.0668498	.1106631	-0.60	0.548	-.2876166	.153917
C55	.4045208	.1125848	3.59	0.001	.1799203	.6291213
_cons	2.807199	.3905832	7.19	0.000	2.028007	3.586391

Table 6. Regression analysis on extent of usage basing on level of education.

Source	SS	df	MS			
				Number of obs	=	34
				F(5, 28)	=	1.11
Model	.921556398	5	.18431128	Prob > F	=	0.3761
Residual	4.63726713	28	.165616683	R-squared	=	0.1658
				Adj R-squared	=	0.0168
Total	5.55882353	33	.168449198	Root MSE	=	.40696

Educationa~l	Coef.	Std. Err.	t	P>|t|	[95% Conf.	Interval]
E61	.0209446	.0788399	0.27	0.792	-.1405516	.1824407
E62	-.0178195	.0809629	-0.22	0.827	-.1836645	.1480254
E63	-.1509568	.1177436	-1.28	0.210	-.3921437	.0902301
E64	-.010674	.0961858	-0.11	0.912	-.2077017	.1863536
E65	.2083121	.0942844	2.21	0.035	.0151792	.4014449
_cons	3.531336	.4031691	8.76	0.000	2.705481	4.35719

The same result with different t-value has shown on Table 7, which give the summary of the analysis basing on job experience of respondents. Check E62, E63 and E65 all had P-Value less than 0.05.

The study generally found that ICT affects the SCM practices by increasing the financial performance of the company. ICT is highly used in Resources Planning and Management and Record tracking and keeping of SCM practices of the Company. And, lastly, the study found that improvement of information availability and visibility and the effectiveness of operation were the highly rated effects of an integration of ICT into SCM.

Table 7. Regression analysis on extent of usage basing on job experience.

Source	SS	df	MS			
				Number of obs	=	79
				F(5, 73)	=	5.50
Model	20.1041493	5	4.02082986	Prob > F	=	0.0002
Residual	53.4148381	73	.73171011	R-squared	=	0.2735
				Adj R-squared	=	0.2237
Total	73.5189873	78	.94255112	Root MSE	=	.8554

Job_experi~e	Coef.	Std. Err.	t	P>|t|	[95% Conf.	Interval]
E61	.1917591	.1161145	1.65	0.103	-.0396568	.423175
E62	-.4027416	.115145	-3.50	0.001	-.6322252	-.1732579
E63	-.4367105	.1712482	-2.55	0.013	-.7780077	-.0954133
E64	-.1182995	.1375066	-0.86	0.392	-.3923498	.1557507
E65	.3642525	.1401544	2.60	0.011	.0849252	.6435797
_cons	4.151079	.5469682	7.59	0.000	3.060973	5.241185

11 Conclusion

The study found that ICT affects the SCM practices by increase the financial performance of the Company. It was further noted that iScala made it easy for accounts and finance related departments to connects and integrate with supplies and logistics activities and that led to overall comfort and stability of the two sections. Nevertheless, increased customer service and satisfaction also expressed the opinions of a significant average of the respondents while the advanced production/power generation came last with the least average of the respondents.

The highest rated challenges that encounter ICT adoption are the issues of security and reliability perception and higher running cost for undertaking the ICT initiatives and paying the workforce. Lack of committed management and running cost represented the opinions of a fairly average of respondents while resistance of people/workers towards change and lack of skilled represented a small number of respondents with small average of all respondents.

Generally the study found that Improvement of Information availability and visibility and the effectiveness of operation were the highly rated effects of an integration of ICT into SCM practices of the Company. Other effects, especially an increase in effectiveness and efficiency of operations and improved supply chain agility represented a rational average of the respondents of the study.

References

Barney, J.B.: Firm resources and sustained competitive advantage. J. Manage. **17**(1), 99–120 (1991)

Coase, R.H.: The Nature of the Firm, pp. 386–405. Economica, N.S. (1937)

Conner, K.: A historical comparison of resource-based theory and five schools of thought within industrial organization economics: Do we have a new theory of the firm? J. Manage. **17**(1), 121–154 (2011)

Davis, F.D.: Perceived Usefulness, Perceived Ease of Use, and User Acceptance of Information Technology. MIS Q. **13**(3), 319–342 (1989)

Graham, D., Manikas, I., Folinas, D.: E-Logistics and E-Supply Chain Management: Applications for Evolving Business, pp. 1, 2, 5–20, Idea Group Inc. (2013)

Lambert, D.M., Cooper, M.C.: Issues in supply chain management. Ind. Mark. Manage. **29**, 65–83 (2010)

Lee, E., Wang, Y.: An integrated resource management view of facilities management. J. Glob. Inf. Technol. Manage. **5**(2), 48–67 (2011). Facilities. Pearson Education: Washington DC

Lee, H.L.: Aligning supply chain strategies with product uncertainties. California Manage. Rev. 44(3) 105–115 (2012)

Lee, H.L.: The triple-A supply chain. Harvard Bus. Rev. **82**(10) 102–112 (2014)

Lee, H.L., So, K.C., Tang, C.S.: The value of information sharing in a two-level supply chain. Manage. Sci. **46**(5), 626–643 (2010)

Levary, R.R.: Better supply chains through information technology. Ind. Manage. **42**(3), 24–33 (2010)

Lim, D., Palvia, P.: EDI in strategic supply chain: effects on customer service. Int. J. Inf. Manage. **21**(3), 193–211 (2011)

Mukhopadhyay, T., Kekre, S.: Strategic and operational benefits of electronic integration in B2B procurement processes. Manage. Sci. **48**(10), 1301–1313 (2012)

Oh, J., Rhee, S.K.: The influence of supplier capabilities and technology uncertainty on manufacturer-supplier collaboration. Int. J. Oper. Prod. Manag. **28**(6), 490–517 (2008)

Olusegun, F., Gabriel, A., Sushil, S., Zhang, J.: Factors affecting the adoption of E-commerce: a study in Nigeria. J. Appl. Sci. **6**(10), 2224–2230 (2016)

Peteraf, M.: The cornerstones of competitive advantage: a resource-based view. Strateg. Manag. J. **14**(3), 179–191 (2013)

Sambamurthy, V., Bharadwaj, A., Grover, V.: Shaping agility through digital options: Reconceptualizing the role of information technology in contemporary firms. MIS Quart. **27**(2), 237–263 (2013)

Waters, D.: Supply Chain Management, An introduction to logistics, second edition. Palgrave Macmillan (2009)

Wernerfelt, B.: A resources-based view of the firm. Strateg. Manag. J. **5**(2), 171–180 (1984)

Williamson, O.E.: The Economic Institutions of Capitalism. Free Press, New York (2015)

Zhu, K., Kraemer, K.: E-commerce metrics for net-enhanced organizations: assessing the value of e-commerce to firm performance in the manufacturing sector. Inform. Syst. Res. **13**(3), 275–295 (2012)

Zhu, K., Kraemer, K.: Post-adoption variations in usage and value of e-business by organizations: Cross-country evidence from the retail industry. Inform. Syst. Res. **16**(1), 61–84 (2015)

Adoption of Employment and Labour Relation Act (ELRA) No. 6 of 2004 by Private Organizations – in Mwanza City Council, Tanzania

D. K. Nziku(✉) and J. M. Lelo

Business Administration Department, College of Business Education - Mwanza Campus, Dar es Salaam, Tanzania
{d.nziku,j.lelo}@cbe.ac.tz

Abstract. Organizations in the world operate under well-defined policies, rules and regulations which are approved by the higher authorities of the particular organizations. The Government of Tanzania (GoT) has set the minimum standards that all the employers should treat their employees with or above the minimum standards as described under ELRA No. 6 of 2004. The study has assessed the magnitude of adoption by private organizations to the act in Mwanza City Council. This study considered few elements of the act such as; working hours, remunerations, leaves, termination procedures, formulation and implementation of trade unions, employer-employee collective bargaining, strikes and proved that private employers are against the act and do not significantly implement at their workplace as required appropriately. The study focused on 32 private companies with a total of 986 employees in which stratified random sampling method was engaged to obtain a sample of 384 respondents. Descriptive statistics involving mean scores were analysed using Statistical Package for Social Sciences (SPSS). Private companies put little consideration to their manpower by utilizing maximally with little payments targeting to maximize output. Private employers need to abide to the act so as to use the platform as motivational strategies to the employees and eventually reduce staff turnover in their organizations.

Keywords: Employee · Employer · Mwanza & Management

1 Introduction

1.1 Background and Functions of Employment and Labour Relations Act No. 6 of 2004

On the basis of an employment contract, usually an employee works for employer as subordinate to the management and supervisor on behalf of the employer. The employer remunerates the employee for his or her work done. An employment relationship often begins with little formal agreements about the tasks and responsibilities the employee will be obligated to carry out. For proper employment standards, an employee must be

J. N. Mojekwu et al. (Eds.): *Sustainable Education and Development*, pp. 321–334, 2021.
https://doi.org/10.1007/978-3-030-68836-3_28

fully contracted with employers so as to put all sides of employment safe in all aspects. The informal nature of such agreements is not good because when disputes arise the court will have little to rely upon when constructing the obligations of each party instead will focus on contract. With poorly defined obligations, determining whether a breach occurred presents a difficult task, as does in choosing an appropriate remedy (MacLeod 2010).

Organizations' staffs are employees whether are working as part-time or full time. The employer must fulfil certain legal responsibilities and obligations to the employees such as saving for their Social Security Fund, treating employees in accordance to the minimum obligations as described by the government of Tanzania under ELRA No. 6 of 2004 and the standing orders as revised in 2007. Malekela (2015), pointed that in Tanzania, labour relations started during plantation agriculture in 1924 and 1935 where railways and roads were built and many people were employed by the colonialist as casual labourers. The railway line from Tanga to Dar es Salaam in 1929, in 1919 was extended to Moshi and in 1934 the Tabora to Kigoma line was extended to Manyoni. At this moment there were palm gown in Kigoma, coffee in Moshi, tobacco in Tabora and Manyoni, sisal in Tanga and Dar es Salaam harbour for exportation. Hence a pioneer labour force was formed in this way. The study further argued that, the state as an active participant of industrial relations (IRs) assumes the role of formulating laws and policies to ensure proper relationship between employees and employers through the medium of legislation and operational rules and regulations. That means there is a wide range and levels of industrial disputes from latent to manifest. A dispute can either be of interest or of right. United Republic of Tanzania [URT], 2004.

1.2 Problem Statement

Traditionally, any organization aims at maximizing profit and its general growth. The minimum working and benefit standards as stipulated by the Government of Tanzania under ELRA No. 6 of 2004 demand employers to exercise rights of employees in many different aspects like daily working hours, remuneration, leaves, termination procedures, strikes, as few to mention. Kersley et al. (2013); assert that, these minimum standards when practiced properly employees become motivated and work efficiently, while when not can make employees to be negative against employment state. Furthermore observed that, some employees in private and informal organizations are working because they have got no alternative, since their employers utilize them effective to maximize returns of the organization while paid low salaries.

This has been reflected in few different aspects of the act. For instance, the act requires employees to work 8 h per day, while the normal working hours in private organization is not less than 9, any other payments are calculated less as stipulated in the act, remuneration is low as compared to duties and responsibilities performed by employees particularly organizations owned and or lead by Hindi, some leaves like maternity, paternity, and sick leaves are somewhat exercised however not satisfactory, termination procedures are not treated as stipulated in the act. Therefore the study on the hand wants to check out reasons for the private organizations not exercising such right vigorously.

Malekela (2015), most of private organizations are not actively aligned to the demands of the act in some sensitive area like failure to submit the deducted amounts from employees to social security funds (particularly National Social Security Fund); rarely, they do it when forced or sued. Employees' long working hours with no or less overtime payments, employees termination without following properly the termination procedures, not entertaining collective bargaining at all, and not allowing any strikes at workplace. All these are against the ELRA No. 6 of 2004. Therefore the study on the hand targeted to assess the important reasons for the private organizations to be against the ELRA No. 6 of 2004 which revealed by common features of the private employees such as, turnover, lack of work's morale, low performance, demotivation and engaging on unethical conduct as summarized in the conceptual framework which influence the researchers to conduct study on an adoption of private companies to ELRA No. 6 of 2004. The objectives of the study are to determine the compliance of ELRA No. 6 of 2004 by private organizations in Mwanza Region and to identify the effects of implementation of the act ELRA No. 6 of 2004 on private organizations.

1.3 Theoretical Framework

Trebilcock (2011) showed that labour relations system incorporates both societal values (e.g., freedom of association, a sense of group solidarity, search for maximized profits) and techniques (e.g., methods of negotiation, work organization, consultation and dispute resolution). Both private and public interests are at stake in any labour relations system. The state is an actor in the system as well, although its role varies from active to passive in different countries. The nature of the relationships among organized labour, employers and the government with respect to health and safety are indicative of the overall status of industrial relations in a country or an industry and the obverse is equally the case. An underdeveloped labour relations system tends to be authoritarian, with rules dictated by an employer without direct or indirect employee involvement except at the point of accepting employment on the terms offered.

Whilst some well-established and a few small- to medium-sized firms consider skilful, committed and motivated personnel as a strategic resource, other firms view the labour force as an easily replaceable commodity and base their operations on contract employees. The predominant form of employment, particularly in newly established firms, is the fixed-term contract or 'contract work'. There is also the open contract, which is commonly referred to as a 'permanent contract' and is prevalent in well-established security firms. One can remain a contract worker for as long as the contract is renewed. One male guard interviewed indicated that he has been on a three-month renewable contract for the last three years. This problem stems from the loopholes in the Labour Act which fails to provide a maximum time limit for fixed-term contracts. A cut-off point is needed in order to minimize the exploitation of workers.

The Employment and Labour Relations Act (ELRA) of 2004 sets fundamental rights at work and regulates hours of work, remuneration, leave, termination of employment, trade unions and employers' organizations, organizational rights, collective bargaining, strikes, and sets dispute resolution under the Commission for Mediation and Arbitration. The labour laws cover all workers, including foreign and migrant workers.

Several legal reforms of the labour market were approved with some improvements in recent years. However, there are some flaws on the labour legislations of the right to organize, right to collective bargaining and right to strike in relation to the international standards. It is still not easy of doing business. A point often overlooked is that the labour regulations are only reaching a relatively small formal sector in practice, which includes the minimum wages. In reality, a large majority (85%) of the total employment is enclosed by a growing informal economy due to insufficient job creation in the formal sector. (Andreoni 2018).

1.4 Theories of Management

Table 1. Summary of management theories in relation to the assessed issues from ELRA No. 6 of 2004

S/N	Name of the theory	Founder of the theory	Concerns of the theory
1	*Scientific management*	*Frederick Winslow Taylor (Taylorism)*	He established how much workers should do with the equipment and materials at hand Workers who were more productive were encouraged to receive or earn higher 'scientifically correct' rates
2	*Administrative management*	*Henri Fayol*	He grouped the core activities of any organization into six (Technical activities, commercial activities, financial activities, security activities, accounting activities, and managerial activities) He is the first one to come up with the functions of management (planning, organizing, leading and controlling Provided a break-down of principles of management, which he thought could be applied to all business organizations, including industries
3	*Bureaucratic school*	Max Weber	He was interested in how management could be more consistent and he believed that bureaucratic structures can help eliminate the variability in managers having different skills, experience and goals He strictly, defined hierarchies in organizations which will be clearly governed by defined regulations and lines of authority for the organization with many employees

(continued)

Table 1. (*continued*)

S/N	Name of the theory	Founder of the theory	Concerns of the theory
4	Theory X and Theory Y	Douglas McGregor	**Assumptions of theory X** Employees inherently do not like work and *whenever possible, will attempt to avoid it.* Because employees dislike work, they have to be forced, coerced or threatened with punishment to achieve goals, Employees avoid responsibilities and do not work fill formal directions are issued, Most workers place a greater importance on security over all other factors and *display little ambition)* Assumptions of theory Y Physical and mental effort at work is as natural as rest or play. People do exercise self-control and self-direction and if they are committed to those goals. Average human beings are willing to take responsibility and exercise imagination, ingenuity and creativity in solving the problems of the organization. That the way things are organized, the average human being's brainpower is only partly used.
5	Need Hierarchy	Abraham Maslow's (1940–1950)	Physiological Needs Security or Safety Needs Social Needs Esteem Needs Need for self-actualization

Source: Geisler and Wickramasinghe (2015)

Management theories are formulated to depict the truth about a specific management aspect or situation. For instance theory X and Y (McGregor) is the one telling about lazy and hard workers in the organization respectively by nature, scientific theory (Taylor) explain about scientific approach in solving organizational problems, administrative theory (Fayol) is stipulated the general practice of managers and the 14 principles to be applied while practicing managerial action, Bureaucratic theory (Weber) highlight the delay of decision and communication due to the disciplinary compliance of chain of command by the employees and need hierarchy (Maslow) reminds managers to be careful when intend to motivate individual employees in the organization. These theories teaches private employers to deal with employees fairly as retention strategies and making them part of the organization in all aspects of decision. The selected components of ELRA No.

6 of 2004 like working hours, remuneration, leaves, termination procedures, involvement of trade unions, collective bargaining, and strikes are less valued by private organization, however if the theories are well adopted by rulers of the private companies would results into better leading manpower and retention strategies in the organization. In the findings and discussion the study managed to assess the effectives of the mentioned parameters relating with theories to test their effective use.

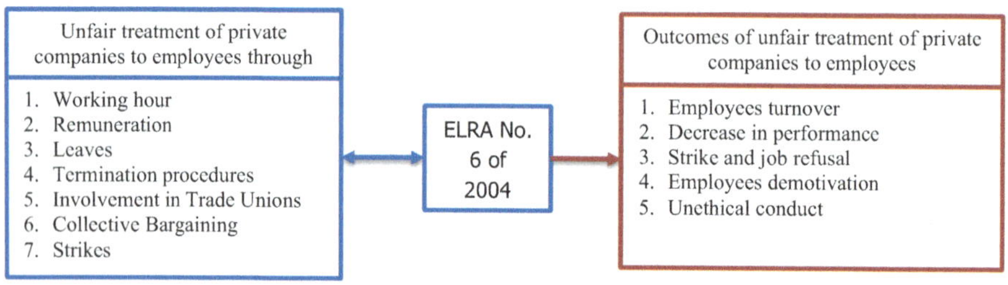

Fig. 1. Conceptual framework indicating the impact of unfair treatment of private organization to employees on the key players of ELRA No. 6 of 2004 Source: Research Construct (2020)

2 Research Methodology

For the purpose of making the methodology to be meaningful, this section has highlighted the research area, research design, target population, sampling techniques, data collection techniques, methods of data analysis and the statistical measurement model guiding in the analysis process.

Due to the nature of the study, the researchers adopted case study design to make easy during analysis of respondent's ideas. The case study is considered appropriate because it is the best method to describe the characteristics, perceptions, general situation and preferences of the organizations under study. It also enabled the researchers to critically analyze information gathered from organizations from both personal and professional points of view.

Bryman and Bell (2016), insert that descriptive studies are done when researchers want to establish the relationship of events without interfering with the purpose of reporting facts as they are. Thus, the design is chosen and considered appropriately for this study since it is able to give room for exploratory and descriptive data. This form of data is important in understanding the devotion of private organization to the minimum employment standards sets by ELRA No. 6 of 2004.

2.1 Research Study Area

The study covered private organization situated in Mwanza City Council. The main concern of the study is to assess the effectiveness use of ELRA No. 6 of 2004 by private organizations, where the focus is on working hours, remuneration, leaves, and termination procedures, involvement of trade unions, collective bargaining, and strikes.

2.2 Sampling Size

A subset of the total population which can act as true representative is known as sample (Oso and Onen 2009). This study adopted stratified random sampling approach. The basis of stratification was on the employees picked from private organizations in Mwanza City Council (MCC) and from each organization simple random sampling was applied to select a total of 384 employees from all organizations. The necessary sample size was derived from the formulae presented by Kothari (2004):

$$n = \left[Z^2\sigma\,(1-\sigma)\right]/e^2 \text{for } z = 1.96,\ \sigma = 0.5,\ \text{and } e = 0.05$$

Thus,

$$n = \left[1.96^2 * 0.5(1-0.5)\right]/0.05^2 = 384$$

Where by:

n - The sample size
z - The Z-score and for the purpose of this study was 1.96 in order to have a 95% confidence level.
σ - The Standard of Deviation and to be safe the decision is to use 0.5 as this ensures that the sample is large enough.
e - The margin of error and for the purpose of this study one construed to give a confidence interval of +/− 5%.

Mathematically from the above formulae the study envisaged that a sample size of 384 respondents is needed to be representative of the population.

2.3 Target Population

The population for the study is mainly made up by private organization situated in Mwanza City Council (MCC). The private organizations in MCC have so many employees, but for the selected private organizations considering only people with formal employment and liable to all statutory deductions, the study captured 32 private companies with total population of 986 employees. Thus, some of them were taken randomly to meet the demands of the study.

2.4 Data Collection

A questionnaire, capturing the variables under the study is prepared. Kothari and Garg (2014). The questionnaires contained only closed and open ended questions. The closed questions were used to limit the respondents to the variables of the study while the open ended questions enabled respondents to freely give their opinions in a more pragmatic way (Kothari and Garg (2014)).

The research instrument is divided into six (6) parts. Part I covered general information, part II, III, IV, and V, covered questions related to compliance of private organizations to ELRA No. 6 of 2004 and part VI focused on other information related to work performance as per employees' views.

2.5 Methods of Data Analysis

Data collected in the course of the research is processed and analysed using. Descriptive analysis in the form of percentages and univariate measures such as mean were used to analyse the data using Statistical Package for Social Sciences (SPSS). After both data have been analysed and presented separately, the interpretation or discussions were presented in such a way that it enabled the researchers to either accept or reject whatever defined idea have about the differences or relationships among variables under study. The main issue is to measure the compliance of private employers to ELRA No. 6 of 2004 and to provide recommendations for both employers and employees.

3 Results and Discussion

3.1 Private Employers' Compliance to the ELRA No. 6 of 2004

The study aimed at assessing the compliance of private employers to ELRA No. 6 of 2004. To make the situation meaningful, the contents were categorized into two important aspects which are; (1) employees opinions on employers' compliance to the act, and (2) Management approach and motivational strategies adapted by employers in private organization, which are summarized into Tables 2 and 3.

Table 2. Private employees' opinions on employers' compliance to ELRA No. 6 of 2004

Employee relations	1	2	3	4	5	Total	Mean
Working hours exceeds that prescribed into ELRA without extra payments				169(676)	215(1075)	1751	4.56
Working hours exceeds that prescribed into ELRA with extra payments	376(376)	0	0	4(16)	4(20)	412	1.07
Working hours exactly the same as prescribed into ELRA	238(238)	131(262)	15(45)	0	0	545	1.42
Employees are paid basing on what they contribute	65(65)	215(430)	38(114)	35(140)	31(155)	904	2.35
All leaves (annual, maternity, paternity & sick) are well treated	127(127)	146(292)	65(195)	19(76)	27(135)	825	2.15
Employees' hiring procedure are legally done	300(300)	31(61)	19(57)	15(60)	19(95)	573	1.49
Employees' termination procedures are legally done	92(92)	292(584)	0	0	0	676	1.76
Employees are allowed to form trade unions and being part of them	165(165)	196(392)	12(36)	8(32)	4(20)	645	1.68

(continued)

Table 2. (*continued*)

Employee relations	1	2	3	4	5	Total	Mean
Employees are involved in organization's decision making	92(92)	253(506)	8(24)	19(76)	12(60)	758	1.97
Employees are involved in collective bargaining	196(196)	157(314)	0	23(92)	12(60)	662	1.72
Strikes are done legally when need arises	88(88)	296(592)	0	0	0	680	1.77

Source: Field Data, 2020

Although job satisfaction is mostly related to employee feelings about the job in general, attention must also be given to satisfaction concerning specific facets, such as supervision, pay, opportunity for advancement and morale (Shields et al. 2015). In sum, the responses brought to bear the view held by Noe et al. (2017), that a satisfying job has the following three features: it has inherently enjoyable features; it presents the opportunity for growth and development; and it makes employees feel efficient in the execution of their duties. Thus, to make the study meaningful as per objectives, employees were asked to give their opinions about the following paramount issues reflecting the acceptability or refusal of the employers to the act.

i. *Working hours and overtimes in private organizations:*
Normal working hours per day as stipulated in the act is 8 h a day, 40 per week, and any extra hours must be treated as overtime case. Respondents were asked to rate on acceptance of their organization on working hours, 100% argued that, they work for a minimum of 9 h a day, 45 h per week and if exceeds two hours per day is termed as overtime with minimal payment rates as voted by 98% of the respondents. The reflection is that, private organizations intend to gain profit through intensive utilization of resources in the organization and thus not aligning to the demands of the act.

ii. *Employees remuneration*
73% of the private employees (respondents) argued that, they work very hard with multiple tasks however they are paid very low wages as compared to public servants. Some of them argued that, Hindi employers utilize them fully; engaging more tasks, duties and responsibilities for about eleven hours per day, and paid low salaries and there is no element of overtime. This is evidencing that, private organizations do not abide to ELRA especially for remunerations and other related payments such as overtimes, extra duties, severance pays, fare for annual leaves, as few to mention.

iii. *Leaves to the employees*
ELRA No. 6 of 2004; states very clear about legal leaves to be granted to employees at work place. Section 31 (1) states the annual leave of 28 days to the employees, section 32 (1) and (2) of the act states how the employer should grand sick leaves to the employees, section 33 (1) to (6) tells more about procedures and situations for maternity leave to female employees, and section 34 (1) (a) and (b) reminds the employers to grand paternity leave to male employees. 71% of the respondents

argued that private employers do abide with the act for annual leave and maternity leave only, other forms leave they are typically against.

iv. *Employees hiring and termination procedures*
For about 86% of the private organizations do not align to the acts regarding hiring procedure of the employees. Respondents' voices emphasized by saying most of the employees therein are hired without formal procedures, they normally call for relatives and friends for employments when needs arise. Respondents further argued that, 100% termination procedures are not observed in private organizations as stipulated in the act that is why when employee is terminated they used to raise a case to Commission of Mediation and Arbitration (CMA) demanding their rights.

v. *Employees' ability to form trade unions and being part of them*
In private organization such situation is there however employers they discourage it a lot to avoid possible frictions between them and employees. 82% of the respondents argued that, private employers they dislike formation and practicing trade unions at work place because brings power to the employees in bargaining capacity. The rejection of trade union resulted into weak or absence of elements of participation in decision making and in collective bargaining for 90% and 92% respectively in the sampled private organization in Mwanza City Council.

vi. *Strikes at workplace*
ELRA No. 6 of 2004; allows lawful strike at work place as described in part (vii) section 75 and 76 of the act. Respondents argued that, 100% the strikes are completely discouraged even when needs arises at workplace.

Table 3. Management styles and motivation strategies to employees in private organization

Management styles	1	2	3	4	5	Total	Mean
Authoritarian management style	15(15)	19(38)	19(57)	211(844)	119(595)	1549	4.03
Democratic (participative) management style	150(150)	138(276)	0	77(308)	19(95)	829	2.16
Paternalistic management style	85(85)	125(250)	12(36)	85(340)	77(385)	1096	2.85
Laissez-Faire management style	184(184)	180(361)	8(24)	8(32)	4(20)	621	1.62
Coercive management style	77(77)	50(100)	0	180(720)	77(385)	1,282	3.33
Coaching management style	272(272)	88(176)	4(12)	12(48)	8(40)	548	1.43
Bureaucratic style management style	157(157)	188(376)	12(36)	15(60)	12(60)	689	1.79

Source: Field Data, 2020

3.1.1 Management Styles Commonly Engaged at Workplace

From the theoretical part of this study, Geisler and Wickramasinghe (2015) analysed very clear the popular management and motivation theories practiced mostly but with different faces in different organizations depending on the situation available at particular time. In private organization powers and orders are more exercised than any other things in management. This has been reflected by the respondents' mean score of 4.03 as authoritarian management style are being engaged in the organizations, where all other management styles like democratic, paternalistic, laissez-Faire, coercive, coaching and bureaucratic management styles recorded insignificant mean scores. Additional information from respondents most of the employers have harsh language when dealing with staff in most circumstances.

3.2 Outcomes of Private Employers to Align Their Operations Towards Minimum Working Standards Set by the Act

The study discussed basing on observable behaviour of the employees developed at work place and its related organizational outcomes. This part is assessed basing on two important aspects (1) employees' feelings at work place and (2) organizational benefits after engagement of the act in their operations, which are summarized into Table 4.

Table 4. Organizational benefits towards proper exercising of ELRA No. 6 of 2004

Organizational benefits	1	2	3	4	5	Total	Mean
Customer satisfaction	61(61)	88(176)	4(12)	154(616)	77(385)	1250	3.26
Growth in revenue and stakeholders returns	46(46)	57(114)	8(24)	165(660)	108(540)	1384	3.60
Increase in profits and market share	42(42)	38(76)	12(36)	215(860)	77(385)	1399	3.64
Improved productivity	46(46)	80(160)	8(24)	173(692)	77(385)	1307	3.40
Enhanced company image	38(38)	177(354)	12(36)	115(460)	42(210)	1098	2.86
Commitment of employees	73(73)	61(122)	8(24)	177(708)	65(325)	1252	3.26
Magnitude of industrial relations in the organization	46(46)	104(208)	12(36)	203(812)	19(95)	1197	3.12

Source: Field Data, 2020

The effects of abiding or not abiding by the employers to the act were also measured. The behaviour of the employees at workplace were the tool helped to measure the effective or ineffective employers' practice of the act while positive direction of the organization as a result of the proper practice of the act is used as a tool to determine the proper treatment of the employees at work place.

Among the benefits an organization will experience when proper exercise of ELRA No. 6 of 2004 is practised the organisation will befits from increase in profits and market share recording a mean score of 3.64 and there will be growth in revenue and stakeholders returns that will be as a result of improved productivity as indicated in Table 4.

3.3 Private Employers' Views on About the Act

This part of the study reported and discussed the findings basing on observed behaviour of the employees at work place and its related organizational outcomes.

Traditionally, employers aim at utilizing fully the available resource to earn more profit in the course of operations. It has been observed that, Hindi owned organizations are the once with practical examples of utilizing human resources at maximum level with very minimal payments as narrated by respondents (employees). Group of employers were asked to provide their views about general aspects of the act and they rated as; 80% is fair to both employers and employees, 25% is fair to only employees, 47% is fair to only employers, 0% is crucial to involve all the employees in the decision making and 100% the involvement of employees in decision making is the source of wearying the company while the remaining percentages of 14%, 67%, 43%, 100% and 100% respectively are the rejection of all circumstances respectively. The average percent of acceptance (50%) is greater than average percent of rejection (44.8%), from there it can be concluded that, private employers are against the act with the reason that would like to avoid employees excuse, utilize them vigorously to generate more incomes of the organization.

3.4 Employees' Voices on Their Employment Condition

The methodology of the study provided an extension of the findings by leaving a parameter in its model so as to hear the views of the employees out of those developed by the researchers. Employees' voices were identified as complains against their employers as following:

i. Majority of the employees from private organizations demands government to intervene the practical operations in private organizations to enforce employers to abide to the act to secure their rights.
ii. Companies lead by foreigners, particularly Hindi, are the ones in fore line for not abiding to the act, they treat employees unfairly at intolerable level.
iii. Private employers engage their employees at work place for an average of ten (10) hours per day, which is total against the act. Private employees' demands government to harmonize this situation to be the same to the public employees.
iv. Overtime payments are not paid on time if is agreed as overtime, or mostly rejected while they are forced to work arrogantly.

From the employees' voice, it is concluded that most of the employees at work place slightly handled with care, despite of their positive commitment in their respective organization. Thus private employers need to oversee on this aspect for productivity improvements.

4 Conclusion and Recommendations

4.1 Conclusion

In private organizations, the commitment of the employees coming from pleasant remuneration, pleasant co-worker relationship coupled with good working conditions, granting all leaves accordingly, involvement of employees in collective bargaining, employees formulation and being part of trade unions, lawful engagement in strikes as well as proper procedural in employees' termination are one of the paramount things getting employees to be satisfied on their jobs and subsequently directly reflecting in their intention to remain committed in the organization. The objective of the study is to measure how ELRA No. 6 of 2004 is effectively adopted by private organizations in their mode of operations. The study's findings reveal that; the selected paramount parameters of the act like leaves, collective bargaining, engagement in strikes, involvement in trade unions, procedural employees termination, remuneration and average working conditions are insignificantly practiced and their outcome and impact in the society have low negative correction value between employers and employees at workplace. The first lesson drawn from the study is that employees would be more committed to private institutions when they are given rewards that are commensurate with responsibility and skills, the second lesson is that, private employers should abide their operations to the act in creating good working atmosphere at workplace and the third aspect is that, employers should act fairly and adopt management theories when leading employees in the organization.

5 Recommendations

Based on this study, it is recommended that; measures have to be put in place not just to increase their salaries but also pay all their emoluments promptly. Changes in compensation packages have associated impact on job satisfaction levels of employees. Again, private employers should devise ways of obtaining adequate facilities to enhance effective career management and try to switch their operations in such a way that will be aligned to ERLA No. 6 of 2004 to exercise both employees' and employers' rights at workplace. From employees' responses, is found that about 58.7% feel dissatisfied and therefore there should be incentive packages for employees who stay at the same post for a considerable number of years or accepts posting to rural areas. There is a positive link between performance and incentive packages, where the incentive may be direct or indirect, or may be when the employers are fully practicing the important requirements as demanded by the act, that will automatically harmonize their efficiency, performance and reduce their turnover. It is also revealed in this study that, private employers must have concrete career development structures as well as retention policies for their staff in order to develop and retain them. The promotion and promotion criteria in private organizations need to be reconsidered in order to enhance the morale of staff so as to put them in their best level to help in achieving organizational goals.

References

Andreoni, A.: Skilling Tanzania: improving financing, governance and outputs of the skills development sector (2018)

Bryman, A., Bell, E.: Social Research Methods (Fourth Canadian). Don Mills, ON (2016)

Geisler, E., Wickramasinghe, N.: Principles of Knowledge Management: Theory, Practice, and Cases: Theory, Practice, and Cases. Routledge (2015)

Kersley, B., Alpin, C., Forth, J., Bryson, A., Bewley, H., Dix, G., Oxenbridge, S.: Inside the workplace: findings from the 2004 Workplace Employment Relations Survey. Routledge (2013)

Kothari, C.R.: Research methodology: Methods and techniques. New Age International (2004)
Kothari, C.R., Garg, G.: Research Methodology and Techniques New Age (2014)
MacLeod, W.B.: Great expectations: Law, employment contracts, and labor market performance (No. w16048). National Bureau of Economic Research (2010)
Malekela, T.: Labour disputes prevention mechanisms and industrial relations: A Case of Wood Industry in Mufindi District, Tanzania (Doctoral dissertation, Mzumbe University) (2015)
Noe, R.A., Hollenbeck, J.R., Gerhart, B., Wright, P.M.: Human Resource Management: Gaining a Competitive Advantage. McGraw-Hill Education, New York, NY (2017)
Oso, W.Y., Onen, D.: A general guide to writing research proposal and report. Jomo Kenyatta Foundation (2009)
Shields, J., Brown, M., Kaine, S., Dolle-Samuel, C., North-Samardzic, A., McLean, P., Johns, R., O'Leary, P., Plimmer, G.: Managing employee performance & reward: Concepts, practices, strategies. Cambridge University Press (2015)
Trebilcock, A.: Labour Relations and Human Resources Management: An Overview. ILO available online at www. ilo. org/iloenc/part iii, Geneva (2011)

Characterization of Palm Oil Mill Wastewater: The Case of Small-Scale Mills in Ghana

E. Awere[1,3](✉), A. Bonoli[1], and P. A. Obeng[2]

[1] DICAM, University of Bologna, via Terracini 28, 40131 Bologna, Italy
eric.awere2@unibo.it

[2] Department of Water and Sanitation, University of Cape Coast, Cape Coast, Ghana

[3] Department of Civil Engineering, Cape Coast Technical University, Cape Coast, Ghana

Abstract. Palm oil production in Ghana is dominated by informal small-scale mills that produces about 80% of the national production. These mills have been noted for violating environmental regulations. This research was aimed at characterizing palm oil mill wastewater produced by small-scale mills in Ghana to better understand the extent of environmental damage. Four processing mills were selected from Abura Aseibu Kwamankese District of Ghana. Wastewater samples were collected from each of the four processing mills in March 2020 (peak production season). Samples were collected in opaque plastic containers and stored under 4 °C. Parameters measured were pH, total solids, TSS, TDS, BOD_5, COD, total nitrogen, phosphorus, potassium and oil and grease using standard analytical methods. The mean characteristics of the wastewater were pH (4.5 ± 0.05), total solids (3,976 ± 1,397 mg/l), TSS (3,976 ± 1,397 mg/l), TDS (358 ± 158 mg/l), BOD_5 (21,877 ± 4,728 mg/l), COD (56,357 ± 3,441 mg/l), COD:BOD_5 (2.6), total nitrogen (246 ± 86 mg/l), phosphorus (60 ± 16 mg/l), potassium (156 ± 24 mg/l), and oil & grease (527 ± 198 mg/l). The mean concentrations of 6 out of the 7 parameters were over 2-orders of magnitude higher than the Ghana effluent discharge standard. The pH, TDS, BOD_5 and COD of the wastewater from boiling were higher than for clarification. The current practice of disposing raw wastewater into the natural environment by the small-scale processing mills is negatively affecting the environment.

Keywords: Characterisation · Ghana · Palm oil mill wastewater · Palm oil processing · Small-scale industries

1 Introduction

The palm oil processing industry of Ghana is dominated by the informal small-scale mills which produces about 80% of the national palm oil production (Angelucci 2013; Osei-Amponsah et al. 2012). Available data indicates that there are more than 400 small-scale palm oil processing units in Ghana (Fold and Whitfield 2012) most of which are sited in small towns and rural communities. The small-scale processing mills have weak milling

The original version of this chapter was revised: The title has been changed. The correction to this chapter is available at https://doi.org/10.1007/978-3-030-68836-3_46

J. N. Mojekwu et al. (Eds.): *Sustainable Education and Development*, pp. 335–344, 2021.
https://doi.org/10.1007/978-3-030-68836-3_29

capacity (Fold and Whitfield 2012; Uckert et al. 2015) and thus are able to process up to 2 tonnes of fresh fruit bunches per hour (MASDAR 2011; Poku 2002). This is partly due to the extensive use of manual processes. As observed during the field survey and also reported by other researchers (Adjei-Nsiah et al. 2012; Osei-Amponsah et al. 2012), the only mechanized processes at the small-scale mills were the digestion of boiled fruits and pressing of the digested fruits to extract the oil. Unlike the large-scale mills that uses technologically up to date processes and machinery, the small-scale mills employ low-efficiency stand-alone machines (MASDAR 2011; Poku 2002) for fruits digestion and pressing.

Irrespective of the level of mechanization of the techniques employed, processing fresh palm fruits into crude palm oil requires high quantities of fresh water (Hassan et al. 2004) and produces significant quantities of wastewater (Chavalparit et al. 2006). In Malaysia for example, an estimated 5.0–7.5 tonnes of water is consumed to produce one tonne of crude palm oil, out of which 50% returns as wastewater (Ahmad et al. 2003). Similarly, findings from field measurements at 21 small-scale processing mills as part of this study showed comparatively lower quantities of water usage and wastewater production. In processing one tonne of crude palm oil, 0.86–2.72 tonnes of water were consumed resulting in 68–82% wastewater. At the large scale mills in Southeast Asia, the palm oil mill wastewater originates from sterilization (17–36%), clarification (60–75%) and hydrocyclone (4–8%) (Department of Environment 1999; Nasution et al. 2018; Prasertsan and Prasertsan 1996). But at the small-scale mills in the study area, the proportions of wastewater from different processes are 42–80% for boiling, 21% for clarification and 11–40% for cleaning. Many studies have characterized palm oil mill wastewater produced mostly in Southeast Asia (Malaysia, Indonesia and Thailand) where palm oil processing is undertaken by at large-scale industry. Review of related literature showed disparities in the results of characterisation of palm oil mill wastewater. For instance, raw palm oil mill wastewater is reported to contain high organic matter content (10,250–43,750 mg/l BOD_3 and 15,000–100,000 mg/l COD) and solids contents (11,500–79,000 mg/l total solids; 5,000–54,000 mg/l suspended solids, and 9,000–72,000 mg/l total volatile solids) (Lam and Lee 2011). In terms of percentage proportions, palm oil mill wastewater is a colloidal suspension with 95–96% water, 0.6–0.7% oil and 2–4% suspended solids (Ma 1999). Palm oil mill wastewater is composed also of high organic substances (Wang Mahmood et al. 2015), making them suitable substrate for biological treatment.

The quality of palm oil mill wastewater is reported to differ based on the processing techniques, processed batches or days, quality of the palm fruits, type of fruits (Ng et al. 1987), quality control of individual mills (Yusof and Ariffin 1996), climate, condition of the palm oil processing (Liew et al. 2015), and cropping season of the oil palm (Wu et al. 2010). Hence, the differences in wastewater production quantities, proportions of wastewater from different processing operations and technological differences in processing techniques between the large and small scale could lead to variations in the characteristics of the wastewater produced.

The small-scale palm oil processing mills in Ghana have been noted for their non-compliance with environmental regulations (MASDAR 2011; Poku 2002). Besides, raw palm oil mill wastewater is discharged into the environment without treatment. To the best of our knowledge, there is limited data in scientific literature on the extent of environmental damage caused by the activities of the small-scale processing mills. This study was aimed at qualitatively assessing the characteristics of palm oil mill wastewater produced by small scale palm oil processing mills in Ghana. Characterizing the palm oil mill wastewater will bring to light the potential environmental damage caused by the operations of the small-scale processing mills. This study is part of an ongoing PhD research to select and test appropriate technologies for wastewater management in the small-scale palm oil extraction industry in Ghana.

2 Materials and Methods

2.1 Study Context

The study was conducted in the Central Region of Ghana. The current population of the region is estimated at 2,563,228 inhabitants (Citypopulation 2019). Based on climate, the region is divided into three agro-ecological zones namely coastal savanna, transitional and forest zones (MOFA 2020). The average temperature ranges between 24 °C and 34 °C with a relative humidity of 50% to 85%. The region is characterized by bi-modal rainfall pattern with major and minor rainy seasons of March-July and September-November respectively (FAO 2005). In terms of palm fruit production, the peak and lean seasons are respectively February-June and July-January (Osei-Amponsah et al. 2012). The average annual rainfall ranges from 800 mm in the Coastal Savanna to 1,500 mm in the forest zone. The main economic activities are agriculture with 80% of the region's total land area considered as cultivable (MOFA 2020).

2.2 Sampling Sources and Preservation

Four (4) small-scale palm oil processing mills employing wet extraction method were selected from Abura Aseibu Kwamankese District, Ghana. The processing mills were part of the twenty-one (21) small-scale processing mills selected for assessing their water consumption and wastewater return factors as part of the PhD research project. The choice of processing mills using wet extraction method was based on their popularity in the study area as observed during our field studies in February to August 2019. For each of the processing mills and production season, palm oil mill wastewater samples were collected separately from boiler and clarification tanks in March 2020 during the peak palm oil production season. Samples were collected in opaque plastic containers and labelled appropriately before transport.

The initial wastewater temperatures of 80–85°C were cooled to reach room temperature before transporting to the Environmental Quality Engineering laboratory of Cape Coast Technical University, Ghana for analysis. During transportation to the laboratory, the samples were protected from light to ensure that the bioactivity of the samples was not altered. At the laboratory, samples were stored under 4°C in a refrigerator to inhibit the microbial activities (Choo et al. 2015) before use in the experiment. Prior to characterization, wastewater samples were kept out of the refrigerator and allowed to reach room temperature.

2.3 Analytical Methods

Parameters measured were pH, total solids (TS), total suspended solids (TSS), total dissolved solids (TDS), chemical oxygen demand (COD), biochemical oxygen demand (BOD_5), total nitrogen, phosphorus, potassium and oil and grease. pH was measured using Portable pH-meters XS Series. Total, suspended and dissolved solids were determined using the gravimetric method. Fats and oils were determined using the Soxhlet extraction method. All the remaining parameters were analyzed using Hanna multi-parameter photometer (HI83399) and associated reagents. All reagents used were of Analytical Grade. Analysis was carried out according to Standard analytical methods prescribed by Standard Methods for Examination of Water and Wastewater (APHA et al. 2017). All analysis was performed in triplicates and the mean value taken.

2.4 Statistical Analysis

Statistical analysis was performed using Microsoft Excel. A test for normality was performed using Jarque-Bera test with significance level of 95%. The mean and standard deviations are recorded for all the data. An unpaired sample T-test ($\alpha = 0.05$) was used to test for statistically significant differences in means. The results are compared to the Ghana Effluent Discharge Standards (GEDS) set by the Ghana Standard Authority (GSA) (GSA 2019).

3 Results and Discussions

3.1 Characteristics of Palm Oil Mill Wastewater

The mean characteristics of wastewater from small-scale palm oil processing in Central Region, Ghana is summarized in Table 1. The wastewater contained solids, oxygen-consuming compounds, nutrients (nitrogen, phosphorus and potassium) and oil and grease. For most of the parameters measured, there were wide disparities in the results as shown by the range of values reported in Table 1. The results of the pH showed that the wastewater is very acidic. Over 90% of the solids content were in the form of suspended solids. Around 13-15% of the total solids and 16% of suspended solids were in the form of oil and grease. The COD:BOD_5 was 2.2−3.1.

Wastewater with COD:BOD $\geq$ 2.5 is characterized as slowly biodegradable organic matter (Henze et al. 2008). The COD:BOD_5 from this study is an indication of the presence of slowly biodegradable organic matter largely attributed to the presence of unrecovered fats and oils in the wastewater as noted by Cisterna-Osorio and Arancibia-Avila (2019). The low pH of wastewater from palm oil processing is also due to the organic acids formed during fermentation of the palm fruits (Rupani et al. 2010). As observed during the field studies, small-scale processing mills store the fresh fruit bunches for 2–6 days for the fruits to undergo fermentation. Suspended solids in wastewater consists of carbohydrates with oil and other organic and inorganic solids (Wood et al. 1979). Most of these constituents of the solids could serve as nutrient sources for microorganisms.

For the oxygen-demanding substances, the results in this study are consistent with literature (Najafpour et al. 2006; Wood et al. 1979). But, the concentration of solids

Table 1. Characteristics of wastewater from small-scale palm oil processing in Central Region, Ghana

Parameter	Mean (SD)	Range	Department of environment (1999)	Wood, Pillai, and Rajaratnam (1979)	Najafpour, et al. (2006)	Ghana effluent discharge standard
	This study					
pH	4.65 (0.047)	4.61–4.74	3.4–5.2		3.8–4.4	6–9
Total solids	3,976 (1,397)	2,569–5,327	11,500–79,000	29,600–55,400	–	–
TDS	358 (158)	211–551		15,500–59,000	–	1,000
TSS	3,618 (1,551)	2,070–5,106	5,000–54,000	14,100–26,400	16,500–19,500	50
BOD_5	21,877 (4,728)	16,172–27,888	10,000–44,000*	17,000–26,700	23,000–26,000	50
COD	56,357 (3,441)	50,391–60,544	16,000–100,000	42,900–88,250	42,500–55,700	250
Total Nitrogen	246 (86)	160–378	180–1,400	500–800	500–700	–
Phosphorus	60 (16)	43–90	180	94–131	–	2
Potassium	156 (24)	126–191	2,270	1,281–1,928	–	–
Oil and grease	527 (198)	321–792	150–1,800	4,400–8,000	4,900–5,700	10

All values are in mg/l except pH *BOD3 at 30 °C
TS-total solids; TDS-total dissolved solids; TSS-total suspended solids

(total and suspended) recorded in this study are lower compared with the results from other studies (Iskandar et al. 2018; Ma 1999; Najafpour et al. 2006). The differences in some of the parameters compared with literature could be attributed to the differences in the processing technologies employed. Similarly, the proportion of oil and grease as a percentage of total solids in this study (13–22%) are higher than those reported by other studies (Iskandar et al. 2018). The results of oil and grease obtained in this study confirms the low oil extraction rate of 12–13% reported for small-scale palm oil processers in Ghana (MASDAR 2011). The peak production seasons coincide with the rainy seasons in Ghana. The impacts associated with discharging raw wastewater in the natural environment could have a wider spatial extent due to runoff.

Comparing the results with the Ghana Effluent Discharge Standard (GEDS) for oil and fat processing, 85% (6 out of 7) of the parameters had mean concentrations far higher than the standard. The only parameter that met the effluent discharge standard was TDS (mean = 727 mg/l; SD = 498 mg/l). The concentrations of most parameters were over 2-orders of magnitude higher than the standard. Using a per capita BOD loading of 54 gBOD/day (Von Sperling 2007) and average daily wastewater production of 474

1 for small-scale palm oil processing mills in Ghana, the population equivalent (PE) for the small-scale industry is about 200 inhabitants. The PE shows that a small-scale palm oil processing mill in Ghana produces wastewater with BOD_5 equal to the average daily BOD_5 produced by 200 people. The results suggest that the current practice of disposing raw wastewater into the natural environment by small-scale processing mills is negatively affecting the environment.

3.2 Characteristics of Different Wastewater Streams

The characteristics of the wastewater from boiling and clarification sampled are presented in Table 2. The main sources of wastewater from small-scale palm oil processing are boiling and clarification. The pH, TDS, BOD_5 and COD of the wastewater from boiling were higher than for clarification. For the remaining parameters (TS, TSS, oil & grease, total nitrogen, phosphorus and potassium) the clarification wastewater was higher than the wastewater from boiling. Apart from BOD_5 and COD, the trend of the results are consistent with the characteristics of individual wastewater streams reported in Malaysia (see Table 3).

Table 2. Characteristics of wastewater from boiling and clarification for peak and lean production seasons

Parameter	Mean (SD)		*p-value*
	Boiling	Clarification	
pH	4.36 (0.08)	3.98 (0.13)	0.054
TS	2,130 (82)	4,708 (81)	0.000**
TDS	1,420 (55)	503 (113)	0.001**
TSS	710 (27)	4,205 (179)	0.000**
BOD_5	26,672 (3,050)	20,935 (1,358)	0.026*
COD	63,503 (2,867)	54,392 (1,932)	0.003**
Total nitrogen	362 (3.1)	393 (55)	0.339
Phosphorus	29 (8.1)	69 (12)	0.003**
Potassium	163 (5.4)	214 (7.1)	0.000**
Oil and grease	276 (19)	980 (147)	0.003**

All values are in mg/l except pH
*Significant at 2% level
**Significant at 1% level

The COD:BOD_5 was 2.4 for wastewater from boiling and 2.6 for wastewater from clarification. The biodegradability of the wastewater from boiling would be better than the wastewater from clarification as noted by Henze et al. (2008). The higher COD:BOD for wastewater from clarification compared to boiling could be attributed to the higher fat and oil content of the wastewater from clarification. The duration (up to 2 h) and method

Table 3. Characteristics of individual wastewater streams in Malaysia (Department of Environment 1999)

Parameter	Sterilizer condensate	Oil clarification wastewater	Hydrocyclone wastewater
pH	5.0	4.5	–
Suspended solids	5,000	23,000	7,000
Dissolved solids	34,000	22,000	100
BOD_3 at 30 °C	23,000	29,000	5,000
COD	47,000	64,000	15,000
Total nitrogen	500	1,200	100
Oil and grease	4,000	7,000	300

All values are in mg/l except pH

of boiling by submerging fruits in water practiced by the small-scale mills may have contributed to the higher BOD_5 and COD concentrations of the wastewater from boiling compared to clarification. The differences in the mean concentrations of parameters between boiling and clarification were statistically significant at 1–2% level. As reported earlier, an average of 64% of wastewater produced by the small-scale processing mills in this study originated from boiling. The characteristics of the different wastewater streams from the small-scale palm oil processing mills in Ghana suggests the need to find appropriate solutions for their management.

Many technologies have been tested and applied to successfully treat palm oil mill wastewater mostly in Asia. These treatment technologies include anaerobic digestion (Ohimain and Izah 2017; Yacob et al. 2005), aerobic systems (Vijayaraghavan et al. 2007), co-composting (Hasanudin et al. 2015), adsorption (Alkhatib et al. 2015), advanced oxidation (Bashiret al. 2017; Ng and Cheng 2016), and membrane filtration system (Wang et al. 2015). Detailed description of different the treatment methods can be found in the works by Liew et al. (2015), Iskandar et al. (2018) and Ohimain and Izah (2017). However, most of the technologies are expensive and may not be adaptable in a resource constraint environment such as pertains in small towns and villages where small-scale mills are located. In addition, downscaling some of the technologies to be applicable to informal small-scale processing mills could increase the unit cost of treatment and affect their acceptance. Based on the characteristics of the palm oil mill wastewater obtained, anaerobic digesters, co-composting and filtration may be considered for adopted. Removing excess oils and pH adjustment are crucial for using palm oil mill wastewater as substrate for biodigesters.

4 Conclusion

This study characterized different palm oil mill wastewater streams and seasons from small-scale processing mills in Central region of Ghana to inform the selection of appropriate management solutions. The characteristics of the palm oil mill wastewater from small-scale processing mills shows variation in wastewater characteristics with source. The wastewater was characterized by low pH, high oxygen consuming compounds (BOD_5 and COD), low solids content, fairly high nutrients (total nitrogen, phosphorus and potassium) and unrecovered fats and oils contents. The mean characteristics of the wastewater were pH (4.5 ± 0.05), total solids (3,976 ± 1,397 mg/l), TSS (3,976 ± 1,397 mg/l), TDS (358 ± 158 mg/l), BOD_5 (21,877 ± 4,728 mg/l), COD (56,357 ± 3,441 mg/l), total nitrogen (246 ± 86 mg/l), phosphorus (60 ± 16 mg/l), potassium (156 ± 24 mg/l), and oil & grease (527 ± 198 mg/l). The wastewater was characterized by slowly biodegradable organic matter ($COD:BOD_5 = 2.5–2.6$). Wastewater from clarification had higher solids and nutrients content but lower oxygen-consuming compounds compared with wastewater from boiling. Discharging the wastewater without treatment will have dire consequences on the natural environment. There is the need to explore 'appropriate' technologies for management palm oil mill wastewater from small-scale industry in Ghana. Particular attention should be paid to the small-scale processing mills which dominates the palm oil production sector. Enforcement of environmental regulations should be extended to the small-scale (cottage) industries to ensure adoption of appropriate wastewater management technologies.

Acknowledgements. The authors acknowledge the support of the following persons during the sampling: Emmanuel Arthur, Ibrahim Adjei and Richard Mensah (past students of Cape Coast Technical University, Ghana). The authors are also grateful to Mr. Emmanuel Kekeli Ekuaku (Technician at the Environmental Quality Engineering laboratory – Cape Coast Technical University) for his assistance during the laboratory work.

References

Adjei-Nsiah, S., Zu, A., Nimoh, F.: Technological and financial assessment of small scale palm oil production in Kwaebibrem district. Ghana J. Agri. Sci. **4**(7), 111 (2012)

Ahmad, A.L., Ismail, S., Bhatia, S.: Water recycling from palm oil mill effluent (POME) using membrane technology. Desalination **157**(1–3), 87–95 (2003). https://doi.org/10.1016/S0011-9164(03)00387-4

Alkhatib, M.F., Mamun, A.A., Akbar, I.: Application of response surface methodology (RSM) for optimization of color removal from POME by granular activated carbon. Int. J. Environ. Sci. Technol. **12**(4), 1295–1302 (2015). https://doi.org/10.1007/s13762-014-0504-4

Angelucci, F.: Analysis of Incentives and Disincentives for Palm oil in Ghana. Technical Notes Series, MAFAP, FAO, Rome (2013)

APHA, AWWA, & WEF. Standard methods for the examination of water and wastewater (Baird, R.B., Eaton,A.D., Rice, E.W., Eds. 23rd ed.). Washington, DC: American Public Health Association (2017)

Bashir, M.J., Wei, C.J., Aun, N.C., Amr, S.S.A.: Electro persulphate oxidation for polishing of biologically treated palm oil mill effluent (POME). J. Environ. Manage. **193**, 458–469 (2017). https://doi.org/10.1016/j.jenvman.2017.02.031

Chavalparit, O., Rulkens, W., Mol, A., Khaodhair, S.: Options for environmental sustainability of the crude palm oil industry in Thailand through enhancement of industrial ecosystems. Environ. Dev. Sustain. **8**(2), 271–287 (2006). https://doi.org/10.1007/s10668-005-9018-z

Choo, J.M., Leong, L.E., Rogers, G.B.: Sample storage conditions significantly influence faecal microbiome profiles. Sci. Rep. **5**(1), 1–10 (2015). https://doi.org/10.1038/srep16350

Cisterna-Osorio, P., Arancibia-Avila, P.: Comparison of biodegradation of fats and oils by activated sludge on experimental and real scales. Water **11**(6), 1286 (2019). https://doi.org/10.3390/w11061286

Citypopulation. Central Region in Ghana (2019). https://www.citypopulation.de/en/ghana/admin/02__central/

Department of Environment. *Industrial Processes and the Environment (Handbook No. 3): Crude palm oil Industry*. Malaysia: Department of Environment (1999)

FAO. *Fertilizer use by crop in Ghana* (2005): http://www.fao.org/3/a0013e/a0013e05.htm#bm05.2

Fold, N., Whitfield, L.: Developing a Palm Oil Sector: The Experiences of Malaysia and Ghana Compared. Danish Institute for International Studies, Copenhagen (2012)

GSA. Environmental Protection - Requirements for effluent discharge. In. Accra, Ghana: Ghana Standard Authority (2019)

Hasanudin, U., Sugiharto, R., Haryanto, A., Setiadi, T., Fujie, K.: Palm oil mill effluent treatment and utilization to ensure the sustainability of palm oil industries. Water Sci. Technol. **72**(7), 1089–1095 (2015). https://doi.org/10.2166/wst.2015.311

Hassan, M.A., Yacob, S., Shirai, Y., Hung, Y.-T.: Treatment of palm oil wastewaters. In: Wang, L.K., Hung, Y.-T., Lo, H.H., Yapijakis, C. (eds.) Handbook of Industrial and Hazardous Wastes Treatment, pp. 776–796. Marcel Dekker, New York (2004)

Henze, M., van Loosdrecht, M.C.M., Ekama, G.A., Brdjanovic, D.: Biological Wastewater Treatment. IWA Publishing, London (2008)

Iskandar, M.J., Baharum, A., Anuar, F.H., Othaman, R.: Palm oil industry in South East Asia and the effluent treatment technology—a review. Environ. Technol. Innov. **9**, 169–185 (2018). https://doi.org/10.1016/j.eti.2017.11.003

Lam, M.K., Lee, K.T.: Renewable and sustainable bioenergies production from palm oil mill effluent (POME): win–win strategies toward better environmental protection. Biotechnol. Adv. **29**(1), 124–141 (2011). https://doi.org/10.1016/j.biotechadv.2010.10.001

Liew, W.L., Kassim, M.A., Muda, K., Loh, S.K., Affam, A.C.: Conventional methods and emerging wastewater polishing technologies for palm oil mill effluent treatment: a review. J. Environ. Manage. **149**, 222–235 (2015). https://doi.org/10.1016/j.jenvman.2014.10.016

Ma, A.: Environmental management for the palm oil industry. Palm Oil Dev. **30**, 1–10 (1999)

MASDAR. Master Plan Study on the Oil Palm Industry in Ghana: Final Report. Retrieved from Hampshire, UK: (2011). http://mofa.gov.gh/site/?page_id=10244

MOFA. Central Region (2020). https://mofa.gov.gh/site/index.php/sports/regional-directorates/central-region

Najafpour, G., Zinatizadeh, A., Mohamed, A., Isa, M.H., Nasrollahzadeh, H.: High-rate anaerobic digestion of palm oil mill effluent in an upflow anaerobic sludge-fixed film bioreactor. Process Biochem. **41**(2), 370–379 (2006). https://doi.org/10.1016/j.procbio.2005.06.031

Nasution, M.A., Wibawa, D.S., Ahamed, T., Noguchi, R.: Comparative environmental impact evaluation of palm oil mill effluent treatment using a life cycle assessment approach: a case study based on composting and a combination for biogas technologies in North Sumatera of Indonesia. J. Clean. Product. **184**, 1028–1040 (2018). https://doi.org/10.1016/j.jclepro.2018.02.299

Ng, K.H., Cheng, C.K.: Photo-polishing of POME into CH4-lean biogas over the UV-responsive ZnO photocatalyst. Chem. Eng. J. **300**, 127–138 (2016). https://doi.org/10.1016/j.cej.2016.04.105

Ng, W., Goh, A.C., Tay, J.: Palm oil mill effluent (POME) treatment—an assessment of coagulants used to aid liquid-solid separation. Biol. Wastes **21**(4), 237–248 (1987). https://doi.org/10.1016/0269-7483(87)90068-1

Ohimain, E.I., Izah, S.C.: A review of biogas production from palm oil mill effluents using different configurations of bioreactors. Renew. Sustain. Energy Rev. **70**, 242–253 (2017). https://doi.org/10.1016/j.rser.2016.11.221

Osei-Amponsah, C., Visser, L., Adjei-Nsiah, S., Struik, P., Sakyi-Dawson, O., Stomph, T.: Processing practices of small-scale palm oil producers in the Kwaebibirem District, Ghana: a diagnostic study. NJAS-Wageningen J. Life Sci. **60**, 49–56 (2012)

Poku, K.: *Small-scale palm oil processing in Africa* (Vol. 148): Food & Agriculture Organization of the United Nations (2002)

Prasertsan, S., Prasertsan, P.: Biomass residues from palm oil mills in Thailand: an overview on quantity and potential usage. Biomass Bioenergy **11**(5), 387–395 (1996). https://doi.org/10.1016/S0961-9534(96)00034-7

Rupani, P.F., Singh, R.P., Ibrahim, M.H., Esa, N.: Review of current palm oil mill effluent (POME) treatment methods: vermicomposting as a sustainable practice. World Appl. Sci. J. **11**(1), 70–81 (2010)

Uckert, G., Hoffmann, H., Graef, F., Grundmann, P., Sieber, S.: Increase without spatial extension: productivity in small-scale palm oil production in Africa—the case of Kigoma. Tanzania. Reg. Environ. Change **15**(7), 1229–1241 (2015). https://doi.org/10.1007/s10113-015-0798-x

Vijayaraghavan, K., Ahmad, D., Aziz, M.E.B.A.: Aerobic treatment of palm oil mill effluent. J. Environ. Manage. **82**(1), 24–31 (2007). https://doi.org/10.1016/j.jenvman.2005.11.016

Von Sperling, M.: Wastewater Characteristics, Treatment and Disposal. IWA Publishing, London (2007)

Wang, J., Mahmood, Q., Qiu, J.-P., Li, Y.-S., Chang, Y.-S., Chi, L.-N., Li, X.-D.: Zero discharge performance of an industrial pilot-scale plant treating palm oil mill effluent. Biomed. Res. Int. **2015**, 9 (2015). https://doi.org/10.1155/2015/617861

Wood, B., Pillai, K., Rajaratnam, J.: Palm oil mill effluent disposal on land. Agri. Wastes **1**(2), 103–127 (1979). https://doi.org/10.1016/0141-4607(79)90046-5

Wu, T.Y., Mohammad, A.W., Jahim, J.M., Anuar, N.: Pollution control technologies for the treatment of palm oil mill effluent (POME) through end-of-pipe processes. J. Environ. Management **91**(7), 1467–1490 (2010). https://doi.org/10.1016/j.jenvman.2010.02.008

Yacob, S., Hassan, M.A., Shirai, Y., Wakisaka, M., Subash, S.: Baseline study of methane emission from open digesting tanks of palm oil mill effluent treatment. Chemosphere **59**(11), 1575–1581 (2005). https://doi.org/10.1016/j.chemosphere.2004.11.040

Yusof, B., Ariffin, D.: The oil palm industry-from pollution to zero waste. Planter **72**(840), 141–165 (1996)

The Effect of Concentration and Heat Treatment on Optical Properties of Zinc Sulphide and Aluminum Doped Zinc Sulphide Thin Solid Films

L. O. Odo(✉)

Department of Physics, Federal College of Education, Eha Amufu, Enugu State, Nigeria

Abstract. Thin films of Zinc sulphide as well as Aluminum doped Zinc sulphide were deposited on microscope slides using the Chemical Bath deposition technique. Zinc sulphate ($ZnSO_4.7H_2O$) and Thiourea [$SC(NH_2)_2$] were used as sources of Zn^{2+} and S^{2-} respectively in alkaline baths. Aluminum chloride ($AlCl_3$) was used as source of Al^{3+}. Ammonia (NH_3) was used as complexing agent while Citric acid ($C_6H_8O_6$) served as oxidizing agent. The precursors were prepared in three different concentrations of Zinc ion and Aluminum ion respectively in; 0.3M, 0.5M, and 0.7M to determine the effect of concentration on the properties to be examined. The thin film samples were annealed at 100 °C, 150 °C and 200 °C respectively. Analysis of transmittance and absorbance data revealed that transmittance and absorbance curves of the as – deposited films decreased with increase in Zinc ion concentration. Increase in Aluminum ion concentration resulted to high increases in % transmittance of the as – deposited films of Al doped Zinc sulphide samples. However there were slight reduction of absorbance spectra with increase in the dopant concentration in the as – deposited Al doped Zinc sulphide samples. Annealing resulted to increases in transmittance and reductions in absorbance with increase in Zn^{2+} and Al^{3+} concentrations. The difference in the effects is that the dopant concentration resulted to higher increases in transmittance and lower values of absorbance than the Zn^{2+} concentration in undoped samples. The dopant (Al^{3+}) concentration did not show significant improvement in the reflection property of the ZnS thin films. There were evidences of reduction in band gap energies with increase in temperature and Zn^{2+} and Al^{3+} concentrations. Doping concentration had little effect on the bandgap of Zinc sulphide films.

Keywords: Concentration · Optical properties · Zinc sulphide thin films · Aluminum doped Zinc sulphide thin films

1 Introduction

The photovoltaic effect is the direct conversion of sunlight into electricity using either an electrochemical junction or a p-n (or p-i-n) junction made using semiconductor materials. The photovoltaic effect was first discovered by Becquerel in 1839 when he found that

J. N. Mojekwu et al. (Eds.): *Sustainable Education and Development*, pp. 345–353, 2021.
https://doi.org/10.1007/978-3-030-68836-3_30

if he illuminated platinum electrodes immersed in a solution of dilute sulphuric acid, a voltage was produced. Solar cells represent the fundamental power conversion unit of a photovoltaic system. Photovoltaic energy conversion relies on the quantum nature of light whereby light is perceived as a flux of particles, photons which carry the energy.

$$\mathrm{Eph}(\lambda) = \frac{hc}{\lambda} \tag{1}$$

Where h is the Planck constant, c is the speed of light and λ is the wavelength of light. Only those photons with energy in excess of the band gap can be converted into electricity by the solar cell. When such a photon enters the semiconductor, it may be absorbed and then it promotes an electron from the valence band to the conduction band. Semiconductors can only conduct electricity if carriers are introduced into the conduction band or removed from the valence band.

Doping makes it possible by exerting a great deal of control over the electronic properties of a semiconductor and lies at the heart of the manufacturing process of all semiconductor devices. The critical role that dopants play in semiconductor devices has stimulated research on the properties and potential applications of semiconductor nano crystals. Aluminum is commonly used as a dopant for silicon. In reasonable concentration it has exactly the same effect on carrier density as Boron since they all have the same number of valence shells.

Zinc Sulphide (ZnS) belongs to group II – VI compounds semiconductor with a wide direct band gap and has a high refractive index (2.35 at 632 nm) (Keskenler et al. 2013). This makes ZnS a ready candidate for application in opto electronics consisting of light emitting diodes with short wavelength, electroluminescent devices and solar cells. Many methods are available for depositing ZnS thin films. These include sputtering, molecular beam, epitaxy, chemical vapour deposition and chemical bath deposition (CBD). Among these, CBD is the most attractive because it is less expensive and can be employed for large area growth without vapour deposition related to physical techniques and free of some inherent problems associated with high temperature deposition.

1.1 Theoretical and Conceptual Framework

Several studies have been carried out using several growth techniques on ZnS for device applications in solar cells as well as possible dopants for high optical and electrical performance of such cells. Oloko and Chukwuocha (2017) studied the optical and solid state properties of zinc sulphide films for possible device applications. The analysis of the transmission spectra of ZnS revealed a maximum value of 75% in the VIS/NIR regions of the spectra. Jinhuo and Wenjin (2014) investigated the performance of ZnS by indium incorporation because the high resistivity of ZnS of about24 ohm cm is too high to meet the demand of solar cells.

Thin film solar cells based on $CuInS_2$, $CuInSe_2$, $Cu(In,Ga)Se_2$, $Cu(In,Ga)(SSe)_2$ and (CIGSSe) utilize cadmium sulphide (CdS) and Zinc sulphide (ZnS) semiconductors as buffer layers (Wei et al. 2013). Although a higher maximum efficiency of 19.9% is attained with CdS buffer layer, the choice of ZnS buffer layer with maximum efficiency of 18.6% in $CuIn_{1\text{-}x}Ga_xSe_2$ thin film solar cell is to avoid cadmium toxicity damage to the environment (Riu and Yen 2016). The challenge therefore is on improving the overall efficiency of ZnS buffer layer in solar cells and at the same time maintaining a clean environment by doing away with cadmium materials in solar cells. For better performance, the ZnS buffer layer requires high optical transmission that allows photons to reach the absorption layer and excite electrons to generate Electron Hole Pairs (EHP). This is why in this research, doping with Aluminum as appropriate material is vital from the effectiveness of Aluminum doping in silicon cells. Concentrations of the precursor and annealing temperatures play significant determinant roles in the materials for buffer layer in modern solar cells.

2 Experimental

2.1 Slide Preparation

The glass slides used as substrates were first cleaned using distilled water and subsequently soaked in trioxonitrate V acid for 48 h. Thereafter, the slides were removed, washed with deionized water severally and then treated with ethanol and rinsed with deionized water in ultrasonic action and dried in air.

2.2 Preparation of Chemicals

Aqueous solutions of 0.3M, 0.5M and 0.7M ZnCl was prepared by dissolving 4.09 g, 6.82 g and 9.54 g of ZnCl salt respectively in 100 ml of distilled water in three containers and stirred constantly during preparation. Aqueous solutions of 0.3M, 0.5M and 0.7M $AlCl_3$ was prepared by dissolving 7.24 g, 12.07 g and 16.9 g of the salt respectively in 100 ml of distilled water and stirred severally during preparation. 0.3M, 0.5M and 0.7M of Thiourea was prepared by dissolving 2.28 g, 3.81 g and 5.33 of the salt respectively in 100 ml of distilled water and stirred. 0.3M, 0.5M and 0.7M of Citric acid was prepared by dissolving 2.28 g, 3.81 g and 5.33 g of the salt respectively in 100ml of distilled water and stirred. Aqueous solutions of 0.3M, 0.5M and 0.7M $ZnSO_4$ was prepared by dissolving 4.85 g, 8.08 g and 11.31 g of $ZnSO_4$ salt respectively in 100 ml of distilled water and stirred.

2.3 Deposition of ZnS Thin Films

The reaction bath for the deposition of ZnS thin films consists of 15ml, 0.3M of $ZnSO_4$, 15ml, 0.3M of Thiourea and 4 drops of ammonia solution. Four glass slides were dipped vertically into the beaker and the deposition was allowed to take place for 3 h at a bath temperature of 60 °C after which the glass slides were removed, rinsed with distilled water and dried in air. The concentration of Zn^{2+} was varied to 0.5M and 0.7M and the process was repeated in each case. The pH was maintained at 8.7 to ensure alkalinity of the bath.

2.4 Deposition of Al-Doped ZnS Thin Films

The reaction bath for the deposition of Al-doped ZnS thin films consists of 10 ml, 0.3M of $AlCl_3$, 10 ml ZnCl, 10 ml, 0.3M thiourea, 7 ml, 0.3M of Citric acid and four drops of ammonia solution. Four glass slides were dipped vertically into the beakers and the deposition time was 1 h at a temperature of 60 °C after which the glass slides were removed, washed and dried in air. The concentration of the Al^{3+}, Zn^{2+} and S^{2-} ions were varied to 0.5M and 0.7M and the process repeated in each case. pH was fixed at 8.7 to ensure uniform alkaline bath.

One side from each category of 0.3m, 0.5m and 0.7m of all deposited films were selected "as deposited" giving a total of 6 slides films. The rest of the 18 films were subjected to annealing in an oven in the range of 100 °C, 150 °C and 200 °C. Time of annealing was maintained as 1 h. The films were characterized to obtain the optical properties. UV-Vis spectrophotometer was used to study the transmittance, absorbance and reflectance of the film samples on their behaviour to light, in the UV, visible and near Infra red regions.

3 Results and Discussion

Figures 1, 2, 3, 4, 5 and 6 show the plots of transmittance as a function of wavelength of ZnS thin films compared with that of AlZnS film at different concentrations of Zn^{2+} and Al^{3+} ions in the range, 0.3M, 0.5M and 0.7M and at different temperatures; as-deposited, 100 °C, 150 °C and 200 °C. It is observed that as the Al^{3+} ion concentration increases, the % Transmittance of the ZnS sample increases for as-deposited and annealed films. Annealing however contributed to slight increases in % Transmittance attributable to a transition of samples from amorphous to polycrystalline as annealing temperature increases Agbo et al. (2016). The fundamental absorption edge experienced red shifts which could be caused by sub band gap absorption, dispersion or scattering on the surface of the nanostructure resulting to an increase in the light free path at the nanostructure Carlos et al. (2015).

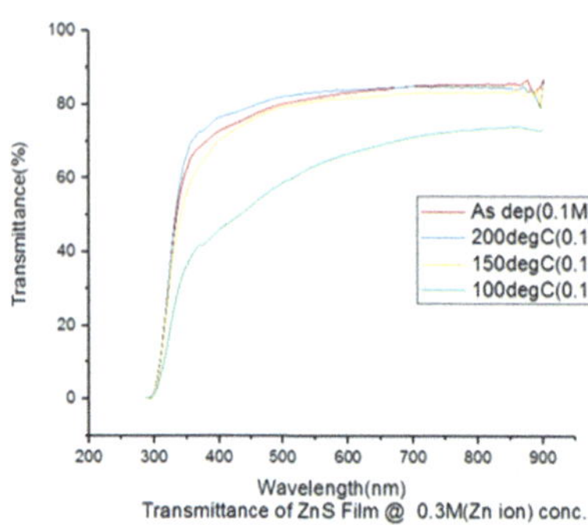

Fig. 1. .

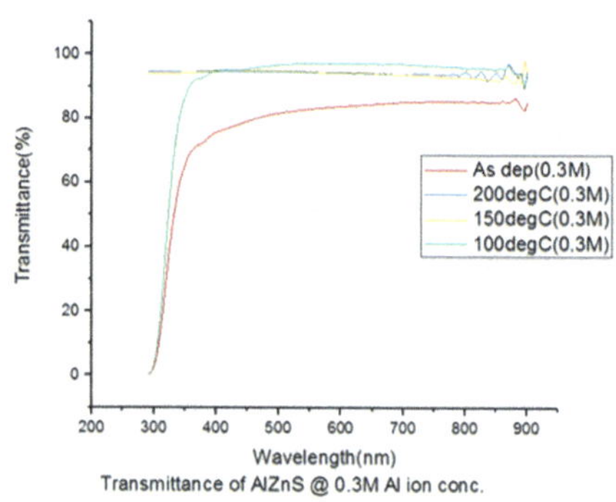

Fig. 2. .

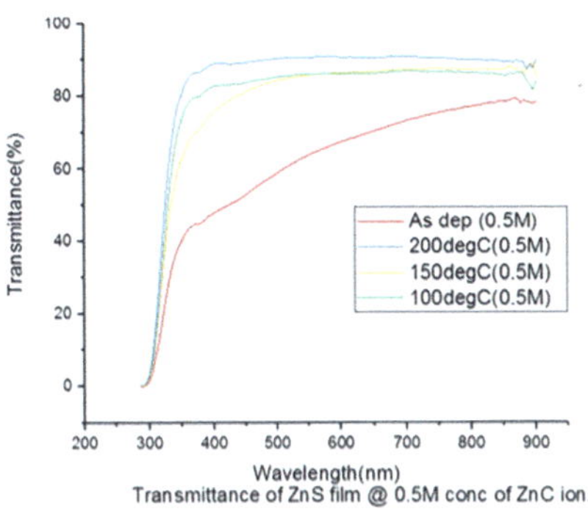

Fig. 3. .

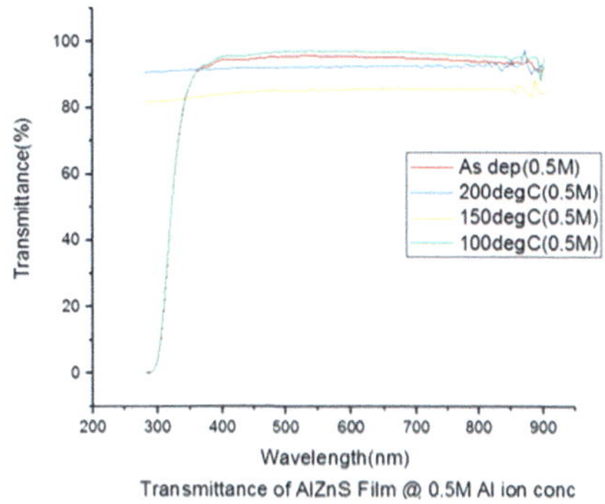

Fig. 4. .

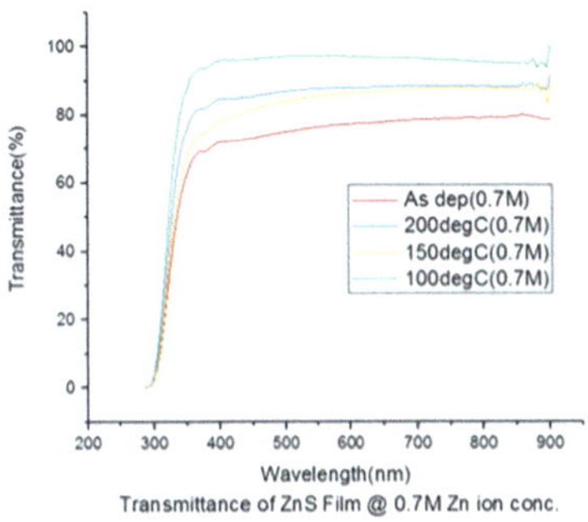

Fig. 5. .

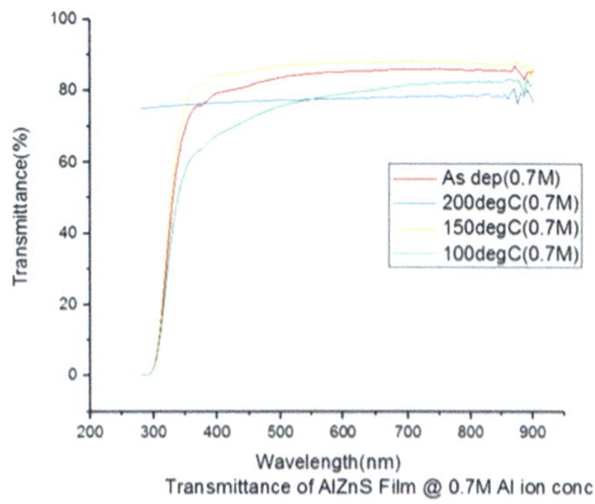

Fig. 6. .

Figure 7, 8, 9, 10, 11, and 12 show the plots of Absorbance as a function of wavelength of ZnS samples compared with that of AlZnS samples at Zn^{2+} and Al^{3+} ions concentrations of 0.3M, 0.5M and 0.7M and at different temperatures; as-deposited, 100 °C, 150 °C and 200 °C. It is observed that the % absorbance decreased slightly especially in the as-deposited films with increase in Al^{3+} ion dopant concentration. Annealing brought about a decrease in % Absorbance and displayed better linear curves.

Figures 13, 14, 15, 16, 17 and 18 show the plots of reflectance as a function of wavelength of ZnS samples at Zn^{2+} and Al^{3+} ions concentrations of 0.3M, 0.5M and 0.7M and at different temperatures; as-deposited, 100 °C, 150 °C and 200 °C. It is observed that the reflectance of the films at short wavelength is higher than at long wavelengths. The dopant (Al^{3+} ion) concentration did not show any visible change in trend in the % Reflectance of ZnS thin films.

Figures 19, 20, 21, 22, 23 and 24 show the plots of $(\alpha h\nu)^2$ Vs $h\nu$ showing the optical band gaps of ZnS samples as against that of AlZnS samples at 0.3M, 0.5M and 0.7M of Zn^{2+} and Al^{3+} ion concentrations at different temperatures; 100°C, 150°C and 200°C. It is observed that band gaps of ZnS thin films are closer to each other at different annealing temperatures unlike the band gaps of Al-doped ZnS thin films which

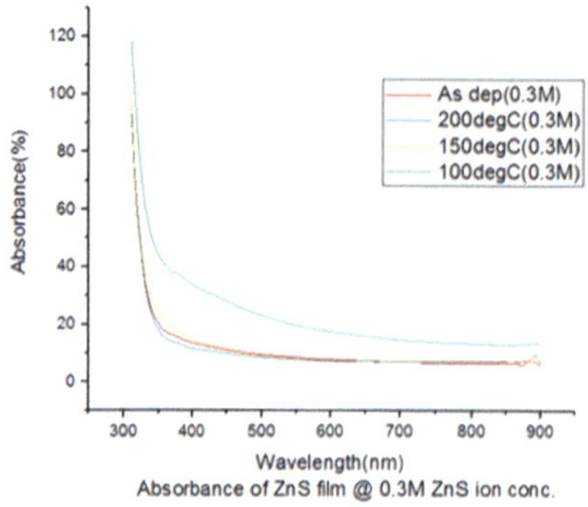

Fig. 7. .

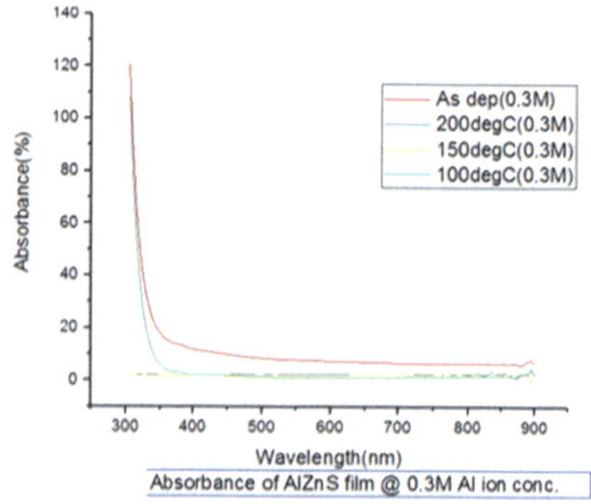

Fig. 8. .

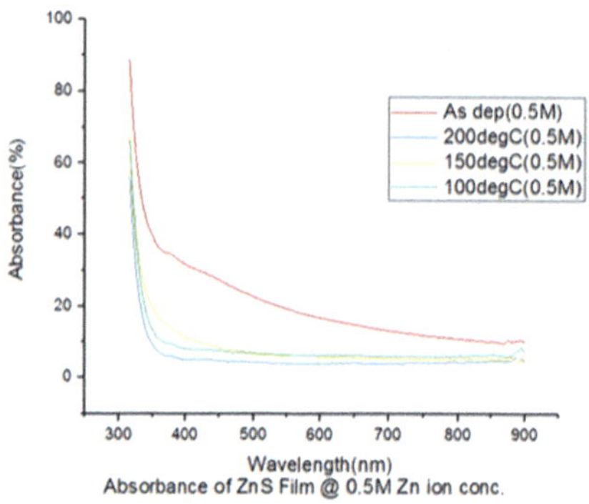

Fig. 9. .

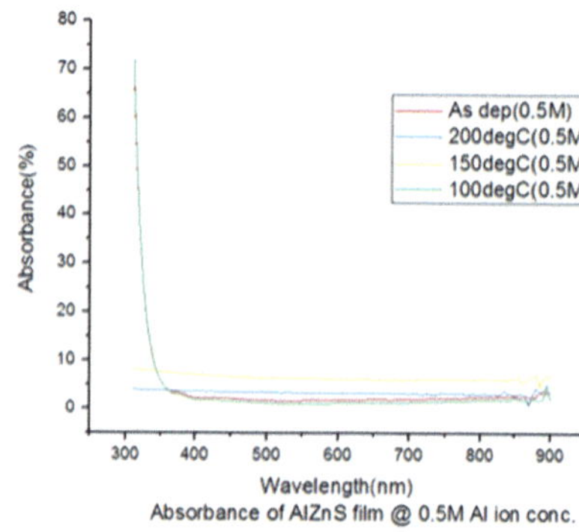

Fig. 10. .

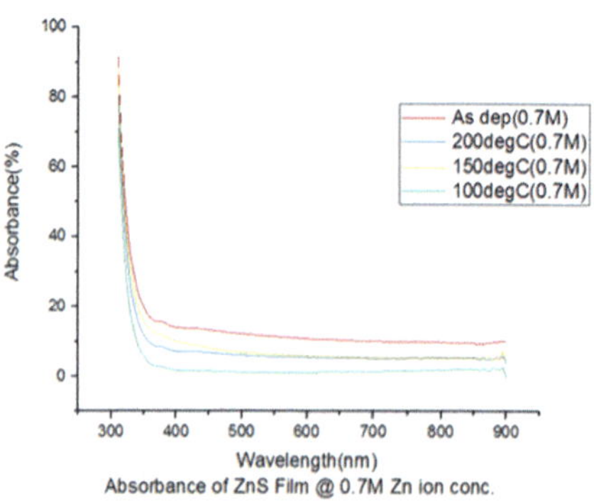

Fig. 11. .

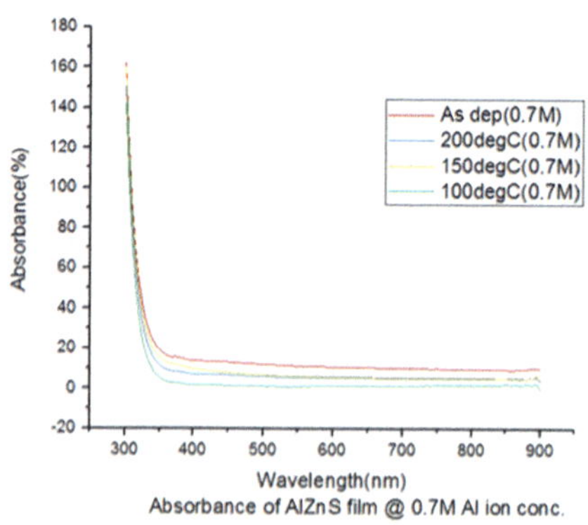

Fig. 12. .

are varying in non-regular pattern with annealing temperatures, showing that doping concentration had irregular effects on band gap of ZnS which could be improved by other deposition procedures.

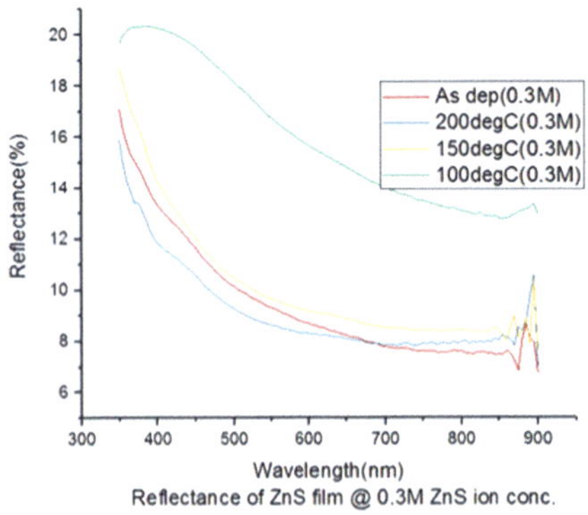

Fig. 13. .

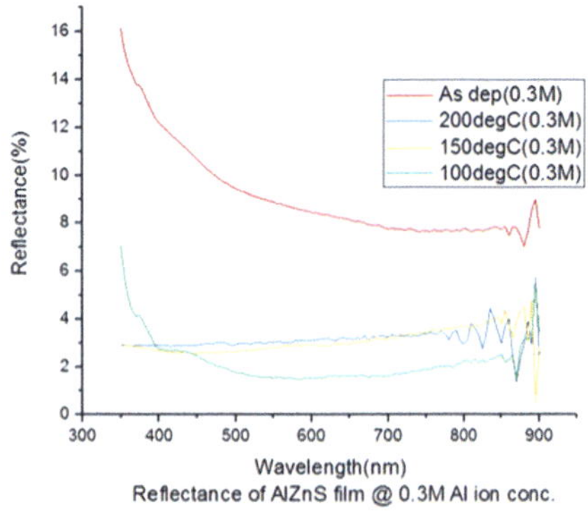

Fig. 14. .

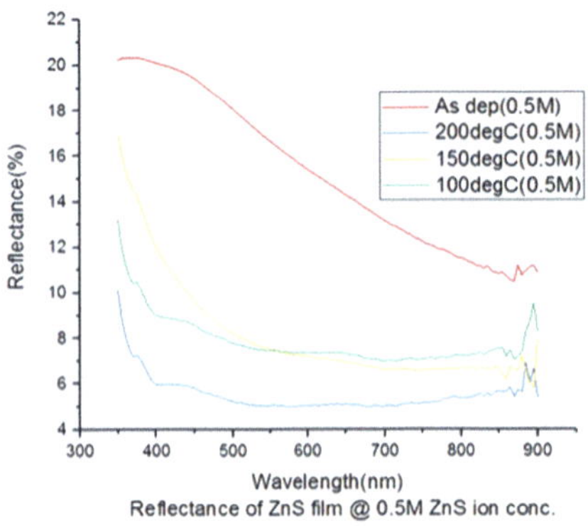

Fig. 15. .

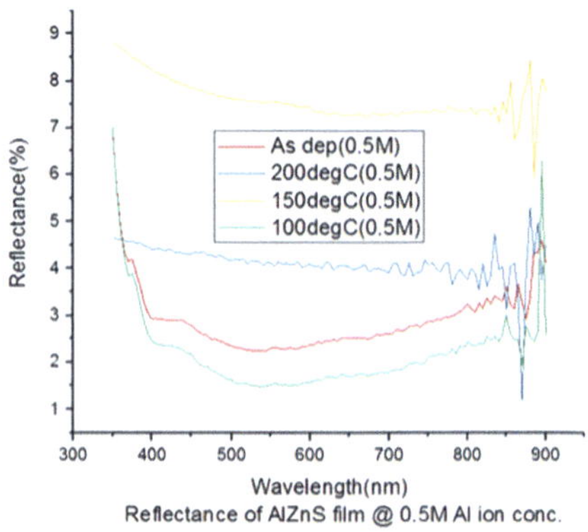

Fig. 16. .

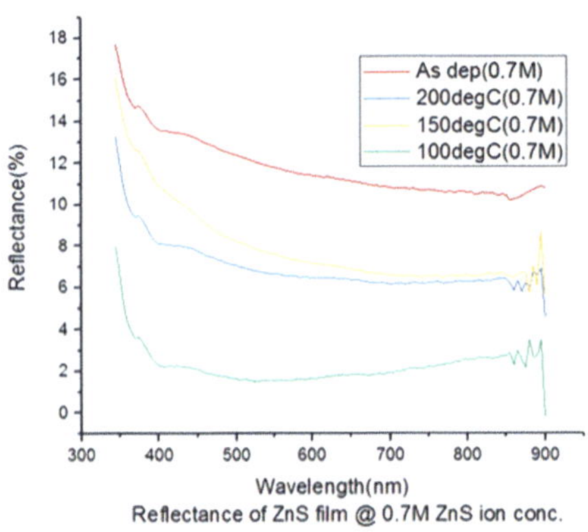

Fig. 17. .

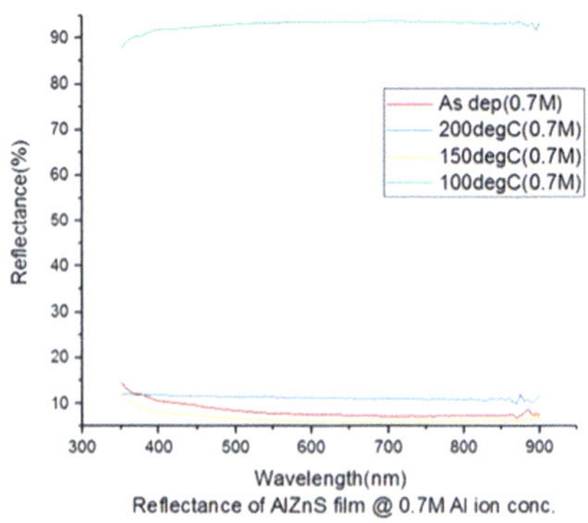

Fig. 18. .

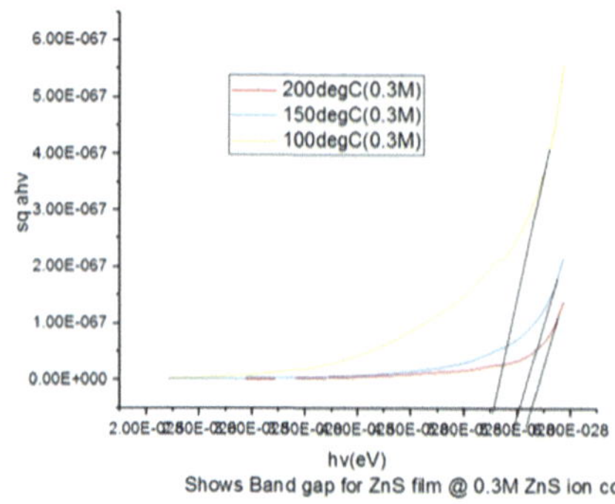

Fig. 19. .

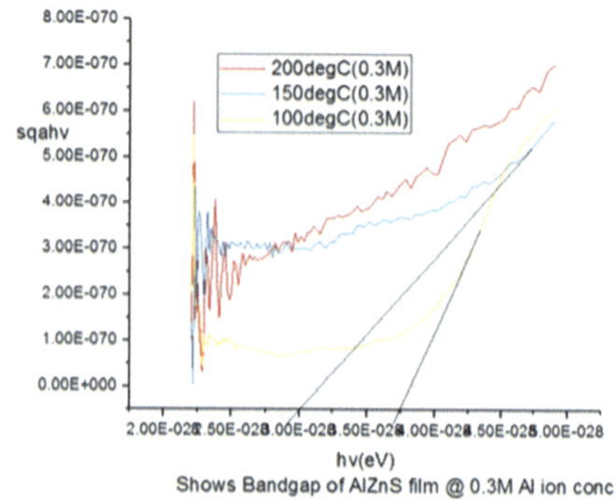

Fig. 20. .

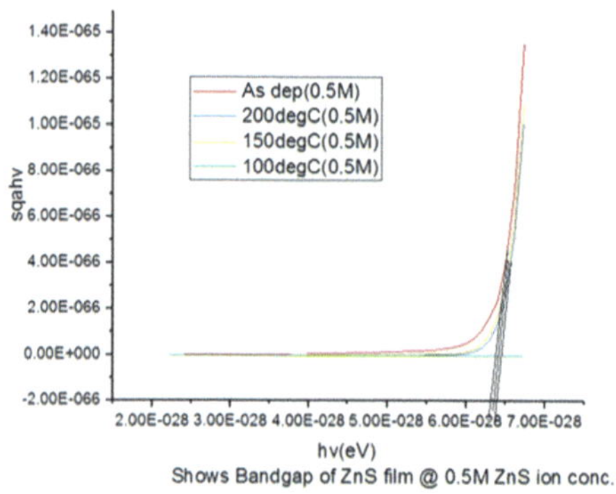

Fig. 21. .

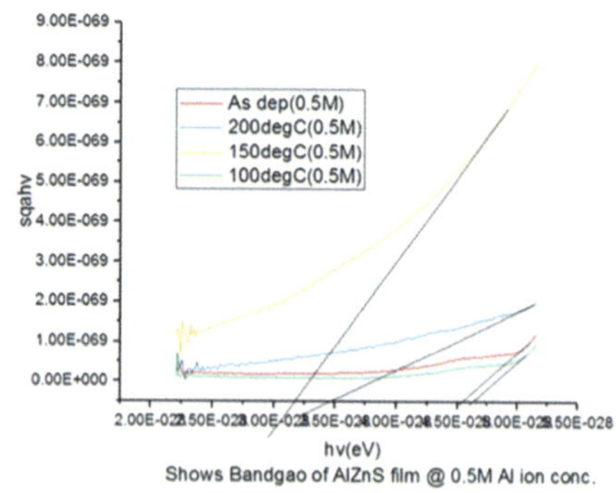

Fig. 22. .

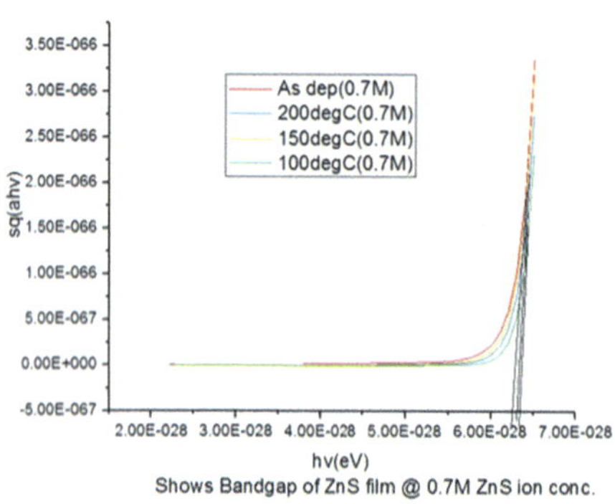

Fig. 23. .

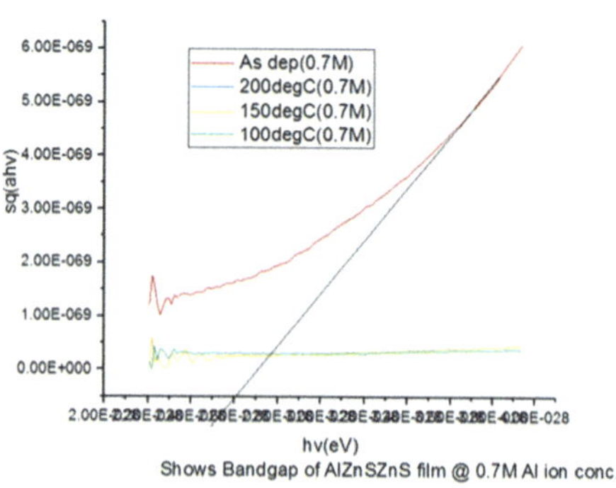

Fig. 24. .

4 Summary and Conclusion

We have successfully deposited thin solid films of ZnS doped with Aluminum impurities in different concentrations. The deposited films were characterized using UV-VIS spectrophotometer where the transmittance, absorbance and reflectance spectra were obtained. The addition of Al^{3+} ion impurities increased the density of the majority carriers as demonstrated by the increase in % Transmittance and lowering of % Absorbance as the impurity concentration increased. Temperature contributed to increase in transmittance and crystallinity of the films but might not have contributed significantly to high conductivity of the doped ZnS sample since Fermi level moves to the middle at high temperatures returning the material to its intrinsic status from literature.

5 Contributions to Knowledge

The results indicated the dependence of the optical properties on the concentrations of Zn^{2+} and Al^{3+} respectively as well as on the annealing temperatures. From the foregoing, the properties determined from the ZnS and the AlZnS films demonstrate the high promise of the materials in thin film growth, making a great impact in developing highly efficient and more environmentally accepted PV solar cells. Further study can be carried out to verify the structural properties of the materials within the concentration and temperature ranges demonstrated in this research.

References

Agbo, P.E., Nwofe, P.A., Odo, L.O.: Post-deposition heat treatments and characterization of dye-sensitized chemically deposited Zinc Sulphide (ZnS) thin films. Ovonic Res. **12**(3), 163–169 (2016)

Carlos, J.P., Ferrer, F., Campo, L., Marotti, R., Martin, F., Leinen, D., Barrodo, R., Ariel, D.: Optical absorption enhancement in sensitized ZnO nano rods for solar cells. Material (Rio J) **30**(3), 747–756 (2015). https://doi.org/10.1590/s1517-7076201

JinHuo, C., Wenjin, L.: Significant improvement in ZnS film electrical and optical performance by indium incorporation. J. Semiconductors **35**(9), 10–20, (ID:093003) (2014)

Keskenler, F., Turgut, G., Ayding, R., Dibber, U.: Electronic, optical and magnetic materials. J. Ovonic Res. **9**(2), 61–71 (2013)

Oloko, R.E., Chukwuocha, E.O.: Chemical bath deposition and characterization of zinc sulphide thin film for possible device applications. Retrieved Afr. J. Online (AJOL) **16**, 2. Accessed 11 Mar 2018 (2017)

Riu, W.Y., Yen, P.E.: Zinc sulphide buffer layer for CIGS solar cells prepared by chemical bath deposition. Adv. Technol. Innov. **2**(3), 95–98 (2016)

Wei, A., Liu, A., Zhuang, M., Zhao, Y.: Preparation and characterization of ZnS thin films prepared by chemical bath deposition. Mat. Sci. Semicond. Process. **16**, 1478–1484 (2013)

The Effect of Bitter Kola (Garcinia) Biodiesel and n-Octanol Additives on Performance, Emission and Combustion Characteristics of Diesel Engines

L. Atepor(✉)

Department of Mechanical Engineering, Cape Coast Technical University, Box AD 50, Cape Coast, Ghana
lawrence.atepor@cctu.edu.gh

Abstract. This paper examines the effect of octanol as an oxygenated additive to reduce emissions and to improve the performance of Bitter Kola biodiesel. Methanol and alkaline catalyst (KOH) were used for the transesterification process to produce the biodiesel. Neat bitter kola biodiesel is blended with octanol and petroleum diesel by volume to create the fuel blends, which are labelled as DCB10, DCB20 and DCB30. The fuel properties are found to be improved on using the octanol as an additive having high energy content, cetane number and are also easily miscible in biodiesel and petroleum diesel. Single cylinder, air-cooled diesel engine was employed in this research using both petroleum diesel and the blends as fuels. Engine tests resulted in lower CO_2 and NO_x emissions. The brake specific fuel consumption reduced and the thermal efficiency increased for the blends when compared with petroleum diesel. The results indicate that octanol can be added to bitter kola biodiesel blends and use effectively as alternative fuels for diesel engines.

Keywords: Bitter kola biodiesel · Octanol · Emissions · Carbon dioxide · Nitrogen oxide

1 Introduction

Diesel fuel is widely employed as a major fuel in industry, power and transportation areas owing to its high efficiency. Pollutants such as carbon monoxide, smoke and hydrocarbons from diesel fuel combustion have a serious impact on human health and the environment. In addition, the consumption of diesel fuels is also increasing the rapid depletion of worldwide petroleum reserves, which are predicted to end in the not too distant future. These reasons have motivated people to conduct research in the area of both edible and non-edible plant oil-based fuel alternatives. In considering lowering these emissions, fuel derived from renewable sources are being sort for (Devarajan et al. 2019). Biodiesels are potential fuels, which could be used in current engines without much alteration (Appavu 2018). These fuels have similar fuel properties to diesel. However,

J. N. Mojekwu et al. (Eds.): *Sustainable Education and Development*, pp. 354–362, 2021.
https://doi.org/10.1007/978-3-030-68836-3_31

neat biodiesel used in diesel engines result in higher viscosity, poor atomization and increased NOx emissions issues (Ganesan 2019). Hence, the viscosity of neat biodiesel should be lowered as far as possible to minimize the drawbacks mentioned.

In this study Bitter Kola *(Garcinia)* seed oil is chosen for obtaining biodiesel due to the abundant availability in Ghana and the West African sub-region, and Bitter Kola oil biodiesel is found to have diesel like properties from a previous research by Ogembi et al. (2019). The trend of using alcohols as a fuel source for SI engine to deliver high power and to lower the emissions has increased over the years. Commonly used alcohols in SI engines are ethanol or methanol which are short chain alcohols. Infusion of alcohols in CI engines has become an area of interest in recent times. In case of CI engines, alcohols having long chain carbon atoms are preferred as blend components. This is because the higher alcohols are distinguished for their high energy content as well as higher cetane number. The alcohols above butanol are found to form blends of diesel and biodiesel without any phase separations due to their hygroscopic nature and low polarity as a result of carbon content (Pramod and Sivanesan 2019). Many studies were attempted by blending the lower carbon–hydrogen (C–H) alcohols such as methanol, ethanol and which resulted in phase separation leading to poor ignition (Kumar and Saravanan 2016; Ramakrishnan et al. 2019). To reduce this drawback, alcohols having longer C–H chains and higher calorific values, namely butanol, pentanol and octanol, are being used as additives to diesel–biodiesel blends (Devarajan 2019; Joy et al. 2019; Devarajan 2018 and Devaraj et al. 2020). Devaraj et al. (2020) have found that the addition of higher C–H alcohols (pentanol) to diesel reduces CO, NOx emissions. Joy et al. (2019) confirmed that pentanol addition lowered biodiesel HC and CO emissions. Pandian et al. (2017) also agreed with the result stating that the addition of pentanol to biodiesel fuel lowers its NOx emissions. Octanol is gaining consideration among the researchers not only due to diesel like properties but also due to development of several method of synthesizing using micro-organisms. Zhang et al. (2015) doped diesel with octanol up to 30% by volume in a CI engine and found reduction in smoke, CO and NOx on comparison to neat diesel. Mahalingam et al. (2018) studied the effect of doping neat mahua biodiesel with varying proportion of octanol on the performance and emission characteristics of a diesel engine. Substantial reduction of all emission parameters was observed at different octanol proportions. Hence the literature review has put forth the feasibility of using octanol as an additive while making blends of biodiesel and diesel to produce alternate fuel source having improved combustion properties and reduced emission characteristics.

Information from previous works show that adding higher alcohols, namely butanol, ethanol, hexanol and octanol, in certain volume proportions to diesel/biodiesel and its blends is an effective way of reducing the associated emissions and improving on the performance of the engine. However, no specific work has been conducted on using Bitter Kola seed oil biodiesel as fuel in compression ignition engine applications. Further, detailed investigations of the effect of Bitter Kola and octanol in Bitter Kola biodiesels have not been attempted before. Hence, this study details the outcome of using octanol as an oxygen donating additive on emissions and performance patterns of Bitter Kola biodiesel in a diesel engine.

2 Engine Test Equipment and Methods

Bitter Kola seeds obtained from the Bitter Kola tree yield raw oil on drying and crushing. The oil obtained from these seeds is nontoxic, free from sulphur and aromatics and biodegradable. It also has a high boiling point, cetane number and flash point, low vapour pressure and high density, which enhance the running of engines. The bitter kola oil was then taken through transesterification process for the biodiesel production, where beakers were used as reactors.

The engine test was carried out in the laboratory using a four-stroke single cylinder victor type air-cooled diesel engine. Table 1 provides the specifications of the diesel engine. Figure 1 depicts the equipment connections for the engine test. The equipment was assembled and procedure followed Maina (2014). The engine (1) was coupled with a dynamometer (2) to provide brake load, while the engine throttling and dynamometer settings were controlled by a computer (8). A pressure transducer (9) was installed in one of the piston cylinders. Cylinder pressure signals from pressure transducer were amplified by a charge amplifier (11), and connected to the SMETech COMBI-PC indication system (7) for data acquisition.

Table 1. Specification of test engine

Manufacturer	Victor diesel engine company Ltd
Engine	Number 42
Type	Single cylinder, 4 stroke, vertical compression, Air cooled, fixed throttle
Cylinder bore	80 mm
Torque arm	10 mm
Stroke	100 mm
Swept volume	0.5 (l)
Fuel	Diesel
Max. speed	1500 rpm
Brake power	2.982 KW at 1500 rpm

The data acquisition system was externally triggered 1024 times in one revolution by an incremental crank angle transducer-optical encoder (10). Fuel was introduced from a fuel tank (3) equipped with flow measurement system. During fuel switching, the fuel tank was drained from the engine fuel filter, new fuel was introduced into the tank until the fuel filter was full, and the engine was then started and allowed to run for a few minutes to clear fuel lines and stabilize. AVL ditest MDS 350 mission analyser station designed for diesel engines (5) was used for measuring (CO, CO2, and HC), (THC), and (NOx) respectively and a smoke meter (6) connected before the oxidative converter at the engine exhaust pipe (4).

The blends were prepared by mixing octanol, bitter kola biodiesel and petroleum diesel together at varying proportions as shown below. For the experiment, three blends

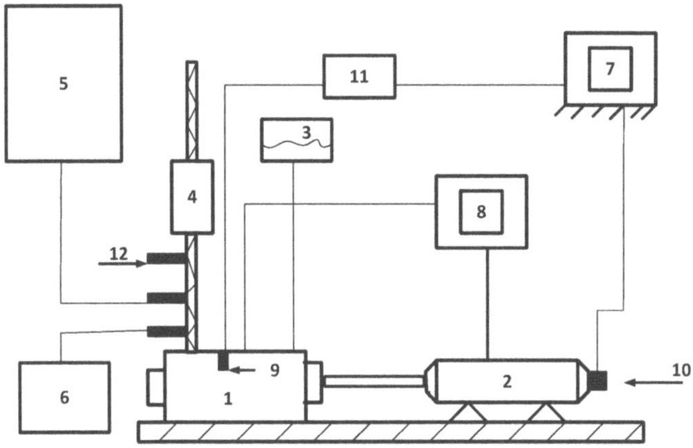

Fig. 1. Experimental Setup (after Maina 2014). 1-Engine, 2-Dynamometer, 3-Fuel Tank, 4-Exhaust Pipe, 5-Gas Analyzer, 6-Smoke Meter, 7-Computer, 8-Computer, 9-Pressure Transducer, 10-Crank Angle Transducer, 11-Charge Amplifier, 12-Temperature Sensor.

of fuel were prepared by mixing octanol (C) and bitter kola biodiesel (B) with petroleum diesel (D) by varying its volume.

- 80% diesel + 10% bitter kola biodiesel + 10% Oct = DCB10
- 70% diesel + 20% bitter kola biodiesel + 10% Oct = DCB20
- 60% diesel + 30% bitter kola biodiesel + 10% Oct = DCB30

3 Results and Discussion

3.1 Emissions

Engine emissions, which were obtained experimentally, are plotted against load and discussed as follows:

3.1.1 Oxides of Nitrogen (NO_x)

The NO_x emissions for the various blends under different load conditions are presented in Fig. 2. NO_x emissions increase with load for all fuels. At higher loads the in-cylinder temperature increases, the mixture gets rich and aids incomplete combustion thus the formation of higher NO_x (Joy et al. 2019). Adding octanol to bitter kola biodiesel lowers its NO_x emission and this trend is consistent with the results of the study by Pramod and Sivanesan (2019) except at the load of 15 N where the blend DCB20 has a higher NO_x emission. The reduction in the NO_x emission levels of the blends may be due to the lower viscosities of the fuel blends, which improves the atomization process and reduces ignition delay. DCB10, DCB20 and DCB30 produced 11.6%, 11.5% and 1.57% lower NO_x emissions respectively at the peak load than the pure petroleum diesel. The DCB10 is found to be the most efficient blend in terms of NO_x emission.

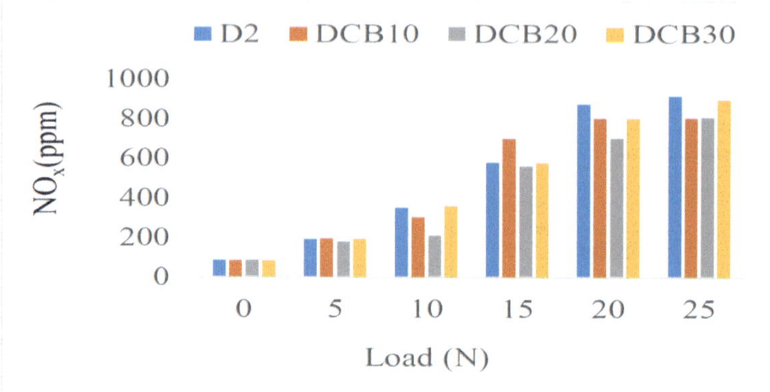

Fig. 2. NO_x emissions for the fuel samples at different loads

3.1.2 Carbon Dioxide (CO_2)

Figure 3 shows the CO_2 emissions for the various blends under different load conditions. The CO_2 emissions are found to increase with the load and this is in consistent with the results in the study by Pramod and Sivanesan (2019). The CO_2 emissions from the blends are considerably lower than petroleum diesel owing to their natural oxygen content and the additional oxygen contributed by the octanol. The oxygen present improves the combustion reaction and lowers the CO_2 emissions (Arulprakasajothi et al. 2018). The DCB20 blend produced relatively the lowest CO_2 emissions.

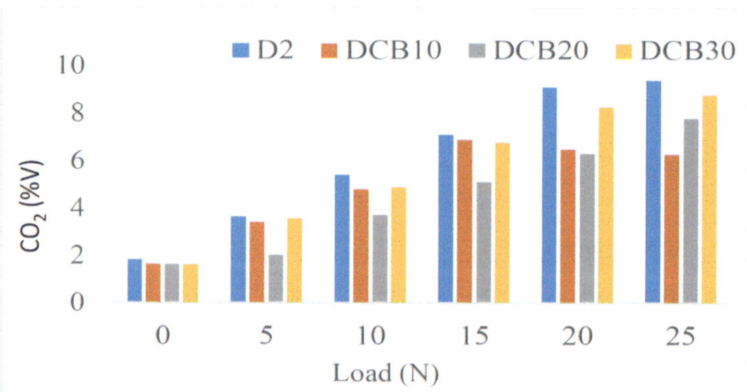

Fig. 3. CO_2 emissions for the fuel samples at different loads

3.2 Brake Specific Fuel Consumption

Figure 4 illustrates the variation of specific fuel consumption with load. The BSFC reduce with load for all test fuels. At low load operations, fuel consumption is higher than at high load operations. This may be due to more fuel required to produce sufficient torque at lower load conditions (Pramod and Sivanesan 2019).

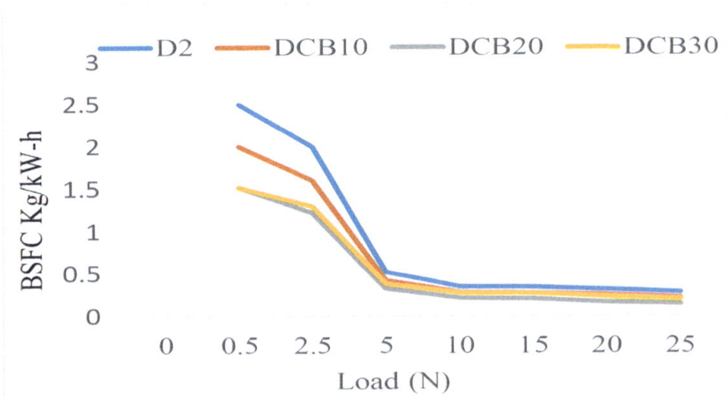

Fig. 4. Variation of specific fuel consumption with load

From Fig. 4 a significant reduction in BSFC is observed for the blends over petroleum diesel despite their lower calorific values. This may be due to the effective fuel combustion because of the additional O_2 content from both the octanol and biodiesel. The blend DCB20 showed lowest BSFC of 50% compared to petroleum diesel.

3.3 Brake Thermal Efficiency

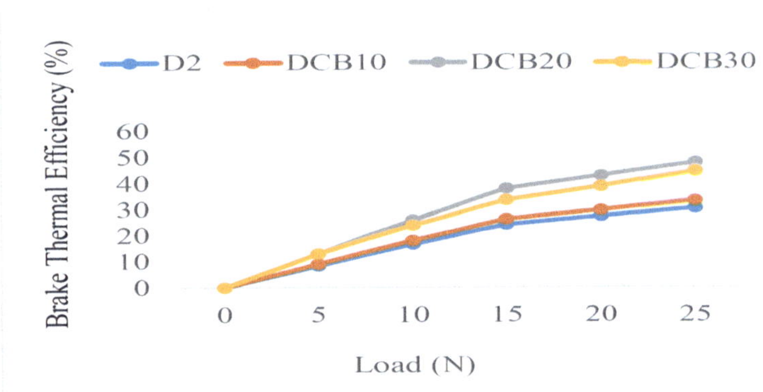

Fig. 5. Variation of brake thermal efficiency with load

Variation of brake thermal efficiency (BTE) with load is shown in Fig. 5. BTE for all the fuels increase with load. The average BTE for DCB20 is higher than all the other blends and petroleum diesel and has a maximum increase of 57.4% compared to the petroleum diesel.

3.4 Exhaust Gas Temperature

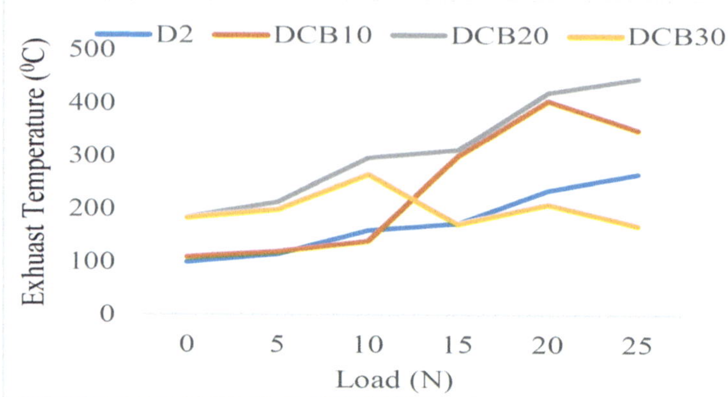

Fig. 6. Variation of exhaust gas temperature with load

Figure 6 shows the variation of exhaust gas temperature (EGT) with load. The EGT is always high for blends contrary to petroleum diesel (Pramod and Sivanesan 2019) except at higher loads of 15N to 25N in this particular study, where the EGTs for DCB30 blend are lower. The high EGTs may be due to the effective combustion of fuel mixtures of the blends coming from the additional O_2 content infused by the octanol/biodiesel blend.

4 Summary and Conclusion

The following are deduced from the experimental results:

- NO_x emissions for the blends are lower compared to the pure petroleum diesel and this is due to the high latent heat of evaporation of octanol, which reduces the in-cylinder temperature slowing the rate of formation of Nitrogen Oxides.
- CO_2 emissions from the blends are lower than petroleum diesel.
- The blend DCB20 has the lowest BSFC of about 50% lower than that of the petroleum diesel.
- The thermal efficiencies of all the blends are higher than that of petroleum diesel.
- Exhaust temperature is high indicating effective combustion of the fuel blends.
- DCB20 demonstrates to be the most efficient fuel blend with better emissions and performance patterns.

From the experiment conducted using a diesel engine fueled with bitter kola biodiesel and octanol additive, it can be concluded that bitter kola biodiesel blended with octanol and petroleum diesel can effectively be used as an alternative renewable fuel to replace pure petroleum diesel. The DCB20 blend was found to be the most efficient in terms of emissions and performance. This could be due to the high oxygen content of the bitter kola biodiesel and the additional oxygen from the octanol.

Acknowledgements. The author would like to acknowledge the support of Mr. Samuel Gariba of Cape Coast Technical University who assisted in the setting up of the experimental rig and the Laboratory Technicians of University of Cape Coast Chemistry and the Ghana Standard Authority laboratories who assisted in various ways in the performance of the analysis.

Conflict of Interest. The author declared no potential conflicts of interest with respect to the research, authorship and publication of this article.

References

Appavu, P.: Effect of injection timing on performance and emission characteristics of palm biodiesel and diesel blends. J. Oil Palm Res. **30**, 674–681 (2018)

Arulprakasajothi, M., Elangovan, K., Chandrasekhar, U., Suresh, S.: Performance study of conical strip inserts in tube heat exchanger using water based titanium oxide nanofluid. Thermal Sci. **22**(1 Part B), 477–485 (2018)

Devaraj, A., Yuvarajan, D., Vinoth Kanna, I.: Study on the outcome of a cetane improver on the emission characteristics of a diesel engine. Int. J. Ambient Energy **41**(7), 798–801 (2020)

Devarajan, Y.: Experimental evaluation of combustion, emission and performance of research diesel engine fuelled Di-methyl-carbonate and biodiesel blends. Atmos. Pollut. Res. **10**(3), 795–801 (2019)

Devarajan, Y., Choubey, G., Mehar, K.: Ignition analysis on neat alcohols and biodiesel blends propelled research compression ignition engine. Energy Sources Part A: Recovery Utilization Environ. Eff. 1–12 (2019)

Devarajan, Y., Munuswamy, D.B., Mahalingam, A.: Performance, combustion and emission analysis on the effect of ferrofluid on neat biodiesel. Process Saf. Environ. Prot. **111**, 283–291 (2017)

Devarajan, Y., Munuswamy, D.B., Nagappan, B., Pandian, A.K.: Performance, combustion and emission analysis of mustard oil biodiesel and octanol blends in diesel engine. Heat Mass Transf. **54**(6), 1803–1811 (2018)

Devarajan, Y., Munuswamy, D., Nagappan, B., Subbiah, G.: Experimental assessment of performance and exhaust emission characteristics of a diesel engine fuelled with Punnai biodiesel/butanol fuel blends. Pet. Sci. **16**(6), 1471–1478 (2019)

Ganesan, S.: Effect of EGR & nanoparticles on performance and emission characteristics of a diesel engine fuelled with palm biodiesel and diesel blends. J. Oil Palm Res. **31**(1), 130–137 (2019)

Ganesan, S., Sivasubramanian, R., Sajin, J.B., Subbiah, G., Devarajan, Y.: Performance and emission study on the effect of oxygenated additive in neat biodiesel fueled diesel engine. Energy Sources A: Recovery Utilization Environ. Effects **41**(16), 2017–2027 (2019)

Joy, N., Yuvarajan, D., Beemkumar, N.: Performance evaluation and emission characteristics of biodiesel-ignition enhancer blends propelled in a research diesel engine. Int. J. Green Energy **16**(4), 277–283 (2019)

Kumar, B.R., Saravanan, S.: Effects of iso-butanol/diesel and n-pentanol/diesel blends on performance and emissions of a DI diesel engine under premixed LTC (low temperature combustion) mode. Fuel **170**, 49–59 (2016)

Mahalingam, A., Devarajan, Y., Radhakrishnan, S., Vellaiyan, S., Nagappan, B.: Emissions analysis on mahua oil biodiesel and higher alcohol blends in diesel engine. Alex. Eng. J. **57**(4), 2627–2631 (2018)

Maina, P.: Investigation of fuel properties and engine analysis of Jatropha biodiesel of Kenyan Origin. J. Energy South Africa **25**(2), 107–116 (2014)

Ogemdi, I.K., Chidubem, E.E., Gold, E.: Production of Biodiesel from Garcinia Kola Seeds Using Trans-Esterification Reaction. Compos. Mater. **2**(2), 55 (2019)

Pandian, A.K., Munuswamy, D.B., Radhakrishana, S., Ramakrishnan, R.B.B., Nagappan, B., Devarajan, Y.: Influence of an oxygenated additive on emission of an engine fueled with neat biodiesel. Pet. Sci. **14**(4), 791–797 (2017)

Pramod, K.P., Sivanesan, M.: Analysis of performance and emission parameters of IC engine fueled with neem biodiesel and n-octanol additives. Int. J. Innov. Technol. Exploring Eng. **8**(8), 2237–2241 (2019)

Ramakrishnan, G., Krishnan, P., Rathinam, S.R.T., Devarajan, Y.: Role of nano-additive blended biodieselon emission characteristics of the research diesel engine. Int. J. Green Energy **16**, 435–441 (2019)

Reddy, V.P.K., Kumar, D.S., Thirumalini, S.: Effect of antioxidants on the performance and emission characteristics of a diesel engine fuelled by waste cooking sunflower methyl ester. In: IOP Conference Series: Materials Science and Engineering, vol. 310, p. 012116 (2018)

Zhang, T., Munch, K., Denbratt, I.: An experimental study on the use of butanol or octanol blends in a heavy duty diesel engine. SAE Int. J. Fuels Lubr. **8**(3), 610–621 (2015)

Decomposing Total Factor Productivity of Non-life Insurance Firms in Tanzania

K. M. Bwana(✉)

Accountancy Department, College of Business Education, P. O. Box 2077, Dodoma, Tanzania

Abstract. The purpose of this study is to decompose the total factor productivity of non-life insurance firms in terms of technical efficiency change (TECH) and efficiency change (EFFCH). The study also focuses on factors deriving productivity change of the insurance sector in Tanzani. Malmquist Productivity Index (MPI) model was employed in 19 non-life insurance firms over the period ***2014/15–2015/16.*** Findings revealed that 94.7% of all firms were experiencing improvement in productivity change by 54.6%, while one firm was experiencing regress in productivity change by 1.2% over the study period. As far as efficiency change and technical efficiency change, only one firm was experiencing deterioration in each category by 5.8% and 1.2% respectively. It was further revealed that in the year ***2014/15–2017/18*** insurance sector was performing better (with productivity improvement of 90.6%) compared to the remaining year under review. The efficiency change largely derived productivity of insurance sector (catch up effect). The study suggests that non-life insurance firms in Tanzania should redesign and improve their existing production technology as it is the leading performance deriving factor. Findings will be useful to insurance managers and regulatory organs who wish to make smart and informed decisions to support policy implementation.

Keywords: Productivity · Non-life insurance · Firms · Tanzania

1 Introduction

As the economy grows in developing countries, the financial sectors also seem to expand hence deriving other subs financial sector such as insurance to grow as well. A well-regulated and robust insurance industry can considerably contribute to economic growth and efficient resource allocation through the transfer of risk and mobilization of saving (Udaibir 2003). Chakraborty and Harper (2017) added that a well-performing insurance sector contributes a significant role in the economic growth of any nation in the modern world. Insurance sector protects institutions from the risk of unforeseen losses, levelling earnings of businesses firms and create value. At the same time, promoting national investment and create jobs and income for operators. Importance of the insurance sector can be seen through its traditional role of managing risk by indemnification, the insurance sector can enhance long term savings and serves as a medium to channel funds from policyholders to investment opportunities including mortgage lending (Hammoud 2008).

Tanzania has witnessed a significant growth of insurance sector from two insurance firms before liberalization to 31 registered insurance companies after liberalization in

J. N. Mojekwu et al. (Eds.): *Sustainable Education and Development*, pp. 363–372, 2021.
https://doi.org/10.1007/978-3-030-68836-3_32

the late 1980s. The country also has 596 insurance agents, 115 insurance brokers and 54 loss adjusters/assessors (TIRA Annual Report 2018). The sector is largely regulated by Tanzania Insurance Regulatory Authority (TIRA) which was established by Act No. 18 of 1996 after the adoption of trade liberalization policy by the government in the late 1980s. Generally, insurance in Tanzania is mainly grouped as general (non-life) insurance and life insurance. General insurance includes motor-private, fire-domestic, motor-commercial, aviation, fire-industrial and engineering, theft, workmen's compensation, marine. According to TIRA report (2017), insurance sector contribution to Gross Domestic Product (GDP) stood at 0.55% which is equivalent to TZS 116,102 billion which signifies relevancy and importance of insurance sector to the country's economy.

Over recent years, several empirical researches have been conducted regarding performance of insurance firms in developing countries, most of which focus on efficiency performance. According to Barros et al. (2010); Cummins and Xie (2008) gauging performance is one of the critical aspects among insurance firms and many studies are focusing on the relative efficiency of the insurance firms. As Bauer et al. (1998) contended performance of insurance companies is considered as the central theme in contemporary research. Being a measure of efficiency, total factors productivity (TFP) is considered to be more appropriate when one wants to gauge and compare the performance of the firms over some time. Therefore the TFP of insurance firms may be defined as the ratio of aggregated outputs over aggregated inputs. Generally, the productivity of any organization has always been one of exciting topics to many researchers and managers. For example, when it comes to non-banking financial institutions such as insurance firms which deal with pooled resources from insured (clients) understanding the factors influencing productivity change has been the priority of managers (Kaur and Aggarwal 2016). Review of literature on insurance productivity confirmed that, there is a little or no attention has been paid to the productivity of non-life insurance companies in Tanzania despite its contribution to the economy. OECD (2015) also added that productivity is the ultimate engine of growth in the global economy. As contended in the study by Bwana (2018) economic system is considered to be relatively efficient than the other only if it can produce more goods (or provide services) without consuming more resources. Insurance sector can develop financial system efficiency by reducing transaction costs, creating liquidity, and facilitating economies of scale in investment (Hammoud 2008). Given the same, it implies that the efficiency of Tanzania economy and the financial system largely depends on the performance of the insurance sector in the country. Therefore, the main objective of this research is to bridge the gap and decompose total factor productivity (TFP) of non-life insurance companies in Tanzania. Specifically, the study aims to:

i) Measure total factor productivity and evaluate technical and efficiency change of non- life insurance companies in Tanzania
ii) Examine major factors deriving total factor productivity change in non-life insurance companies in Tanzania.

The study is crucial since it intends to disclose the productivity of non-life insurance companies in Tanzania, part of the financial services sector, which is not yet fully tapped in terms of research. The remaining part of this paper is organized as follows: Sect. 2

describes the data and methodology where variable employed in the study and techniques engaged in the analysis are explained, Sect. 3 narrates the findings and discussion where by results obtained from the analysis are presented and discussed, Implications of the results is also pointed out in this part. Conclusion and recommendations regarding the findings is presented in Sect. 4.

2 Methodology

Data was extracted from annual reports of 19 non-life insurance companies operating in Tanzania. The sample was drawn from 31 registered life and non-life insurance companies in the country. The study involves secondary data which was extracted from Tanzania Insurance Regulatory Authority (TIRA) published annual reports for the period covering 2014/15–2017/18. The insurance companies under scrutiny included: Alliance, UAP, ZIC, Reliance, Britam, IGT, NIC, Phoenix, and Sanlam General. Others are Bumaco, Maxinsure, Mgen, First, Tanzania, Icea Lion, Mayfair, Mo as well as Star General, Milembe.

2.1 Inputs and Outputs Variables

Inputs variables are resources which are employed in the production process to produce outputs. These resources may differ from one firm (or sector) to another depending on the nature of activities. In this study *commission paid* and *management expenses* were employed as inputs. *Commission Paid* – is an amount of money paid to a broker (agent) or insurance salesperson as a percentage of the policy premium. The variable was also employed in the study by Norma et al. (2006) which was conducted in Malaysia. *Management expenses* - Include expenses, commission, brokerage and remuneration to agents and to intermediaries, charged to the revenue.

Outputs variables are the outcome of the production process, in the insurance sector the most widely seen outputs involve *premium* and *income from investment* activities, in this study two outputs (premium is written and net investment income) have been employed. *Premium written* - money an individual or entity pays for an insurance policy. It also represents a liability, as the insurer must provide coverage for claims being made against the policy. The variable was also employed in the study by Hawang and Kao (2006) in Indonesia. *Net investment income* - Income derived from its investments as opposed to its operations. The variable was also employed in the study by Hawang and Kao (2006) in Indonesia. According to Avkiran (1999), the correlation between inputs and outputs can be used to test the correctness of variables. Analysis of the correlation between inputs and outputs is positive, implying that the variables move in a positive direction. The result signifies the need to increase inputs such as premium in order to be able to cover more risks. General analysis of the insurance characteristics shows that the sector has heterogeneity characters since standard deviation is higher than mean; the same result was revealed in the study by Jackson (2012) in Kenya. However, based on the DEA approach heterogeneity in the scale of operation of the underlying DMU does not affect the analysis (Coelli et al. 2005).

2.2 DEA-Based Malmquist Productivity Index Model

Malmquist productivity index was first developed by Malmquist (1953) a Swedish economist, he introduced quantity index as the ratio of the distance function. The model was initially used in the analysis of consumer theory. The model was later advanced by Caves et al. (1982) after defining the Malmquist Total Factors Productivity Index (MTFPI), they referred to the original paper of Malmquist and allowed their proposed productivity index to go by the name of Malmquist. Farrell (1957) calculated Malmquist index-based distance function on which the index is based and which depends on the technical efficiency measures proposed by Farrell (1957). Therefore, Fare et al. (1989) managed to link technical efficiency, Data Envelopment Analysis by Charnes et al. (1978) and Malmquist Productivity Index by Caves et al. (1982) to introduce a DEA based Malmquist Productivity Index. According to Fare et al. (FGLR-Model) (1992) total factor productivity index can be decomposed into technical change and efficiency change. In the work of Fare et al. (1994) it was added that efficiency change can further be decomposed into pure efficiency change and scale efficiency change.

Malmquist index of total factor productivity measures changes in total outputs relative to the change in total inputs (Sakar 2006). This study adopts a non-parametric approach which is a DEA-based Malmquist index suitable for panel data, the result of which will tell the productivity changes between two different periods for a given set of non-life insurance companies. The main reason for employing a DEA- based Malmquist index technique is because we are the missing price of output and inputs. Input orientation model shows how the firm can minimize inputs without changing output quantity, while output orientation determines how the firm can maximize the output without altering the input quantities (Bwana 2015). As contended in the study by Griffel-Tatje and Lovell (1995) Malmquist TFP may not accurately measure TFP changes when the variable return to scale model is assumed. Therefore this study adopts constant return to scale (CSR) model. This study further builds on the Alirezaee and Afsharian (2013). on the argument that the Malmquist productivity index is one of crucial and widely index for gauging relative productivity change of firms (decision-making units). Further, we employed the DEA-based Malmquist Productivity Index to measure relative productivity change of insurance firms because it has also been used in the majority of existing papers (Cummins et al. 1999).

This means that productivity and efficiency measurements must consider the extent to which the outputs can be expanded without affecting (altering) the quantity of inputs (Jacobs et al. 2006). A relevant tool in analyzing this would be output distance function, which for a period t, is defined as:

$$D_0^t\left(x^t, y^t\right) = \inf_\theta\left\{\theta > 0 : \left(x^t, y^t/\theta\right) \in s^t\right\} \tag{1}$$

It should be noted that $D_0^t\left(x^t, y^t\right) \leq 1$ if and only if $\left(x^t, y^t\right) \in s^t$, additionally $D_0^t\left(x^t, y^t\right) = 1$ if and only if $(\left(x^t, y^t\right)$ is on the (output) isoquant or frontier of technology, the terminology was proposed by Farrell (1957), it occurs when production is technically efficient. We can define the MPI by intertemporal extension of Eq. (2), the extension gives us:

$$D_0^T\left(x^s, y^s\right) = \inf_\theta\left\{\theta > 0 : \left(x^s, y^s/\theta\right) \in s^T\right\}, \ T, S \in \{t, t+1\} \tag{2}$$

Whereby when T = S we get Eq. (1), while when $T = t, S = t + 1$ we get the distance function $D_0^t(x^{t+1}, y^{t+1})$ Measuring the maximum proportional change in inputs required to make (x^{t+1}, y^{t+1}) onto frontier technology at the previous period t. Similarly, when $T = t, S = t + 1$ we obtain the distance function $D_0^{t+1}(x^t, y^t)$ estimating (measuring) the maximum proportional change in outputs required to make (x^t, y^t) onto the frontier of technology at *t + 1*. From the intertemporal measures, we follow Caves et al. (1982) in defining the output-oriented Malmquist productivity index (MPI) as follows:

$$M_o\left(x^t, y^t, x^{t+1}, y^{t+1}\right) = \left[\frac{D_o^t(x^{t+1}, y^{t+1}) + D_o^{t+1}(x^{t+1}, y^{t+1})}{D_o^t(x^t, y^t)\ D_o^{t+1}(x^t, yt)}\right]^{1/2} \quad (3)$$

Moreover, from Färe et al. (1994) the MPI is decomposed into efficiency change (ECH) and technology change (CTH) as follows:

$$M_o\left(x^t, y^t, x^{t+1}, y^{t+1}\right) = \frac{D_o^{t+1}(x^{t+1}, y^{t+1})}{D_o^t(x^t, y^t)}\left[\frac{D_o^t(x^{t+1}, y^{t+1}) + D_o^t(x^t, y^t)}{D_o^{t+1}(x^{t+1}, y^{t+1})\ D_o^{t+1}(x^t, y^t)}\right]^{-1/2}$$
$$= ECH \times TCH \quad (4)$$

The efficiency change term **(ECH)** is equivalent to the ratio of Farrell technical efficiency in period *t + 1* divided by Farrell technical efficiency in period *t*. the technological change **(TCH)** implies the geometric mean of the shift in technology as observed at (x^{t+1}, y^{t+1}) (the first ratio in the bracket) and shift in technology observed at (x^t, y^t) (the second ratio inside bracket). The ECH component is more significant than, equal to, or less than unity depending on whether the efficiency of the evaluated DMUS improves (catching the frontier effect), stagnates, or declines. This will depend on the case. However, the TCH may also take a value greater than, equal to or less than unity to make the technological change positive, zero, or negative, respectively. Malmquist has been previously used in the insurance study by Cummins et al. (1999), Mahlberg and Url (2003).

3 Findings and Discussion

According to Färe et al. (1994), DEA-based Malmquist index approach allows decomposing TFP changes into two major components. The first specific objective of this study was to decompose the total factor productivity change into *(i)* a catching-up term or efficiency change (EFFC) that reflecting movements towards the efficient frontier, and *(ii)* a frontier shift or technical change (TECH) reflecting technological advancement or innovations. According to Grosskopf (2003) demand for a decomposition, TFP demonstrates the ability to disentangle TFP changes into components associated with factors proven to be the most critical application of these indexes, this reflect the second objective of this study (Table 1). Generally, efficiency change greater than one (EFFCH > 1) implies a movement closer to the frontier, which also reflect how well the firm is utilizing its resources to catch up with the best performance, on the other hand efficiency change less than one (EFFCH < 1) implies falling behind or poor performance in terms of resources utilization and administration in general. Technical change (TECHCH) innovation or progress in technology, a value greater than 1 implies an increase (progress in technological advancement), while a value less than 1 reflect deterioration in innovation. TFP with value greater than one indicates total productivity growth between two periods.

Result revealed that the best three performing insurance firms in terms of efficiency change and TFP change are *First (1.929)*, followed by *Tanzindia (1.855) and Sanlam General (1.819)*, three firms have recorded an improvement of 92.9%; 85.5% and 81.9% respectively over the study period. On the other hand, *Bumaco (0.942)* experienced a regress of 5.8% in terms of efficiency change. In terms of innovation (technological change) Alliance (1.395) records the best performance compared to other companies, recording technological progress of 39.5%. On the other hand, Milembe (0.988) experienced a regress in innovation (technological advancement) by 1.2% over the study period. As far as TFP is concern First (2.412) recorded the best improvement in productivity change while Milembe (0.988) experienced decline in productivity by 1.2%. Analysis of components of TFP after Decomposition indicates that improvement of the

Table 1. Malmquist index summary of firm means

Insurance firms	Efficiency change	Technical change	Pure efficiency change	Scale efficiency change	TFP change
1	1.065	1.340	1.065	1.000	***1.427***
2	1.001	1.395	1.001	1.000	***1.396***
3	1.117	1.280	1.117	1.000	***1.430***
4	1.459	1.342	1.459	1.000	***1.957***
5	1.286	1.221	1.459	1.000	***1.570***
6	1.081	1.331	1.286	1.000	***1.438***
7	1.377	1.316	1.081	1.000	***1.812***
8	1.208	1.309	1.377	1.000	***1.582***
9	1.819	1.319	1.208	1.000	**2.398**
10	0.942	1.298	1.819	1.000	***1.223***
11	1.157	1.298	0.942	1.000	***1.300***
12	1.383	1.123	1.157	1.000	***1.714***
13	1.929	1.251	1.383	1.000	**2.412**
14	1.855	1.160	1.929	1.000	**2.153**
15	1.348	1.188	1.855	1.000	***1.601***
16	1.071	1.074	1.348	1.000	***1.150***
17	1.111	1.100	1.071	1.000	***1.223***
18	1.367	1.055	1.111	1.000	***1.442***
19	1.000	0.988	1.367	1.000	***0.988***
AVERAGE	**1.265**	**1.222**	**1.265**	**1.000**	***1.546***

productivity of best performing firm (First) was attributed mainly by efficiency change of 92.9% while regress in the productivity of Milembe was primarily contributed by deterioration in technological aspect (innovation) by 1.2%. The analysis, concludes that the performance of the insurance sector in Tanzania is mostly dominated or derived by how well the firm is using existing production technology (catch up effect). The argument is based on the fact that ranking shows that nine out the best ten companies the deriving factor was efficiency change.

Generally, efficiency change (EFFCH) or catch up effect indicates productivity change through more efficient use of available production technology, where Technical change (TECHCH) reflect the *geometric mean of the shift in technology between two periods* and can be regarded as innovation; as it was in the case of EFFCH a value greater than 1 implies an increase (progress in technological advancement), while a value less than 1 reflect deterioration in innovation. TFP with a value greater than one indicates total productivity growth between two periods, which implies in the second period, the same quantity of input produces more output. By contrast, a decline of total productivity change is presented by TFP less than one (TFPCH < 1) which implies in the second period the same quantity of inputs produces less outputs.

Table 2. Malmquist productivity annual means

Year	EFF change	TECHN change	Pure EFF change	Scale EFF change	TFP change
2014/15–2015/16	1.372	1.390	1.372	1.000	***1.906***
2015/16–2016/17	1.308	0.985	1.308	1.000	***1.287***
2016/17–2017/18	1.127	1.335	1.127	1.000	***1.505***
Mean	***1.265***	***1.222***	***1.265***	***1.000***	***1.546***

Findings revealed that during the year 2014/15–2015/16 TFP was 1.906 which is greater than one, this implies that productivity of non-life insurance companies improved during 2014/15–2015/16 by 90.6%. Findings further records that the insurance sector continue to experience improvement in productivity change in the subsequent years whereby in the year 2015/16–2016/17 and 2016/17–2017/18 productivity improved by 28.7% and 50.5%, respectively. Mean for the TFP change over the study period is 1.546, which implies an improvement of total productivity in the insurance sector by 54.6%. The analysis shows that improvement observed was primarily attributed by 22.2% progress in technical change and 26.5% of efficiency change (Table 2). The finding is contrary to the result obtained in the study by Jackson (2012) where the total factor productivity change of non-life insurance companies in Kenya progressed by 2.7% over the study period (2005–2009) the growth of which was attributed by technical progress of 11.4% while efficiency change was deteriorating by 7.8%. The result also contravenes findings by Cummins and Turchetti (1996) in which it was revealed that Italian insurance industry manifested 3.5% decline in TFP for the period 1985–1993. Findings revealed that in the year 2014/15–2015/16 insurance sector in Tanzania experienced the highest level of improvement in all aspects (both efficiency change and technical progress). In contrast, in the year 2015/16–2016/17, the sector experienced the lowest level of efficiency progress as well as deterioration in the technological progress (Table 2). Result also reflects unsystematic changes in the components of total factor productivity over the study period as some line graphs do cross and overlap at a different point. For example, a line graph representing technical change (innovation) cross at the lower and upper end of the pure efficiency change (catching up effect).

4 Conclusion and Recommendations

This study examined non-life insurance in Tanzania and decomposed total factor productivity change into efficiency change and technical change using a DEA-based Malmquist productivity index, the study period covers the period of 2014/15–2017/18. Finding divulge that in general non-life insurance firms in Tanzania were performing good both in the aspect of resource utilization (efficiency change) and technological change (innovation). Looking at the specific year, non-life insurance experienced a slight regress of innovation in the year 2015/16–2016/17. However, the performance of the insurance firms in Tanzania is primarily derived by the extent to which the firm utilizes the existing production technology, which implies how well insurance firm is striving to get close to frontier (catch up effect). In terms of ranking findings revealed that first, Sanlam General and Tanzidia were the most performing insurance firms. At the same time, Alliance was manifested poor performance in terms of productivity over the study period. The study recommends that more improvement of innovation is highly needed as regress in innovation tends to erode improvement accruing from operational efficiency. It was evident that several decades after deregulation of the insurance sector in the country competition among insurance firms has increased, which calls for innovation for the firm to survive. The natural extension of this study, should focus on how exogenous factors affect the performance of the non-life insurance firm in Tanzania. To provide a platform for comparison of result based on the methodology it would be useful to apply stochastic frontier analysis and DEA during the extension of this study.

References

Alirezaee, M., Afsharian, M.: Measuring the effect of the rules and regulations on global Malmquist index. In: Optimizing, Innovating, and Capitalizing on Information Systems for Operations, pp. 215–229. IGI Global (2013)

Avkiran, N.K.: The evidence on efficiency gains: the role of mergers and the benefits to the public. J. Bank. Financ. **23**(7), 991–1013 (1999)

Barros, C.P., Nektarios, M., Assaf, A.: Efficiency in the Greek insurance industry. Eur. J. Oper. Res. **205**(2), 431–436 (2010)

Bauer, P.W., Berger, A.N., Ferrier, G.D., Humphrey, D.B.: Consistency conditions for regulatory analysis of financial institutions: a comparison of frontier efficiency methods. J. Econ. Bus. **50**(2), 85–114 (1998)

Bwana, K.M.: Measuring technical efficiency of faith based hospitals in Tanzania: an application of data envelopment analysis (DEA). Res. Appl. Econ. **7**(1) (2015)

Bwana, K.M.: Investigating efficiency based on the hospitals size. Afr. J. Appl. Res. (AJAR) **4**(1), 106–119 (2018)

Caves, D.W., Christensen, L.R., Diewert, W.E.: The economic theory of index numbers and the measurement of input, output, and productivity. Econometrica J. Econometric Soc. 1393–1414 (1982)

Chakraborty, K., Harper, R.K.: Dynamic productivity analysis of insurance firms–the effect of firm-specific and macroeconomic characteristics. Int. J. Appl. Econ. **14**(2), 37–55 (2017)

Charnes, A., Cooper, W.W., Rhodes, E.: Measuring the efficiency of decision making units. Eur. J. Oper. Res. **2**(6), 429–444 (1978)

Coelli, T.J., Rao, D.S.P., O'Donnell, C.J., Battese, G.E.: An Introduction to Efficiency and Productivity Analysis. Springer, Heidelberg (2005)

Cummins, J.D., Turchetti, G.: Productivity and technical efficiency in the Italian insurance industry (No. 96–10). Wharton School Center for Financial Institutions, University of Pennsylvania (1996)

Cummins, J.D., Xie, X.: Mergers and acquisitions in the US property-liability insurance industry: productivity and efficiency effects. J. Bank. Financ. **32**(1), 30–55 (2008)

Cummins, J.D., Weiss, M.A., Zi, H.: Organizational form and efficiency: the coexistence of stock and mutual property-liability insurers. Manag. Sci. **45**(9), 1254–1269 (1999)

Cummins, J.D., Weiss, M.A.: Analyzing firm performance in the insurance industry using frontier efficiency and productivity methods. In: Dionne (ed.) Handbook of Insurance. Kluwer Academic Publishers, Boston (1999)

Fare, R., Grosskopf, S., Norris, M., Zhang, Z.: Productivity growth, technical progress, and efficiency change in industrialized countries. Am. Econ. Rev. **84**, 66–83 (1994)

Fare, R., Färe, R., Fèare, R., Grosskopf, S., Lovell, C.K.: Production Frontiers. Cambridge University Press, Cambridge (1994)

Färe, R., Grosskopf, S., Lindgren, B., Roos, P.: Productivity developments in Swedish hospitals: a Malmquist output index approach. In: Data Envelopment Analysis: Theory, Methodology, and Applications, pp. 253–272. Springer, Dordrecht (1994)

Farrell, M.J.: The measurement of productive efficiency. J. R. Stat. Soc. Ser. A (General) **120**(3), 253–281 (1957)

Grifell-Tatjé, E., Lovell, C.K.: A note on the Malmquist productivity index. Econ. Lett. **47**(2), 169–175 (1995)

Grosskopf, S.: Some remarks on productivity and its decompositions. J. Prod. Anal. **20**(3), 459–474 (2003)

Hammoud, V.A.: Promoting the growth and competitiveness of the insurance sector in Arab World. Makati city, Philippines (2008)

Hwang, S.N., Tong-Liang, K.: Measuring managerial efficiency in non-life insurance companies: an application of two-stage data envelopment analysis. Int. J. Manag. **23**(3), 699 (2006)

Jacobs, R., Smith, P.C., Street, A.: Measuring Efficiency in Health Care: Analytic Techniques and Health Policy. Cambridge University Press, Cambridge (2006)

Kaur, R., Aggarwal, M.: Mathematical modelling of malmquist TFP index as applicable in banks: a study of its origin and development. J. Bus. Manag. 2070–2075 (2016)

Mahlberg, B., Url, T.: Effects of the single market on the Austrian insurance industry. Empirical Econ. **28**(4), 813–838 (2003)

Malmquist, S.: Index numbers and indifference surfaces. Trabajos de estadística **4**(2), 209–242 (1953)

Mdoe, J.: Mtotal factor productivity change in the non-life insurance sector. Published Masters dissertation, Kenyata University, Kenya 2005–2009 (2012)

OECD: The Future of Productivity. OECD Publishing, Paris (2015). https://doi.org/10.1787/9789264248533. Accessed 4 May 2020

Sakar, B.: A study on efficiency and productivity of Turkish Banks in Istanbul stock exchange using Malmquist DEA. J. Am. Acad. Bus. **8**(2) (2006)

Saad, N.M., Majid, M.S.A., Yusof, R.M., Duasa, J., Rahman, A.A.: Measuring efficiency of insurance and Takaful companies in Malaysia using data envelopment analysis (DEA). Rev. Islamic Econ. **10**(2), 5 (2006)

Tanzania Insurance Regulatory Authority: Annual Insurance Market Performance Report (2017). https://www.tira.go.tz/content/annual-insurance-market-performance. Accessed 20 Apr 2020

Tanzania Insurance Regulatory Authority: Annual Insurance Market Performance Report (2018). https://www.tira.go.tz/content/annual-insurance-market-performance. Accessed 20 Apr 2020

Udaibir, S.D.: Insurance and Issues in Financial Soundness/Udaibir S Das, Nigel Davies, Richard Podpiera. IMF Working Paper WP/03/138, July 2003. 40 p.

Value Chain Factors Influencing the Adoption of Improved Bean Varieties Among Smallholder Farmers in Misenyi District, Tanzania

S. N. Justus[1], A. D. Mchopa[2(✉)], and I. E. Kazungu[2]

[1] Department of Local Government Accounting and Finance Local Government Training Institute (LGTI), Dodoma, Tanzania

[2] Department of Marketing, Procurement and Supply Management, Moshi Co-operative University (MoCU), Kilimanjaro, Tanzania

ABSTRACT. Common Bean has been regarded as the most produced food crop by the smallholder farmers in Sub-Saharan Africa. As a result, a number of value chain initiatives targeting bean value chain have been designed and implemented in order to improve bean varieties. Unlike the traditional recycled bean seeds, improved bean varieties have more potentials for enhancing productivity and increase yields. Despite the initiatives, literatures indicate that smallholder farmers have been reluctant to adopt the improved bean varieties. Therefore, the study aimed to examine value chain factors influencing the adoption of improved bean varieties among smallholder farmers' households. A cross sectional research design supported by mixed methods approach guided the study whereby data was collected using household survey administered to 166 smallholder farmers. Also, 5 key informant interviews were conducted with value chain experts at district and village levels respectively. Qualitative data were analysed using content analysis while quantitative data were analysed using multiple response analysis, chi square and binary logistic regression. Findings indicated that among the predictors, presence of seed suppliers (wald = 3.900; p = 0.048), availability of pesticides (wald = 41.626; p = 0.000) and provision of extension services (wald = 4.583; p = 0.032) had a significant influence. Therefore, the study concluded that value chain factors have a significant influence on the adoption of improved been varieties though not singlehandedly. As the diffusion of innovation theory holds, the pull and push factors towards adoption need to be considered in order to deal with the phobia among smallholders. Also, continued provision of basic and advanced trainings on the production of improved varieties is vital for improved productivity and spread of varieties.

Keywords: Value chain · Adoption · Bean · Factors · Smallholder farmers

1 Introduction

Agricultural sector plays a very important role in the socio-economic development of Tanzania because most of the population who live in rural areas are heavily dependent

J. N. Mojekwu et al. (Eds.): *Sustainable Education and Development*, pp. 373–382, 2021.
https://doi.org/10.1007/978-3-030-68836-3_33

on agriculture for their livelihood. Also, the sector (agriculture) has a reasonable contribution to the Gross Domestic Product (Chongela 2015) with 29.1% in 2016 (Deloitte 2017) though of late, its contribution is declining while the service sector is picking up. In order to revive the sector, a number of initiatives have been done by the government including establishment of agricultural research and innovations institutes. In view of that it is expected that dissemination of research outputs, innovations and technologies in agriculture plays a major role in enhancing food security and improving the livelihoods of the poor since they are associated with improved nutritional status, higher earnings among households and increased employment opportunities. Thus, agricultural innovations no matter how well developed, would be perceived as useless if not well adopted and disseminated (Gathecha et al. 2012).

Access to improved seed varieties is an integral juncture towards stimulating agricultural technologies uptake and increasing productivity. The adoption process attracts considerable attention since it provides the basis for increasing production and household income mostly in rural areas. Despite the importance, agricultural technologies are often adopted slowly and several aspects of adoption remain poorly understood despite being a vital route for livelihood improvement (Mwangi and Kariuki 2015). Majority of smallholder farmers are reluctant and overly on traditional methods of production which has lowered productivity because of low yields potentials. (Mwangi and Kariuki 2015). Thus, more innovative extension and advisory systems are also needed to facilitate farmer learning and adapt techniques and technologies to local environmental and social conditions (Monela 2014).

Among the pronounced agricultural innovations is the improvement of crop seeds potential for improving productivity since they respond to farmers' needs towards meeting the rising demands (Challa and Tilahun 2014). Common bean (*Phaseolus vulgaris L.)* is among the most demanded and produced food crop by the smallholder farmers in the Eastern and Great lakes Region of Africa (Binagwa et al. 2016; Birachi et al. 2011). In Tanzania, it is the most important food legume for direct consumption and as a source of farm income (NBS 2012). The beans are vital sources of micronutrients, such as iron, and can help reduce iron deficiency caused by the lack of diversity in the starch-based diets of the poor (Larochelle et al. 2016). As a result, a number of value chain initiatives targeting bean value chain have been designed and implemented by stakeholders in order to improve productivity and yields among smallholder farmers. Amongst the initiatives is the production and distribution of quality declared seed designed to make the best use of limited resources though the production is not good compared to Kenya and Uganda, which gradually increased seed production from less than 1000 to more than 3000 tones (Kaguongo et al. 2014).

Despite decades of agricultural policies that promoted the adoption of fertiliser and hybrid seed technologies as ways of improving productivity in the agricultural sector, there have been low rate of adoption of improved seeds among smallholder farmers in Tanzania (Monela 2014). The decisions to adopt or reject agricultural technologies depends on smallholder farmers perceptions on constraints as well as cost and benefit accruing to it (Million and Belay 2004). Smallholder farmers encounter multiple socioeconomic and value chain constraints such as inadequate information about new production technology as well as inadequate capital to acquire the inputs and supplies

(Birachi et al. 2011). As a result, smallholder farmers in the value chain are mostly hesitant to adopt improved bean varieties and recommended practices due to constraining agronomic factors (Ayalew 2011). Therefore, the study aimed to examine value chain factors influencing the adoption of improved bean varieties among smallholder farmers' households.

2 Theoretical and Conceptual Framework

The study was underpinned by Diffusion of Innovation Theory (Rogers 2003;1976) which deals with the process of innovation and provides the principle foundations for understanding diffusion in terms of relationship between technological innovations and social relations (Petry et al. 2019). As a result of dynamisms in production and marketing, smallholder farmers face an increasingly dynamic and complex decision-making scenarios which demand a range of different agricultural innovations. Adoption and diffusion of agricultural innovations and technologies comprehend a certain degree of complexity in the decisions taken by small-scale farmers (Petry et al. 2019) due to lack of certainty with relation to the benefits of such technologies before they are adopted. Mostly, innovations are diffused from its source to the smallholder farmer through an intermediary frequently via extension services (on and off farm trainings). As a process which an innovation is communicated, diffusion consists of a mental process of acceptance of an idea or new practices which passes through stages of awareness, interest, evaluation, trial, and adoption (Rogers 2003). Among the mostly pronounced puzzling decisions among smallholder farmers is the adoption of improved or modified seeds and farming technologies due to limited knowledge and adverse peer influence based on myths. Therefore, adoption and diffusion of improved seeds (as an innovation in agriculture) is influenced by a number of socio-economic and value chain factors in the context of smallholder farmers at individual and household level.

Based on the theoretical assumptions and empirical reflections, the study hypothesised that the adoption of improved bean varieties by households of smallholder farmers is influenced by a number of factors social, economic and value chain factors. For the purpose of this paper, the focus was more on the value chain factors unlike previous studies that focused more on household factors and social factors. Therefore, a conceptual framework was developed to provide the hypothesised causal relationship between the Independent Variables (IVs) and Dependent Variable (DV) as shown in Fig. 1 below. The framework was guided by the theoretical assumptions and literature reflections. The Figure shows that the adoption process is influenced by a number of value chain factors including availability of farm inputs and supplies, presence of extension services and the farming practices implemented by the households of smallholder farmers in the respective locality since they are not uniform. Some of the practices are indigenous while the rest are more contemporary as a result of exposure to the best production techniques and practices.

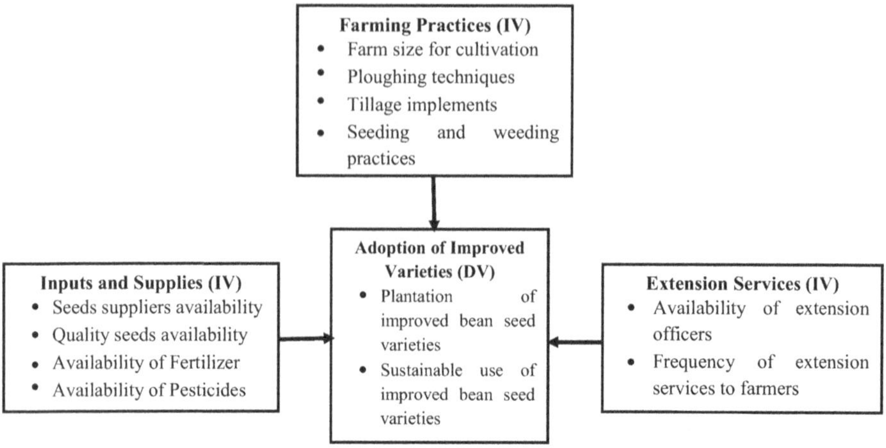

Fig. 1. Conceptual framework

3 Methodology

The study adopted a cross sectional research design since it allowed the researcher to collect data for multiple variables from a representative sample with varied characteristics in order to detect variables' patterns of associations as observed by Bryman (2012). The design allowed data to be collected rigorously within a specified time in order to draw inferences with regard to the key variables of the study. Also, a mixed methods approach was adopted to guide the study in order to provide a complete understanding of a research problem than either approach alone as recommended by Creswell (2014). Hence, both qualitative and quantitative data were collected, analysed and cross-discussed respectively to complement each other and corroborate findings. Data were collected from Misenyi District which is one among the 8 Districts of the Kagera Region. The District was purposely selected because it is the leading in bean production with yields of about 95000 Metric tons per year despite a limited land size compared to other Districts in the Region (District Agricultural Statistics 2016). The study used mixed methods approach hence; triangulation of data collection methods was important as it allowed corroboration of results within the study. A combination of Household Survey (HS) and Key Informant Interviews (KIIs) were used to collect quantitative and qualitative data respectively. The survey questionnaire was administered to all 166 respondents while a total of 5 KIIs were done with 1 District Agricultural Extension Officer, 3 Village Agricultural Extension Officers and 1 Input Supplier who had knowledge relating to bean value chain and adoption of improved variety.

Data were collected from smallholder farmers both the adopters (treated group) as well as non-adopters (control group) of improved bean variety for comparison purposes. The total sample size was 166 respondents including adopters (147) and non-adopters (19) selected using simple random technique using lottery technique. Qualitative data recorded in the field notes and recorded audio conversations were transcribed, categorised, coded and thereafter grouped into themes with reference to the study objectives. Thereafter, constant comparison technique was done through comparing incidents applicable to each category of theme and delimiting data to the theoretical assumptions. Binary logistic regression was used to analyse the influence of value chain factors on the adoption of improved beans varieties. The model was selected since the dependent variable (adoption) was dichotomous (1 = adopted while 0 = otherwise).

$$\text{Logit}(P_i) = \log\left(\frac{p(x)}{1 - p(x)}\right) = \alpha + \beta_1 x_1 + \beta_2 x_2 + \beta_3 x_3 + \ldots\ldots\ldots\ldots\ldots\ldots \beta_p x_p + \varepsilon$$

Logit (Pi) = Y is a binary dependent variable (1 = adopted; 0 = otherwise).
α = intercept of the equation.
β_1 to β_p = predictor variables regression coefficients.
x_1 to x_p = predictor variables.
ε = error term (Table 1).

Table 1. Variable matrix

Variable	Definition	Expected sign
X_1 Experience in farming	Years	−
X_2 Farm size	Acres	−
X_3 Availability of pesticides	1 = available; 0 = unavailable	+
X_4 Availability of fertilizer	1 = available; 0 = unavailable	+
X_5 Extension services	Frequency of services	+
X_6 Availability of seeds	1 = available; 0 = unavailable	+
X_7 Tillage implements	1 = improved; 0 = traditional	+
X_8 Yields (last season)	Kilograms	+

4 Findings and Discussion

4.1 Demographic Characteristics

Participation in bean cultivation involves adults of all ages and findings (Table 2) indicate that among the adopters, majority (35.4%) were aged between 34 to 41 years followed by those aged 26 to 33 years (34.7%) while those aged above 49 years accounted for 5.4%. The case of non-adopters is different since the majority were those aged 42 years and above (84.2%) while those aged between 26 and 33 years accounted for 5.3%. Hence, findings indicate that majority (74.1%) of adopters of improved bean varieties were aged between 18 and 41 years unlike non-adopters where the majority (84.2%) were within the age range of 42 years and above. This implies that the adopters of improved bean varieties in the value chain were relatively younger than non-adopters since the youth are more likely to try new technology compared to the elderly. The youth are more amenable to new ideas and risk but also willing to spend more time to obtain information on improved technologies compared to older farmers as observed by Adeogun et al. (2010).

The study further made assessment of household heads in terms of their sex whereby findings in Table 2 indicate that out majority of adopters were male headed households compare to the female headed ones. Among the adopters' households, male headed accounted for 65.9% while female headed ones accounted for 34.1% which indicate that sex of the household head had an influence on adoption of improved bean variety. Male had an advantage due to socio-cultural settings which favor them (to dominate the most cash generating economic activities) compared to females in terms of exposure to knowledge and techniques mostly provided by Agricultural Extension Officers. During an interview, one of the key informants pointed out that "*...when we conduct village meetings or trainings on improved agricultural technologies, most of participant are male which enable them to be more knowledgeable and exposed on improved practices in agriculture unlike most women who remain at home doing domestic works...*" Similarly, Venance et al. (2016) observed that common bean business has preponderantly attracted male smallholder farmers since it generates significant income.

Table 2. Age and sex of household heads (n = 166)

Variable	Categories	Adopters		Non-adopters	
		Frequency	Percent	Frequency	Percent
Age of household head	18–25	20	13.6	0	0
	26–33	51	34.7	1	5.3
	34–41	52	35.4	2	10.5
	41–49	16	10.9	8	42.1
	Above 49	8	5.4	8	42.1
Sex of household head	Female	50	34.1	11	57.9
	Male	97	65.9	8	42.1

The level of education matters a lot towards the adoption of agricultural technologies. The study assesses the education level of household heads and findings in Table 3 indicate that among the adopters, 59.2% had attended primary school while 40.1% had secondary education compared to their counterparts where the majority (57.9%) had no formal education. Hence, having the basic education level gave adopters an advantage in terms of the ability to comprehend instructions through reading the best practices through training materials provided by Agricultural Extension Officers. Education is not only an important determinant of adoption of innovations, but also an instrument for successful implementation of innovation since it enables smallholder farmers to easily understand concepts taught in the trainings and consequently adopt new technologies with ease unlike those without formal education (Venance et al. 2016). Similar results were found by Mwangi and Kairuki (2015) and Tahirou et al. (2015) that the more educated the households are, the greater the tendency to adopt improved varieties. Likewise, Bruce et al. (2014) found that formal education helps farmers to understand the information which in turn facilitates the adoption since it gave them the ability to perceive, interpret and respond to new information much faster.

Table 3. Education level of smallholder farmers (n = 166)

Education level	Adopters		Non-adopters		Total		χ^2	sig.
	Freq.	Percent	Freq.	Percent	Freq.	Percent		
No formal education	12	7.2	12	7.2	12	7.2	0.000	0.000
Primary education	94	56.6	94	56.6	94	56.6		
Secondary education	60	36.2	60	36.2	60	36.2		

5 Value Chain Factors Influencing Adoption of Improved Bean Varieties

The overall significance of the model was assessed using an Omnibus tests of model coefficients which produced the Chi-square of 64.262 and p-value of 0.000 as well as the Hosmer and Lemeshow test with Chi-square equals to 13.361 and p-value equals to 0.100. The two measures together indicate that the model was more suitable to the data. The 2log likehood of 153.128, Cox & Snell R^2 of 0.327 and Nagelkerke's R^2 was 0.443 indicate a strong relationship between prediction and grouping. A total of 8 variables were tested in order to determine their influence on adoption of improved bean varieties. Among the variables, only 5 (five) were found to have a significant influence at $p < 0.05$ which include availability of pesticides, presence of extension services, availability of fertilizers, tillage implements and availability of seed suppliers as presented in Table 3.

Smallholder farmers participation in the value chain mostly starts with sourcing for seeds either from those preserved from last season or purchasing from suppliers. Hence, presence of improved bean seeds and timely availability is essential in the diffusion process. The study tested the influence of availability of seed suppliers towards influencing adoption and findings indicate presence of a significant influence (P = 0.048; Wald = 3.900; Exp (B) = 4.057). Findings imply that when availability of seed suppliers increase in the locality by 4 the odds ratio is 1.401 that smallholder farmers are more likely to increase the adoption of improved bean varieties. The diffusion of improved bean varieties highly depends on the availability of the respective seeds in the locality conveniently. During focus group discussion smallholder farmers pointed out that they obtain improved bean varieties from the licensed seed suppliers at the District and Farmer Groups/Associations. The two were the mostly trusted sources due to the compliance requirements by the regulators which bind them to sell Quality Declared Seed (QDS).

Frequency of extension of services was found to be a significant for adoption of improved bean varieties at p = 0.032, Exp (B) = 0.052 and Wald = 4.583 as indicated in Table 3. The findings imply that when the frequency of extension of services increase by 0.052 causes the odds ratio to be 2.958 times towards influencing households to adopt improved bean varieties. Through interview, a Village Agricultural Extension Officer pointed out that "*...provision of extension services in the villages enabled most of the smallholder farmers to be aware of the improved bean varieties and how to grow them* *successfully...*" This suggests that the availability of extension services significantly increased the adoption of improved bean varieties among smallholder farmers. Similarly, Akinbode and Bamire (2015) reported that households that had regular contacts with extension agents were more enlightened through advisory services and therefore appreciate more the benefits of new technology whereas an increase in frequency of contact with extension agents also increased the intensity of use of improved varieties as found by Siri et al. (2016).

Availability of fertilizer was also among the significant factors (P = 0.049; Wald = 0.458; Exp (B) = 0.735) influencing adoption of improved bean varieties as indicated in Table 3. Improved bean varieties have specific requirements including timely application of the right fertilizer type in order to increase crop yield per unit area basis. Hence, availability of the required fertiliser in the proximity of smallholder farmers influenced the adoption of improved bean varieties since it increased the probability of yield per area and quality of grains as observed by (Morgado and Willey 2003). Findings imply that an increase of fertilizer availability to smallholder farmers, the odds ratio is 0.307 that smallholder farmers will increase adoption of improved bean varieties. However, the response to the type of fertilizer and rate of application vary widely with climate and soil type in the locality (Table 4).

Table 4. Value chain factors and adoption of improved bean varieties (n = 166)

Variables	B	S.E	Wald	df	Sig	Exp (B)
Availability of seed suppliers	1.401	0.709	3.900	1	0.048	4.057
Experience in farming	−0.016	0.196	0.007	1	0.934	0.984
Extension services	−2.958	1.382	4.583	1	0.032	0.052
Availability of fertilizers	−0.307	0.454	0.458	1	0.049	0.735
Availability of pesticides	−3.212	0.498	1.626	1	0.000	0.040
Farm size	−0.228	0.459	0.246	1	0.620	0.796
Tillage implements	−0.422	0.177	5.661	1	0.017	0.656
Last season yields	0.000	0.002	0.004	1	0.949	1.000
Constant	4.779	1.789	7.134	1	0.008	18.987

Pesticides are among the essential inputs to smallholder farmers in the production node of the value chain hence; timely availability highly determine the yields mostly. The study tested the influence of availability of pesticides towards influencing adoption of improved bean varieties among other factors in the value chain. Findings in Table 3 indicate that there is a significant influence of pesticides availability on adoption of improved bean varieties at p = 0.000, Wald = 1.626 and Exp (B) = 0.040. Common beans like any other food crops are prone to pest and diseases attack(s) which require(s) producers to provide special care for the plants. Thus, as the availability of pesticides from suppliers increases by 0.040, smallholder farmers are likely to increase adoption of improved bean varieties by odds ratio 3.212 since pesticides availability increases the probability of bean plants to grow without pest, disease and weeds attacks. Similar findings were obtained by Department of Agriculture and Fisheries (2013) that farmers need to apply insecticides, fungicides and herbicides to manage insects, diseases and weeds which can damage flowering and pod development stages which are more critical since damaged pods cannot be marketed.

6 Conclusion and Recommendations

Adoption of agricultural technologies and innovations such as improved bean varieties, is a continuous process and influenced by a number of factors among households of smallholder farmers. Based on the findings, it is concluded that among others, value chain factors such as availability of pesticides, presence of extension services, availability of fertilizers, tillage implements and availability of seed suppliers have an influence towards the adoption of improved bean varieties among households of smallholder farmers. However, since some household characteristics have shown a significant association with adoption, it is evident that the adoption of improved been varieties is also associated with multiple socio-economic factors at household level. Despite some predictors being significant, there is a need for continued efforts to strengthen the availability of quality declared seed (improve varieties), fertilizer and pesticides which are critical in the earlier nodes of the value chain in order to guarantee the expected results in terms of yields and/or productivity. Frequency of extension services was among the significant predictors though it is apparent that not all smallholder farmers possess proper skills and knowledge on improved bean varieties husbandry. Therefore, dissemination of improved bean varieties should go hand-in-hand with strengthening of farmers' training sessions on improved beans varieties management practices in terms of improving quality and availability of extension services within the proximity of smallholder farmers farmsteads.

References

Adeogun, S.O., Olawoye, J.E., Akinbile, L.A.: Information sources to cocoa farmers on cocoa rehabilitation techniques (CRTs) in selected states of Nigeria. J. Media Commun. Stud. **2**(1), 9–15 (2010)

Akinbode, W., Bamire, A.: Determinants of adoption of Improved Maize Varieties in Osun State Nigeria. J. Agric. Extension Rural Dev. **7**(3), 65–72 (2015)

Binagwa, H., Bonsi, K., Msolla, N., Ritte, I.: Morphological and molecular identification of Pythium spp. isolated from common beans (Phaseolus vulgaris) infected with root rot disease. Afr. J. Plant Sci. **10**(1), 1–9 (2016)

Birachi, E., Ochieng, J., Wozemba, D., Ruraduma, C., Niyuhire, M.: Factors influencing smallholder farmers' Bean production and supply to market in Burundi. Afr. Crop Sci. J. **19**(4), 335–342 (2011)

Bruce, A., Donkoh, S., Ayamga, M.: Improved rice variety adoption and its effects on farmers output in Ghana. J. Dev. Agric. Econ. **6**(6), 242–248 (2014)

Bryman, A.: Social Research Methods. Oxford University Press, Oxford (2012)

Challa, M., Tilahun, U.: Determinants and impacts of modern agricultural technology adoption in West Wollega: The case of Gulliso district. J. Biol. Agric. Healthc. **4**(20), 63–77 (2014)

Chongela, J.: Contribution of agriculture sector to the Tanzanian economy. Am. J. Res. Com. **3**(7), 57–70 (2015)

Creswell, J.: Research Design: Qualitative, Quantitative, and Mixed Methods Approaches. SAGE Publications, Thousand Oaks (2014)

Deloitte.: Tanzania Economic Outlook. Deloitte and Touche (2017)

Gathecha, C., Bowen, M., Silim, S., Kochomay, S.: The diffusion of agricultural innovations: the effectiveness of communication channels used in the improved Pigeonpea varieties in Makueni County, Kenya. In: Proceeding of the International Conference on Agriculture, Chemical and Environmental Sciences held at Dubai, 6–7 October 2012

Kaguongo, W., Kyotalimye, M., Waithaka, M., Ronoh, M., Ng'ang'a, N.: Enhancing adoption of harmonised seed standards, regulations and procedures in Eastern and Central Africa. In: CTA 2014: Seed Systems, Science and Policy in East and Central Africa, pp. 8–14 (2014)

Larochelle, C., Asare-Marafo, D., Birol, E., Alwang, J.: Assessing the Adoption of Improved Bean Varieties in Rwanda and the Role of Varietal Attributes in Adoption Decisions. HarvestPlus Working Paper No. 25, p. 25 (2016)

Monela, A.: Access to and Adoption of Improved Seeds by Smallholder Farmers in Tanzania: Cases of Maize and Rice Seeds in Mbeya and Morogoro Regions. Sokoine University of Agriculture Research Repository (2014). https://suaire.suanet.ac.tz:8080/xmlui/handle/123456789/601

Morgado, L., Willey, R.: Effect of plant population and Nitrogen fertilizer on yield and efficiency of Maize\Bean intercropping. Pesq. Agropec. Bras., Brasilia **38**(11),1257–1264 (2003)

Mwangi, M., Kariuki, S.: Factors determining adoption of new agricultural technology by smallholder farmers in developing countries. J. Econ. Sustain. Dev. **6**(5), 208–216 (2015)

Pelmer, P.: Agriculture in the developing world: connecting innovation in plant breeding research to downstream applications. Proc. National Acad. Sci. **102**(44), 15739–15746 (2005)

Petry, J., Sebastiano, S., Martins, E., Barros, P.: Innovation and the diffusion of technology in agriculture in floodplains in the state of Amazonas. J. Contemp. Adm. **23**(5), 619–635 (2019)

Rogers, E.M.: New product adoption and diffusion. J. Consum. Res. **2**(4), 290–301 (1976)

Rogers, E.M.: Diffusion of Innovation (5th ed.). Free Press (2003)

Siri, B.N., Martin, N., Samuel, B.E., Martin, F., Mboussi, M., Celestine, N., Laurent.: Factors Affecting Adoption of Improved Common beans (Phaseolus Vulgaris L.) Varieties in the Western Highlands of Cameroon (2016)

Tahirou, A., Bamire, A., Oparinde, A., Akinola, A.: Determinants of Adoption of Improved Cassava Variables among Farming Households in Oyo, Benue and Akwa Ibom state of Nigeria, Harvest Plus Working paper, No. 20 (2015)

Venance, S., Mshenga, P., Birachi, E.A.: Factors influencing on-farm common bean profitability: the case of smallholder Bean farmers in Babati district. J. Econ. Sustain. Dev. **7**(22), 196–201 (2016)

Prediction of Financial Distress of Listed Commercial Banks in Tanzania and Kenya: A Comparative Study

O. J. Ally[1(✉)] and K. M. Bwana[2]

[1] Department of Accountancy, College of Business Education, P. O. Box 1968, Dar es Salaam, Tanzania

[2] Department of Accountancy, College of Business Education, P. O. Box 2077, Dodoma, Tanzania

Abstract. The main objective of the Study is to predict financial distress of the listed commercial banks in Kenya and Tanzania. we employed fifteen (15) listed commercial banks from Kenya and Tanzania. Study period covers 2014–2018. Multi Discriminant Analysis (MDA) was adopted to consolidate all ratios measuring the critical aspects of Banks' financial health. Findings revealed that none of listed commercial banks has been in safe financial health over the study period. Comparatively, the financial health of CBK was relatively higher compared to its peers, while NMB ranks the second. Significant growth of sales, total assets, EBIT and retained earnings contributed mainly to the performance of CBK and NMB. In contrast, stagnation in working capital and an increase in total liability affected the financial health of commercial banks. The result holds that in 2015 commercial banks required close monitoring to make sure they are not financially distressed, while in the subsequent years there was no significant improvement in the financial health, which implies the risk of being under financial distress was increasing. The Study recommends that the management of listed commercial banks should focus on the effective management of working capital and its components as it plays a very important role in day-to day activities and operating cycle of the bank. The natural extension of this research should focus on the use of the alternative model of bankruptcy predictions to confirm the validity of the findings of this Study

Keywords: Prediction · Financial distress · Commercial banks · Kenya · Tanzania

1 Introduction and Background of the Study

Financial distress refers the situation when a borrower is unable to meet short term financial obligations to lenders and other creditors whenever they are coming due. It also refers to the situation where 'firms' financial responsibilities are met with difficulty. Outecheva (2007) defined financial distress as the incapability of the firm to pay its financial responsibilities as they mature. In a more common and basic logic, financial

J. N. Mojekwu et al. (Eds.): *Sustainable Education and Development*, pp. 383–393, 2021.
https://doi.org/10.1007/978-3-030-68836-3_34

distress is a lessening in financial efficacy that results from a shortage of cash (Korteweg 2007). In most cases the firm facing financial distress possess the following: *Firstly,* its earnings before Interest and Tax, Depreciation and Amortization (EBITDA) are lower than its financial expenses for two consecutive years, leading the firm into a situation in which it cannot generate enough funds from its operation activities to comply with its financial obligations. *Secondly* a fall in its market value occurs between two consecutive periods. A firm is then said to be financially distressed in the year following the occurrence of these two events (Pindado et al. 2008). According to Betz et al. (2014), distress in financial institutions include Bankruptcy, liquidation and failure to meet obligations. Constantin et al. (2018) defined financial distress as a situation in which a firm has solvency problems at different stages that prevent it from carrying out its business without external support and reduce its value until it reaches Bankruptcy and therefore has to exit the market.

1.1 Financial Distress and Bankruptcy as Experienced in Different Countries

Many firms worldwide have fallen due to financial distress, the number of bankruptcy proceedings across the world have been filed, for example, Swissair and Asea Brown Boveri (ABB) in the USA. In Ghana, recent cases of business failures include the Gateway Broadcasting Services, Ghana Co-operative Bank, Bank for Housing and Construction, National Savings and Credit Bank (Appiah 2011). Research undertaken in recent years indicated that the annual flow of business failure of companies is increasing significantly during the periods of the financial crisis (Sami 2013). The particular example can be seen on Enron Corp, WorldCom, Xerox, Lehman Brothers, AIG, and Freddie.

In Ghana, recent cases of business failures include the Gateway Broadcasting Services, Ghana Co-operative Bank, Bank for Housing and Construction, National Savings and Credit Bank (Appiah 2011). In Kenya, recent cases of corporate failure include Uchumi Supermarket as shown in the Study by Kipruto (2013) as well as (Shisia et al. 2014). Tanzania financial sector intermediation and deepening have improved quite appreciably with the number of banks increasing from 3 before the 1990s to 53 in December 2018. It should be borne in mind that the concept of financial distress needs analysis of financial 'institutions' current and future financial problems.

1.2 Performance of the Banking Sector in Tanzania and Kenya

During the fiscal year ended June 2018 Tanzania banking sector comprised 53 deposit-taking banks and financial institutions, consisting of 40 commercial banks, 6 community banks, 2 development finance institutions and 5 microfinance banks and out of 40 commercial banks 5 banks are listed at the stock market, despite being at nascent stage banking sector continued to maintain steady growth with total assets reaching TZS 30,215.9 billion at the end of December 2018 from TZS 29,804.9 recorded in December 2017 with the contribution to nominal Gross Domestic Product (GDP) contributed by the commercial banks stand at 25.7% at the end of year 2018 (BOT Annual report, 2018). Banking sector in Kenya started in the early 19th century. The first bank was National bank of India in Mombasa. According to Central Bank of Kenya (CBK) report (2018) as at June 30, 2018, the Kenyan banking sector comprised 42 commercial banks,

1 mortgage finance company, 13 microfinance banks, 9 representative offices of foreign banks, 74 foreign exchange bureaus, 19 money remittance providers and 3 credit reference bureaus out of 42 commercial banks 11 are listed at Nairobi stock exchange market. Kenya banking industry is growing and maintained steady growth with total assets reaching to KES 4,408.59 billion in December 2018 compared to KES 4,002.74 billion in December 2017, which is equivalent to 10.14%. Commercial banks play a vital role in economic resource allocation of a country; since they channel funds from depositors to investors (or from surplus unit to deficit unit) continuously. To manage this and sustain to the business operation, they should generate necessary earnings to cover the operational cost they incur. Their financial performance should be monitored closely as they have impacted the economic growth of the country. Sound financial performance rewards investors for their investment. This, in turn, motivates additional investment and brings about economic growth. Likewise, poor banking performance can lead to banking distress and financial crisis which have negative impacts on the economic development of the country (Ongore and Kusa 2013). Banking sector is one of the vital industry in the economic role of a government, it performs two unique functions; banking business as well as stabilizing the state financial atmosphere. With the challenges indicated above regarding the performance of banking sector in Tanzania and Kenya; this Study wants to predict financial distress of listed commercial banks in Tanzania and Kenya by using Altman Z – Score model and compare the financial health of commercial banks in the two countries.

1.3 The objective of the Study

Although predicting the firm's financial distress has received a lot of attention in recent years but to our understanding, the prediction of commercial banks' financial distress is far from complete. There are two gaps in the literature that the Study is trying to cover. Firstly, Study aimed at predicting the financial distress of listed commercial banks in Tanzania and Kenya for a period between 2014 to 2018, the main reason for picking Tanzania and Kenya is that the two countries are considered as the emerging economy in East Africa Community. Therefore the economic strength of the two countries is almost the same. Secondly, the Study will compare the financial distress of listed commercial banks between countries to establish relative financial health of listed commercial banks in the two countries. Literature indicated that less attention had been given on comparative analysis of financial distress of listed commercial banks between two countries in East Africa, particularly between Tanzania and Kenya. Therefore, the main objective of this research is to predict the financial distress of listed commercial banks in Tanzania and Kenya. Specifically, the study intended:

i. To determine the financial health and compare level of distress of listed commercial banks in Tanzania and Kenya
ii. To evaluate internal and external bank-specific factors contributing to poor financial health

Findings from this Study will be useful as it intends to reveal the financial status of listed commercial banks in Tanzania and Kenya, relevancy of this Study is built on the fact that the two countries have been undergoing some economic reforms which may have general impact on the performance of economy, banking sector is one of the important sector of the economy. According to Kinyariro (2016), banking distress and failure, on the one hand, uncover the shortcomings of the existing monitoring system of the financial sector. Therefore, the Study will be beneficial to regulators such as central banks as it would uncover existing weaknesses on the part of the management, and would add on the basis for necessary intervention if needed. The findings will contribute to the existing body of knowledge and literature as this Study will attract and replicate more studies on financial distress from different angles.

2 Review of Literature

This Study has been built on the Entropy theory or the Balance Sheet Decomposition Measure theory which explains that; it is possible to detect the potential risk of financial distress by carefully observing changes in their balance sheet (Aziz and Dar 2006a). According to this theory, if a firm is not capable of maintaining equilibrium state in their balance-sheet component (Asset and liability) and is not able to control shortly, it is more likely to face financial distress (Aziz and Dar 2006b). The theory employs Multiple Discriminate Analysis (MDA) in examining changes in the structure of balance sheets. MDA is a statistical analysis whereby more than one variable is analyzed at the same time (Slotemaker 2008). In their studies, Aziz and Dar (2004); Sayari (2013); Sun and Li (2008), as sighted in (Kinyariro et al. 2016), have employed entropy theory as the hypothetical foundation for investigating studies on financial distress. Predicting financial distress brings benefits to investors by providing early warning signs to stakeholders of firms. As pointed out by Ray (2011), financial distress prediction assist the manager in making a close follow up on firm's performance in a period and act proactively in identifying essential needs.

Similarly, Stepanyan (2014) used the model to analyze the US Airline business and found the model to be very useful. A study conducted by Samarakoon and Hasan (2003) tested the original Altman's Z-score models and find out that the third version model (Z-score model) gives the highest overall accuracy rate. It seems that Z-score models have an outstanding potential in predicting financial distress of firms in developing markets, but with a declining overall accuracy at the two consecutive years before distress. This Study offers evidence that Altman's Z-score model is an appropriate analytical tool for firms in predicting financial distress. Basing on that conclusion of Nanyakkara and Azeez (2013) their Study develops a model specific to Sri Lanka with a predicting ability of financial distress for three years in advance using the 'Altman's Z" score model.

Ijaz et al. (2013) conducted research in Pakistan over the period 2009–2010. The main objective of the study was to test the reliability of the Z-score and current ratio in predicting financial distress among the 35 listed companies of the Karachi Stock Exchange. Findings indicated that current ratio and Altman's Z-score are useful tools for evaluating the financial health of sugar industry listed companies of Karachi Stock Exchange. Pam (2013) conducted a study in the banking industry of Nigeria and found that liquidity, profitability, operating efficiency and total assets turnover which are main variables of the Altman's Z-score are a significant tool in determining the financial distress of a bank. The research focused on two failed banks and two banks, which were very strong. Research by Alexia (2008) pointed out that Altman's Z-score model performs well in predicting failures for up to 5 years earlier. His study was based on whether Z-score could predict failures. Ephrem (2015) researched to ascertain the determinants of financial distress based on six commercial banks, using Altman Z-score, which deviates from what it has to be. Research shows that descriptive analysis has been applied in reporting the findings of the Altman Z-score model. In study conducted by Mohamed (2013) using descriptive analysis and was used to present the result from the Altman Z-score model, which was conducted on listed Kenyan firms. In another similar study by Kariuki (2013) & Mamo (2011), Shisia et al. (2014) and (Mohamed 2013) Altman Z-score model was used in testing financial distress of listed companies in Kenya. Shisia et al. (2014) researched with the objective of Altman failure prediction model in predicting financial distress in Uchumi Supermarket in Kenya. Secondary data was used for five years from 2001–2006. The research found that Altman failure prediction model was appropriate for Uchumi supermarket as it recorded declining Z-score values indicating that it was suffering financial distress.

3 Research Methodology

The study used panel data generated from 15 listed commercial banks over the period 2014–2018. The sample was drawn from a population of 17 listed commercial banks. Purposive sampling technique was employed to select commercial banks which meet requirements of the study. Two listed commercial banks were dropped since they did not meet the need, for example, one was cross-listed both in NSE and DSE while the second was dropped because it was listed in 2015, therefore, data for the year 2014 were missing.

3.1 Data Collection

The data were collected from the financial statements of the annual report of fifteen (15) listed banks in Dar es Salaam Stock Exchange and Nairobi Security Exchanges respectively, for the period of five years started from 2014 to 2018. Mwalimu Commercial Bank and Mufindi Community Bank were excluded from the study due to the fact that banks were not listed in year 2014 in DSE and data was not available. Panel data was applied in this research descriptive study was used to present the result. A descriptive study has been described by Cooper & Schindler (2001) as a study that is typically structured with the clearly stated investigative objective. This design was applied by Ally and Bwana (2019) in their study on predicting financial distress in Tanzania, listed Manufacturing firms. The MDA technique has been used by Kariuki (2013) and Mamo (2011) in analyzing financial distress of the banking industry in Kenya using the Z-score, Shisia et al. (2014) studied financial distress in Uchumi Supermarkets using the Altman Z-score model with positive results.

3.2 Altman Z-Score and Its Application in Financial Distress

The financial distress of the firm, can be tested using different techniques such as Financials strength index (FSI) and Altman Altman Z-score model. However, the FSI was designed specifically for hospitals (Bwana 2018). Altman (1968) studied 22 common financial ratios to determine their predictive ability. According to Altman's Z score model, a company is considered to have good financial health if the Z score exceeds 2.99. While the score lower than 1.81, implies that the company is in financial distress. If a Z value lies in between, then it is said the company to be the on grey zone and it needs to be closely monitored. Discrimination zones can further be summarized as followed: *Z > 2.99, "Safe" zone; 1.81 < Z < 2.99 "Grey" zone and Z < 1.81 "Distress" zone.* The model has been widely applied for the past two decades by auditors, management consultants, courts of law and even used in database systems used for loan evaluations. According to Ally and Bwana (2019), for the adoption of the MDA it is crucial to determine how the sample and the variables of the model were selected. The Z-score value computed is a binary variable used in the classification of equally exclusive projects. Independent variables under this study are *X1, X2, X3, X4 and X5* together with their corresponding coefficients value which remains unchanged, and this is according to the Altman Z score model.

$Z = 1.2X1 + 1.4X2 + 3.3X3 + 0.6X4 + 1.0X5$ *Where:*

X1 - is the ratio of working capital to total assets (WC/TA)

The working capital to total assets ratio is a measure of net liquid assets of the firm to total capitalization. Liquidity is significant in operationalizing new projects (Bwana 2018a). Positive working capital implies the firm is capable of meeting its short financial obligations while negative working capital indicates the difficulties of the firm in honouring short term financial obligations.

X2 - is the ratio of retained earnings to total assets (RE/TA)

Retained earnings are an internal source of finance used to facilitate the growth of companies (Triumalaisamy 2013). Retained earnings are funds retained by the firms for investment and therefore not paid out as dividends to the owner of the business. The higher the ratio of retained earnings to total assets, the better is for the firm.

X3 - is the ratio of earnings before interest and tax to total assets (EBIT/TA)

This ratio measures a firm's ability to generate profits from its assets before deducting interest and taxes. The measure indicates whether management can effectively utilize assets to develop a reasonable return for a business; the lower the ratio implies the firm is not using efficiently its assets to generates more profits.

X4 - is the ratio of the market value of owners' equity to book value of total liabilities (MC/TL).

Altman (1968) explains that the ratio "shows how much the firm's assets can decline in value (measured by the market value of equity) before the liabilities exceed the assets and the firm becomes insolvent." These ratios include the aspect of market dimension to assist in predicting financial distress.

X5 - is the ratio of sales to total assets (S/TA)

This ratio measures a firm's efficiency in managing its assets with comparison to the revenue generated. Palepu and Healy (2008) as cited in Bwana (2019) contended that a firm might generate a relatively high profit if applies efficiency management of its assets.

4 Findings and Discussion

Findings presented in Table 1 indicates that out of 15 commercial banks only one commercial bank (HF Group) from Kenya manifested a Z score above 2.99 in the year 2018, which implies that the bank had good financial health compared to other commercial banks under review. For Tanzania commercial banks, none of them has good financial health since all banks have Z-score less than 2.99. Findings also revealed that only a few banks had Z-score ranging between $1.81 < Z < 2.99$ which implies 'gray zone', the gray zone indicate that the banks need to be closely monitored. From Tanzania for example, in the year 2015 only NMB, DCB, ABSA, DTB and EQUITY scored the z-score which lies between $1.81 < Z < 2.99$ this implies that the in the year 2015 the said banks needed close monitoring while in the remaining years all listed commercial banks from Tanzanian manifested score below 1.88 which indicates that the banks were facing financial distress. On the other hand, I&M, KCB, STANDARD and CBK from Kenya had Z score ranging between $1.81 < Z < 2.99$, indicating the said banks require monitoring during the same year (2015). In the subsequent years 2016–2018 all listed commercial banks under review both from Kenya and Tanzania experienced financial distress except for HF Group in the year 2018.

Findings further revealed that during the period under review listed commercial banks experienced the highest performance in the year 2015 where the average Z-score performance of banks under scrutiny was 1.96 compared to the year 2016 where the banks manifested the lowest performance with average Z-score of 0.52. This finding implies that in the year 2015 almost all listed commercial banks required close attention even though they were not experiencing financial distress, on average during the remaining years the banks were experiencing difficulties in financial health. Analysis of the listed bank by country indicates that financial health of the NMB (the top-performing commercial bank in this Study) was mainly derived mainly by the growth in sales and total assets from TZS 417,603,000; 3,889,995,000 to TZS 601,638,000; 5,680,984,000 in the year 2014 and 2018 respectively. The two variables (sales and total assets) gauge the ability of the firm (commercial bank in this Study) to use its assets to generate revenue and fight competition. Further decomposition of the NMB's findings indicates that the bank was also experiencing an increase in profitability, earnings before interest and tax (EBIT) provide evidence of this growth as in the year 2014 NMB had EBIT of TZS 471,530,000 which grew to TZS 550,594,000 in the year 2018. Increase in EBIT indicates how well the bank utilized its assets efficiently to generate a return (profit) and it further shows the supply of cash available to lenders, shareholders and government.

As far as the analysis financial health of CBK from Kenya is concerned findings indicate that the bank experienced significant growth in sales and total assets from KSH 27,126,063; 282689,097 to KSH 332,597,365; 408,303,625 from the year 2014 to 2018 respectively. This implies CBK.'s ability to generate revenue and withstand competition using its assets. There was also a growth of retained earnings from KSH 31,264,374 to KSH 52,376,127 which when linked to significant growth in total assets the two variables (retained earnings and total assets) it implies accumulative profitability and ability of the firm to finance its assets using internal sources. The higher the ratio between the variables means higher earning power and the healthier the bank financially. Unlike in other eight listed commercial banks from Kenya, CBK managed to increase its working

Table 1. Z-score of Listed commercial banks in Kenya and Tanzania

YEAR	CRDB	NMB	DCB	MKOMBOZI	ABSA	DTB	EQUITY BANK	HFGROUP	I&M BANK	KCB	NBK	NIC	STANBIC	STANDAD	CBK
2014	0.45	1.10	0.57	0.66	0.84	0.84	1.07	0.42	0.71	0.98	0.20	0.71	0.37	1.03	0.90
2015	1.64	2.61	2.04	1.41	2.64	2.23	2.72	1.05	2.64	2.33	0.35	1.13	1.47	2.61	2.47
2016	0.34	0.88	0.14	0.37	0.67	0.56	0.41	0.52	0.83	0.48	0.13	0.57	0.36	0.74	0.80
2017	0.31	0.91	0.68	0.42	0.57	0.60	0.40	0.24	0.82	0.51	0.20	0.43	0.24	0.69	0.82
2018	0.31	0.71	0.55	0.32	0.38	0.63	0.31	3.56	0.95	0.75	0.10	0.50	0.47	0.86	1.55
AVERAGE-Z	**0.61**	**1.24**	**0.80**	**0.64**	**1.02**	**0.97**	**0.98**	**1.16**	**1.19**	**1.01**	**0.20**	**0.67**	**0.58**	**1.19**	**1.31**

capital from KSH 10,407,673 in the year 2014 to KSH 30,212,141 in the year 2018, when linked to total assets the two ratios tell the ability of the bank's liquidity assets about capitalization. Based on the comparative analysis of individual average Z-score of listed commercial banks in Kenya and Tanzania, findings indicate that the most three performing commercial bank during the period under review are CBK from Kenya followed by NMB from Tanzania and I&M Bank from Kenya. On the other hand, NBK and STANBIC experienced difficulty in financial health during the same period under review.

5 Conclusion and Recommendations

This Study aimed at predicting financial distress fifteen (15) listed commercial banks from Kenya and Tanzania during 2014–2018, the Study considered only those banks listed at Dar es salaam stock exchange and Nairobi Stock Exchange. Generally, based on the average Z-score of the individual bank, the findings record that during the study period, none of listed commercial banks in Kenya and Tanzania has been in safe financial health. Comparatively, CBK from Kenya was relatively higher compared to its peer, while NMB from Tanzania ranks the second. It was further noted that significant growth of sales, total assets, EBIT and retained earnings contributed mainly to the performance of CBK and NMB. On the other hand, stagnation and decline in working capital affected the financial health of many listed commercial banks in Kenya and Tanzania. By considering the annual average score, the result holds that in the year 2015 all listed commercial banks were not in financial distress; instead the banks require close monitoring to make sure they are not distressed financially. Analysis of average performance also indicates that in the subsequent years (2016–2018) there was no significant improvement in the financial health of the listed commercial banks, which implies that if not well handled the banks could face the risk of being under financial distress. The Study recommends that management and board of directors of listed commercial banks should focus on the effective management of working capital and its components as it plays a very important role in day today activities and operating cycle of bank, this is due to the fact there was a mixed result indicating stagnation and decline of working capital for some banks in some of years under review. The Study also suggests that regulators should pay attention to the total liabilities of the listed commercial bank as it is linked to market capitalization, it reflects the extent to which the assets must decline in value before being rendered insolvent. The natural extension of this research, should focus on the use of the alternative model of bankruptcy predictions to confirm the validity of the findings of this Study. The use of a qualitative model in the future similar study is also recommended. The Study also suggests that future similar study could broaden the study areas and other east African countries inclusive.

References

Alexia, P.: Altmans Z-score model and prediction of business failures. Int. J. Monetary Econ. Finan. **1**(4) (2008)

Ally, O., Bwana, K.: Testing financial distress of manufacturing firms in Tanzania: an application of Altman Z-score model. Bus. Educ. J. (BEJ) **2**(2), 13 (2019)
Altman, E.I.: Financial ratio analysis, discriminant analysis and the prediction of corporate bankruptcy. J. Finan. **23**(4), 589–609 (1968)
Appiah, K.O.: Corporate failure prediction: some empirical evidence from listed firms in Ghana. China-USA Bus. Rev. **10**(1), 32–41 (2011)
Aziz, J., Dar, H.: Predicting corporate financial distress: where do we stand? Corp. Gov. **6**(1), 18–33 (2006)
Aziz, M.A., Dar, H.A.: Predicting corporate Bankruptcy: where we stand?. Corp. Governance Int. J. Bus. Soc. (2006)
Betz, F., Oprică, S., Peltonen, T.A., Sarlin, P.: Predicting distress in European banks. J. Bank. Finan. **45**, 225–241 (2014)
Bwana, K.M.: Financial performance of council designated hospitals (CDHs) and volunteering agency hospitals (VAHs) in Tanzania. Bus. Educ. J. **1**(2)(2019)
Bwana, K.M.: Evaluating the financial strength of council designated hospitals (CDHS) in Tanzania using financial strength index (FSI) model. Afr. J. Appl. Res. **4**(2), 32–44 (2018)
Constantin, A., Peltonen, T.A., Sarlin, P.: Network linkages to predict bank distress. J. Financ. Stab. **35**, 226–241 (2018)
Cooper and Schindler: Business Research Methods, 7th edn. Irwin/ McGraw- Hill, New York (2001)
Ephrem, G.: Determinants of financial distress conditions of commercial banks in Ethiopia: a case study of selected private commercial banks. J. Poverty Investment Dev. **13**, 59–73 (2015)
Hellen, N.K.: The effect of financial distress on financial performance of commercial banks in Kenya. Master's Thesis (2013)
https://www.bot.go.tz/Publications/Economic and Operations Annual Reports.pdf. Accessed May 11 2020
https://www.centralbank.go.ke/uploads/annual_reports.pdf . Accessed May 11 2020
https://www.thecitizen.co.tz/magazine/index.html
Ijaz, M.S., Hunjira, A.I., Hameed, Z., Maqbool, A.: Assessing the financial failure using the Z-score and current ratio: a case of sugar sector listed companies of Karachi stock exchange. World Appl. Sci. J. **23**(6), 863–870 (2013)
Kariuki, H.N.: The effect of financial distress on the financial performance of commercial banks in Kenya. Unpublished MBA Research Project, University of Nairobi (2013)
Kinyariro, D.K., Meeme, M.M., Maina, J.N., Muriithi, M.J.:Implications of Basel III accord adherence on financial distress status of commercial banks in Kenya (2016)
Kipruto, E.K.: The validity of Altman's failure prediction model in predicting Corporate financial distress in Uchumi Supermarket in Kenya. Unpublished MBA Project, University of Nairobi (2013)
Korteweg, A.G.: The costs of financial distress across industries. Available at SSRN 945425 (2007)
Mamo, A.Q.: Applicability of Altman (1968) model in predicting financial distress of commercial banks in Kenya. Unpublished MBA Research Project, University of Nairobi (2011)
Mohamed, S.: Bankruptcy prediction of firms listed at the Nairobi Securities Exchange. Unpublished MSc Research Project, University of Nairobi (2013)
Mohammed, S.: Bankruptcy prediction by using the Altman Z-score model in oman: a case study of Raysut cement company SAOG and its subsidiaries. Australas. Acc. Bus. Finan. J. **10**(4), 70–80 (2016). https://doi.org/10.14453/aabfj.v10i4.6
Nanayakkara, K.G.M., Azeez, A.A.: Predicting financial distress of quoted public companies in Sri Lanka; special reference to Z-score model. In: Conference proceedings of International Conference on Business & Information, Faculty of Commerce and Financial Management, University of Kelaniya, Sri Lanka (2013)

Ongore, V.O., Kusa, G.B.: Determinants of the financial performance of commercial banks in Kenya. Int. J. Econ. Financ. Issues **3**(1), 237 (2013)

Outecheva, N.: Corporate Financial Distress: An Empirical Analysis of Distress Risk. Unpublished Doctorate Dissertation, University of St. Gallen (2007)

Pam,W.B.: Discriminant Analysis & Prediction of corporate Bankruptcy in the Banking sector of Nigeria. Int. J. Finan. Acc. 319–325 (2013)

Pesola, J.: Banking fragility and distress: An econometric study of macroeconomic determinants. Bank Finland Res. Discuss. 13 (2005)

Pindado, J., Rodrigues, L., de la Torre, C.: Estimating financial distress likelihood. J. Bus. Res. **61**(9), 995–1003 (2008)

Samarakoon, L.P., Hasan, T.: Altman's Z-Score models of predicting corporate distress: evidence from the emerging Sri Lankan stock market. J. Acad. Finan. **1**, 119–125 (2003)

Sami, B.J.: Financial distress and bankruptcy costs. In: Dincer, H., Hacioglu, U. (eds.) Global Strategies for Banking and Finance, pp. 369–379. IGI Global, United States (2013)

Shisia, A., Sand, W., Okibo, W.B.: An in-depth analysis of the Altman's failure Prediction model on corporate financial distress in Uchumi supermarket in Kenya. Eur. J. Bus. Manage. **6**(23), 27–41 (2014)

Slotemaker, R.: Prediction of Corporate Bankruptcy of Private Firms in the Netherlands (A Master's Thesis, Erasmus University, Rotterdam, Netherlands) (2008)

Statement Analysis (FSA) Approach: Research J. Finan. Acc. **5**(5), 81–90

Stepanyan, A.: Altman's Z-score in the airline business. case study of major U.S carriers. Int. J. Adv. Manage. Econ. (2014). ISSN: 2278–3369

Thriumalasamy, R.: Firm growth and retained earnings behavior. a study on Indian firms. Eur. J. Bus. Manage. **5**(57), 40–57(2013)

The Determinants of Non-performing Loans in Commercial Banks

D. Pastory(✉)

Department of Accountancy, College of Business Education, Mbeya, Tanzania

Abstract. The maintenance of asset quality, efficiency and profitability is a vital requirement for the survival and development of banks. Loans are the main asset class from which banks generate their major portion of income and also signify the greatest risk to banks. Commercial banks are very important financial institutions in the financial system and the global economy. However, in their course of lending, commercial banks are confronted with non-performing loans (NPLs) that tend to escalate into financial crisis when left unresolved. Non-performing loans (NPLs) is a worldwide issue that affects financial markets stability in general and banking industry's viability in particular. Over last 5 years, the country has witnessed a tremendous increase in the ratio of nonperforming loans. This study examines determinants of non-performing loans in Tanzania. The study is stimulated by the assumption that both the bank specific variables and macroeconomic variables have an effect on NPLs. The study applied explanatory research design and employed both primary and secondary data. Primary data were collected through questionnaire from 63 respondents from 5 branches of CRDB bank in Dar es Salaam while secondary data on the banking sector were obtained from Bank of Tanzania, the Central Bank of Tanzania (BOT) and World Bank reports. The data was analyzed using regression model. Findings indicate that, macroeconomic variables (i.e. effective tax rate, unemployment rate, inflation rate and lending rate) and bank specific variables (i.e. poor credit appraisal, insider lending, inadequate market information and compromised integrity) have statistically significant impact on the NPL rate. On the other hand, exchange rate, poor credit monitoring and poor credit policy had a statistically insignificant relationship with NPLs. The study recommends continuous monitoring of banks by BOT as it can help to improve the loan performance in commercial banks.

Keywords: Non-performing loans · Macroeconomic variables · Bank specific variables

1 Introduction

The significant role of commercial banks in any economy cannot be undermined. They play an intermediary function in the sense that, they collect money from those who have excess and lend it to others who need it for their investment (Badar, Javid, & Zulfiquar, 2013). Providing credit to borrowers is one means by which banks contribute to the growth of economies. Commercial banks play a vital role in the economic resource allocation of countries. They channel funds from depositors to investors continuously. They

J. N. Mojekwu et al. (Eds.): *Sustainable Education and Development*, pp. 394–409, 2021.
https://doi.org/10.1007/978-3-030-68836-3_35

can do so, if they generate necessary income to cover operational cost they incur in the due course. In other words for sustainable intermediary function, banks need to be profitable. Beyond this function, the financial performance of banks has critical implications for economic growth of countries (Ongore & Kusa, 2013). Lending represents the heart of the banking industry. Loans represent 80% portion of the total assets in commercial banks in Tanzania (Mchopa, 2013). Lending remains the mainstay in banking as it is the main source of bank returns. However, bank lending in developing countries suffers from increasing Non-Performing Loans (NPLs) risks (Mataba, 2018). This is more true to emerging economies like Tanzania where capital markets are not well developed (Richard, 2011). Firms in Tanzania on one hand are complaining about lack of credits and the stringent requirements set by banks, while banks on the other hand have suffered large losses on bad loans (Richard, 2011). The percent of non-performing loans in Tanzania reflect the health of the banking system. A higher percentage of such loans shows that banks have difficulty in collecting interests and principals on their credits. That may lead to less profit for the banks and possibly, bank closures. The situation was experienced in 2017 when licenses for five community banks were revoked. Such banks were the Covenant Bank for Women (Tanzania) Ltd, Efatha Bank Ltd, Njombe Community Bank Ltd, Kagera Farmers' Cooperative Bank Ltd and Meru Community Bank Ltd.

Despite the presence of number of studies conducted in Tanzania (Richard, 2011, Mchopa, 2013; Mataba, 2018) on the same subject, commercial banks are still facing the problem of non-performing loans. Considering the fact that the earmarked studies were done in the past and before instituting a number of new directives, has created a need for a study to investigate the current determinants of non-performing loans. Likewise due to rapid expansion of banking institutions in Tanzania, it is better to conduct this investigation to ensure their continuous operation. Non-performing loans could rise further with the ongoing deceleration in economic activity. This gives a reasonable concern for scholars to examine determinants of nonperforming loans in commercial bank in the current times. The study mainly intends to examine the determinants of non-performing loan of commercial banks in Tanzania specifically examining bank specific determinants, macro-economic determinants and trends of non-performing loans (NPLs) at the study area.

Research Hypothesis

In this section, the authors reviewed a number of literature as a result testable hypotheses was developed to examine the relationship between different determinants of NPL. Amon these include, bank specific and macroeconomic determinants nonperforming loans of commercial banks. Thus, based on reviewed related literatures, the researcher developed the following hypotheses to estimate the sign relationship of bank specific and macroeconomic determinants with nonperforming loans of commercial banks based on empirical evidence reviewed in the literature parts. Accordingly, the following hypotheses are tested.

H1. Inflation rate (INFR) has positive relation with Nonperforming loans (NPLs) banks.
H2.Lending rate (LR) has positive relation with Nonperforming loans (NPLs) of banks.

H3.Effective tax rate (ETR) has negative relation with Nonperforming loans (NPLs) banks.
H4.Unemployment rate (UR) has negative relation with Nonperforming loans (NPLs) of banks.
H5.Exchange rate (ER) has negative relation with Nonperforming loans (NPLs) banks.
H6. Compromised Integrity (CIT) has positive relation with Nonperforming loans (NPLs) of banks.
H7. Poor credit policy (PCP) has positive relation with Nonperforming loans (NPLs) banks.
H8.Poor credit monitoring (PCM) has positive relation with Nonperforming loans (NPLs) of banks.
H9. Poor credit appraisal (PCA) has positive relation with Nonperforming loans (NPLs) banks.
H10. Inadequate Market Information (IMI) has positive relation with Nonperforming loans of banks
H11. Insider loans (IL) has negative relation with (NPLs) banks

2 Theoretical Framework

2.1 The Theory of Asymmetric Information

The theory of asymmetric information informs that, it might be difficult to distinguish well from bad borrowers (Auronen, 2003) in (Richard, 2011), which may result into adverse selection and moral hazards problems. The theory explains that in the market, the party that possesses more information on a specific item to be transacted (in this case the borrower) is in a position to negotiate optimal terms for the transaction than the other party (in this case, the lender) (Auronen, 2003) in (Richard, 2011). The party that knows less about the same specific item to be transacted is therefore in a position of making either right or wrong decision concerning the transaction. Adverse selection and moral hazards have led to significant accumulation of non-performing loans in banks (Bofondi & Gobbi, 2003) and Dickson (2002)

2.2 A Review of Related Empirical Literature

There are various studies that have been conducted across the world on issues related to non performing loans. Studies including those of (Dimitrios, Helen & Mike, 2016; Makri, Tsagkanos & Bellas, 2014; Beck, Jakubik & Piloiu, 2013; Klein, 2013; Messai & Jouini, 2013). Despite their active research in the field of banking on non-performing loans. These studies have been focused on the Eurozone and American economies. Similarly, the earmarked researches only considered general determinants, thus did not find which determinant is more significant than the other. The wide spread of studies in this phenomena results from the reality that loans mean 80% of the entire assets of commercial banks and the life of the bank as well. Thus studying about NPL is of paramount importance for sustainability of banks. Besides a number of research on NPL, little has been done with a focus on developing economies. Further, studies focusing on which determinant has great significance on NPL are scanty. See the following,

Vogiazas & Nikolaidou (2011), Bofondi & Ropele (2011) and Skarica (2013) conducted a study on the determinants of non-performing loans external debt to GDP, unemployment and inflation rate, construction and investment expenditure and money supply influence the credit risk of country's banking system. Further they argued that macroeconomic determinants of bad loans. The study found that non-performing loans are positively associated to the lending rates, unemployment rates, and negatively associated with the growth domestic product rate. Also the study utilized loan growth, real GDP growth rate, market interest rate, unemployment and inflation rate as determinants of NPLs. The study found that GDP growth rate and unemployment rate have statistically significant negative association with NPLs with justification of rising recession and falling during expansions and growth has an impact on the levels of NPLs

With a similar intention of studying about the Non performing loans, a study by Saba, Kouser, & Azeem (2012) with an intention of looking on determinants of Nonperforming Loan in the US banking sector, examined the bank specific and macroeconomic variables of nonperforming loans from 1985 to 2010 period using OLS regression model. They considered total loans, lending rate and Real GDP per capital as independent variables. The finding revealed that, real total loans have positive significant effect, whereas interest rate and GDP per capital have negative significant association with NPLs.

The study of Louzis, Vouldis & Metaxas (2011), Makri, Tsagkanos, & Bellas (2014 on Macroeconomic and bank-specific determinants of non-performing loans. The finding reveals that loan to deposit ratio, solvency ratio and credit growth have no significant effect on NPLs. However, inflation and lending rate has positive significant effect whereas ROE and ROA has negative significant effect on NPLs. In another study by Farhan, Sattar, Chaudhry, & Khalil (2012) on the Economic Determinants of Non-Performing Loans and specifically on Perception, the study utilized both primary and secondary data. Correlation and regression analysis was carried out to analyze the impact of selected independent variables. The variables included were interest rate, energy crisis, unemployment, inflation, GDP growth, and exchange rate. The study found that, interest rate, energy crisis, unemployment, inflation and exchange rate had a significant positive relationship whereas GDP growth has insignificant negative relationship with the non-performing loans. Also their findings reveal strong correlations between *NPLs* and various macroeconomic (public debt, unemployment, annual percentage growth rate of *GDP*) and bank-specific factors (capital adequacy ratio, rate of nonperforming loans of the previous year and *ROE*). Precisely, they found statistically significant and negative correlation between NPLs and *ROE*. They also found statistically significant and positive relationship between *NPLs* and its lagged value; *NPLs* and public debt; and *NPLs* and the unemployment. Akinlo & Emmanuel (2014) studied the relationship between NPLs and economic variables in Nigeria, and their empirical analysis confirmed that, in the long run, economic growth is negatively related to NPLs. On the other hand, unemployment, credit to the private sector and exchange rate exerted positive influence on NPLs in Nigeria. They further established that, in the short run, credits to the private sector, exchange rate, lending rate and stock market index were the main determinants of NPLs. Fofack (2005) conducted a study on non-performing loans in sub Saharan Africa after which he concluded that economic growth, real exchange rate appreciation, the real interest rate, net interest margins, and inter-bank loans are significant determinants of non- performing loans in these countries. The author attributed strong association between the macroeconomic factors and non-performing loans to the undiversified nature of some African economies.

Nkusu (2011) conducted a study on twenty-six (26) advanced economies over the period 1998–2009. The study investigated the determinants of NPL ratio and of the first difference of the NPL ratio. The results showed that adverse macroeconomic development in particular a contraction of real GDP, a high unemployment rate, high interest rates, a fall in house prices and a fall in equity prices negatively affected NPLs. Tsumake (2016) conducted the study on determinants of NPL in Botswana. The study covered the period 2005–2014 using a linear multiple regression analysis model. The study concluded that inflation, real interest rates, real GDP, unemployment, profitability, industry size and credit growth have a statistically significant effect on the level of NPLs. However, the results of the regression model also revealed that there is an insignificant effect of capitalization and diversification on the level of NPLs in Botswana for the period under consideration.

Wangui (2010) conducted a study on causes of NPLs in Kenyan banks. Using exploratory design, and collecting data from 43 commercial bank in Kenya. According to the study, causes included; the national economic downturn which led to depression for business in general; reduced buying ability of consumers; insider lending and owner concentration; inadequate procedures for credit risk assessment and credit management; misuse of the loan; and legal delays. The study concludes that, NPLs have greater effects on the bank's profitability and are likely to cause profitability crisis to most Commercial banks.

Richard (2011) identified the factors That Cause Non– Performing Loans in Commercial Banks in Tanzania, findings suggest that factors controllable by commercial banks to be the major contributor to non-performing loans specifically, the diversification of funds and weak credit analysis. It was highlighted that there is a need of developing mechanism to ensure that banks solve capital related problems and provide financial related advice to borrowers to ensure that money borrowed is used for the intended cause. It further suggests banks to keep a close follow up on their borrowers so as to keep them intact and in track. Mataba (2018) conducted a study on determinants on non-performing loans in Tanzania commercial banks, the findings indicate that both bank specific and macro-economic factors impacted on NPLs in community banks. The effect of Net interest margin and gross loans to deposit ratio were positive and significant. The effect of capitalization ratio on NPLs was negative, consistent with the moral hazard hypothesis, and with the agency theory. The effect on NPLs ratio was positive and significant.

Mchopa (2013) conducted a study on assessment of the causes of non-performing loans and found that non-performing loans in Tanzania commercial Banks are caused by both factors related to bank operations and factors related to customers operations. Factors related to bank operation identified were poor credit appraisal, poor credit policy, frauds from bank officials, competition from other financial institutions and long queue in banking halls. Factors related to customers operations identified are inadequate general business management skills, inadequate of financial services skills, and inadequate accounting and book keeping skills.

A number of studies have been presented and most of which show that NPLs are a threat to the wellbeing and sustainability of most commercial banks. However, the presence of different findings regarding which determinants had a positive or negative influence on NPLs, considering the fact that most of the studies were carried in the developed economies, and those carried in the developing economies were carried some years back, forms a right moment for another study to identify determinants of NPLs in the Tanzanian context and confirm which ones have positive or negative influence on the NPL in the contemporary Tanzanian context.

2.3 Conceptual Framework

The main objective of this study is to examine the determinants of NPLs in commercial banks in Tanzania. Based on the objectives of the study, literature surveyed, the following conceptual model is framed. As previously discussed in the related literature review parts, nonperforming loans are affected by both bank specific and macroeconomic factors. Macroeconomic factors are interest/lending rate, inflation rate, public debt, exchange rate, money supply, real GDP growth and unemployment rate. Bank specific factors are profitability, Capital adequacy Ratio, ROE, ROA, liquidity, diversification, bank size, poor credit assessment, failed loan monitoring, underdeveloped credit culture, lenient credit terms and conditions, compromised integrity, willful defaults by borrower and their knowledge limitation and capital structure. The author need to state the addition of the factors that have not been considered by the theories reviewed (Fig. 1).

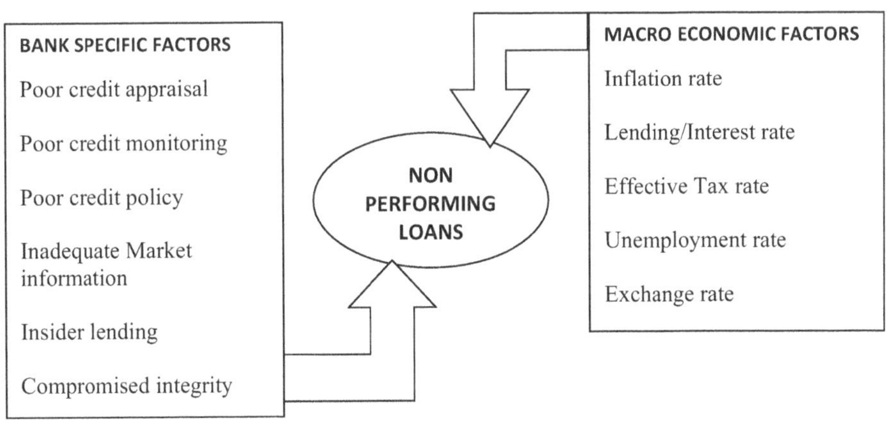

Fig. 1. Conceptual framework. Source: developed by the author (2019)

3 Research Methodology

The study was conducted at CRDB bank in Dar es Salaam because of being a business capital with many CBRD branches than any other region. Explanatory research design was employed to examine the cause and effect relationships between nonperforming loans and its determinants. Purposive sampling and simple random sampling techniques were employed with the target respondents of 29 employees and 34 loan defaulters respectively. Secondary data were collected from World Bank reports, Central Bank of Tanzania and CRDB bank official documents, annual reports and financial statements. Data collected through questionnaires from 63 respondents from 5 branches of CRDB bank in Dar es Salaam were subjected to SPSS version 26 for analysis. The regression model was applied through SPSS and it helped to explain the relationship between NPLs of commercial banks and its determinants.

4 Findings and Discussions

4.1 Result of Regression Analysis

The Results are Based on Analysis of Regression Model as Discussed here Under
The model used to examine the determinants of NPLs of commercial banks in this study was:

NPLit = $\beta_0 + \beta_1$(INFR)it + β_2(LR)it + β_3(ETR)it + β_4(UR)it + β_5(ER)it + β_6(CIT) it + β_7(PCP)t + β_8(PCM)it + β_9(PCA) it + β_{10}(IMI)it + β_{11}(IL)it + εit

Where;

NPL = nonperforming loan ratio of bank ‘*i*’ in year *t*
INFR = represent inflation rate of bank ‘*i*’ in year *t*
LR = represent lending rate of bank ‘*i*’ in year *t*
ETR = represent effective tax rate of bank ‘*i*’ in year *t*
UR = represent unemployment rate of bank ‘*i*’ in year *t*
ER = represent exchange rate of bank ‘*i*’ in year *t*
IT = represent compromised integrity from the bank staff of bank ‘*i*’ in year *t*
PCP = represent poor credit policy of bank ‘*i*’ in year *t*
PCM = represent poor credit monitoring of bank ‘*i*’ in year *t*
PCA = represent poor credit appraisal of bank ‘*i*’ in year *t*
IMI = represent inadequate market information of bank ‘*i*’ in year *t*
IL = represent insider lending of bank ‘*i*’ in year *t*
$\beta 0$ = an intercept,

β1, *β2, β3, β4, β5, β6, β7, β8, β9, β10 and β11*, = estimated coefficient of explanatory variables for bank ‘i’ in year *t* εit = the error term for error terms for intentionally/unintentionally omitted or added variables. It has zero mean, constant variance and non-auto correlated.

As shown in the above Table 1, coefficient of determination was 68.3% revealing that 68.3% of variation in NPLs ratio is explained by the selected explanatory variables (lending rate, inflation rate, effective tax rate, unemployment rate, exchange rate, poor credit appraisal, poor credit monitoring, poor credit policy, insider lending, inadequate marketing information and integrity of the bank staffs). This is an initial indication that the selected variable have an influence on the NPLs Table 2.

Table 1. The model summary

Model summary				
Model	R	R Square	Adjusted r square	Std. error of the estimate
1	.827[a]	.683	.615	.46231
a. Predictors: (Constant), CIT, UR, PCA, ER, PCM, PCP, LR, IL, IMI, ETR, INFR				

Table 2. Anova

ANOVA[a]						
Model		Sum of squares	Df	Mean square	F	Sig.
1	Regression	23.513	11	2.138	10.001	.000[b]
	Residual	10.900	51	.214		
	Total	34.413	62			
a. Dependent Variable: NPL						
b. Predictors: (Constant), CIT, UR, PCA, ER, PCM, PCP, LR, IL, IMI, ETR, INFR						

Furthermore, since F-statistics is designed to jointly test the impact of explanatory variables on dependent variables, F-statistics of this model has a p-value of 0.000 indicating rejecting of the null hypothesis as shown in the Table 3. This implies all selected variables can affect the level of NPLs in common.

Accordingly, Table 3 below presents the result of the regression model made to examine the impact of explanatory variables on NPLs. Hence, NPLs ratio is a dependent variable whereas inflation rate, lending rate, effective tax rate, unemployment rate, exchange rate, compromised integrity, poor credit policy, poor credit monitoring, poor credit appraisal inadequate market information and insider loans are explanatory variables. Thus, the regression result in the following table demonstrates both coefficients of explanatory variables and corresponding p-values as follows.

Thus based on the Table 3, the following model was developed to examine the determinants of NPLs in this study.

$$NPL = 3.200 + 0.681LR + 0.762INFR - 0.64ETR - 0.464UR + 0.089ER + 0.349PCA + 0.205PCM + 0.047PCP - 0.369IL - 0.611IMI + 0.748CIT + \varepsilon$$

The researcher examined the impact of both bank specific and macroeconomic factor on the levels of NPLs based on the regression result provided in Table 3 by examining

Table 3. Results of the regression model

Coefficients[a]					
Model	Unstandardized coefficients		Standardized coefficients	T	Sig.
	B	Std. error	Beta		
(Constant)	3.200	.687		4.659	.000
LR	−.681	.231	−.425	−2.952	.005
INFR	.762	.297	1.062	2.563	.013
ETR	−.640	.183	−.941	−3.496	.001
UR	−.464	.174	−.650	−2.674	.010
ER	.089	.107	.104	.835	.408
PCA	.349	.125	.347	2.806	.007
PCM	.205	.136	.250	1.514	.136
PCP	.047	.108	.064	.435	.666
IL	−.369	.119	−.458	−3.097	.003
IMI	−.611	.140	−.685	−4.371	.000
CIT	.748	.133	1.333	5.637	.000

a. Dependent Variable: NPL

Source: own computations Via SPSS 20 from the study area

coefficients of explanatory variables and significance level. Each of the explanatory variable is discussed in the subsequent sections.

Lending Rate/Interest Rate (LR) The regression result in Table 3 above is inconsistent with hypothesis developed in this study. The study hypothesized that there is a positive association between lending rate and NPLs of commercial banks. Unlike the findings of Farhan *et al.* (2010), Bofondi & Ropele (2011) and Louzis *et al.* (2011). The results of the model in the table indicate a statistically significant negative impact of lending rate on NPLs. It implies that for one unit change in the bank lending rate had resulted 0.68 units change on the levels of NPLs in opposite direction. The finding of this study confirms the finding of Saba *et al.* (2012) and Nkusu (2011) who argue that there is a negative effect of lending rate on the NPLs of banks. The main reason for this negative association between lending rate and NPLs is due to the fact that, higher rate curtail ability to borrow, decreases the amount of loan and then reduce NPLs. Thus, higher lending rate enables individuals with excess funds to save their money in banks so that they earn from it but investors with profitable projects feel unwilling to borrow and invest, Dickson (2012)

Inflation Rate (INFR)
Table 3 indicate consistence of inflation rate with the hypothesis developed in the study.

The study hypothesized that there is positive association between inflation rate and NPLs of commercial banks. Thus, consistent with the hypothesis, the estimated coefficients and test statistics of inflation rate were 0.76 and 0.13 respectively. This implies that everyone unit change in inflation rate, had resulted into 0.76 units change in the levels of NPLs in the same direction. The result of this study confirms the arguments of Farhan *et al.* (2012), Skarica (2013), Louzis *et al.* (2011) and Vogiazas and Nikolaidou (2011) that there is positive relationship between NPLs and inflation rate. This positive impact of inflation rate on NPLs of commercial banks results indicate that as high inflation may pass through to nominal interest rate, it reduces the borrower's capacity to repay their debt. Inflation causes firms to increase their costs of changing prices, as it causes individuals to hold less cash and make more trips to banks since inflation lowers the real value of money holdings. Furthermore, increased inflation can also erode the loan payment capacity of the borrowers by decreasing the real income when salaries or wages are sticky (Tsumake, 2016).

Effective Tax Rate (ETR)

Effective tax rate has been revealed to possess a negative association with NPLs. The regression result in the Table 3 indicate that there is consistence between results of the regression modal and the hypothesis developed. The study hypothesized that, there is negative association between effective tax rate and NPLs of commercial banks. Thus, consistent with the hypothesis, the estimated coefficients and test statistics of effective tax rate was −0.64 and 0.01 respectively showing statistically significant negative impact of effective tax rate on the level of NPLs. This implies that, for every one unit change in effective tax rate, keeping other factors constant had resulted into 0.64 units change on the levels of NPLs in the opposite direction. Unlike the findings of Khan *et al.* (2011) and Gezu (2014) who attest that NPLs gets higher during high income tax rate as bank shift its tax burden to borrowers by increasing fees, other commission and lending rate on loans. The borrowers pay this tax burden for the banks as compensation and as their own obligatory tax to the government. Thus borrowers who facing this double burden are unable to pay their debt. High tax burden enable the banks to shift the tax burden either by increasing lending rate and fees or paying low interests on deposits. Thus, the bank is capable of transferring the tax costs to its customers by raising fees and interest spreads (Khan et al., 2011).

Unemployment Rate (UR)

The regression results in the Table 3 are consistent with hypothesis developed in this study. The study hypothesized that there is a negative association between unemployment and NPLs of commercial banks. Unlike the findings of different scholars, (Akinlo & Emmanuel, 2014; Makri *et al.,* 2014; Farhan *et al.,* 2012; Vogiazas & Nikolaidou, 2011; Nkusu 2011), result of the model in Table 3 indicates a statistically significant negative impact of unemployment rate on NPLs. This negative sign indicates an inverse relationship between unemployment rate and NPLs. It implies that for one unit change in the unemployment rate, keeping other factors constant result into 0.46 units change on the level of NPLs in opposite direction. The finding of this study confirms the finding of Skarica (2013) and Tsumake, (2016) who also report the presence of a negative effect of unemployment rate on the NPLs in Commercial banks. Unemployment rate negatively affects an individual's income to pay their loan installments henceforth increasing their debt burden.

Exchange Rate (ER)
The international competitiveness of an economy also has an impact on NPLs. The regression result in Table 3 is inconsistent with the hypothesis developed in the study. The study hypothesized that there is negative association between exchange rate and NPLs of commercial banks. The estimated coefficients and test statistics of exchange rate were 0.09 and 0.41 showing statistically insignificant positive impact of exchange rate on the level of NPLs of commercial banks. Fofack (2005) reveals that the real effective exchange rate has a positive impact on NPLs in several Sub-Saharan African countries with fixed exchange rates. The study discussed that currency appreciation increases the value of goods and services produced in the country thus reducing the competitiveness of export-oriented firms and negatively affecting their ability to service their debt. The findings of Akinlo and Emmanuel (2014) also support that an appreciation of the exchange rate worsens the performance of export-oriented sectors, contributing to a deterioration of bank portfolios. Badar, Javid and Zulfiquar (2013) suggest that the, exchange rate depreciations might lead to a higher level of NPLs in countries with un-hedged borrowers who lend more in foreign currencies. Therefore, since their incomes are usually in local currency, borrowers face more difficulties in paying their debts.

Poor Credit Appraisal (PCA)
There is a need to appraise borrowers and the way they plan to use the credit. In this study, it has been revealed that credit appraisal is associated to NPLs. The regression result in Table 3 show that there positive association between Poor Credit appraisal and NPLs. This is similar to the study's hypothesis that there is positive association between poor credit appraisal and NPLs of commercial banks. The estimated coefficients and test statistics of poor credit appraisal were 0.35 and 0.007 respectively, showing statistically significant positive impact of poor credit appraisal on the level of NPLs in commercial banks. The result of this study confirms the arguments given by different researchers (Mchopa, 2013; Wangui, 2010; Aballey, 2009) who had earlier said that there is a positive relationship between NPLs and poor credit appraisal. This positive and statistically significant impact of poor credit appraisal on NPLs of commercial banks reflects loan repayment capability problems from their creditworthiness of the borrowers. Banks need to cautious to carry the credit appraisal. They can do this by employing unique objective, subjective, financial and non-financial techniques to evaluate the creditworthiness of their customers. Borrowers total income, age, repayment capability, work experience and job stability, nature of employment, amount spent each month, future liabilities, taxes paid, assets/ business owned and the capital structure of the business (debt or equity) should be considered during appraisal process.

Insider Lending (IL)
Insider lending has a negative association with NPLs. This has been affirmed by the regression model run in this study. The regression result in Table 3 provide that in for any variations in NPLs is negatively inversely caused by insider lending. The findings lead us to accept the hypothesisi developed earlier that, there is a negative association

between insider lending and NPLs of commercial banks. Unlike the findings of Wangui, (2010) that there is a positive association between insider lending and NPLs, results of this model indicate a statistically significant negative impact of insider lending on NPLs. This negative sign indicates an inverse relationship between insider lending and NPLs. It implies that for one unit change in insider lending, keeping other factors constant results into 0.37 units change on the levels of NPLs in the opposite direction. Insider lending has the potential to bring about the collapse of the bank (Nkusu, 2011). However, managers often challenge the set regulations and offer better credit terms to their staff. Consequently, insider lending has been identified to be an influential factor determining the level of non-performing loans for many banks (Tsumake, 2016). Richard (2011) observes that insider loans are one of the key reasons for the failure of many banks. The main reason why insider loans fails is because loans are being issued under different terms than those given to outsiders; loans obtained from insider lending are also invested in speculative projects with high propensity for failure such as real estate development (Tsumake, 2016). Besides, the loans are often invested in huge extended projects that are less likely to generate returns in the short-term.

Poor Credit Monitoring (PCM)

The regression result in Table 3 gave results that are inconsistent with the hypothesis developed in the study. The study hypothesized that there is positive association between poor credit monitoring and NPLs of commercial banks. The estimated coefficients and test statistics of poor credit monitoring were 0.21 and 0.14 showing there is no statistically significant impact of poor credit monitoring on the level of NPLs of commercial banks. The results of this study differ from the arguments of Aballey (2009) who, according to his study, attest that, there is a positive relationship between NPLs and poor credit monitoring.

Poor Credit Policy (PCP)

It has been discovered in this study that credit policies have no association with NPLs. Through the regression results in Table 3, the estimated coefficients and test statistics of poor credit policy were 0.05 and 0.67. Such data indicate that there is no statistically significant impact of poor credit policy on the level of NPLs of commercial banks. This is inconsistent with the hypothesis developed in the study. The study hypothesized that there is positive association between poor credit policy and NPLs of commercial banks. Such results of this study differ from those of Mchopa (2013) whose arguments after a conclusion from his study confirm that, there is a positive relationship between NPLs and poor credit policy.

Compromised Integrity (CIT)

Integrity forms a greatest segment of the banks' operation. Observance of integrity means a lot to the bank. It determines smooth running of operations and contributes positively and negatively towards loan status and bank profitability. The regression result in the Table 3 indicate that there is an association of compromised integrity with NPLs. It was revealed that the estimated coefficients and test statistics of compromised integrity was 0.75 and 0.00 respectively showing statistically significant positive impact of compromised integrity on the level of NPLs. This leads us to accept the earlier developed hypothesis that there is positive association between compromised integrity and NPLs of commercial banks. This implies that for every one unit change in compromised integrity, keeping other factors constant resulted into 0.75 units change on the levels of NPLs in the same direction. The result of this study confirms the arguments of Mchopa, (2013) that there is positive relationship between NPLs and compromised integrity. This suggests that unfaithfulness of the bank staff increase the level of NPLs and the general profitability of banks.

Inadequate Market Information (IMI)

Information about what is taking place in the market is key. It might affect the performance of loans in both directions. In this study, basing on the regression model run, it was revealed that the estimated coefficients and test statistics of inadequate market information were −0.61 and 0.00 respectively. This shows a statistically significant negative impact of inadequate market information on the level of NPLs in commercial banks. This implies that for every unit change in inadequate market information, keeping other factors constant had resulted 0.61 units change on the levels of NPLs in an opposite direction. The regression result in Table 3 is consistent with the hypothesis developed in the study. The study hypothesized that there is negative association between inadequate market information and NPLs of commercial banks. Results of this study confirms the arguments of Mchopa, (2013) and Dickson (2013) that there is positive relationship between NPLs and inadequate market information. The negative relationship between NPLs and inadequate market information suggests that, both parties (borrowers and lenders) should be informed fully about the loan product and loan transactions to reduce NPLs risks.

5 Conclusion and Recommendations

The NPL rate is a key factor that reflects the sound nature of a banking sector. The study intended to identify both macroeconomic and bank specific determinants of NPLs in commercial banks. The study concluded that inflation rate, real interest rates, effective tax rate, unemployment rate, poor credit appraisal, insider lending, compromised integrity and inadequate market information have a statistically significant effect on the level of NPLs. However, the results of the regression model also revealed that there is an insignificant effect of exchange rate, poor credit monitoring and poor credit policy for the period under consideration. In this study results suggests that the lending rate has a negative impact on NPLs. As expected, effective tax rate and unemployment rate significantly affect NPLs concluding that an improvement in the economic health of the country is vital for the reduction of NPLs. Moreover, inflation rate had a positive significant relationship with NPLs concluding that increased inflation erode the loan payment capacity of the borrowers by decreasing the real income when salaries or wages are sticky. Moreover poor credit appraisal increases the chances of loan defaults to borrowers. Insider lending has been identified to be an influential factor determining the level of NPLs because it is provided to lenders on different terms from those of given to outsiders. Compromised integrity has a positive relationship with NPLs which suggests that when bank staff become unfaithful increases the risk of creating troubles when it comes to NPLs. The study also finds a negative relationship between NPLs and inadequate market information which suggest that researching on one another's information and what is taking place in the market is a key to ensuring that NPLs are reduced. Furthermore, real exchange rate, poor credit monitoring and poor credit policy had a statistically insignificant relationship with NPLs. The findings have several implications in terms of policy and regulation. Specifically, the macroeconomic significant variables identified may serve as leading indicators of credit risk deterioration.

Recommendation

In order to improve asset quality, specifically loans, it is strongly recommended that bank management and loan officers should always give a serious attention to the health of asset quality of banks specifically loan performance. Lending rate has an influential impact on the level of NPLs. The degree of increasing and decreasing the level of lending rate has its own limit as per the regulatory authorities of the country set by the BOT. Since high interest rates makes it hard for the borrowers to service their loans that increase the levels of NPLs. It is imposed to overcome different costs. In case, it is better for the bank management to use moderate lending rate and overcome its costs via increasing fees and commission charges on current account and ATM withdrawal charges which are very important to reduce NPLs level as per the result of this study. The author finds that insider lending has a negative effect on NPLs of commercial banks, since banks are exposed to many risks, including financial risk, due to the unique nature of their operations and their customers. Thus it is advised that commercial banks should follow up on their unchecked insider advances and loans.

References

Aballey, F.B.: Bad loans portfolio: the case of ADB. (Doctoral dissertation). (2009)

Akinlo, G., Emmanuel, M.: determinants of nonperforming loans in Nigeria. Account. Taxation **6**(2), 21 (2014)

Auronen, L.: Asymetric information: theory and applications. In: Paper presented in the Seminar of Strategy and International Business as Helsinki University of Technology, May, 21st 2003. (2003)

Badar, M., Javid, A.Y., Zulfiquar, S.: Impact of macro economic forces of nonperforming loans an empirical study of commercial banks in Pakistan. Trans. Bus. Econ. **10**(1), 40–48 (2013)

Beck, R., Jakubik, P., Piloiu, A.: Non-performing loans: What matters in addition to the economic cycle? (2013)

Bofondi, M., Gobbi, G.: Bad loans and entry in local credit markets. Bank of Italy. Bank of Italy (2003)

Bofondi, M., Ropele, T.: Macroeconomic determinants of bad loans: evidence from Italian banks (2011)

BOT. Monentary Policy Statement. Governor Bank of Tanzania (2018)

Calice, P.: Resolving nonperforming loans in Tunisia: coordinated private sector approach. J. Afr. Econ. Brief **3**, (2012)

Chimkono, E.E., Muturi, W., Njeru, A.: Effect of nonperforming loans and other factors on performance of commercial banks in Malawi. Int. J. Econ. Commer. Manage. **4**, 1–5 (2016)

Creswell, J.W., Plano Clark, V.L., Gutmann, M.L., Hanson, W.E.: Advanced mixed methods research designs. In: Tashakkori, A., Teddlie, C. (eds.), Handbook o mixed methods in social and behavioral research, pp. 209–240 (2003)

Dimitrios, A., Helen, L., Mike, T.: Determinants of non-performing loans: evidence from Euro-area countries. Finance Res. Lett. **18**, 116–119 (2016)
Dickson, P.: Bank profitability of commercial banks in Tanzania. Int. J. Bus. Manage. (2002)
Dickson, P.: Comparative Analysis of Commercial Banks Liquidity Position in Tanzania. Int. J. Bus. Manage. **7**(10) (2012)
Dickson, P., Marobhe, M.: The influence of capital adequacy on asset quality position of banks in Tanzania. Int. J. Econ. Finance **5**(2) (2013)
Djiogap, F., Ngomsi, A.: Determinants of bank long-term lending behaviour in the central african economic and monetary community (CEMAC). Rev. Econ. Finance **2**, 107–114 (2012)
Farhan, M., Sattar, A., Chaudhry, A.H., Khalil, F.: Economic determinants of non-performing loans: perception of Pakistani bankers. Eur. J. Bus. Manage. **2**(6), 1–11 (2012)
Fofack, H.: Non-performing loans in Sub-Saharan Africa: Causal analysis and macro-economic implications. World Bank policy research working paper, No. WP 3769 (2005)
Gezu, G.: Determinants of nonperforming loans: empirical study in case of commercial banks Ethiopia. (Doctoral dissertation) (2014)
Khan, F., Ahmed, A.M., Guan, L.C., Khan, H.: Determinants of bank profitability in Pakistan; case study of Pakistan Banking Sector. World Appl. Sci. J. **15**(10), 1484–1493 (2011) ISSN 1818–4952
Klein, N.: Non-Performing Loans in CESEE: Determinants and Impact on Macroeconomic Performance. International Monetary Fund, No. 13–72 (2013)
Kimei, C.: Non Performing Loans at CRDB. Dodoma, Tanzania (2018)
Kothari, C.R.: Research Methodology: Methods and techniques. New Age International, New Delhi (2004)
Louzis, D.P., Vouldis, A.T., Metaxas, V.L.: Macroeconomic and bank-specific determinants of non-performing loans in Greece: A comparative study of mortgage, business and consumer loan portfolios. J. Bank. Finance (2011)
Makri, V., Tsagnakos, A., Bellas, A.: Determinants of non-perfoeming loans: the case of eurozone. Panoeconomicus **61**(2), 193–206 (2014)
Mataba, L.: Determinants of non-performing loans in Tanzania community banks. J. Coop. Bus. Stud. (JCBS) **1**(1), 1–20 (2018)
Messai, A.S., Jouini, F.: Micro and macro determinants of non-performing loans. Int. J. Econ. Fin. Issues **3**(4), 852–860 (2013)
Mchopa, P.S.: An assessment of the causes of non performing loans in Tanzania commercial banks: A case of NMB Bank Plc. (Doctoral dissertation, Mzumbe University) (2013)
Nkusu, M.: Nonperforming loans and macrofinancial vulnerabilities in advanced economies. Int. Monetaru Fund (IMF) 11–161 (2011)
Msinjili, T., Marandu, M., Ayub, A.: Bank of tanzania Circular on NPLs. Retrieved November 16, 2018 (20 March 2018) from www.mondaq.com: http://www.mondaq.com/x/684574/Financial+Services/Bank+Of+Tanzania+Circular+On+NPLs
Ongore, V.O., Kusa, G.B.: Determinants of financial performance of commercial banks in Kenya. Int. J. Econ. Financ. Issues **3**(1), 237–252 (2013)
Richard, E.: Factors that cause non-performing loans in commercial banks in Tanzania and strategies to resolve them. J. Manage. Policy Pract. **12**(7), 16–23 (2011)
Saba, I., Kouser, R., Azeem, M.: Determinants of non-performing loans: case of US banking sector. Rom. Econ. J. **44**(6), 125–136 (2012)
Saunders, M., Lewis, P., Thornhill, A.: Research methods for business. London, Pitman, pp. 124–126 (2007)
Shingjergji, A., Shingjergji, I.: An analysis of the nonperforming loans in the Albanian banking system. Int. J. Bus. Commer. **2**(6), 1–11 (2013)
Skarica, B.: Determinants of nonperforming loans in central and eastern European countries. Fin. Theor. Pract. **38**(1), 37–59 (2013)

Tsumake, G.K.: What are the determinants of non-performing loans in Botswana? Doctorial dissertation, University of Cape Town (2016)
Vogiazas, S.D., Nikolaidou, E.: Investigating the determinants of nonperforming loans in the Romanian banking system: an empirical study with reference to the Greek crisis. Econ. Res. Int. (2011)
Wangui, G.E.: A survey of the causes of non-performing loans of commercial banks in Kenya. An Executive MBA thesis (2010)

Barriers to Good Governance for Maize Farmers' Groups in Southern Highlands of Tanzania

E. J. Munishi(✉)

Department of Business Administration, College of Business Education, P.O. Box 1968, Dar es Salaam, Tanzania
e.munishi@cbe.ac.tz

Abstract. Despite the critical role played by good governance in organisations, as well as the various initiatives undertaken to enhance this role. Good governance is not effectively practiced among the maize farmers' groups in Southern highlands of Tanzania. Moreover, the available studies on good governance have not adequately examined governance barriers in grassroots organisations. This study examines barriers to good governance for the maize farmers' groups in southern highlands of Tanzania and proposes strategies for overcoming the barriers. The study was conducted in three regions of Tanzania; notably Iringa, Mbeya and Ruvuma from December 2018 to January 2019, whereby around 100 respondents from 60 groups were purposefully selected and interviewed. Qualitative design was adopted and data were collected using in-depth interviews, Focus Group Discussion (FGD) and observations. Findings indicated that barriers to good governance for the Maize farmers' groups were lack of relevant good governance structures and policies, lack of education and awareness on good governance, lack of leadership skills and ethics, poor technology, poor records keeping, inadequate communication skills and use of foreign languages in specific. Other barriers include poverty and lack of financial resources in particular, disability of some group members as well as cultural beliefs that impeded participation. Accordingly, strategies for ensuring good governance of the groups are institutionalisation of relevant policies and structures, training on leadership, good governance and communication skills, records keeping skills, economic and technological empowerment of group leaders and members.

Keywords: Barriers · Good governance · Strategies · Southern highlands · Tanzania

1 Introduction and Background

Governance is commonly defined an exercise of power or authority by leaders for the well-being of their people or simply a way in which organizations are managed and the systems for doing it based on statutory or regulatory requirements, organisational culture, ethics and behaviours (HIMSS 2017; Srivastava 2009). Governance may as well be understood as structures and processes designed to ensure accountability, transparency,

J. N. Mojekwu et al. (Eds.): *Sustainable Education and Development*, pp. 410–424, 2021.
https://doi.org/10.1007/978-3-030-68836-3_36

responsiveness, rule of law, stability, equity and inclusiveness, empowerment, and broad-based participation of members (International Bureau of Education 2019, p. 1). To this end, Governance represents the norms, values and rules of the game through which public [organisational] affairs are managed in a manner that is transparent, participatory, inclusive and responsive (International Bureau of Education 2019, p. 1). The importance of governance in both public and private sectors cannot be overemphasised. Governance promotes participation by ensuring that members of an organisation have a voice in decision-making, directly or indirectly through representation (Nurdin et al. 2011; Solihah et al. 2017). In this way, Good governance is also consensus oriented as it serves to bring different interests for the sake of establishing complete consensus regarding what is best for the community groups, especially in formulating policies and procedures (Nurdin et al. 2011; Solihah et al. 2017; Glawcal 2018).

Transparency basically means ensuring free flow of information in a manner that organisational information is accessible to all stakeholders, and the information provided is sufficient as well as effectively understood and monitored (Glawcal 2018; Solihah et al. 2017). Good governance promotes equality; a situation that ensures that all citizens have the opportunity to improve or maintain their well-being (Solihah et al. 2017). It also promotes accountability whereby organisational decision-makers are responsible both to society and to the institutions concerned (Solihah et al. 2017). Thus good governance facilitates responsiveness which basically entails effective customer care to stakeholders through equitable receptiveness of institutions and in a manner that whole organisational process serves all stakeholders (Solihah et al. 2017). Ultimately, good governance ensures effectiveness and efficiency in an organisation, meaning that the institutions of the organisation will produce results according to the needs of society and citizens by using existing resources in an optimal way possible (Solihah et al. 2017).

At the international level, good governance is considered critical in discharging various socio- economic development agenda. The United Nations (UN) Millennium Declaration for example considers aspects of good governance such as human rights and democracy as important for discharging its mandate (Wouters and Ryngaert 2004). This aspect is also well observed in the European Union (EU) where good governance is critically considered in preventing as well as resolving conflicts among the member states; emphasising that good governance is imperative for achieving balanced and sustainable development. On the other hand, the OECD specifically is determined to fight against corruption as a barrier to good governance by establishing a directorate that focuses exclusively on corruption since corruption respects no borders, knows no economic distinctions and infects all forms of government [aspects of good governance] (Wouters and Ryngaert 2004). Needless to say, the World Bank is said to be the first international organization to address the issues of good governance when it first attributed it to the African development crisis of governance in 1990s through introduction of Structural Adjustment Programmes ('SAPs'), and later on introduction of Poverty Reduction Strategy Papers ('PRSPs') that aimed at ensuring good governance in the borrowing countries (Wouters and Ryngaert 2004).

In Tanzania the government is committed to ensure good governance of resources, and especially land, water and forests especially among its citizens, farmers' groups inclusive in order for the country to reach a middle income country by 2025 (URT

2014). The need to empower stakeholders in the governance was listed as important in ASDS 2001 and it still stands valid to date (URT 2014). The government also cherishes improved governance of farmers' organizations which include but not limited to promoting good use of constitutions, support women in leadership positions, as well as ensuring democratic elections in the organizations (URT 2014).

Despite the important role played by good governance to organisations as well as efforts invested in ensuring good governance practice in organisations, still some organisations do not seem to be practicing good governance effectively, leading to a number of negative consequences. Indeed, previous studies have informed that, lack of good governance in organisations evidenced by inadequate participation, poor responsiveness, lack of transparency, lack of democracy, presence of corruption, double responsibility and lack of members' awareness are responsible for weak organisational performance (Dayanandan 2013; Solihah et al. 2017).

Indeed, failure to practice good governance has seriously jeopardised delivery of service by public sector by failing to properly tailor the needs to customers (Ali 2013; Lubuva 2008). Lack of good governance has also led to major setbacks to the efficient running of the public organizational system that include lack of employee motivation, poor accountability and accumulated debts due to unethical and inadequate formulation and implementation of policies governing these organizations (Ali 2013; Lubuva 2008). Recent evidence shows that even when resources are allocated for provision of services, a good amount of it never reaches the intended public (Ali 2013; Lubuva 2008). Moreover, despite broad plans and massive injections of international and domestic resources, public services delivery is still poor in Tanzania (Ali 2013). This is primarily due to poor funds management which is an apparent indicator of poor governance in the country's public institutions (Ali 2013).

Based on the foregoing discussion it is therefore clear that, despite the critical role played by good governance in organisations, and various initiatives undertaken to enhance this role, good governance is not effectively practiced among the maize farmers' groups in the Southern highlands of Tanzania. The available studies on good governance have inadequately examined governance barriers by focusing on public sector as well as ignoring specific components of good governance. This study examines barriers to good governance for the maize farmers' groups in southern highlands of Tanzania and proposes strategies for overcoming the barriers.

The basic components of good governance examined in the context of this paper are Rule of Law, Accountability, Transparency, Participation and Responsiveness. Rule of law relates to the existence of legal frameworks and their fair enforcement (Nurdin et al. 2011). Accountability and responsibility means that decision-makers are accountable and responsible to the organisational stakeholders, through meetings and provision of periodic reports demonstrating the extent to which they fulfil responsibilities assigned to them (Ali 2013). Transparency means that institutions and information should be directly accessible to those concerned, and enough information should be provided to render them understandable and monitored (HIMSS 2017). Participation means that all men and women in the organisation should have a voice in decision-making, directly or through legitimate representation (Ali 2013; Dayanandan 2013). Ultimately responsiveness means that all institutions and process effectively serve stakeholders well-being (Ali 2013).

2 Theoretical Framework

There are a number of good governance theories, but only few of them are discussed here that demonstrate a significant relevance to the problem at hand. One cluster of theories is suggested by (Mintzberg 1996) who firstly perceives governance as a machine dominated by rules, regulations, and standards of all kinds. The theory also sees governance as-network of models, an intertwined system, a complex network of temporary relationships, fashioned to work out problems as they arise and linked by informal channels of communication. Thirdly it perceives governance as the performance-control model that functions as business, assuming that the overall organization consists of business units, which are assigned performance targets for which their managers are held accountable. On the other hand, (Peters 2001), models suggest four interrelated aspects. One is the market model, according to which the private sector can provide better services than the traditional public sector. Second is the participatory state model, which puts more emphasis on greater individual and collective participation by segments of government organizations that have been commonly excluded from decision-making. Third is the flexible governance model, which dictates that organisation should be contextual and flexible in order to face environmental challenges and changes, and to meet the people's demands, adding that appropriate and suitable policies should be made prevail in the government/organisation. Number four is the deregulated governance aspect, which focuses on less bureaucratic control, more managerial freedom, and recommendation. Generally, the above discussed theories emphasise that good governance essentially constitutes of Rule of Law, participation, consensus oriented, equity and Inclusiveness, effectiveness and efficiency, accountability, transparency, Responsiveness. The absence of good governance on the other hand is manifested through corruption, inadequate democracy, violation of human rights, lack of decision making and communication mechanism, ineffectiveness and inefficiency. Accordingly, this situation is caused by the barriers to good governance including but not limited to ineffective communication, lack of transparency and accountability, inadequate leadership skills, bureaucracy and inadequate institutions (Kaufmann et al. 2000). This paper therefore concentrates on discussing barriers to governance and recommend strategies for alleviating the barriers as detailed in the subsequent section.

3 Barriers to Good Governance

Literature avails a number of barriers to good governance in both public and private organisations which include but not limited to ineffective communication, lack of transparency and accountability, inadequate leadership skills by the organisational officials, bureaucracy as well as lack of proper institutions for enhancing good governance to mention just a few. While some barriers are general others are specific to certain aspects of good governance as further discussed in the subsequent paragraphs.

Accordingly, one of the critical barriers to good governance in organisations relates to lack of effective communication in organisations notably poor communication between leaders and subordinates. This is to say that there is a significant relationship between communication on the one hand and adherence and practicing of governance on the other hand. This further indicates that lack of communication structures subsequently leads to poor sharing of governance messages and the vice versa (Argentino de Medeiros Sousa et al. 2017). There is therefore a need for investing in effective communication in organisations if good governance is to flourish there (Argentino et al. 2017). Another category of literature further opens up the debate and suggests barriers to implementing good governance as relating to inadequate funds, poor staff's competency, and ambiguity of policy implementation system (Wee et al. 2017).

Moreover, the other good governance barrier widely cited by the literature relates to the presence of poor governance structures meaning that organizations either lack or possess inadequate institutional structures that can support rule of law, accountability, transparency, participation as well as responsiveness. This is to say that poor or weak institutions are at times ill-conceived and organizations may as well not have the capacity nor the resources to implement the policies and procedures as required (Mardiasmo et al. 2008); This subsequently, further suggests that efficient and effective institutions form the backbone of a successful development and governance process (Mardiasmo et al. 2008). Another barrier closely related to the above is lack of governance and accountability mechanism within the organizations meaning that organizations lack effective systems to hold the civil servants accountable for their actions (Wee et al. 2017). Thus, disciplinary proceedings are hardly initiated against delinquent public or private officials (Wee et al. 2017). Moreover, performance evaluation systems within government have not been effectively structured (Dayanandan 2013). Another barrier has been related to poor perception and lack of knowledge on governance among both the organizational officials and members (Nurdin et al. 2011; Price 2017). This is further related to lack of knowledge on good governance or simply poorer perception on good governance by the leaders (Srivastava 2009). This basically means that leaders have poor knowledge and attitude on governance or simply leaders are insensitivity and indifference to the needs of citizens or group members (Wakuru 2016). In this case leaders may end up regarding themselves as dispensing favours to citizens rather than serving them or solving their problems (Srivastava 2009; Wakuru 2016).

Another barrier to good governance has to do with inadequate awareness of group members about their rights (Solihah et al. 2017). Such lack of awareness of civil rights among the organizational members prevent the members from effectively holding their leaders responsible to various principles of good governance in discharging their daily matters (International Bureau of Education 2019). Moreover, when members' servants are unware of their rights or existing institutions they themselves exhibit low levels of compliance of rules as well as to good governance in general. This follows the logic that awareness of rights and adherence to duties are two sides of the same coin (Solihah et al. 2017; Wouters and Ryngaert 2004). Moreover, ineffective implementation of Laws and Rules has also been captured as one of the barriers to practicing good governance in organizations (Wee et al. 2017; Wouters and Ryngaert 2004). Effective implementation of these laws creates an environment which would improve the welfare of all citizens and at the same time, encourages each citizen to contribute his or her best towards the development of society (Argentino et al. 2017; Wee et al. 2017). On the other hand, weak implementation can cause a great deal of hardships to citizens and even erode the faith of the citizenry in the government [or organizational] machinery (Price 2017). Furthermore bureaucratic factors have also been earmarked as among the barriers to implementing good governance in organizations (Solihah et al. 2017). At times the existing rules and procedures become ill conceived and cumbersome and, therefore, do not serve their purpose (Solihah et al. 2017). Also, government servants [and organizational workers] sometimes become overly pre-occupied with rules and procedures and view these as an end in themselves (Wee et al. 2017). This is often the root cause of corruption as well [which is the prime enemy to good governance] (Price 2017).

Lack of strong governance institutions in organizations are repeatedly cited as yet another barrier to good governance. Some organizations do not have the necessary policies, rules, regulations and structures that can support aspects of good governance such as transparency, accountability and rule of law. These are cases where organisations lack feedback and communication mechanisms as well as policies that force people to be accountable or transparent. This idea is supported by (Mardiasmo et al. 2008), who noted that lack of good Governance System particularly well-defined management departments, policies and regulations are among the constraints towards practicing good governance. Another factor that is put forward as being responsible for poor governance is lack of skilled Human Resource when it comes to issues of good governance (Mardiasmo et al. 2008). This means that leaders and other people entrusted with responsibilities do not understand the ABCs of good governance and therefore it becomes difficult for them to implement it (Mardiasmo et al. 2008). Poverty and low income is also captured as another barrier responsible for poor governance in organizations suggesting that remuneration and welfare for the employee involved in discharging good governance is too low to the extent that it forces them to ignore good governance practices (Mardiasmo et al. 2008). Consequently, workers and officials involve themselves in corrupt practices and other less decent practices that do not support good governance (Mardiasmo et al. 2008). Another strand of literature notes that one of the barriers to good governance relates to lack of participation and transparency, presence of corruption, low educational level, poor responsiveness and poor sense of ownership among the organization members (Dayanandan 2013). Other factors impeding good governance are cited as lack of cooperative democracy, poor leadership skills for both top and mid management, lack of consensus as well as double responsibility leading to conflicts of interests (Dayanandan 2013; Nurdin et al. 2011).

It can basically be argued that the surveyed literature has unveiled a good number of barriers to good governance in organizations which practically provides significant light to the subject matter under study. Basically, the literature has unveiled social, economic and political hindrances to good governance in organizations. However, the literature is not aligned to specific good governance components notably rule of law, accountability and responsibility, transparency, participation and responsiveness. Moreover, the literature is general in the sense that it covers all continents and it is neither tied to Africa and Tanzania in particular nor is it specified to the private sector. It is also not specific especially when studying such barriers among farmers' groups. Therefore, more specific data specifying barriers to each component of good governance focusing on the private sector notably on farmers' groups in the context of Africa and Tanzania in specific is required. This is the essence of the current study.

4 Methodology

This study adopted qualitative design owing to the sensitive nature of the problems at hand and some governance aspects such as transparence, responsiveness and participation that can hardly be captured quantitatively given their complex nature. Data were collected using in-depth interviews, focus group discussion (FGD) and observations. The study was conducted in three regions of Tanzania markedly in Iringa, Mbeya and Ruvuma from December 2018 to January 2019. Purposive sampling was mainly utilized to get the respondents with first-hand information and those who were willing to participate in the discussion. Data were collected from around 100 respondents from 60 groups were purposefully selected and interviewed in-depth. Accordingly, recruitment of farmers for interviews proved sensitive as farmers seemed to be mobile and unpredictable due to the fact that agricultural season was ongoing and so were the related activities. Before participating in the interviews, research ethical considerations were made clear to the informants based on the qualitative research ethical guidelines (Master and Smith 2014). It was stipulated that participants were free to engage and withdraw from the research at any time and that every kind of information they shared would be treated confidential as per qualitative research ethics (Master and Smith 2014).

During data collection, a number of challenges were encountered including confusion between the ages of participants, some respondents mistaking out the data collection exercise with listing them for loans as well as failing to meet farmers timely due to the unpredictable nature of their activity. Moreover, the process of tracing farmers was a big challenging, especially considering the fact that it was during farming seasons therefore taking them out of farm activities proved sensitive. This could have jeopardized trustworthiness of the data. Consequently, trustworthiness of data was maintained through triangulation in which data was collected from various sources using various methods including interviews notably Focus Group Discussion, observation and review of secondary data. Other aspects considered for reliability and validity of data include, member checking, analysis of negative cases, peer debriefing as well as daily discussion and reflection on data (Master and Smith 2014). The collected data were nicely transcribed, Swahili transcriptions were translated into English (by a qualified language translator) and handwritten transcripts were typed and saved as documents in rich text format. Content analysis of the transcriptions was done in MAXQDA 10 [VERBI Software, Marburg, Germany]. Data were grouped accordingly; codes were generated, leading to categories and themes. Quantitative data were analysed using the mixed method function of MAXQDA 10 software.

4.1 Findings and Discussion

A: Barriers to Good Governance for the Maize Farmers' Groups
This section presents and discusses the findings on the various barriers to good governance faced by the maize group farmers. It focuses on the barriers to the selected components of good governance notably the Rule of law, accountability & responsibility, transparency, participation as well as responsiveness.

Barriers to the Rule of Law Faced by Farmer's Groups: The first component of good governance examined under this study were barriers to Rule of law in the farmers' groups. Accordingly, it was noted that groups failed to observe rule of law due to the absence of relevant documents related to the rule of law such as polices, rules and regulations e.g. the constitutions which would guide them in their day to day organisational activities. Another constraint closely related to this was absence or inadequate availability of necessary structures to support rule of law such as specified departments, personnel as well as relevant forums designated for handling issues related to the rule of law such as leadership and meetings to mention just a few. Indeed, further investigation proved that respondents were not logical as well as exhaustive enough in explaining how they made use of relevant documents such as the constitution in the context of their groups. Moreover, most of the respondents [organisation leaders] were unware of the content of their constitutions including how various sections of the constitutions apply to different decision making process of the organisations though they claimed to use the constitution as they were interviewed. Constraints such absence or inadequate availability of necessary structures to support rule of law have also generally been associated to poor governance even though specifically associated with the rule of law (Ali 2013; Mardiasmo et al. 2008). Another factor mentioned was lack of education and awareness about the rule of law by the group members. More than ¾ of the members attested to have not been aware of the rule of law as well as expressed the dire need for being sensitised on the same. Respondents argued that they had not been using a constitution and other guidelines to guide their day to day activities. Adding these documents were critical for deliberation of their various group matters such as recruitment of new members, election of leaders, determining number of meetings to be held and the meeting schedules, handling of groups' revenues and expenditure issues, as well as instituting disciplinary measures. Equally, factors related to lack of education and awareness about the rule of law in organisations as barriers to practicing rule of law in organisation's have also been partly captured by (HIMSS 2017; Nurdin et al. 2011), suggesting that this current work contributes to the current debate on good governance

Barriers to Accountability and Responsibility: One of the barriers to accountability and responsibility cited by the respondents was mental as well as physical disabilities by some leaders noting that leaders with physical disabilities could not effectively serve the group members as some of them could not walk or hear appropriately. Another barrier is lack of education and awareness on accountability and responsibility by both the leaders and members of the groups. Leaders demonstrated a significant degree of lack of knowledge on accountability and responsibility noting that they had not received this kind of education before and that they needed it. In this case they could not practice something that they were not aware of. This was coupled with lack of effective mechanism or environment for practicing accountability and responsibility in the groups e.g. rules, regulations, policies and mechanisms that could enable the leaders practice accountability as well as those that would incline the members to demand for accountability from their leaders. For example, members would need forums like meetings to demand accountability, but there were no regular meetings. The other reason was related to lack of financial and physical resources for initiating and implementing accountability in groups such as financing members to attend meetings and workshops. Through these meetings members would be enlightened more on the ways of demanding for accountability e.g. writing, reports, and policies. Associated to this was poor and ineffective communication skills by organisational leaders particularly skills related to effective writing, speaking and listening that could enable them initiate and implement the accountability in the organisation. This significantly jeopardised accountability and responsibility. Indeed, most of the foregoing discussed barriers to accountability & responsibility in organisation particularly mental as well as physical disabilities by organisational officials, lack of education and awareness on accountability and responsibility by both the leaders and members of the groups seem to be well captured in the existing literature (Ali 2013; Lubuva 2008; Nurdin et al. 2011). Barriers to accountability and responsibility are summarised in Table 1. Most of the respondents mentioned more than one barriers to accountability & responsibility in groups so the percentages do not add up to 100% but are calculated based on how many respondents mentioned the responses as can be observed in the following table.

Table 1. Summary, barriers to accountability & responsibility in the groups

Barriers to accountability	Frequency in %
Mental and physical disabilities by group leaders	**20**
Lack of awareness and knowledge on accountability	55
Lack of good governance mechanism/environment	61
Inadequate financial and physical resources	71
Leaders ineffective communication skills	56

Source: Field Data (2019)

Barriers to Transparency: One of the barriers to transparency mentioned is inadequate knowledge and awareness on transparency by leaders. Leaders did not understand the meaning as well as the importance of transparency in the context of their respective groups. It follows that, they could not implement something that they did not know. Another barrier was lack of effective communication mechanism. Communication is essential in ensuring transparency of various information. However, there hardly existed necessary mechanism for ensuring transparency nor did the leaders possess necessary communication skills for sharing the information in a transparent manner. In addition, respondents mentioned lack of leadership skills in general and participatory leadership in particular as another barrier to transparency. Moreover, respondents informed that lack of necessary institutions e.g. policies for ensuring transparency another barrier to transparency in their groups. This explicitly means that groups did not have proper mechanisms for ensuring transparency. To some extent the few existing transparent mechanisms such as meetings were also limited and not given deserved priority. It was further noted that lack of records keeping served as critical impediment to transparency as group leaders could not keep as well as retrieve records related to, financial records such as income and expenditure, meeting minutes as well as groups assets when required. To this end barrier to transparency in organisations include, inadequate knowledge and awareness on transparency by leaders, lack of effective communication mechanisms and skills, lack of leadership as well as lack of necessary transparency institutions at organisational level. These findings are partly supported by (Glawcal 2018; International Bureau of Education 2019). The only difference at this particular point is that the reviewed literature does not specifically associate these points with the aspect of transparency but generally associate them with good governances. Associating them to this particular aspect sounds a specific contribution of this paper to the realm of governance. Accordingly, summary for barriers to transparency are summarised in Table 2. As may be observed in the table many respondents mentioned more than one barriers to transparency in groups so the percentages do not add up to 100% but are calculated based on how many people mentioned the responses.

Table 2. Summary, barriers to transparency

Barriers to transparency	Frequency in %
Inadequate knowledge and awareness on transparency by leaders	22
Lack of effective communication mechanism	55
Lack of Participatory leadership	51
Lack of necessary transparency institutions	61
Lack of/inadequate records keeping	50

Source: Field Data (2019)

Barriers to Participation: Accordingly, this study noted that one of the key barriers to participation had to do with lack of necessary mechanisms and infrastructures for participation. It was noted that, there were no forums such as meetings and other meaningful gatherings such as meetings that would bring people together and participate in decisions making exercise. For example, respondents were required to provide dates for the last meeting as a proof that they had been holding meetings. Results were as indicated here under, which basically shows that there were less frequent meetings in the group (Table 3).

Secondly, there was a communication barrier that emanated from the use of unfriendly languages such as foreign languages. Respondents argued that some documents that contained important messages pertaining maize production were written

Table 3. Dates for the last meeting in the organisation

Less than a month	Month ago	2 months and above
5	49	6

Source: (Field Data, 2019)

in English and they could not be translated in a friendly language in a timely manner. Also, a few old people said that they could not understand Kiswahili very well even though Swahili was a medium of communication at the group. Some individuals were incapable of reading and writing in general. Therefore, they could not participate directly in decision making. Another critical impediment mentioned by the respondents was the existence of some cultural practices or perceptions that hindered some groups to participate effectively. Such cultural practices did not allow women to participate effectively in leadership as well as decisions making forums such as meetings. Consequently, some people said that in some instances either women were excluded or they themselves declined to participate in some decisions making events such as meetings. Another barrier was fear and insecurity. Some members stated that they were afraid of making their contribution in various decision making forums such as in the meetings or whenever required to do so due to fear of being victimised by the authorities or some influential group leaders.

Another critical barrier to participation was income poverty by some group leaders and members. According to the respondents, some group members were so poor to the extent that they spent more of their time on raising income rather than participating in various decisions making forums. Another constrain was lack of good leadership and management knowledge and skills. This inclined the group leaders to always practice top down leadership approach that subsequently deny the members the opportunity to participate in various decision making events. Concluding the above point, it can be said that barriers to participation in organisations include the use of unfriendly/foreign languages, oppressive cultural practices, fear and insecurity, income poverty as well as lack of good leadership and management skills. Most of these factors have been captured by previous literature notably (Argentino et al. 2017; Dayanandan 2013), except aspects related to oppressive cultural practices as well as fear and insecurity. Therefore, the two points on oppressive cultural practices as well as fear and insecurity can be said to be unique contribution of this particular work in the topic related to barriers of good governance in organisations.

Summary of barriers to participation in farmers' groups is provided in Table 4. As can be observed in the table many respondents mentioned more than one barriers to participation in groups so the percentages do not add up to 100% but are calculated based on how many respondents mentioned the responses.

Barriers to Responsiveness: Lastly, the study examined some specific barriers to responsiveness in the context of farmers' groups. Accordingly, one of the specific barriers to responsiveness is lack of communication and life skills by leaders. Leaders were unresponsive to some group matters due to their inability to express themselves clearly,

Table 4. Summary barriers to participation

Barriers to participation	Frequency in %
Lack mechanisms for participation	57
Use of unfriendly/foreign languages	66
Oppressive cultural practices	51
Fear and insecurity	67
Income poverty	55
Lack of good leadership and management skills	63

Source: Field Data (2019)

courtesy, as well as displaying customer service and customer care elements. Another is lack of Interpersonal skills such using derogatory language which does not please the members, lack of effective communication between leaders and members themselves, inadequate mechanisms and institutions to enforce responsiveness in the group context. This was fuelled by lack of training on the responsiveness specifically how to implement it at the group level. Another barrier was lack of knowledge and awareness about responsiveness. Finally, barriers to responsiveness are summarised as inadequate listening skills, poor interpersonal skills, inadequate possession of negotiation skills, lack of sound mechanisms and institutions, lack of knowledge and awareness about responsiveness. These barriers correspond well with those in the existing literature of (Glawcal 2018; Nurdin et al. 2011; Price 2017). This suggests that the current work supports and contributes to the existing and ongoing debates in the area of constraints to good governance and responsiveness in particular. Just like in the previous components of governance summary of barriers to responsiveness is displayed in Table 5. As can be noticed many respondents mentioned more than one barriers to responsiveness in groups so the percentages do not add up to 100% but are calculated based on how many people mentioned the responses as can further be observed in the subsequent table.

Table 5. Summary, barriers to responsiveness

Barriers to responsiveness	Frequencies in %
Lack of listening skills	53
Lack of interpersonal skills	71
Lack of negotiation skills	81
Lack of sound mechanisms and institutions	61
Lack of knowledge and awareness about responsiveness	67

Source: Field Data (2019)

B: Policy Recommendations: Strategies for Ensuring Good Governance for Farmers' Groups Accordingly, the following strategies should be taken into account in ensuring good governance among the Maize Farmers' Groups in the South Eastern Zone of Tanzania.

- In the first place group leaders are supposed to be empowered and sensitized on the various components of good governance notably the Rule of law, accountability & responsibility, transparency, participation as well as responsiveness. This is because they have proved to be unware of them and that this constituted as a constraint to practicing good governance in the Maize Farmers Groups.
- Moreover, groups have to ensure existence of good policies, rules and regulations that can initiate and support the implementation and enforcement of good governance in groups such as rule of law.
- Indeed, groups should invest in good leadership which means electing good, morally upright leaders who can facilitate institutionalisation of good governance such as rule of law as well as ensure effective enforcement of other components of good governance
- Further, groups should ensure effective communication in the organisations. This is to say that, in order to effectively practice good governance in an organisation, information must be passed in a uniform manner, without generating noise, because the communication process can directly impact the understanding of the message that must be passed by the organization
- Moving forward, groups should put in place proper mechanisms for the disabled to participate in various decisions making matters. This will enhance all aspects of governance notably participation, rule of law, accountability and responsiveness
- On the other hand, groups should get rid of all cultures, traditions and beliefs that prevent the members from effectively and meaningfully participating in various decisions making events and forums.
- Alongside the above point, both the group leaders and members should be educated on the importance of and better ways of enforcing participation in their groups. Closely related to this, organisations should put in place proper mechanisms for ensuring effective and meaningful participation among the members. These include meetings, committees, policies preparation etc.
- Group members should be empowered economically. This is because one of the barriers to participation was related to income poverty. Some group members were so poor to the extent that they spent more of their time on raising income rather than participating in various decisions making forums
- Sensitization and capacity building on financial, assets and meeting records management for group leaders and members will contribute to raising levels of accountability, responsibility and transparency.

5 Conclusion

Conclusively, this study examined barriers to good governance for the maize farmers' groups in southern highlands of Tanzania and proposes strategies for overcoming the barriers. The study was conducted in three regions of Tanzania notably Iringa, Mbeya and Ruvuma from December 2018 to January 2019, whereby around 100 respondents from 60 groups were purposefully selected and interviewed. Findings indicated that barriers to good governance for the Maize farmers' groups were inadequate good governance structures and policies, lack of education and awareness on good governance, lack of leadership skills and ethics, lack of records keeping skills, poor technology and inadequate communication skills and use of foreign languages in specific. Other barriers include poverty and lack of financial resources in particular, disability of some leaders and members as well as cultural beliefs that impeded participation. Accordingly, strategies for ensuring good governance of the groups are institutionalisation of relevant policies and structures, training on leadership, good governance and communications skills, economic and technological empowerment of group leaders and members.

References

Ali, S.A.: The Role of Good Governance Practices in Enhancing Service Delivery in Public Institutions in Tanzania: The Case Study of the Tanzania Electric Supply Company Ltd. A Dissertation Submitted in Partial Fulfilment of the Requirements for the Degree of Master of Business Administration. The Open University of Tanzania (OUT) (2013). Dar es Salaam. http://repository.out.ac.tz/1809/1/DISSERTATION_-_SAADA_FINAL.pdf

Argentino, L.G., de Medeiros Sousa, J.L., Nose, E.T., Petraglia, I.C., Rosini, A.M.: Barriers and difficulties in the process of implementing corporate governance in companies: a study of the management process and the disclosure of information. J. Innov. Sustain. RISUS **8**(1), 106–129 (2017)

Dayanandan, R.: Good governance practice for better performance of community: organizations - myths and realities. J. Power Polit. Governance. **1**(1), 10–26 (2013). www.aripd.org/jppg

Glawcal. The Importance of Good Governance for The Development of Institutions: Glawcal Comment#123 (2018). http://www.glawcal.org.uk/glawcal-comments/the-importance-of-good-governance-for-the-development-of-institutions

HIMSS. The Importance of Good Governance: August. 31, 2017; updated March 12, 2019 (2017) https://www.himss.org/resources/importance-good-governance

International Bureau of Education. Concept of Governance (2019). Geneva. http://www.ibe.unesco.org/en/geqaf/technical-notes/concept-governance

Kaufmann, D., et al.: Aggregating governance indicators, World Bank policy research paper (2000). http://wwwwds.worldbank.org/servlet/WDSContentServer/WDSP/IB/1999/10/23/000094946_99101105050593/Rendered/PDF/multi_page.pdf. Accessed 22 Apr 2020

Lubuva, K.: The effect of motivation on the performance of public and private organizations in Tanzania. A comparative analysis of Tanzania Posts Corporation: FEDEX, SCANDINAVIA and DHL. (Masters Dissertation). Open University of Tanzania, Dar es Salaam (2008). https://journalissues.org/wp-content/uploads/2017/05/Mollel-et-al.pdf

Mardiasmo, D., Barnes, P.H., Sakurai, Y.: implementation of good governance by regional governments in Indonesia: the challenges. In: Brown, K.A., Mandell, M., Furneaux, C.W., Beach, S., (eds.) Proceedings Contemporary Issues in Public Management: The 12th Annual Conference of the International Research Society for Public Management (IRSPM XII), pp. 1–36,. Brisbane, Australia (2008)

Master, Z., Smith, E.: Ethical Practice of Research Involving Humans: Environmental Health and Sustainability: Environmental Health and Sustainability (2014). https://www.researchgate.net/publication/273059362

Mintzberg, H.: Managing government, governing management. Harv Bus Rev **74**(3), 75–83 (1996)
Nurdin, N., Stockdale, R., Scheepers, H.: Understanding organizational barriers influencing local electronic government adoption and implementation: the electronic government implementation framework. J. Theor. Appl. Electron. Commer. Res. **6**(3), 13–27 (2011). https://scielo.conicyt.cl/scielo.php?script=sci_arttext&pid=S0718-18762011000300003
Peters, B.G.: The future of governing. University. Press of Kansas, Lawrence (2001)
Price, N.J.: Importance of Corporate Governance in an Organization (2017). https://insights.diligent.com/corporate-governance/importance-of-corporate-governance-in-an-organization
Solihah, R., Djuyandi, Y., Witianti, S., Herdiansah, A.G., Ganjar, A.: The importance of good governance implementation in the legislative institutions. Adv. Sci. Lett. (2017).https://doi.org/10.1166/asl.2017.8917
Srivastava, M.: Good Governance - Concept, Meaning and Features: A Detailed Study (2009). https://papers.ssrn.com/sol3/papers.cfm?abstract_id=1528449
URT. Agricultural Sector Development Strategy – II 2015/2016 – 2024/2025: United Republic of Tanzania. Dar es Salaam (2014)
Wakuru, M.: Ushirika na Ujenzi wa Uchumi wa Kisasa: Kulikoni na tufanyeje? (Toleo la kwanza,). Dar es Salaam: Safi Publihers Trading Co. Ltd (2016)
Wee, S.T., Abas, M.A., Mohamed, Z., Kai Chen. G.K., Zainal, R.: Good governance in national solid waste management policy (A case study of Malaysia) implementation: a case study of Malaysia. In: AIP Conference Proceedings, vol. 1891, p. 020128 (2017). https://doi.org/10.1063/1.5005461 Published Online: 03 October 2017 (2017). https://aip.scitation.org/doi/pdf/10.1063/1.5005461
Wouters, J., Ryngaert, C.: Good Governance: Lessons from International Organizations: Institute for International Law. (Working Paper No. 54 - May 2004). Leuven (2004). Retrieved from Leuven Faculty of Law website: https://www.law.kuleuven.be/iir/nl/onderzoek/working-papers/WP54e.pdf

Economic Burden of Non-communicable Diseases and Poverty in Nigeria: A Cross-sectional Study

C. O. Ibukun(✉) and A. A. Adebayo

Department of Economics, Faculty of Social Sciences, Obafemi Awolowo University, Ile-Ife, Nigeria
{cibukun,bayoade}@oauife.edu.ng

Abstract. Efforts to alleviate poverty and ensure sustainable development are recently being sabotaged by the remarkable loss of productivity, income, and human capital aggravated by Non-communicable Diseases (NCDs). While a considerable amount of literature in developed countries is concerned with the connection between NCDs and poverty, comparable studies for developing countries are sparse. Using a mixed-method research approach, this study assessed the level of poverty among those with NCDs, the out-of-pocket (OOP) expenses incurred on NCDs while considering the probability of NCDs inducing catastrophic health expenditure and impoverishment. Quantitative as well as qualitative data were obtained from individuals with NCDs and key personnel's distributed across 9 referral hospitals in Southwestern Nigeria. The result showed that 25% of the respondents were multidimensionally poor, while 72% had no health insurance coverage. The findings further indicated that the median out-of-pocket cost on NCDs was N10,750 monthly and being multidimensionally poor increased the probability of incurring catastrophic health expenditure, meanwhile having a health insurance coverage reduced the probability of impoverishment due to NCD by 3% ($p < 0.05$). This implies that NCDs induced health expenditure is notably associated with economic distress that can aggravate poverty. Hence, there should be a strategic sensitization of Nigerians on the benefits of health insurance and social security should be provided for individuals with NCDs in order to reduce the burden on households.

Keywords: Non-communicable diseases · Poverty · Out-of-pocket expenditure · Catastrophic health expenditure · Impoverishment

1 Introduction

The global Multidimensional Poverty Index (MPI) estimate of Nigerians living in poverty is over 100 million (Multidimensional Poverty Peer Network, n.d) making her one of the poorest countries in the world. Meanwhile, poverty is intricately connected to health because it can be both a cause and consequence of poor health, and it can also serve as a barrier to accessing quality healthcare when necessary (World Bank 2014).

J. N. Mojekwu et al. (Eds.): *Sustainable Education and Development*, pp. 425–444, 2021.
https://doi.org/10.1007/978-3-030-68836-3_37

The traditional challenge affecting the health of Nigerian's and the health sector has been the scourge of infectious diseases, also known as communicable diseases (such as HIV/AIDS, Malaria, Cholera, Tuberculosis, Diarrhoea, and so on). Although, Nigeria is still besieged with the emergence and re-emergence of these infectious diseases and other high impact ones such as Lassa Virus; there has been an upward trend, and increasing prevalence of non-communicable disease as well. Non-communicable diseases (NCDs), equally known as chronic diseases, are basically slow progressing and long duration diseases that cannot be transferred from one human to another (WHO 2018). They explain an enormous number of deaths worldwide and contribute immensely to the financial burden of diseases in Low-and-Middle Income Countries (LMICs). Hence, they are considered a paramount threat to human health, productivity and sustainable development in the 21st century (Niessen et al. 2018).

The dominant types of NCDs, which are of concern in this study are; diabetes, cardiovascular diseases (such as heart attacks, high blood pressure, and stroke), chronic respiratory diseases (such as asthma and chronic obstructive pulmonary disease (COPD)), and cancers of various forms (WHO 2018). The financial burden of these diseases is increasing all around the world, particularly, in resource-poor settings, with many individuals and households rolling into poverty.

Nigeria unlike other lower-middle-income countries such as Kenya and Ghana contributes a very small amount of its Gross Domestic Product (GDP) to the health sector, as it allocates less than 6% of its total budget to health yearly (the highest percentage was in 2012 when 5.95% of the budget was allotted to health). This is evidently lower than the 2001 WHO Abuja declaration that governments should allocate 15% of their budgets to the health sector. It also contradicts the World Health Report of 2010, which remarked that it is laborious to get close to universal health coverage with less than 4–5% of GDP investment into health (WHO 2011). Hence, the Nigerian health sector is under-funded, which suggests that the burden of healthcare will shift to individuals and households.

Studies globally have focused on NCDs and they (Abegunde et al. 2007; Engelgau et al. 2012; Wang et al. 2016; Kien et al. 2017; Datta et al. 2018) have established the huge cost burden of these diseases and their possibility of inducing catastrophic health expenditure and impoverishment. Empirical evidence from Nigeria (Onoka et al. 2011; Adisa 2015; Aregbesola and Khan 2017) indicates that at least about 10% of households face catastrophic health expenditure due to various diseases. However, studies that have focused on NCDs in Nigeria (Onyeneonoro et al. 2016) established a high prevalence of NCDs in Nigeria unlike other countries but noted that only about 20% of people with NCDs seek formal health care services. Janssens et al. (2016) extended this research by focusing on health care utilization and expenditure while Owoeye and Olaniyan (2015) focused only on the economic cost of tobacco-related diseases. Other Nigerian studies on NCDs (Ogha et al. 2013; Yiltok et al. 2017) buttressed the increasing prevalence of NCDs; but did not consider the economic implications of these diseases. More recently, Okediji et al. (2017) addressed the economic impact of chronic illness on patients in Ile-Ife, Osun state Nigeria but the study like Onyeneonoro et al. (2016) focused on prevalence, risk factors and direct cost without examining its effect on poverty, therefore, creating a gap for the present study.

The purpose of this study was to identify the proportion of the poor and non-poor that seek appropriate healthcare for NCDs, their out-of-pocket expenses and to examine the extent of catastrophic health expenditure and impoverishment incurred due to NCDs in the context of Nigeria with emphasis on the Southwestern part. Such evidence is germane for policymakers and stakeholders particularly with respect to resource allocation to this sector.

2 Methodology

2.1 Study Setting

This study was conducted in Southwestern Nigeria, which comprises of 6 states with an estimated population of about 40 million (City Population 2018). In this study, 3 states namely Lagos, Osun and Ekiti were purposively selected as these included both industrialised and inland sates. Thereafter 9 referral healthcare facilities were also purposely selected. The hospitals comprised three Federal teaching hospitals, three State teaching hospitals and three private hospitals. The choice of these facilities is based on their capacity to handle NCD cases. The Federal healthcare facilities were Lagos University Teaching Hospital, Obafemi Awolowo University Teaching Hospital, and Federal Teaching Hospital Ido-Ekiti; the State healthcare facilities were Lagos State University Teaching Hospital, Ladoke Akintola University Teaching Hospital, and Ekiti State University Teaching Hospital; while the private healthcare facilities were Promise Specialist Hospital, Our Lady of Fatima Catholic Hospital, and Afe-Babalola University Teaching Hospital all of which are located within Lagos, Osun, and the Ekiti States respectively.

2.2 Data

This was a facility-based cross-sectional study collected on a sample of 1320 individuals diagnosed with NCDs, after giving consideration to their composition and geographical disparities. The primary outcomes are poverty, the incidence of financial catastrophe, and impoverishment due to NCD expenses. Individuals who had been diagnosed with an NCDs for over 3 months, and receiving medications or treatment for any of the NCDs were included in the study. Meanwhile, individuals younger than 16 years old were excluded from the study.

2.3 Sample Size and the Study Time Frame

Given an NCD prevalence of 29% in Nigeria (WHO 2019), a 95% confidence interval (that is, $Z_{1-\alpha} = 1.96$), and a 5% margin of error, the Kish (1965) formula where n = z2pq/d2 was employed in obtaining the minimum sample size of approximately 390 after applying a 20% non-response rate. While envisaging data collection challenges due to privacy, disruption and lack of consent, the application of stratification based on equal allocation across the three selected states produced an estimate of 1170 individuals with NCDs. For the qualitative data, 27 persons (18 individuals with NCDs and 9 healthcare professionals, particularly consultants attending to respondents with NCDs) were purposively selected. Making three from each facility. These respondents were selected between August to September 2019 in order to avoid the problem of double counting.

2.4 Data Collection

This study made use of a standardized instrument in data collection which was administered by trained graduate personnel, with a good grasp of the local language. Information about the socio-demographic characteristics of the respondents and their households such as age, gender, marital status, occupation, educational attainment, household income, occupation and education of the household head amongst others were collected. Data on household assets, income, and expenditure were also retrieved in order to ascertain the individual and household poverty status. The cost of NCDs to individuals and their caregivers was unravelled while exploring questions on the direct and indirect cost of disease (in terms of consultation, medication, transportation, productivity loss, etc.).

2.5 Definition of the Study Variables

The following definitions were employed in capturing poverty, catastrophe and impoverishment of the households during the analysis of data

Poverty: This was measured using the multidimensional poverty index (MPI). The framework of Alkire and Santos (2014) was adopted and their algorithms of deprivation were employed in separating the poor from the non-poor. This encompasses the health dimension, education dimension, and household living standards such as the floor, improved sanitation, water, cooking materials, electricity, and assets. Households with a multidimensional poverty index (MPI) of more than 0.33 were considered multidimensionally poor and households with less than 0.33 were classified as multidimensionally non-poor.

As a robustness check, the asset-based wealth index and global monetary poverty were constructed using household assets and income respectively. The wealth index was constructed through PCA on a list of 26 variables of a household asset, meanwhile, variables that include more than 95% or 5% of the households were dropped. Variables were categorized as dummies and varimax (orthogonal) rotation was employed to enhance the interpretation of components. These results were classified and participants were grouped as poor if they fell in the bottom 40% of the distribution (Mirelman et al. 2016). On the other hand, the global monetary poverty of the household was estimated using the average monthly income from all sources, equalized by the household size. To determine the Naira per adult equivalent monthly, the OECD Modified Equivalence scale $AE = 1 + 0.5(N_{adults} - 1) + 0.3N_{children}$ was employed. Poor households were constructed based on the World Bank's PPP (2010), which is living below $3.20 poverty line for low middle-income countries.

Out-of-Pocket Health Expenditure (OOP): this included the sum of direct and the indirect cost of care. The direct cost comprised of both the direct medical and non-medical costs such as the consultation fees, diagnostic/laboratory tests, drugs, medical aids and disposables, and the cost of transportation directly associated with all healthcare-seeking events incurred over the one-month recall period. The indirect cost encompassed the time and income cost to the individual and caregiver, Since the county's applicable minimum wage for 2011–2019, was N18,000 monthly, this was multiplied by the lost work time reported, in order to estimate the average minimum income lost and obtain the monthly OOP.

Catastrophic Health Expenditure: This occurs when a household's out-of-pocket health expenditure exceeds or equals the household's capacity to pay, and the household cannot maintain its customary standard of living. That is when OOP spending exceeds (between) 5% to 40% of a household's income since various thresholds have been employed in the literature (Wagstaff and Doorslaer 2003; Russell 2004)

Impoverishment: This occurs when a household becomes poor or is pushed further into poverty after the OOP expenses on healthcare have been made. This study employed the international poverty line of $1.90 and $3.20 daily per person living in low-and-middle-income countries. The household income was equalized using the modified OECD scale in order to account for different financial requirements of various types of households. This was then converted this into the local currency using the official 2019 purchasing power parity exchange rate.

2.6 Analysis

The data analysis for this study was conducted in two phases. The first phase involved the analysis of quantitative data which was coded into EPI DATAb3.0 and was downloaded into STATA 16.1 for analysis. Descriptive statistics of all variables was first conducted and the households were classified as poor and non-poor. The dependent variables were dummy variables on catastrophic health expenditure and impoverishment due to healthcare payment. Probit regression was used to explore their covariates amongst the poor and non-poor. The independent variables include the household characteristics, health insurance status, poverty status and the type of NCD. The second phase involved the analysis of the qualitative data. The qualitative data gathered during the interview sessions were transcribed, edited, organized, interpreted verbatim and others that were conducted in the local language (Yoruba) were translated into English.

Note taken and memos were employed to augment the information recorded on audio recorders. The analysis was conducted using NVIVO 11 after the coding of transcripts and the reduction of these into smaller categories. The coding was also tested for reliability by a qualitative expert. This did not only deepen the understanding of the themes that emerged from the data, but the qualitative finding also augmented the findings from quantitative data.

2.7 Ethical Consideration

This study obtained ethical clearance from the health research and ethics board of all the following hospitals; Lagos University Teaching Hospital, Obafemi Awolowo University Teaching Hospital, Federal Teaching Hospital Ido-Ekiti, Lagos State University Teaching Hospital, Ekiti State University Teaching Hospital and Ladoke Akintola University Teaching Hospital, while the Chief Medical Directors of the private hospitals (Promise Specialist Hospital, Our Lady of Fatima Catholic Hospital and Afe-Babalola University Teaching Hospital) also provided ethical clearance. For both quantitative and qualitative component of this study, written informed consent was obtained from all participants after explaining to them the objectives of the study and assuring them of confidentiality of all information provided.

3 Result

3.1 Descriptive Statistics of the Study Participants

Quantitative

Figure 1 presents a summary of 1156 individuals with NCD cases that were included in the quantitative phase of this study. 35% of the study population had diabetes, 32% had cardiovascular diseases, about one-quarter had chronic respiratory diseases and less than 10% had cancer. In general, the individual characteristics of the participant showed no clear discrepancy due to gender. That is, the percentage of males and females in the study population was roughly 50%. Over three-quarter, (85%) of respondents were in the age bracket 16 to 69 with a mean of 52 years and a standard deviation of $\pm$16 years. By implication, the majority of the study population were adults of working age. This, therefore, suggests that NCDs are more prominent among the elderly than the young. Also, about 64% of the population had tertiary education and above, while 14% had only completed secondary education during the period of data collection. About 10% had just primary education, 6% had some secondary education while about 7% of the sample had not gone through any formal education. A consideration of the employment status of participants depicted in Table 1 showed that the majority ($\approx$76%) were either in paid employment or self-employed, while over 8% were unemployed and another 8.1% had retired. 6% of the respondents were searching for employment, while about 1.5% were homemakers. Surprisingly, just a little over one-fourth of the respondents had health insurance cover, while the majority (72%) have no health insurance coverage. This supports the discussion that majority of Nigerians are not covered by health insurance which exposes them to huge healthcare expenses.

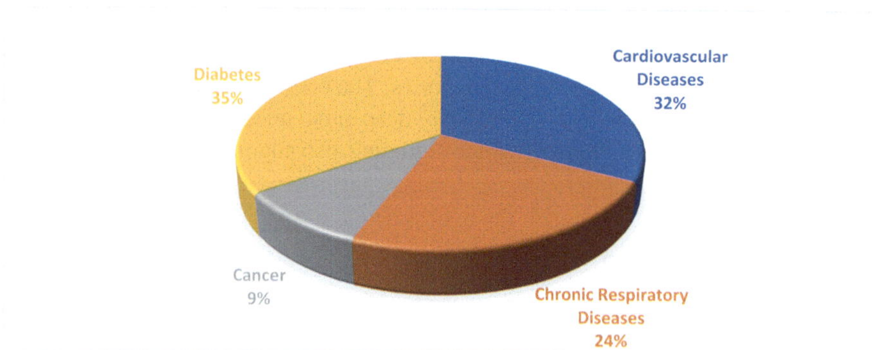

Fig. 1. Distribution of NCDs within the study group Source: Fieldwork (2019)

Qualitative

A total of 27 one on one interviews were conducted (18 with individuals with NCDs and 9 with health providers). The average duration of the interviews was 15 min, most of the healthcare providers interviewed were below the age of 50 (89%) while most of the respondents with NCD (67%) were above 50 years old. Regarding marital status, over two-third of both the participants with NCD (89%) and the healthcare provider (66%) were married, while 33% of the healthcare providers were single. The level of education of healthcare providers was highly skewed because all of them had tertiary education and above while 33% of those with NCDs only completed secondary school education.

Table 1. Socio-demographic and economic characteristics of the study population

Variable	Text description		Sample size	Mean	Std. Dev.
Panel A: Individual characteristics					
Sex	A binary variable for whether or not the respondent is male or female	Male	587 (50.74)	1.49	0.50
		Female	569 (49.26)		
Age	Continuous, but categorized variable for age as at last birthday	16–29 years	138 (11.94)	51.57	16.14
		30–49 years	276 (23.88)		
		50–69 years	570 (49.31)		
		70 years and above	172 (17.88)		
Marital status	Categorical variable for the current marital status of an individual with NCD	Single	273 (23.62)	1.94	0.73
		Married/Civil partner	735 (63.60)		
		Widowed	108 (9.36)		
		Separated	23 (2.01)		
		Divorced	16 (1.40)		
Education	Categorical variable of the highest attained level of schooling	No formal Education	76 (6.57)	4.42	1.48
		Primary	110 (9.50)		
		Some secondary	74 (6.39)		
		All secondary	160 (13.85)		
		Tertiary and above	736 (63.68)		
Religion	Categorical variable indicating the specific religion of the respondent	Islam	266 (23.04)	1.77	0.43
		Christianity	885 (76.52)		
		Traditional religion	5 (0.44)		
Ethnicity	Categorical variable reflecting the major ethnic groups in Nigeria	Hausa	32 (2.75)	2.12	0.68
		Yoruba	1005 (86.94)		

(continued)

Table 1. (*continued*)

Variable	Text description		Sample size	Mean	Std. Dev.
		Igbo	111 (9.59)		
		Others	8 (0.71)		
Employment status	Categorical variable indicating whether the respondent is employed or not	Paid Employment	564 (48.84)	2.42	1.58
		Unemployed	97 (8.38)		
		Currently Seeking	71 (6.17)		
		Self Employed	311 (26.88)		
		Retired	94 (8.09)		
		Home maker and Others	19 (1.64)		
Health insurance status	Categorical variable indicating if the respondent is covered by health insurance or not	Yes	322 (27.77)	1.72	0.44
		No	835 (72.23)		

Note: in Table 1 figures are frequencies and percentages are in parenthesis.
Source: Fieldwork (2019)

3.2 Poverty Outcomes of the Study Population

The three measures of poverty captured in this study provide complementary but different pictures of household poverty as presented in Table 2. Here, the percentage of the poor varied with the measures utilized. For the MPI, 25% of the participants were classified as belonging to poor households, 40% were categorized as poor using the asset-based index while 16% were considered to be monetarily poor. Hence the majority of those who sought healthcare for NCDs in these facilities were not poor, which is understandable because 76% of the participants of this study were employed. Qualitative findings also buttress this as expressed below

> *"Quite a number of people here are not extremely poor because healthcare in Nigeria is not cheap. The extreme poor will not come to the hospital because insurance is minimal, although some may come when it is life-threatening."*
>
> ***(A 42 years old female consultant at OAUTHC)***
>
> *"Many poor people reside in the villages, where you will not find tertiary healthcare facilities, and they usually cannot even afford the cost of transportation to the cities every month to make consultations. They would either visit the primary healthcare facility or seek alternative care. So, there is a limited number of very poor people here unless it is severe."* ***(A 32 years old male registrar at EKSUTH)***

Table 2. Poverty outcomes

S/N	Poverty outcome	Description	Percentage poor (SE)	Gender of household head	
				Male (poor %)	Female (poor %)
1.	Multidimensional Poverty Index (MPI)	Based on education, health and living standards	0.25 (0.43)	23.88	28.07
2.	Asset-Based Poverty index (API)	Based on 26 durable household assets	0.40 (0.49)	39.74	44.74
3.	Global Monetary Poverty Index (GMPI)	Based on household income	0.16 (0.36)	15.81	15.35

This finding is in agreement with Akawu and Agum (2018) who discovered that poverty has a negative and significant effect on access to healthcare facilities in Nigeria, hence a limited proportion of the poor were found at the selected healthcare facilities.

3.3 Out-of-Pocket Expenses

Table 3 describes the direct and indirect cost component of NCDs which contributes to the out-of-pocket cost monthly, given the median, mean, and mode of the different components. The median is focused on because of the possibilities of outliers skewing the mean. It was discovered that medication cost contributed significantly to the cost of illness at about N5000 monthly, followed by diagnostic tests, consultation/registration and transportation cost which differed considerably across NCDs, individuals and facilities. The cost of hospitalization varied rapidly across illness, facility utilized and severity, even though the median cost was 30000 Naira. The cost of transportation ranged from less than a hundred Naira to about eighty thousand Naira as some people took flights from the Northern part of Nigeria to access healthcare in the Southwest while some others merely took motorcycles or trekked to their healthcare facilities. For the direct cost, the mode could not be given because values varied largely across respondents.

For the indirect cost of illness, the median of the time loss to individuals and carer was minute because most of the participants did not lose up to a day from work/school or didn't involve or make use of any carer whether voluntary or paid. However, for those who incurred indirect cost due to time loss, a mean of two working days was lost to the individual weekly and the carer which amounts to over seven thousand Naira monthly using current Nigeria's Minimum wage of eighteen thousand Naira. This constitutes about 40% lost productivity for the individual and the carer monthly. This is consistent with Okediji et al. (2017) who found about 20% productivity loss for individuals with NCDs and the carers.

The median out-of-pocket costs due to these diseases were therefore around eleven thousand Naira, while the mean was thirty-eight thousand Naira monthly. This finding is consistent with Janssens et al. (2016) whose study showed that over nine thousand Naira is spent as out-of-pocket cost monthly on NCDs and eight hundred Naira is spent on NCD induced transportation averagely in Nigeria. It is also in agreement with the findings of Okediji et al. (2017) which discovered that twenty-three thousand Naira was spent on the average on drugs, approximately seven thousand on laboratory investigations and over ten thousand is spent on NCD induced admission monthly. Furthermore, the findings of this study are in tandem with Owoeye and Olaniyan (2015) whose study estimated laboratory test of over four thousand Naira for lung cancers and about three thousand six hundred for COPD (a type of chronic respiratory disease) monthly. Consultation cost was less than a thousand naira in both cases and an average of over twenty-two thousand and seventeen thousand Naira respectively was spent monthly on these diseases in Southwestern Nigeria (Table 3). Hence, having an NCD has serious financial implications on the individuals as well as their households.

Table 3. Out-of-pocket cost on NCDs

S/N	Type of payment	Cost of NCD			
		Median	Mean	Mode	Standard deviation
1	Registration/Consultation	1,000.00	1,780.29	1,000.00	2,246.60
2	Medication	7,000.00	13,743.36	5,000.00	16,685.25
3	Hospitalization	30,000.00	63,277.22	1,500.00	129,183.60
4	Diagnostic/Laboratory tests	5,000.00	20,719.40	5,000.00	50,148.53
5	Transportation	1,350.00	3,208.19	2,000.00	6,115.09
6	Direct cost $(N1 + N2 + N3 + N4 + N5)$	8,450.00	35,782.75		99,061.12
7	Time loss to individual (days)	<1.00	8.56	<1.00	5.53
8	Time loss to carer (days)	0.00	9.52	0.00	29.67
9	Indirect cost of NCDs	0.00	2,707.27	1,200.00	18,517.91
10	Out-of-pocket cost $(N6 + N9)$	10,750.00	38,490.01		102,320.00

Note: in Table 3, estimates are monthly and values are expressed in Naira.
Findings from the qualitative analysis also indicate the amount spent by people with NCDs monthly as explained below;

Findings from the qualitative analysis also indicate the amount spent by people with NCDs monthly as explained below;

"I have spent over a hundred thousand this month alone, doing several tests. With this hard economy, money is not very easy to come by, but for my children who have been of financial assistance" ***(A 72 years old male with Diabetes)***

"The tests we are being asked to do is too much, and they are all very expensive. There is no small spending in this place, from one test to another. One just has to do them because one has no choice. I have spent about eighty thousand Naira." ***(A 69 years old female with Cancer)***

3.4 Poverty and Catastrophic Health Expenditure

The catastrophic effect of NCDs was examined in the study using three different thresholds to account for the difference in economic status. The findings in Fig. 2 showed the percentage distribution of households who incurred catastrophic health expenditure at 10%, 25% and 40% threshold. This showed that as the threshold increases, the incidence of CHE declines across socioeconomic quintiles. At 10% threshold, about 50% of all households incurred CHE, and at the 25% threshold, the general percentage of households who incurred CHE declined drastically to about 26% of all households on the average. A further increase in the threshold to 40% reduced the number of households who incurred CHE with about 23% in the poorest quintile and 16% per cent in the richest quintile. By implication, as the wealth quintile improved the incidence of CHE declined and about 20% of all households incurred CHE on the average. This implies that one in every five households with members having NCDs incur CHE monthly, hence a need for urgent economic intervention. This is in agreement with the findings of Xu et al. (2003) and Li et al. (2012) that poorer households are at a higher risk of CHE than wealthier households. It is also in conformity with Tagoe (2014) and Mwai (2014) whose study showed that NCD induced financial catastrophe is aggravated when the household is already in the lowest socio-economic class or is experiencing financial inhibitions.

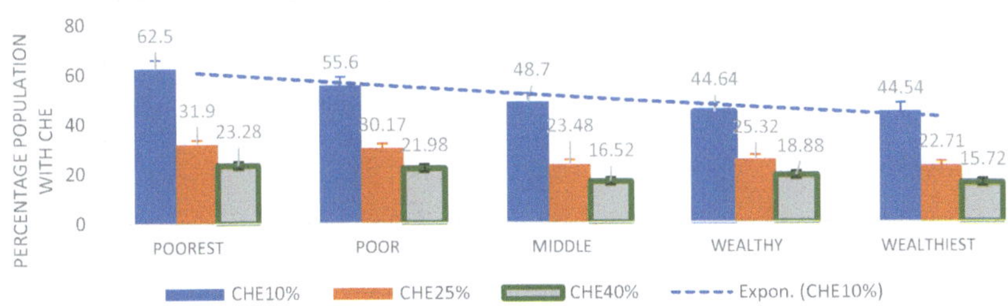

Fig. 2. Catastrophic out-of-pocket (OOP) expenditure across socio-economic quintiles Source: Fieldwork (2019)

To buttress the information above, the factors determining the occurrence of CHE in the entire sample was discussed in Table 4. This showed that at 10% threshold, the probability of incurring catastrophic health expenditure only significantly decreased with an increase in the wealth quintile *ceteris paribus* while utilizing a state healthcare facility or a private healthcare facility significantly increased the probability of incurring CHE when compared with seeking healthcare at a Federal healthcare facility. This suggests that the cost of healthcare services delivered at state healthcare facilities are relatively higher. After disaggregating the sample into those who are multidimensionally non-poor and those who are not, factors such as gender of the household head, household wealth quintile and the choice of healthcare facility significantly influenced the probability of incurring CHE for the poor at the 10% threshold. Meanwhile, the household's wealth quintile and the healthcare facility used were the only factors that significantly influenced the probability of incurring CHE for the multidimensionally poor, when holding other factors constant.

At the 25% threshold, having cancer and chronic respiratory disease increased the probability of incurring CHE by 22% and 7% respectively, which is consistent with Kavosi et al. (2014) and Leng et al. (2019) whose findings showed that having over 80% of people with cancer incur CHE and that health insurance does not adequately compensate for it. Similarly, households of persons with NCDs who are above 50 years of age or married were more likely to incur CHE, while households with above five members were 7% more likely to incur CHE at the 25% threshold. Other factors like the wealth quintile and the healthcare facility also showed statistical significance. Among the multidimensionally poor in this category, when the individual with NCD has at least a tertiary level of education, the probability of household incurring CHE reduced while having a female-headed household increased the probability of incurring CHE for poor households. On the other hand, health insurance and improved wealth quintile reduced the probability of incurring CHE by the poor.

At the 40% threshold, having a household member with cancer still increased the probability of incurring CHE by 21%, and an increase in household size also increased the probability of incurring CHE by 7%. On the other, having a member with NCD who has tertiary education reduced the probability of incurring CHE by 7%. Similar to the findings from the other threshold levels are the effects of an improved wealth quintile and seeking healthcare at a state healthcare facility. Table 5 also showed that for the multidimensionally poor, at 40% threshold, having a large household size and a female-headed household increases the probability of incurring CHE by 7% each, while having health insurance reduced the probability of incurring CHE by 56%.

3.5 Impoverishment

The findings on NCD-related impoverishment depicted in Figs. 3 indicated that less than one percent of the participants lived below the international poverty line of $1.90 daily. However, about 16% of households with NCD patients lived below the World Bank poverty line for lower-middle-income countries defined as $3.20 daily after adjusting for the current exchange rate of (1$ = N360) and the household size. This proportion increased to 28% and 55% respectively after deducting NCD-related out-of-pocket expenditure, while about 45% were not affected after considering their monthly cost of illness. By implication, at least 25% of the households with members having NCDs were pushed into poverty monthly due to their out-of-pocket payment. This is expected because even without capturing the cost of illness, over 50% of Nigerians live below

Table 4. Factors influencing CHE at different thresholds

Characteristics	10% CHE			25% CHE			40% CHE		
	Entire sample	Non-poor	Poor	Entire sample	Non-poor	Poor	Entire sample	Non-poor	Poor
Chronic respiratory	−0.188 (−0.060)	−0.192	−0.227	0.227 (0.072)*	0.272*	0.317	0.147 (0.040)	0.169	0.429
Cancer	0.243 (0.068)*	0.349*	−0.002	0.637 (0.216)***	0.736**	0.179	0.665 (0.208)***	0.697***	0.387
Diabetes	0.074 (0.022)	0.113	−0.209	0.014 (0.004)	0.023	0.066	−0.074 (−0.018)	−0.066	0.055
Age	0.011 (0.003)	0.005	0.026	−0.036 (−0.011)**	−0.043**	−0.020	−0.019 (−0.005)	−0.040*	0.035
Age squared	<0.001 (< 0.001)	<0.001	<0.001	<0.001 (< 0.001)*	<0.001**	<0.001	<0.001 (< 0.001)*	<0.001)**	<0.001
Marital status	−0.202 (−0.060)	−0.312	0.038	0.718 (0.225)***	0.793***	0.377	0.772 (0.207)***	0.891***	0.479*
Educational status	−0.046 (−0.014)	−0.122	−0.048	−0.147 (−0.046)	−0.075	−0.601*	−0.276 (−0.074)*	−0.134	−0.988**
Employment status	−0.100 (−0.030)	−0.104	−0.135	−0.147 (−0.046)	−0.116	−0.268	−0.124 (−0.033)	−0.028	−0.266
Household size	0.138 (0.041)	0.098	0.338	0.223 (0.070)**	0.084	0.760***	0.244 (0.066)**	0.124	0.671***

(*continued*)

Table 4. *(continued)*

Characteristics	10% CHE			25% CHE			40% CHE		
	Entire sample	Non-poor	Poor	Entire sample	Non-poor	Poor	Entire sample	Non-poor	Poor
Gender of household head	−0.230 (−0.069)	−0.414***	0.249	0.221 (0.069)	0.118	0.568**	0.139 (0.037)	0.005	0.678**
Education level of HH	0.086 (0.026)	0.082	0.216	−0.013 (−0.004)	−0.103	0.27	0.109 (0.029)	−0.001	0.45
Employment status of HH	−0.026 (−0.008)	−0.159	0.328	0.061 (0.019)	−0.073	0.465	0.197 (0.053)	0.149	0.296
Health insurance status	0.076 (0.023)	0.164	−0.193	−0.083 (−0.026)	−0.002	−0.590**	−0.060 (−0.016)	0.01	−0.564**
Wealth quintile									
Poor	−0.139 (0.041)	0.113	0.106	−0.387 (−0.128)**	−0.421**	−0.067	−0.287 (−0.084)*	−0.137	−0.098
Neither poor nor wealthy	−0.103 (0.031)**	−0.098	−0.053	−0.533 (−0.17)***	−0.493**	−0.602*	−0.51 (−0.139)***	−0.229**	−1.033**
Wealthy	−0.023 (0.007)***	−0.006*	−0.220*	−0.214 (−0.073)**	−0.154**	−0.418**	−0.172 (−0.052)**	−0.060**	−0.535
Wealthiest	−0.104 (−0.033)**	−0.115***	−0.151*	−0.424 – 0.140)**	−0.462**	−0.107	−0.371 (−0.106)**	−0.227*	0.012

(continued)

Table 4. *(continued)*

Characteristics	10% CHE			25% CHE			40% CHE		
	Entire sample	Non-poor	Poor	Entire sample	Non-poor	Poor	Entire sample	Non-poor	Poor
Healthcare facility									
State facility	0.375 (0.115)***	0.355***	0.598**	0.425 (0.138)***	0.480***	0.451*	0.360 (0.097)***	0.434***	
Private facility	0.334 (0.104)**	0.323**	0.557*	−0.030 (−0.009)	0.072	−0.218	0.179 (0.045)	0.302*	
Multidimensional poverty	0.277 (0.083)**			−0.040 (−0.013)			0.026 (0.007)		
Constant	0.385**	0.874*	−0.260	−0.051	0.112	−0.483	−1.058**	−0.991*	−1.786*
Wald chi2(18)	40.31	36.44	14.32	91.31	78.78	34.78	81.44	69.87	35.32
Prob > chi2	0.0046	0.0093	0.0844	<0.001	<0.000	0.0149	<0.001	<0.001	0.0128
Log pseudolikelihood	−446.252	−355.84	−83.866	−463.678	−348.001	−101.282	−400.876	−297.165	−87.0965

Note: in Table 4 Probit regression coefficients are given and their average marginal effects are in parenthesis. *,**,*** indicate significance at 10%, 5% and 1% respectively. HH represents the household head. The reference category of marital status is unmarried. Reference category for educational status are those who are unemployed. The reference category for gender is male, while that of household size is below six members. Health insurance status represents being covered and MDPS represents being multidimensionally poor. Meanwhile, the wealth quintile is referenced against the lowest quintile (poor).

the international poverty line (World Bank, n.d) while Aregbesola and Khan (2018) established that over 90% of Nigerians are live below the poverty line.

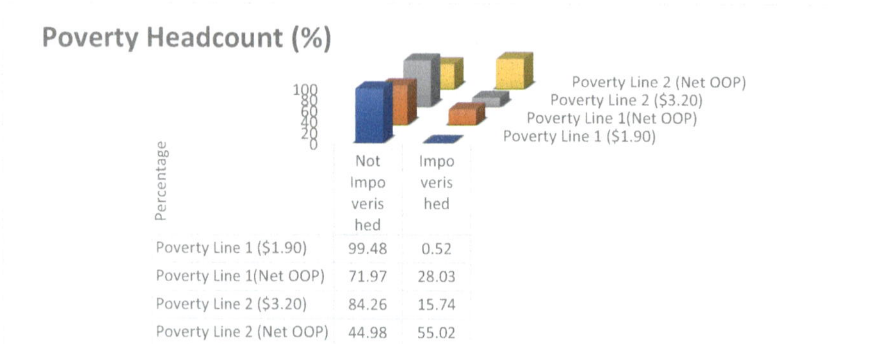

Fig. 3. Percentage of the population living below the poverty line Source: Fieldwork (2019)

Further analysis of the correlates of impoverishment (Table 5) among those with NCDs suggest that a unit increase in the household size above 5 will increase the probability of impoverishment by 27% while having a female-headed household increased the probability of being impoverished by 8%. Furthermore, having an insurance cover reduced the probability of being impoverished by 3% and an increase in the wealth quintile of the household decreased the probability of being impoverished. This is in tandem with Minh and Tran (2012) who asserted that the insurance has a modest influence on impoverishment since co-payment is involved.

Some of the participants in the in-depth interview explained their view as reported below

"The drugs I am asked to buy cost between 6000 and 7000. Just drugs! Sometimes it may not even last me for the whole month. As a pensioner who retired from a state where our pension has not been paid for so long, it is serious. Even though it is not supposed to be big money if the economy was good and things are normal, but in truth, this is where we have found ourselves" ***(A 65 years old female with Asthma)***

"Health insurance makes a lot of things cheap for me. I collect the drugs at almost no cost, even when I pay 1000, it doesn't even matter because I know the drugs that I am given cost much more than that. The other day, they didn't have the drugs I wanted, when I got to a pharmacy outside and I bought it with my money, then I realized I how much I have been enjoying." ***(A 51 years old female with Hypertension)***

Overall, NCDs induce catastrophic health expenditure and lead to impoverishment particularly for households in the lowest socio-economic quintile.

Table 5. Factors associated with impoverishment headcount

Explanatory variables	Coefficient	Marginal effect	Robust std. error	95% CI
Chronic respiratory	−0.002	−0.001	0.041	(−0.082 0.080)
Cancer	0.321	0.108**	0.054	(0.002 0.214)
Diabetes	−0.087	−0.030	0.038	(−0.104 0.044)
Gender of household head[a]	0.217	0.075*	0.025	(0.059 0.158)
Household size[b]	0.786	0.272***	0.032	(0.122 0.005)
Education of HH[c]	−0.122	−0.042	0.040	(−0.004 0.154)
Employment of HH[d]	0.094	0.032	0.027	(0.219 0.324)
Insurance status[e]	−0.077	−0.027*	0.037	(0.114 0.029)
MDP status[f]	−0.042	−0.015	0.040	(−0.046 0.111)
MDPS#Age (non-poor)[g]	−0.508	−0.108	0.033	(−0.039 0.092)
MDPS#Age (poor)[g]	−0.014	−0.059	0.038	(−0.089 0.060)
Poor	0.094	0.032	0.047	(−0.060 0.123)
Neither poor nor wealthy	−0.261	−0.091*	0.052	(−0.193 0.012)
Wealthy	−0.278	−0.097*	0.052	(−0.199 0.005)
Wealthiest	−0.548	−0.192***	0.052	(−0.295−0.090)
State facility	0.458	0.160***	0.034	(0.093 0.227)
Private facility	0.231	0.082**	0.041	(<0.001 0.163)
Constant	−0.200			
Wald Chi2	149.03			
Prob > chi2	<0.001			
Log pseudolikelihood	−576.851			

Note: in Table 5, reference categories a, b, c, d, e, f, g represents having a female household head, having less than five members of the household, household having at least secondary education, unemployed household head, uninsured household, and multidimensionally non-poor respectively.
Source: Fieldwork (2019)

4 Strengths and Limitations

This study employed a facility-based approach of data collection in assessing the economic burden of NCDs and poverty in Southwestern Nigeria, hence it was able to capture the burden of the prominent NCDs directly. However, unlike household surveys there was no comparison of cost between those who exhibited appropriate healthcare behaviour and those who did not. Secondly, the prevalence cost of illness approach (cost of illness measured at a point in time) was conducted in this study, hence, the cost of illness over the individual's lifetime (the incidence approach) was not captured.

5 Conclusion and Recommendation

The summary of the study underscores that a significant proportion of the people with NCDs are elderly and uninsured and a remarkable number of those who sought healthcare at these facilities are not poor. Also, a considerable proportion of households face catastrophic health expenditures and are impoverished as a result of NCDs. Therefore, NCD induced health expenditure is significantly associated with economic distress that can aggravate poverty. Based on the findings of the study which underscore that majority of the people who sought healthcare for NCDs were not extremely poor; there is a need to provide affordable healthcare facilities with the capacity to handle NCDs in strategic locations which will spur accessibility to healthcare for the poor. Additionally, given that a remarkable population of people with NCDs were adults of working-age, and less than 30% of the individuals with NCDs were covered by health insurance, there is a need to strategically sensitize Nigerians on the benefits of subscribing to the health insurance which has the potential to reduce out-of-pocket cost on NCDs and ameliorate appropriate healthcare-seeking behaviour.

Compliance with Ethical Standards

Conflict of Interest: The authors declare hat they have no conflict of interest.

Ethical Approval: All procedures performed in this study involving human participants were in accordance with the ethical standards of the Health Research Ethics Committee defined in the ethical clearance obtained from the of all nine hospitals.

Informed Consent: Informed consent was obtained from all participants after explaining to them the objectives of the study and assuring them of confidentiality of all information provided. The data collection process was non-invasive and participants were also allowed to withdraw from the survey at any time.

Funding: No external funding was obtained.

References

Abegunde, D.O., Mathers, C.D., Adam, T., Ortegon, M., Strong, K.: The burden and costs of chronic diseases in low-income and middle-income countries. Lancet **370**, 1929–1938 (2007)

Adisa, O.: Investigating determinants of catastrophic health spending among poorly insured elderly households in urban Nigeria. Int. J. Equity Health **14**, 79 (2015). https://doi.org/10.1186/s12939-015-0241-4

Akawu, F.A., Agum, C.: Impact of poverty on access to healthcare facilities and services in nigeria: a study of Nasarawa state. J. Econ. Sustain. Dev. **9**(6), 1–9 (2018)

Alkire, S., Santos, M.E.: Measuring acute poverty in the developing world: robustness and scope of the multidimensional poverty index. World Dev. **5**, 251–274 (2014)

Aregbesola, B.S., Khan, S.M.: Determinants of catastrophic health expend Nigeria. Euro. J. Health Econ. (2017). https://doi.org/10.1007/s10198-017-0899-1

Aregbesola, B.S., Khan, S.M.: Out-of-pocket payments, catastrophic health expenditure and poverty among households in Nigeria. Int. J. Health Policy Manage. **7**(9), 798–806 (2018). https://doi.org/10.15171/ijhpm.2018.19

Bryman, A., Cramer, D.: Quantitative Data Analysis for Social Scientists. Taylor & Frances/Routledge, Florence, KY, US (1990)

City Population. Nigeria: States and Cities - Population Statistics, Maps, Charts, Weather and Web Information (2018). https://citypopulation.de/Nigeria-Cities.html

Datta, K.B., Husain, M.J., Husain, M.M., Kostova, D.: Non-communicable disease-attributable medical expenditures, household financial stress and impoverishment in Bangladesh. Popul. Health **6**, 252–258 (2018)

Engelgau, M.M., Karan, A., Mahal, A.: The economic impact of non-communicable diseases on households in India. Glob. Health **8**, 9 (2012). https://doi.org/10.1186/1744-8603-8-9

Janssens, W., Goedecke, J., Bree, G.J., Aderibigbe, S.A., Akande, T.M., Mesnard, A.: The financial burden of non-communicable chronic diseases in rural Nigeria: wealth and gender heterogeneity in health care utilization and health expenditures. PLoS ONE **11**(11), 121–166 (2016)

Kavosi, Z., Delavari, H., Keshtkaran, A., Setoudehzadeh, F.: Catastrophic health expenditures and coping strategies in households with cancer patients in Shiraz Namazi hospital. Middle East J. Cancer **5**(1), 13–22 (2014)

Kien, V.D., Minh, H.V., Ngoc, B.B., Phuong, T.B., Ngan, T.T., Quam, M.B.: Inequalities in household catastrophic health expenditure and impoverishment associated with non-communicable diseases in Chi Linh, Hai Duong. Vietnam Asia Pac. J. Public Health **29**(5S), 35S–44S (2017)

Leng, A., Jing, J., Nicholas, S., Wang, J.: Catastrophic health expenditure of cancer patients at the end-of-life: a retrospective observational study in China. BMC Palliat. Care. **18** (43), 1–10 (2019)

Li, Y., Wu, Q., Xu, L., Legge, D., Hao, Y., Gao, L., Ning, N., Wan, G.: Factors affecting catastrophic health expenditure and impoverishment from medical expenses in China: policy implications of universal health insurance. Bull. World Health Organ. **90**, 664–671 (2012)

Minh, H.V., Tran, B.X.: Assessing the household financial burden associated with the chronic non-communicable diseases in a rural district of Vietnam. Glob. Health Action **5**, 18892 (2012)

Mirelman, A.J., Rose, S., Khan, J.A.M., Ahmed, S., Peters, D.H., Niessen, L.W., Trujillo, A.J.: The relationship between non-communicable disease occurrence and poverty—evidence from demographic surveillance in Matlab. Bangladesh Health Policy Plan. **31**(6), 785–792 (2016)

Multidimensional Poverty Peer Network (MPPN, n. d). National Multidimensional Poverty Index for Nigeria. https://mppn.org/nigeria-national-mpi/. Accessed 20 Jan 2020

Mwai, N.D.: Non-Communicable Diseases in Kenya: Economic Effects And Risk Factors (Ph.D Thesis) (2014). http://erepository.uonbi.ac.ke/bitstream/handle/11295/77585/%20MwaiNon%20communicable%20diseases%20in%20Kenya%3A%20economic%20effects%20and%20risk%20factors.pdf?sequence=1&isAllowed=y. Accessed 15 Jan 2019

Niessen, L.W., Mohan, D., Akuoku, J.K., Mirelman, J., Ahmed, S.Y., Koehlmoos, T.P., Peters, D.H.: Tackling socioeconomic inequalities and non-communicable diseases in low-income and middle-income countries under the Sustainable Development agenda. *The Lancet Taskforce on NCDs and economics*. Retrieved indicate the date it was retrieved from. http://doi.org/10.1016/S0140-6736(18)30482-3

Ogha, O.S., Madukwe, O.O., Chukwuonye, I.I., Onyenoro,U. U., Ukegbu, A.U., Okpechi, I.G.: Prevalence and determinants of hypertension in Abia State Nigeria: results from the Abia State Non-Communicable Diseases and Cardiovascular Risk Factors Survey. Ethn. Dis. **23**(2): 16–1-7 (2013)

Okediji, P.T., Ojo, A.O., Ojo, A.I., Ojo, A.S., Ojo, O.E., Abioye-Kuteyi, E.A.: The economic impacts of chronic illness on households of patients in Ile-Ife. South-W. Niger. Cureus **9**(10), (2017)

Onoka, C.A., Onwujekwe, O.E., Hanson, K., Uzochukwu, B.S.: Examining catastrophic health expenditures at variable thresholds using household consumption expenditure diaries. Trop. Med. Int. Health **16**(10), 1334–1341 (2011)

Onyeonoro, U.O., Ogah, O.S., Ukegbu, A.U., Chukwuonye, I.I., Okechukwu, O.M., Moses, A.O.: Urban–rural differences in healthcare-seeking pattern of residents of Abia state, Nigeria, and the implication in the control of NCDs. Health Serv. Insights **9**, 29–36 (2016). https://doi.org/10.4137/HSI.S31865

Owoeye, O.B., Olaniyan, O.: Economic Cost of Tobacco-Related Diseases in Nigeria: a Study of three Hospitals in Ibadan, Southwest Nigeria. Health Policy Training and Research Programme, Department of Economics University of Ibadan, Nigeria (2015)

Russell, S.: Illuminating cases: understanding the economic burden of illness through case study household research. Health Policy Plan. **20**(5), 277–289 (2004). https://doi.org/10.1093/heapol/czi035

Tagoe, H.A.: Urban Poverty and Household Non-Communicable Disease Burden in Ghana: A Case Study Of Ashiedu Keteke Sub-metropolitan Area (Ph. D Thesis) (2014). http://ugspace.ug.edu.gh/handle/123456789/8176. Accessed 15 Aug 2019

Wagstaff, A., Doorslaer, V.E.: Catastrophe and impoverishment in paying for healthcare: with applications to Vietnam, 1993–98. Health Econ. **12**, 921–934 (2003)

Wang, Q., Brenner, S., Kalmus, O., Banda, H.T., Allegri, M.: The economic burden of chronic non-communicable diseases in rural Malawi: an observational study. BMC Health Serv. Res. **16**, 457 (2016). https://doi.org/10.1186/s12913-016-1716-8

World Bank. Poverty and Health (2014). https://www.worldbank.org/en/topic/health/brief/poverty-health

World Bank (n.d). Nigeria, Poverty Headcount. Retried from http://povertydata.worldbank.org/poverty/country/NGA

World Health Organization (WHO, 2011). https://www.who.int/healthsystems/publications/abuja_report_aug_2011.pdf?ua=1. Accessed 10 June 2019

World Health Organization (WHO, 2018). Non-communicable Disease. Key Facts. https://www.who.int/news-room/fact-sheets/detail/noncommunicable-diseases

World Health Organization (WHO, 2019). Nigeria fulfils commitment, launches Plan for the Prevention and Control of Non-Communicable Diseases| WHO| Regional Office for Africa. https://www.afro.who.int/news/nigeria-fulfils-commitment-launches-plan-prevention-and-control-non-communicable-diseases

Xu, K., Evans, D.B., Kawabata, K., Zeramdini, R., Klavus, J., Murray, C.J.L.: Household catastrophic health expenditure: a multi-country analysis. Lancet **362**, 111–117 (2003)

Yiltok, A., Adedeji, H.O., Ofakunrin, I.A., Ejeliogu, A.O., Okpe, E.: Prevalence and pattern of non-communicable diseases in children in Jos, Nigeria. Br. J. Med. Med. Res. **19**(5), 1–7 (2017)

Vendors' Willingness Drivers for Participation in Public Electronic Procurement System, Ilala District, Tanzania

Meshack Siwandeti[1](✉), Camilius Sanga[2], Abswaidi Mfanga[3], and Faustine Panga[4]

[1] Procurement and Supplies Management Department, College of Business Education, P.O. Box 3168, Mwanza, Tanzania
[2] Informatics Centre for Information and Communication Technology (ICT) Department, Sokoine University of Agriculture (SUA), P.O. Box 3000, Chuo Kikuu, Morogoro, Tanzania
sanga@sua.ac.tz
[3] Information and Communication Technology (ICT) Department, Moshi Co-operative University (MoCU), P.O. Box 474, Moshi, Tanzania
[4] Marketing, Procurement and Supply Management Department, Moshi Co-operative University (MoCU), P.O. Box 474, Moshi, Tanzania

Abstract. Vendors' participation in public e-procurement system termed as a means for government to achieve her objectives on procurement operations. However, little is known about vendors' willingness drives to participate in public e-procurement system. This paper investigates vendors' willingness drivers for participation in public e-procurement system. The objective was to identify the drivers with influence on vendors' willingness for participation in public electronic system. The study adopted a cross-sectional research design. The study was conducted in Ilala District due to concentrations for eligible vendors. The study randomly sampled 300 vendors eligible to participate in public e-procurement system. Public Procurement Regulatory Authority, Government Procurement Services Agency and Medical Stores Department were purposively selected to provide key informants. Quantitative data were collected using structured questionnaire and Key Informants Interview (KIIs) guide used for qualitative data. Quantitative data were analysed by multiple regression for vendors' willingness drivers' influence on public electronic procurement system participation. Qualitative data were analysed using content analysis by thematic approach. The study found significant at $p < 0.05$ on transparent, corruption practice, paper work and perceived usefulness as drivers for vendors' willingness for participation in public e-procurement system. The study concludes that, vendors are willing to participate in public e-procurement system subjective to significant willingness' drivers. The study therefore recommends that, the public e-procurement system's stakeholders must improve on transparent and corruption free zone with awareness creation to attract more vendors to participate. The practical implication is that transparency and corruption free is crucial concern for vendors' willingness drivers to participate in public electronic procurement system.

Keywords: Vendors' willingness drivers · Participation · Public electronic procurement

J. N. Mojekwu et al. (Eds.): *Sustainable Education and Development*, pp. 445–454, 2021.
https://doi.org/10.1007/978-3-030-68836-3_38

1 Introduction

Procurement has attracted attention in many countries due to its significant contribution to the economy. The World Bank estimated public procurement accounts around one-fifth of global gross domestic product, also estimated expenditure on public procurement to account approximately from 15% to 20% of the Gross Domestic Product (GDP) in developing countries (World Bank 2016). Thus, public procurement has to be a critical area where resources can be properly managed and give a significant improvement to the economy, unfortunately, public procurement has been experiencing corruption and mismanagement, leading to inefficient procurement functions under traditional procurement (Mole 2015). In order to improve procurement efficiency, public electronic procurement system has been adopted as one of important strategy, including encouraging vendors participation as the key partner in public procurement (Makoba et al. 2017; Seo and Mehedi 2016).

In Tanzania, the expenditure on public procurement range from 41% to 75% of the total government budget (URT 2018). As a part of its advocacy strategies toward enhanced transparency and fairness practices, competitive bidding, value for money and modern procurement, Public Procurement Regulatory Authority (PPRA) based on the public procurement laws, has developed the Tanzania National e-Procurement System (URT 2014). This is a full-fledged e-procurement system, supporting the entire public procurement circle – from planning to contract management. Where, according and in line with Regulation 343 of GN No 446, the system comprises features like: User registrations; e-Tendering; e-Purchasing; e-Auction; e-Payment and e-Contract management (Mlinga 2018). The public e-procurement system requires public bidding process and its related functions between procuring entities (PEs) and vendors to implement online procurement through public e-procurement system (Ahimbisibwe et al. 2016).

Despite the effort to integrate public procurement functions and its proceedings between vendors and PEs into public e-procurement system, there is reluctance particularly on the vendors' side, resulting into late implementation of public e-procurement system where the PEs has to be forced to use incompetent suppliers due lack of competent suppliers in the database for the required competition (URT 2018). Vendors' willingness drivers for participating in public e-procurement system plays important role toward commitment and trustfulness on the use and achievements of associated benefits of e-procurement by the government (Barsemoi et al. 2014). Until August 2018, only 400 responsive vendors out of 9740 eligible vendors, equivalent to 4.1% registered and used the system for their procurement process with PEs which is significantly low compared to effort government invested on promoting the system to them (Daoud and Ibrahim Daoud and Ibrahim, 2017; Mlinga 2018). Scholars including Zhou et al. (2018); Altayyar and Beaumont-Kerridge (2016); Cousins et al. (2011), anticipated factors that attract vendors' participation in e-procurement in connection with Information Communication Technology (ICT) infrastructures, where: Information Technology (IT) experts, financial aspects, trust, habit, cost saving, usefulness and ease of use as guided by Diffusion of Innovation theory (DOI), but does not reflect willingness toward vendors' participation in public e-procurement system.

Scholars like De Coninick et al. (2018); Flynn and Davis (2016), concentrated on implementation, policy compliance and factors for adoption of e-procurement in public procurement like procurement process, a community built around digital sphere and company culture, while the vital angle on vendors' willingness drivers for participation in public e-procurement system left behind. While, Seo et al. (2018); Altayyar and Beaumont-Kerridge (2016), supported argument that, effective implementation of e-procurement system by public depends much on vendors' willingness, commitment and readiness to participate in public e-procurement system. Moreover, despite the undisputable benefits of public e-procurement, the understanding toward vendors' willingness to engage in public e-procurement system is limited as proved from current rate for registered vendors in Tanzania National electronic Procurement system, on the study financial year 2018/2019, less than 20% of eligible vendors only participated willingly (URT 2018).

Therefore, this study examined vendors' willingness drivers influence for participation in public e-procurement system. The study specific objective was: To determine influence of vendors' willingness drivers in public e-procurement system participation.

2 Theoretical Review

The study was guided by Diffusion of Innovation Theory (DOI) by Rogers (2003) as the main theory and Participation Theory by Midgley et al. (1986) as supportive theory. The main reason of using two theories was the nature of the study which measures the acceptance and diffusion of innovation and on the other side, measure readiness on engaging in development projects willingly for beneficiaries of both involved sides.

2.1 Diffusion of Innovation Theory (DOI)

The theory of Diffusion of Innovation (DOI) insists that technology adoption is a function of a variety of factors including relative advantage and ease of use which both termed as drivers' for willingness. Scholars' review across a range of disciplines led also to conclude that the diffusion process displayed patterns and regularities, across a range of conditions, cultures and innovations, the influence of the spread of new idea: innovation itself, time, communication channel and social system, where mainly relies on human capital (Rogers 2003).

The DOI theory developed new framework with five stages: Knowledge, Persuasion, Decision, Implementation and Confirmation; however, the individual may reject the previous decision if he or she encounters difficulties in adapting to the innovation. Thus, the willingness on innovation-decision process involves searching for information that can be used to reduce uncertainty about the innovation (Rogers 2003).

Main criticism is lacking of cohesion, which leave the theory stagnant with difficult to apply in consistency to new problems (vendors' willingness drivers). Therefore, Participation theory was adopted in order to provide measurable construct relative advantage (drivers) for willingness to participate in a given government project.

2.2 Participation Theory

The participation theory helped the world community to recognize that, suffering on lack development was due to poor involvement in development decisions, implementation and benefits (Store 1999). This study is using participation theory to backup vendors' willingness drivers aspects in participation of public e-procurement system project, where the theory suggest that, acceptance for involvement in certain project depend on a efficiency of use and benefits to be acquired from it (Altayyar and Beaumont-Kerridge 2016).

The theory criticized by traditional inherent were decisions based on top-down approaches, that focused on single disciplines and reductionist paradigms (Agrawal and Gibson 1999), but the advanced participatory approach marked the weakness and made emphasis for popular participation as the remedy of these shortcomings, and proved that, if an individual (vendor) is willing for participation in given project, then it possible to make unique contributions for better implementation of that project (Mompati and Prinsen 2000) (Fig. 1).

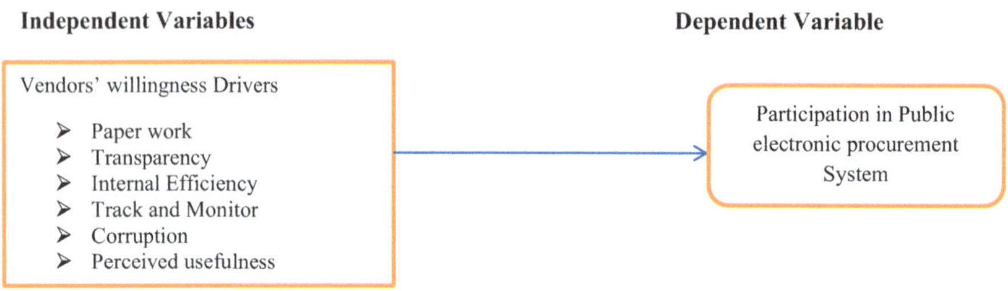

Fig. 1. Conceptual model of the study

3 Methodology

The study adopted cross-sectional research design since it allowed the collection of data with interaction of one variable over another at a time. Data was collected once, hence, allowed the use of variety of analytical techniques, and use of different methods for data collection (Flick 2011; Creswell 2009).

The study was conducted in Ilala District in Dar es Salaam region due to the presence of 1110 vendors with full access of supportive infrastructures (like Internet, reliable power supply) out of 9740 eligible vendors countrywide (URT 2018). The sample size was 300 respondents adjusted from minimum sample size obtained as per Comrey and Lee 1992 (Lingard and Rowlinson 2006). The minimum sample size reached by the use of Cochran' finite population formula (Cochran 1977). Get n_0 from infinite first:

$$n_0 = \frac{z^2pq}{e^2} = \frac{(1.96)^2(0.5)(0.5)}{(0.05)^2} = 384 \quad (1)$$

Cochran (1977) formula for finite population was used to determined sample size for vendors

$$n = \frac{no}{1 + ((no - 1)/)N} = \frac{384}{1 + \left(\frac{384-1}{1110}\right)} = 286 \quad (2)$$

Simple random sampling technique was used to obtain respondents whereby the list for vendors obtained from GPSA in framework agreement contract under Financial Year (FY) 2018/2019. Purposive sampling technique used to pick one system expert as Key Informant from pioneer system institutions, which are Public Regulatory Authority, Government Procurement Service Agency and Medical Stores Department.

Qualitative data were collected using Key Informants Interviews (KIIs). Three (3) key informants obtained government institutions, tasked the main operation to introduce and control the system where empowered to work closely with vendors doing business with the government. Done obtained here were analysed stage-wise: recorded, transcribed, categorised, coded and grouped into themes (vendors willingness' drivers) for public e-procurement system participation and then analysed by content analysis technique.

Quantitative data were collected using structured questionnaire and analysis done by using multiple linear regressions for determining vendors' willingness drivers' influence toward participation in public e-procurement system. Vendors' willingness drivers were scaled by using factor analysis by Principal Component Analysis (PCA) method for the reason to get the most prevalent drivers which influencing vendors' willingness toward public e-procurement system participation, for the best principle of parsimony (Occam's razor). Threshold of KMO and bartlett' test spherity, eigenvalue considered, where 6 out 12 drivers, extracted and retained for further statistical analysis. Thereafter, in order to determine the influence of these extracted drivers on vendors' willingness for participation in public e-procurement system, a multiple regression model was used. The model was selected because the dependent variable (Public e-procurement system participation) was a continuous variable.

Outliers were checked for both independent and dependent variable through the standardised residual values and none of them had values less than −3.3 or above 3.3 as recommended by Tabachnick and Fidell (2007), thus, there were no outliers. Multicollinearity was tested by observing Variance Inflation Factors (VIF) as indicated in Table 3, where VIF should be far from 10 said to be affected and not independent. The test done found none of variable inter-correlation equal or above 0.8 thus, no multicollinearity (Fidell 2009). Normality assumption where tested using histogram where the bell shape required cutting through 0 and ranging between −3 to 3 found. Lastly, linearity assumption was observed (there linear relationship between the independent variable and dependent variable) as tested using scatter plots.

Sample size adequacy, was tested using formula proposed by Tabachnick and Fidell (2007), that a minimum sample size is given by $50 + 8$ (m), where "m" is number of variable in the model and there should be 20 respondents per variable at least. As per Table 1, extracted numbers drivers on vendors' willingness in public e-procurement participation were 6, minimum sample size was $50 + 8(6) = 98$ required, and the current study has sample size of 300 respondents, hence assumption satisfied. Examining assumption of independence, the Durbin Watson test used, where statistic value close to 2 suggest lack of serial correlation while value far from 2 suggest serial correlation, and from the current study, Durbin Watson is 1.827, thus assumption satisfied.

The multiple regression model used was:

$$Y = \beta_0 + \beta_1 X_1 + \beta_2 X_2 + \ldots + \beta_6 X_6 + e \quad (3)$$

Table 1. Factor Analysis for vendors' willingness drivers, reliability and validity

Aspect	Factor loading	Eigenvalues % of Var	Cumulative variance	Cronbach's Alpha	AVE	CR	KMO	Bartlett's Test
			63.671%	0.860	0.800	0.913	0.893	P < 0.001
Track and monitor	0.878	63.671						
paper work	0.851	10.135						
Internal efficiency	0.808	8.390						
Transparency	0.764	8.084						
Perceived usefulness	0.754	5.476						
Corrupt free	0.720	4.244						

NB: Determinants for the correlation matrices was > 0.00001 indicating absence multicolinearity, AVE = Average Variance Extracted, CR = Composite Reliability.

Where:
Y = Participation mean score, X_1, X_2,..... X_6 = The independent variables
$\beta_0, \beta_1, \ldots \beta_6$ = regression coefficients
e = error term

4 Findings and Discussions

4.1 Vendors' Willingness Drivers and Public e-procurement System Participation.

The vendors' willingness in public e-procurement participation was measured by using drivers which were contribution of the system to vendors. Results on vendors' willingness drivers show that perceived usefulness, reduce paper work, ensure transparency, improve internal efficiency, corrupt free and enable work track and monitor, all lie within agree mean, which implies that, vendors willingness are driven by presence of these vital contribution from the system to their business, therefore, vendors are willing to participate in public e-procurement system if their assured on achieving these highlighted benefits, see Table 2.

4.2 The Influence of Vendors' Willingness Drivers on Public e-procurement System Participation

To determine vendors' willingness drivers influence on participation in public e-procurement system, multiple regression was run. The overall result on the model shows r square as 0.297 implying that vendor' willingness drivers predicted system participation by 30%. P value was less than 0.05 indicating that vendors' willingness drivers had a strong significant influence with public e-procurement system participation. The results

Table 2. Descriptive Statistics on vendors' willingness drivers (n = 300)

	Mean	S.D	Median	Mode
Public e-procurement participation	4.41	0.746		
Perceived usefulness	4.0733	0.97526	4	4
Reduce paper work	4.2233	1.05697	4	5
Ensure transparency	4.6200	0.63002	5	5
Improve internal efficiency	4.2100	0.99794	4	4
Corruption free	4.2433	0.99032	4	5
Enable track and monitor	4.0567	0.94327	4	4

also revealed that Durbin Watson was 1.827, which was not higher than 2.5; hence, the model was a good fit. Further, Analysis of Variance (ANOVA), disclosed (p = 0.000) implying that the model was a good fit for study. Degrees of freedom were 6 while F test was 20.668 reflect the adequacy on sample size used.

The influence of vendors' willingness drivers toward public e-procurement system participation was measured by the results from multiple regression analysis on Table 3. The model shows that perceived benefits, (p = 0.000), t value was 5.281; B was 1.688 meaning that there were evidence against the null hypothesis, and data fit in the given model, Variance inflation factor (VIF) was all far below 10 and tolerance is below 1 which meant that there was no serious multicollinearity with variables.

Table 3. Multiple regression results on vendors' willingness drivers influence on participation in public e-procurement system

	Unstd. coefficients			Std. coefficients			
Variables (Drivers)	β	S.E	β	t-value	P-value	Collinearity tolerance	Statistics VIF
(Constant)	1.688	0.320		5.281	0.000***		
Perceived usefulness	0.147	0.049	0.193	3.031	0.003***	0.594	1.683
Track and monitor	0.059	0.043	0.074	1.359	0.175	0.805	1.243
Paper work	0.098	0.046	0.139	2.116	0.035***	0.555	1.802
Transparency	0.125	0.06	0.105	2.081	0.038***	0.934	1.070
Internal efficiency	0.063	0.052	0.083	1.212	0.226	0.507	1.973
Corruption free	0.148	0.048	0.198	3.101	0.002***	0.588	1.700

*** means Significant at $p < 0.05$

The variables such as perceived usefulness ($\beta = 0.147$; $t = 3.031$; $p = 0.003$) paper work ($\beta = 0.098$; $t = 2.116$; $p = 0.035$), transparency ($\beta = 0.125$; $t = 2.081$; $p = 0.038$) and corruption free ($\beta = 0.148$; $t = 3.101$; $p = 0.002$) were significant ($p < 0.05$). This implies that, significant vendors' willingness drivers were capable to influence participation in public e-procurement system. And this only possible if the system can promise and consider being useful with associated benefits, combat corruption by spread of information equally to all vendors, being transparent and reduce the use of papers-work system in procurement process, so vendors can see worthiness to participate. Finding also show that, internal efficiency ($\beta = 0.063$; $t = 1.212$; $p = 0.226$) and track and monitor ($\beta = 0.059$; $t = 1.359$; $p = 0.175$) were not significant vendors' willingness drivers for participation public e-procurement system. This implies that, vendors are not willing to participate in public e-procurement system for their internal operations which they can cater using their own policies rather willing to participate, so that they can cure external hurdles, which there internal policies cannot control them. The findings results were supported by the key informants for the argument provided below:

> "Vendors' willingness to participate in the system (public e-procurement system) derived by reduced clerical work (paper work), and control of unfair treatment from corrupt official (transparency & corruption free), but also they want the system to be more friendly and with long return on its investment (perceived usefulness)" (MSD' TANePS personnel, 7th May, 2019)

Furthermore, the study finding correspond with studies done by Mensah and Mi (2019), Seo et al. (2018); Belokrylov and Belokrylova (2017), proved that, vendors are willing to participate once conditions (drivers) fulfilled, like trust, transparent, fairness of competitions (corruption free). These clearly connect with argument from key informant on vendor's acceptance for the system:

> "Vendors are full involved on every stage, and we as project coordinator, never experienced hardship on rejection of the system, it real give us courage to speed-up our setup for full automation to all our stakeholders" (PPRA' TANePS coordinator, 8th May, 2019)

The arguments from key informants implies that, vendors' willingness to participate in public e-procurement system, were highly derived when transparency on the system development stages were maximized with vendors involvement, also supported by the participation theory as one of promising benefit of it.

4.3 Implications of the Findings on the Guiding Theories

The theoretical implication of the study is that, though the study used the Diffusion of Innovation theory (DOI) and participation theory as its basis, the naming of some variable apart from perceived usefulness, was relative advantages for innovation for participation in given project (public e-procurement system), were transparent, paper-work system, corruption, internal efficiency and tracking and monitoring, clearly supported by the both theories as main drivers for individual (vendor) to diffuse and participate in given innovation.

5 Conclusion and Recommendations

The willingness of vendors to participate and use public e-procurement system found vital on ensuring success of public projects from supply side to the government. Thus, the question on drivers lead vendors' willingness for participation in public e-procurement system was unavoidable.

The study found the vendors' willingness drivers: corrupt free, transparent, perceived usefulness and paper-work system were highly influence on public e-procurement system participation. Therefore, the study concluded that, vendors' willingness drivers have significant impact on the vendors' participation in public e-procurement system. The study therefore recommends that, system developers should engage vendors in all stages on developing public e-procurement system and make sure that, the system fulfills the expected benefits in order to maximize vendors' willingness in participation. This can be done through creating awareness and sensitization on importance and benefits of participating in the system and competitive advantage in doing business with government.

References

Ahimbisibwe, A., Wilson, T., Ronald, T.: Adoption of E-procurement technology in Uganda: Migration from the manual public procurement systems to the internet. J. Supply Chain Manag. **3**(1), 71–94 (2016)

Agrawal, A., Gibson, C.C.: Enchantment and disenchantment: the role of community in natural resource conservation. World Dev. **27**, 629–649 (1999)

Altayyar, A., Beaumont-Kerridge, J.: External factors affecting the adoption of e-procurement in Saudi Arabian's SMEs. Procedia Soc. Behav. Sci. **229**, 363–375 (2016)

Barsemoi, H., Mwangagi, P., Asienyo, B.O.: Factors influencing procurement performance in private sector in Kenya. Int. J. Innov. Appl. Stud. **9**(2), 620–632 (2014)

Belokrylov, K.A., Belokrylova, O.S.: Transparency of the governmental procurement for civil society and the factors of their efficiency. Revista ESPACIOS **38**(31), 2–6 (2017)

Cochran, R.N., Horne, F.H.: Statistically weighted principal component analysis of rapid scanning wavelength kinetics experiments. Anal. Chem. **49**(6), 846–853 (1977)

Comrey, A.L., Lee, H.B.: Interpretation and application of factor analytic results. Comrey AL, Lee HB. First Course Factor Anal. **2**, 1992 (1992)

Cousins, P.D., Lawson, B., Petersen, K.J., Handfield, R.B.: Breakthrough scanning, supplier knowledge exchange, and new product development performance. J. Prod. Innov. Manag. **28**(6), 930–942 (2011)

Creswell, J.W.: Research Design: Qualitative, Quantitative and Mixed Methods Approaches, 3rd edn. SAGE Publications Inc., Thousand Oaks (2009)

Daoud, L., Ibrahim, M.: A conceptual model of factors affecting e-procurement usage and impact among Jordanian listed firms: the moderating role of environmental uncertainty. J. Adv. Res. Bus. Manag. Stud. **9**(1), 36–44 (2017)

De Coninck, B., Viaene, S., Leysen, J.: Public procurement of innovation through increased startup participation: the case of Digipolis (Research-in-progress). In: Proceedings of the 51st Hawaii International Conference on System Sciences (2018)

Flick, U.: Introducing Research Methodology, p. 271. TJ International limited, Britain (2011)

Flynn, A., Davis, P.: Firms' experience of SME-friendly policy and their participation and success in public procurement. J. Small Bus. Enterp. Dev. **23**(3), 616–635 (2016)

Lingard, H.C., Rowlinson, S.: Sample Size in Factor Analysis: Why Size Matters. University of Hong Kong, Hong Kong (2006)
Makoba, N., Nyamagere, G., Eliufoo, H.: E-Procurement risks and mitigation: the case for tanzania construction companies. Int. J. Constr. Eng. Manag. **6**(4), 180–186 (2017)
Mensah, I.K., Mi, J.: Computer self-efficacy and e-government service adoption: the moderating role of age as a demographic factor. Int. J. Public Adm. **42**(2), 158–167 (2019)
Midgley, J., Hall, A., Hardiman, M., Narine, D.: Community participation, social development and the state, Methuen, London, New York (1986)
Mlinga, R.S.: E-procurement in Tanzania and journey toward industrialization. In: 8th PSPTB annual conference 2017. Theme: Nurturing Industrilization for Economic Transformation: Held at Arusha International Conference Centre (AICC), pp. 94–111 (2018)
Mole, S.: Introduction to Procurement and Value for Money: The Financial Regulations and Procedures: The Financial Regulations and Procedures (2015). www.campus.manchester.ac.uk/finance/, Accessed 13 Aug 2018
Mompati, T., Prinsen, G.: Ethnicity and participatory development methods in Botswana: some participants are to be seen and not heard. Dev. Pract. **10**(5), 625–637 (2000)
Rogers, E.M.: Diffusion of Innovation, 3rd edn. New York Free press, New York (2003)
Seo, J.W., Mehedi, H.M.G.: E-government efforts against corruption in Bangladesh: what we have done and what we have to do. Int. J. Polit. Sci. Diplomacy **1**(4), 107–127 (2016)
Seo, D., Tan, C.W., Warman, G.: Vendor satisfaction of E-government procurement systems in developing countries: an empirical research in Indonesia. Inf. Technol. Dev. **3**(2), 1–28 (2018)
Store, D.: Issues of integration, participation and empowerment in rural development: the case of leader in the Republic of Ireland. J. Rural. Stud. **15**, 307–315 (1999)
Tabachnick, B.G., Fidell, L.S.: Using Multivariate statistics, 5th edn., p. 1008. Peason Education, Boston (2007)
URT. The Public Procurement Regulations, (pR 2013). Government notice No. 446 published on 20/12/2013. Printed by the Government Printer, Dar es Salaam by Order of Government (2014). ISSN 0856 – 034X
URT. Notification of award to successful tenderers of framework agreements. GPSA under Ministry of Finance and Economic Affairs, pp. 1–187 (2018)
World Bank Group. World development report 2016: digital dividends. World Bank Publications (2016)
Zhou, W., Chong, A.Y.L., Zhen, C., Bao, H.: E-supply chain integration adoption: examination of buyer-supplier relationships. J. Comput. Inf. Syst. **58**(1), 58–65 (2018)

Transforming the e-waste Management Sector in Ghana: Progress on Regulatory and Institutional Strengthening

E. Awere(✉) and A. Bonoli

Department of Civil, Chemical, Environmental and Materials Engineering (DICAM), University of Bologna, via Terracini 28, 40131 Bologna, Italy
eric.awere2@unibo.it

Abstract. Informal recycling of e-waste in Ghana particularly at Agbogbloshie has attracted global attention. The environmental and health impacts of open burning of e-waste have been well researched. To avert the unsound management practices, Ghana has received extensive support from NGOs, development partners and research Institutions. This paper discusses Ghana's progress in transforming the e-waste management sector with particular emphasis on policy, regulatory and institutional strengthening. Data was collected through the review of scientific literature, local media and NGO reports. In addition, informal discussions were held with some informal e-waste recyclers at the Agbogbloshie e-waste site. E-waste specific policy/regulatory frameworks are the Hazardous and Electronic Waste Control and Management Act, 2016 (Act 917), Hazardous, Electronic and other Wastes Control and Management Regulations, 2016 (LI 2250) and Technical Guidelines on Environmentally Sound E-waste Management in Ghana. One of the greatest achievements in terms of institutional strengthening is the selection of Société Générale de Surveillance (SGS) for the collection of advance eco levy pursuant to Sect. 21 of Act 917. Amid these achievements, the following gaps require immediate attention: formalizing the e-waste sector, enforcing e-waste regulations and guidelines, intensifying public education and promoting public private partnership.

Keywords: E-waste · Formalization · Ghana · Waste management · Regulations

1 Introduction

In recent years, the consumption of electrical and electronic equipment (EEE) has increased mostly in developed countries due to increased domestic and industrial utilization (Prakash et al. 2010), falling prices and the relatively shorter replacement cycles of EEE equipment (Baldé et al. 2017). This has led to the generation of large volume of different electrical and electronic waste (e-waste) streams on a daily basis. E-waste encompasses EEE and its parts that have been discarded by its owner as waste without the intent of re-use (Step Initiative 2014). There is an increase in the global e-waste generation with most coming from the industrialized countries. Specifically, e-waste generation

J. N. Mojekwu et al. (Eds.): *Sustainable Education and Development*, pp. 455–465, 2021.
https://doi.org/10.1007/978-3-030-68836-3_39

globally increased from 33.8 Million metric tons in the year 2010 to 44.7 Million metric tons in 2016 and is expected to increase to 52.2 million metric tons in 2021 (Baldé et al. 2017) with most coming from Asia (Baldé et al. 2015).

Although Africa contributes less than 5% of the global annual e-waste generated, an estimated 75% to 80% of e-waste generated globally is shipped to Africa countries to be re-used, recycled, and disposed (CEHRT Environmental Consulting 2015; Diaz-Barriga 2013). In Ghana for example, it was estimated in 2009 that over 300 importers and distributors of EEE (formal business and informal importers) were imported up to 150,500 tonnes (70% of total imports) of second hand EEE (Amoyaw-Osei et al. 2011). About 15% of all the imports were reported to be unusable joining the recycling stream. This was attributed to the lack of e-waste laws, little to no enforcement of existing e-waste laws coupled with limited technology for sound and sustainable management of e-wastes thus presenting a major challenge for the continent. Ghana has therefore been cited as one of the African countries where e-wastes are dumped for recycling through bad practices (Amoyaw-Osei et al. 2011). Agbogbloshie, the notable e-waste hub in Ghana, is globally identified as one of the major informal e-waste recycling sites in World (Heacock et al. 2016; McElvaney 2014; Srigboh et al. 2016). The recycling practices at Agbogbloshie is horrific and threatens the fundamental human rights of workers, vulnerable population, innocent citizens and ultimately the achievement of the Sustainable Development Goals (SDGs). The technologies used to recycle the e-waste posses a lot of risk to the environment (air, land, water bodies, plants and animals) and public health (Awere et al. 2020). From resource viewpoint, improper management of e-waste leads to a loss of valuable and scarce raw materials. For instance, it is estimated that e-waste contains about 7% of the world's gold (World Economic Forum 2019). Implementation of proper e-waste management is linked to the achievement of six (6) SDGs (Goals 3, 6, 8, 11, 12 and 14) (Baldé et al. 2017). Following the global interest in the informal e-waste recycling activities in Ghana, particularly, at the Agbogbloshie e-waste site in Accra, the Government of Ghana with support from Non-Governmental Organisations (NGOs), Development Partners and Research Institutions has implemented interventions to minimize the negative impacts of the informal recycling activities.

This paper looks at the progress made in transforming the e-waste sector in Ghana. The paper focuses on Ghana's progress on policy, regulatory and institutional strengthening.

2 Overview of e-waste Management Process

E-waste collection, recycling and final disposal is performed by both the formal and informal sectors. The visible and prominent activities of the informal sector have overshadowed the formal sector. Activities of informal sector are divided into collection, refurbishments and reuse, recycling and final disposal (Oteng-Ababio 2012a).

2.1 Collection

Traditionally, waste picking is considered a job for the most marginalized members of society. Informal e-waste collectors execute door-to-door collection of e-waste from private, corporate and institutional consumers freely or at little fee. Others also scavenge for parts at solid waste dump sites. They in turn sell them to recyclers or sometimes recycle themselves. The amount earned by collectors depends on the volume of e-waste collected and sold (Yamoah, 2014). The formal sector players do not have their own house-to-house collection networks (Oteng-Ababio and Amankwaa 2014) but some companies like RLG Communications Ltd, Kassapa (Expresso) and Nokia operate some sort of take-back system (Manhart et al. 2014; Oteng-Ababio and Amankwaa 2014) but it is poorly patronized. Oteng-Ababio (2012b), reports that the informal sector collects 95% of the e-waste while the remaining 5% is collected by the formal sector.

2.2 Repairs/Refurbishment

Non-functioning EEE are repaired and sold in the Ghanaian second-hand electronics market. In certain cases, parts of dismantled e-waste are used to refurbish others. The repairers/refurbishers are strategically located for easy accessibility by EEE users to patronize their services (Amoyaw-Osei et al, 2011). They are scattered across the country even in towns where informal e-waste recycling is non-existent. Some repairers have formed associations depending on specialities. Two (2) of such associations reported are Ghana Electronic Service Technicians Association (GESTA) (with estimated membership of 1,200 nationwide) and the National Refrigeration Workshop Owners Association (NARWOA) for repair of refrigerators and air-conditioners. Not all the repairers/refurbishers belong to the associations. Expert opinion suggests that about 80% of the businesses in the refurbishing/repair sector do not belong to any association (Pwamang 2013). An estimated 111,000 tonnes of EEE are repaired yearly extending the life of these EEE by a couple of years (Amoyaw-Osei et al. 2011).

2.3 Recycling

Recyclers dismantle e-waste in separate fractions for subsequent recovery of valuable materials (such as copper, aluminium, etc.) for export or sale to middlemen in Ghana. Informal e-waste recycling is performed by scavengers and dismantlers who use rudimentary recycling methods. The recycling processes involve dismantling electrical and electronic devices with simple equipment such as chisel, hammers, pliers and screw drivers without any personal protective equipment (PPE) (Oteng-Ababio 2012a). In most cases, open burning (with polyurethane and/or old car tyres as fuels) is used to recover economically valuable materials such as copper, gold, etc. Even though the processes used by the informal sector is rudimentary, unsound and illegal, they handle a larger proportion of the e-waste stream. For example, in 2009 alone, 171,000 tons of e-waste was recycled by the informal sector (Amoyaw-Osei et al. 2011). The informal recyclers do not have environmental permits unlike the formal recyclers. The process flow diagram for informal e-waste recycling in Ghana is presented in Fig. 1. Some of the formal e-waste recyclers are City Waste Management Company Limited (Amoyaw-Osei et al. 2011; Pwamang 2013), Blancomet Recycling Company (Oteng-Ababio and Amankwaa 2014), Environwise Waste Systems, Waste Recycling Ghana Limited (Amoyaw-Osei et al. 2011), Presank Enterprise Limited, Goldline Ghana Limited, Atlantic Recycling International Systems and FIDEV Recycling (Atiemo et al. 2016).

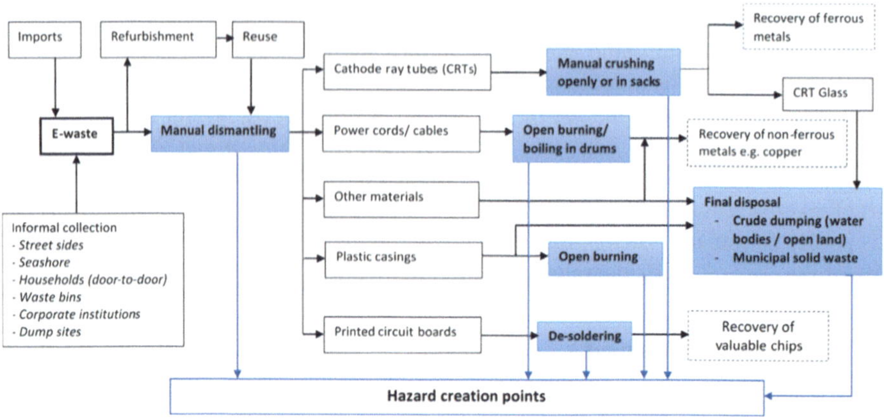

Fig. 1. Process flow diagram for informal e-waste recycling in Ghana (Awere et al. 2020)

2.4 Final Disposal

Materials of no perceived economic value are disposed in large areas at the disposal sites and periodically burnt by the informal recyclers to reduce the volume (Huang et al 2014) without recourse to their effect on the environment and health of humans. Amoyaw-Osei et al. (2011) reported the disposal of non-valuable fractions of e-waste into the Odaw River draining the Agbogbloshie catchment. At other recycling sites, non-valuable fractions and residues from burning (such as ashes) are disposed together with municipal solid waste. The environmental and health impact of these disposal methods have been well researched and documented in scientific literature.

3 Methodology

A large body of knowledge relating to the e-waste sector in Ghana exists (Daum et al. 2017). In this study, scholarly literature, local media and non-governmental organisation (NGO) reports on the Ghanaian e-waste management was thoroughly and comprehensively reviewed. The review focused on the progress of e-waste management in Ghana following the passage of the Hazardous and Electronic Waste Control and Management Act, 2016 (Act 917).

4 Results and Discussion

Following the global interest in the e-waste recycling activities in Ghana, particularly, at the Agbogbloshie e-waste site in Accra, the Government of Ghana with support from development partners, non-governmental agencies (NGOs) and Research Institutions has implemented interventions to formalize the activities of informal recyclers and to minimize the negative impacts of the e-waste recycling activities on both the workers and the environment. From both the literature review, observation and informal interviews, the following sections discusses the results. The discussion of the results focuses on the policy formulation and institutional strengthening.

4.1 E-Waste-Specific Policies and Regulations

Three (3) e-waste specific regulatory instruments have been passed since 2016. Firstly, a Hazardous and Electronic Waste Control and Management Act (Act 917) was passed by the Parliament of Ghana in August 2016. The Act aims to provide control, management and disposal of hazardous waste in general and specifically e-waste. Key aspects of the policy are (i) registration and issuing of permits to importers and exporters, (ii) imposition of advance eco-levy on importers or manufacturers, (iii) setting up of an "Electrical and Electronic Waste Management Fund" to finance environmentally sound management and research on e-waste (iv) Manufacturers, Distributors or Importers of EEE (both used and new) to take-back used or discarded EEE for recycling (Government of Ghana 2016). The Management Fund is required by the Act to be used, among others, for the:

- construction and management of e-waste recycling plant and associated facilities (40% of the funds);
- collection of e-waste and collection centres (20% of the funds);
- Research and development in public awareness creation, education and sensitization (5% of the funds);
- monitoring activities (3.5% of the funds); and Capacity building of key trade associations and manufacturers of electrical and electronic equipment (1% of the funds).

The implementation of the eco levies which started in October 2018 is expected to generate 100 million USD annually (Awusah 2018). With the expected funds from the advance eco levy, the President of Ghana in August 2018, launched a comprehensive plan to construct a state-of-the-art e-waste recycling plant at Agbogbloshie (Asante et al. 2019).

Secondly, for effective implementation of the e-waste Act, a Hazardous, Electronic and Other Wastes Control and Management Regulations (LI 2250) was passed in 2016. The legislative instrument is meant to give meaning to Act 917. Finally, Technical Guidelines on Environmentally Sound E-Waste Management for Collectors, Collection Centres, Transporters, Treatment Facilities and Final Disposal in Ghana was launched on 15th February 2018 by the Ministry of Environment, Science, Technology (MESTI) and the EPA of Ghana. Following the launching of the Technical Guidelines, Ghana has been cited as the first country in Africa to develop a technical guideline to be used to enforce the regulations regarding recycling of e-waste (Sustainable Recycling Industries 2018). It was developed by the EPA with support from Sustainable Recycling Industries (SRI) and funded by the Swiss State Secretariat for Economic Affairs (SECO). These guidelines are mandatory in compliance with Act 917 (Hazardous and Electronic Waste Control and Management Act, 2016), Act 328 (Factories, Offices and Shops Act, 1970) and LI 2250 (Hazardous, Electronic and other Wastes Control and Management Regulations, 2016) with respect to every undertaking operating in the field of collection, storage, transport, treatment and final disposal of e-waste in Ghana (Environmental Protection Agency & Sustainable Recycling Industries 2018).

The e-waste Act and associated regulations have created the legal framework for Ghana to build international and local partnerships for the sound and sustainable management of e-waste.

4.2 Institutional Strengthening

4.2.1 Environmental Protection Agency (EPA)

EPA is the governmental Institution mandated to regulate, coordinate and manage the environment (including e-waste) in Ghana. They have offices in all the regional capitals across the country and derives its mandate from the Environmental Protection Agency Act, 1994 (Act 490). The functions of EPA include but not limited to:

- Advising the Minister responsible for Environment on the formulation of policies on the environment;
- Prescribing standards and guidelines relating to the pollution and the discharge and control of toxic substances;
- Coordinating activities and control the generation, treatment, storage, transportation and disposal of industrial wastes;
- Controlling the volumes, types, constituents and effects of waste discharges, emissions, deposits or other sources of pollutants and/or substances which are hazardous or potentially dangerous to the quality of life, human health and the environment;
- Acting in liaison and cooperation with government agencies, District Assemblies and any other bodies and institutions to control pollution and generally protect the environment.

Aside the Environmental Protection Agency Act, 1994 (Act 490), the Hazardous and Electronic Waste control and Management Act, 2016 (Act 917) also places the management of electronic and hazardous wastes specifically under the remit of the EPA. Companies or organisations that want to do business relating to e-waste are required by law to register with EPA and obtain permit for their operations. Financial provision of 25% of all e-waste management funds have been allocated to EPA for e-waste specific activities including capacity building.

4.2.2 External Service Provider

The Hazardous and Electronic Waste Control and Management Act, 2016 (Act 917) requires the Minister responsible for Environment in consultation with the Minister responsible for Finance to select an External Service provider (ESP) to collect advance eco-levy from importer or manufacturer of EEE before they are imported into Ghana (Government of Ghana,= 2016). Pursuant to Sect. 21 of Act 917, Government selected Société Générale de Surveillance (SGS) as the ESP for the collection of advance eco levy on behalf of Government of Ghana. SGS was appointed based on their presence in 200 countries where the EEE originates from (Andoh 2018).

5 The Way Forward

Past, present and future initiative are aimed at creating the enabling environment for sustainable e-waste management in Ghana. The aim will remain a mirage if issues are not addressed holistically. Amidst the current interventions into the sound management of e-waste in Ghana, there exist gaps what require urgent attention.

5.1 Formalize the e-waste Sector

In most developing countries, the informal sector collects majority of the e-waste. In the Ghana situation, the informal sector collects and recycles about 95% of the e-waste (Oteng-Ababio 2012b). The achievement of the overall objective of sustainable e-waste management in Ghana will depend on how the informal sector is integrated into the overall e-waste management system. Through the mandatory registration and licensing of importers and distributors, integration of informal sector into the management process, and creation of formal collection networks with informal sector involvement, the e-waste sector is in the process of being formalised and regularised. Daum et al. (2017), argues that formalising the e-waste sector entails increased border control and regulation and integrating the informal e-waste workers into the formal economy. Some projects are exploring ways of integrating the informal sector into the formal economy. In this regard, lessons from countries like China and India (Parajuly et al. 2018) will be very useful in the process of formalizing the informal sector. As has been mentioned by Herat and Agamuthu (2012), the integration process should be thoroughly investigated to ensure a trade-off between environmental and socio-economic benefits. Formalising and regularising the informal sector will also promote job security and protect the health and safety of the e-waste workers.

5.2 Enforce e-waste Policies, Regulations and Guidelines

The e-waste legal and regulatory instruments should be strictly enforced to ensure compliance. This role should be performed by all stakeholders particularly, EPA and Customs Division of the Ghana Revenue Authority (GRA). Stricter boarder control to ensure that appropriate advance eco levy for the importation of EEE (including e-waste) should be prioritized by Customs Division of GRA so that the nation derives maximum benefit from it. Other areas needing enforcement is the recycler certification system and take-back system enshrined in the Hazardous and Electronic waste Management Act (Act 917).

The ability of EPA and Customs to perform their functions effectively depends on their capacity. The capacity of EPA as a regulator, should therefore be strengthened. This could be achieved through continuous capacity building of EPA staff at the national, regional and district level. Currently, capacity building is focused on the national and some regional level staff. Aside EPA, there is established in each metropolitan, municipal or district assembly the waste management department. The staff in these departments must be trained to support the EPA in the towns and cities. With enhanced capacity, they would ensure that different actors adhere to the laid down legal and regulatory instruments.

5.3 Intensify Public Education

The sustainable management of e-waste is a collective responsibility of government, the citizenry and the private sector businesses. Sense of responsibility of the citizens is key. Citizens' knowledge level influences their choice of product and their end-of-life management. Until recently, the public knowledge on e-wastes (material types, economic, environmental and human health impacts) was very limited. What materials constitute e-waste and how to dispose them is still not well known in the public domain. This notwithstanding, a large percentage of the people in other urban areas are still ignorant on the e-waste issues trending. This is because e-waste management projects have focused more on Agbogbloshie. But, e-waste activities have been reported in Ashaiman and Pantang (Daum et al. 2017), Tema (Amoyaw-Osei et al. 2011), Koforidua (Agyei-Mensah and Oteng-Ababio 2012; Brigden et al. (2008); Takoradi (Atiemo et al. 2016; Yamoah, 2014) and Obuasi (Atiemo et al. 2016). Intensive education and sensitization of the citizenry on the e-waste management and processes is crucial.

The sensitization and awareness creation (for different target groups) should be a continuous process and should start right from the inception of the transformation process. It is argued that, children are the best agents of change. Therefore, issues on e-waste control and management must be integrating in the educational curriculum right from basic school level.

5.4 Promote Private-Public Partnership and Extended Producer Responsibility

Globally, the role of private sector in the management of waste has been found to be increasing. In the developed countries, management of wastes has been ceded to the private sector whiles government plays a regulatory role. The Switch-Africa Green project (HEMOD) is facilitating the private sector to build recycling plants and refurbishment centres across the country (Switch Africa Green 2017). Additional ways of involving local and foreign private sector into the e-waste management process must be explored. Lessons must be learnt from other developing countries.

In recognition of the extended producer responsibility implemented in other developed countries, the Hazardous and Electronic Waste Control and Management Act (Act 917) require manufacturers, distributors or wholesalers of EEE to take back used or discarded EEE manufactured or sold by it for recycling. The SRI and HEMOD Projects are developing Extended Producer Responsibility (EPR) mechanisms for the sustainability of the recycling business (Asante et al. 2016; Pwamang 2013). As stated earlier, some EEE companies (such as RLG Communications Ltd, Kassapa or Expresso telecommunication company and Nokia) are already practicing some take-back system. With proper incentive scheme in place, individuals and organisations will be more willing to dispose their e-waste appropriately.

6 Conclusion

The e-waste recycling is a very promising business sector in Ghana. The lives of hundreds of people depend on this sector while contributing immensely to the economy of the country. Ghana e-waste problem and global notoriety necessitated attention. This paper sought to identify the progress made in transforming the e-waste sector and discuss existing gaps that requires urgent attention.

A lot of progress has been made in relation to policy and regulatory framework for controlling and managing the e-waste sector. Perhaps the greatest is the passage of the Hazardous and Electronic Waste Control and Management Act, 2016 (Act 917) and the associated legislative instrument – Hazardous, Electronic and other Wastes Control and Management Regulations, 2016 (LI 2250). The Act and regulatory instruments have created the needed legal footing for regulating and transforming e-waste activities in Ghana. With the implementation of the advance eco levy from October 1, 2018, Government of Ghana is expected to obtain US$100 million annually into the Electrical and Electronic Waste Management Fund for managing e-waste in the country. To achieve this, enforcement is crucial, and the responsibility lies on EPA (the regulatory agency), Customs, Excise and Preventive Services (CEPS), and SGS (the External Service Provider). Work on a $30 million e-waste recycling facility at Agbogbloshie is expected to commence soon with funding from the e-waste management fund. All these and other expected achievements will remain a dream if intensive public awareness and education on Act 917 and other regulations are not carried out immediately. It took the country three years to get Act 917 and LI 2250 in place and about one and half years to produce the Technical Guidelines on Environmentally Sound E-Waste Management for Collectors, Collection Centres, Transporters, Treatment Facilities and Final Disposal in Ghana. Admittedly, formulating the right laws for implementation constitute half of the solution but the country should not wait long enough to setup the necessary structures and full-scale implementation.

References

Agyei-Mensah, S., Oteng-Ababio, M.: Perceptions of health and environmental impacts of e-waste management in Ghana. Int. J. Environ. Health Res. **22**(6), 500–517 (2012). https://doi.org/10.1080/09603123.2012.667795

Amoyaw-Osei, Y., Agyekum, O.O., Pwamang, J.A., Mueller, E., Fasko, R., Schluep, M.: Ghana e-waste country assessment. SBC e-waste Africa project, Dubendorf (2011)

Andoh, D.: Work on $30m e-waste recycling facility at Agbogbloshie to begin this year. Graphic Online (2018). https://www.graphic.com.gh/business/business-news/work-on-30m-e-waste-recycling-facility-at-agbogbloshie-to-begin-this-year.html

Asante, K.A., Amoyaw-Osei, Y., Agusa, T.: E-waste recycling in Africa: risks and opportunities. Curr. Opin. Green Sustain. Chem. **18**, 109–117 (2019). https://doi.org/10.1016/j.cogsc.2019.04.001

Asante, K.A., Pwamang, J.A., Amoyaw-Osei, Y., Ampofo, J.A.: E-waste interventions in Ghana. Rev. Environ. Health **31**(1), 145–148 (2016). https://doi.org/10.1515/reveh-2015-0047

Atiemo, S., Faabeluon, L., Manhart, A., Nyaaba, L., & Schleicher, T.: Baseline assessment on e-waste management in Ghana. Accra, Ghana (2016). https://www.sustainable-recycling.org/wp-content/uploads/2016/07/Sampson_2016_SRI-Ghana.pdf

Awere, E., Obeng, P.A., Bonoli, A., Obeng, P.A.: E-waste recycling and public exposure to organic compounds in developing countries: a review of recycling practices and toxicity levels in Ghana. Environ. Technol. Rev. **9**(1), 1–19 (2020). https://doi.org/10.1080/21622515.2020.1714749

Awusah, B.: Government targets $100m from imported e-waste annually. Myjoyonline (2018). https://www.myjoyonline.com/business/2018/august-10th/govt-targets-100m-from-imported-e-waste-annually.php

Baldé, C.P., Forti, V., Gray, V., Kuehr, R., Stegmann, P.: The global e-waste monitor 2017: Quantities, flows and resources, Geneva, Bonn, Vienna (2017). https://collections.unu.edu/eserv/UNU:6341/Global-E-waste_Monitor_2017__electronic_single_pages_.pdf

Balde, C. P., Wang, F., Kuehr, R., Huisman, J.: The global e-waste monitor 2014: Quantities, flows and resources, Geneva, Bonn, Vienna (2015)

Brigden, K., Labunska, I., Santillo, D., Johnston, P.: Chemical contamination at e-waste recycling and disposal sites in Accra and Korforidua, Ghana. In. Amsterdam: Greenpeace (2008)

CEHRT Environmental Consulting. Technical Report on the Sustainable Management of E-Waste in Ghana (2015). https://greenadgh.com/images/documentsrepository/EwasteTechnicalReport WorldBank.pdf

Daum, K., Stoler, J., Grant, R.: Toward a more sustainable trajectory for e-waste policy: a review of a decade of e-waste research in Accra, Ghana. Int. J. Environ. Res. Public Health **14**(2), 135 (2017). https://doi.org/10.3390/ijerph14020135

Diaz-Barriga, F.: Evidence-based intervention programs to reduce children's exposure to chemicals in e-waste sites (2013)

Environmental Protection Agency, & Sustainable Recycling Industries. Technical guidelines on environmentally sound e-waste management for collectors, collection centres, transporters, treatment facilities and final disposal in Ghana. Accra, Ghana Environmental Protection Agency (2018). https://www.sustainable-recycling.org/ewaste-guidelines-ghana_2018_epa-sri/

Government of Ghana. Hazardous and electronic waste control and management Act of 2016 (Act 917). Accra, Ghana: Government of Ghana (2016). https://greenadgh.com/images/documents repository/HazardousandElectronicWasteControl.pdf

Heacock, M., Kelly, C.B., Asante, K.A., Birnbaum, L.S., Bergman, Å.L., Bruné, M.-N., Huo, X.: E-waste and harm to vulnerable populations: a growing global problem. Environ. Health Perspect. **124**(5), 550 (2016). https://doi.org/10.1289/ehp.1509699

Herat, S., Agamuthu, P.: E-waste: a problem or an opportunity? REVIEW of issues, challenges and solutions in Asian countries. Waste Manag. Res. **30**(11), 1113–1129 (2012). https://doi.org/10.1177/0734242X12453378

Huang, J.Y., Nkrumah, P.N., Anim, D.O., Mensah, E., Whitacre, D.M.: E-waste disposal effects on the aquatic environment: Accra, Ghana. Rev. Environ. Contam. Toxicol. **229**, 19–34 (2014). https://doi.org/10.1007/978-3-319-03777-6_2

Manhart, A., Schleicher, T., Degreif, S.: Global Circular Economy of Strategic Metals - The Best-of-two-Worlds Approach (Bo2W), Germany (2014)

McElvaney, K.: Agbogbloshie: The world's largest e-waste dump - in pictures (2014). https://www.theguardian.com/environment/gallery/2014/feb/27/agbogbloshie-worlds-largest-e-waste-dump-in-pictures

Oteng-Ababio, M.: Electronic waste management in Ghana-issues and practices. In Sustainable Development-Authoritative and Leading Edge Content for Environmental Management. IntechOpen Limited, London (2012a)

Oteng-Ababio, M.: When necessity begets ingenuity: E-waste scavenging as a livelihood strategy in Accra. Ghana. Afr. Stud. Q. **13**(1/2), 1 (2012b)

Oteng-Ababio, M.M., Amankwaa, E.F.: The e-waste conundrum: balancing evidence from the north and on-the-ground developing countries' realities for improved management. Afr. Rev. Econ. Finan. **6**(1), 181–204 (2014)

Parajuly, K., Thapa, K.B., Cimpan, C., Wenzel, H.: Electronic waste and informal recycling in Kathmandu, Nepal: challenges and opportunities. J. Mater. Cycles Waste Manag. **20**(1), 656–666 (2018). https://doi.org/10.1007/s10163-017-0610-8

Prakash, S., Manhart, A., Amoyaw-Osei, Y., Agyekum, O.O.: Socio-economic assessment and feasibility study on sustainable e-waste management in Ghana. In: Accra: Ghana: Öko-Institut eV in cooperation with Ghana Environmental Protection Agency (EPA) & Green Advocacy Ghana, Ministry of Housing, Spatial Planning and the Environment, VROM-Inspectorate (2010)
Pwamang, J.A.: Government policy and initiatives on e-waste in Ghana. In: Paper presented at the Proceedings of the 3rd Annual Global E-Waste Management (GEM) Network Meeting, San Francisco, CA, USA (2013)
Srigboh, R.K., Basu, N., Stephens, J., Asampong, E., Perkins, M., Neitzel, R.L., Fobil, J.: Multiple elemental exposures amongst workers at the Agbogbloshie electronic waste (e-waste) site in Ghana. Chemosphere **164**, 68–74 (2016). https://doi.org/10.1016/j.chemosphere.2016.08.089
Step Initiative. One global definition of e-waste, Bonn, Germany (2014). https://www.step-initiative.org/files/step/_documents/StEP_WP_One%20Global%20Definition%20of%20E-waste_20140603_amended.pdf
Sustainable Recycling Industries. Ghana's way towards sustainable e-waste recycling – First country in Africa to officially launch guidelines for environmentally sound e-waste management (2018). https://www.sustainable-recycling.org/ghanas-way-towards-sustainable-e-waste-recycling-first-country-in-africa-to-officially-launch-guidelines-for-environmentally-sound-e-waste-management/
Switch Africa Green. Hanisa e-waste model (HEMOD) (2017). https://www.switchafricagreen.org/index.php?option=com_k2&view=item&id=316:hanisa-e-waste-model-hemod&Itemid=824&lang=en
World Economic Forum. A New Circular Vision for Electronics: Time for a Global Reboot, Geneva (2019). https://www3.weforum.org/docs/WEF_A_New_Circular_Vision_for_Electronics.pdf
Yamoah, S.B.: E-waste in developing country context-Issues, challenges, practices, opportunities: Addressing the WEEE challenge in Ghana. (Master of Science), Aalborg University (2014)

An Appraisal of Electric Energy Supply Security in Residential Estates of Ado-Ekiti, Nigeria

S. E. Okosun[1](✉), J. O. Fasakin[2], J. O. Basorun[2], I. O. Olamiju[2], and E. A. Aluko[2]

[1] Department of Geography, Federal University Lokoja, Lokoja, Nigeria
[2] Department of Urban & Regional Planning, Federal University of Technology, Akure, Nigeria

Abstract. In recent time, increasing attention of academic and political discussion is directed at issues of energy security. Energy security has assumed a global phenomenon which stands at the center of global efforts (of governments, non-governmental organizations, and individuals) and the survival of humanity. The increasing attention has produced a new order of electricity supply in Nigeria urban centres. There is a noticeable variation of poor access to clean, modern, reliable, affordable and available electricity supply in the residential estates of Ado-Ekiti. This research appraises the energy supply security theme and challenges (cost) of electricity supply in Ado-Ekiti using three residential estates randomly selected, with a view to promoting energy security. With the use of GIS and IKONOS Imagery, the total number of buildings in the three estates was 1,879 (Egbewa, 315; Falegan, 1,079 and Federal Housing, 482) out of which 20 percent, representing 375 household heads in the residential buildings were sampled. The probabilistic approaches of the simple and systematic random sampling techniques were used in selecting the units for questionnaire administration in the selected estates. The Pearson Product Moment Correlation (PPMC) test revealed a significant correlation between electricity sources and availability of household energy supply and use of public electricity. Conversely The Spearman Correlation test revealed that there was no correlation between electricity supplied to households, the quantity of electricity consumption in kilowatts-hours (kWh) by households and electricity bills distributed to households at the end of the month in monetary terms. Policy measures of the government encouraging entrepreneurs and individuals to invest in cleaner household energy such as solar PV were set forth, hence will fill the vacuum created due to rising debate on electricity bill.

Keywords: Ado-Ekiti · Appraisal · Electricity · Energy supply security · Residential estates

1 Introduction

Household energy is a cardinal requirement in the 21st century human habitat and global city transformation. Residential household energy supply, is a form of domestic fuel resulting from the existence of charged particle necessary to energize machinery for cooling, heating, cooking and lighting appliances in the residential communities or estates. The United Nations Development Programme (UNDP) in 2001, 2016 noted that access

J. N. Mojekwu et al. (Eds.): *Sustainable Education and Development*, pp. 466–479, 2021.
https://doi.org/10.1007/978-3-030-68836-3_40

to affordable and reliable modern energy services particularly for domestic (household activities) is fundamental to human livelihood and sustenance. The International Energy Agency (IEA) in 2009 simply defines energy security as the affordable access to reliable power supply. As argued by Ikeme (2008), energy security does not only entail sufficient power supply reserve or potentials; but access to affordable and reliable sources of power. The growth in human population has not only dramatically increased mankind's ability to harness energy from nature (World Energy Council 2013) but equally gives rise to greater demand and debate for global energy supply security (Uyigue 2007; Etiosa 2009; Africa Progress Panel 2015). In this study, energy supply security is seen as the ability of the electrical system to provide affordable, reliable, and ensure availability of electricity to end-users with a specified level of continuity and quality in a sustainable manner. The study of keseke & Hosking (2011) highlighted that electricity energy supply is key to the development of any nation; energy use is correlated with healthy economic growth. Nigeria, no doubt is endowed with enormous energy resources both renewable (solar, biomass, wind, hydropower) and non-renewable (crude oil, natural gas, coal) that can be used to generate electric power (Sambo 2008; World Cities Report 2011/2010). Despite these potentials, the World Bank report in 2013 confirmed that Nigeria had 10% of the world population with no access to electricity. Poor access to electricity has been a major impediment to Nigeria's economic growth (World Bank, 2012) and Ado-Ekiti inclusive. The creation of Ado-Ekiti as the divisional headquarters of Ekiti Division in 1945 and with the creation of the old Ondo State in 1976, made the town continue to expand; this expansion become significant with the creation of Ekiti State in 1996. The resultant expansion had caused a change in the demand and supply of electricity in the residential neigbourhood because various forms of people, goods and services found their way into the town, thus causing energy insecurity and making it more intense, with the resultant population growth, which now pose electricity sufficiency challenges in the town (Akintan, 2014; Oginni et al. 2017). Conversely, the rapidly increasing population in the city (NPC 2006) needs more secure, stable, reliable and affordable electric power supply.

This research therefore is designed to study the electricity supply challenges (cost) in the residential estates of Ado-Ekiti, Nigeria with a view to promoting energy security. The broad objectives of this study are to assess the socio-economic characteristics of households in the residential estates vis-à-vis the hours/duration of electricity supply, electricity bill per month, identify types of housing, opinion on the cost of electricity bills, and assess the challenges to the regularity of power supply in the study area.

2 Situation Perspective to Electricity Demand and Supply in Nigeria

Electricity is key to the development of any nation. Limited access to reliable, affordable and available electric energy utilization in developing countries like Nigeria has remained an unresolved scourge in the nation especially the residential sector (Azodo 2014). A considerable number of literature search buttressed that electricity is one of the most important basic necessities for living (Sambo 2008; UND 2015; IEA 2016). Its use in the residential estates has a number of varying factors contributing to the quantity of electricity used by each household, such as income, price of electricity, uncertainty about product quality due to a lack of standardization and population variables (Azekhumen 2016). Other factors such as household size, age and climatic condition of an area also contribute to the household's electricity consumption (Joskow 2008; Chuku, & Effiong, 2011). The UN-Energy (2014) submitted that electricity demand and supply mismatch is now a widespread challenging issue; nations of the world strive for efficient and effective power sector that will meet the ever increasing electricity demand (UN-Energy 2014). In contrast to international concerns, Nigeria, a country blessed with a lot of energy resources (wind, biomass, crude oil, natural gas, solar and coal) has not made notable progress in the provision of accessible electric power supply sources for cooking, heating and lighting domestic household utilities (OECD/IEA 2011; IEA, 2017). Therefore, Nigerians are encouraged to develop an electric power supply strategy – which is crucial in achieving the SDGs (IEA 2016).

Prior to the enactment of the Electricity Power Sector Reform Act (EPSRA, 2005), the Federal Government of Nigeria (FGN) was responsible for policy formulation; regulatory, operational, and investment in the Nigerian power sector (Nigeria Sustainable Energy Programme, 2015). In 2015, Country Report on Nigeria Energy System, highlighted that solar photovoltaic, wind and other sources of renewable energy hold mixed thrilling prospects and challenges.

Orazulike (2013) echoed that due to incessant power electricity failure, about 70% of the industries in Nigeria are dead, 10% are dying and 20% are trying to survive. Despite endemic blackouts, customers (users of public electricity) are billed for services not rendered; this has partially resulted into widespread vandalism of power theft in Nigeria, coupled with the problem of payment of electricity bill. This prompted the privatization of the Power Holding Company of Nigeria (PHCN) formally known as National Electric Power Authority (NEPA) with the expectation for increased stability in the Nigeria. Electricity transmission and distribution remain the exclusive responsibility of the Federal Government of Nigeria (FGN) under the absolute control of PHCN. The state government on its part (for instance Ekiti State), only intervenes on the provision of power distribution infrastructure due to PHCN's lackluster performance in connecting towns and communities to the national grid or maintaining existing power supply networks to meet growing increasing users' demands. There are only 14 generating stations in Nigeria (3 hydro and 11 thermal stations). Out of the approximated 8,039 MW of installed capacity in Nigeria, not more than 4,500 MW is supplied (Sambo, 2009). The Nigeria electricity is characterized by unstable power supply and price fluctuations (Orazulike 2013). In Ado-Ekiti, one of the most prevalent residential household problems is the incessant electricity power failure (Ado-Ekiti Medium Term Fiscal Framework 2016). The cost of electricity in Ado-Ekiti, on metering and charging method as well as household tax on electricity tariffs are highly controversial, because the current charges on electricity used in the residential buildings are not based on metered reading but fixed estimated monthly billings (N5,000 – N9,000 per building). This approach presents significant challenges in electric supply affordability among residential communities/estates in Ado-Ekiti (Leadership Nigeria Newspapers, 2018). Residents of Ado-Ekiti are vulnerable to various electric power supply security threats, forcing them to choose the electric power supply strategies that ensure domestic electric supply security.

3 The Research Methodology

The research was limited to the residential neigbourhood of Ado-Ekiti. In the area, three (3) residential estates were selected randomly; these are Egbewa, Falegan, and Federal Housing Estates. The study focused purposely on these areas in order to examine the electricity energy supply in the residential estates with a view to promoting its energy security for necessary planning and policy intervention. Ado-Ekiti the case study is a traditional Nigeria city like other traditional Yoruba towns in the country. The city is in south-western Nigeria and is the largest city and capital of Ekiti State. The city has a population of 308,621 persons as at 2006 population census (NPC, 2009), as at 2017, the estimated population figure was 438,749 persons using a growth rate of 3.25%. Geographically, Ado-Ekiti occupies the area lying approximately between Latitude 7°30′16″ North of the equator and longitude 5° 15′27″ East of the Greenwich Meridian. It is about 400 m above the sea level in the south-eastern part of Ireje stream and 500m above sea level in the northeast, and has a land area of 265 km^2 (Ogunleye 2013). The town is situated in the tropical rainforest zone in Nigeria Ado-Ekiti (Ogunleye 2013). Ado-Ekiti, being the capital city of Ekiti State, made the town to witness immense growth from immigration, transportation, and commercial activities, all which attracted investors (banks, industries, and educational institutions) and people into the city. As such, different categories of people and households are found within the city, including the poor, and the non-poor households that are connected and/or wish to be connected to the electrical energy grid. As the city continues to grow in population, household electricity energy demand and supply in the town became a major challenge in the area of affordability (cost), reliability and availability. These issues is expected to be a major challenge in the future as the city continue to grow in building development, together with the expected rapid economics and industrial growth.

4 Data Collection Method

The three residential neigbourhoods chosen constitute the sample frame for questionnaire administration for the study. This comprises of Egbewa, Falegan and Federal housing estates. The three neigbourhoods were chosen for ease of data collection, and because the three estates represents three different classes of density zones in Ado-Ekiti, which are, the low, middle and high density zones respectively. Grid method was employed to divide each estate into equal squares. Total number of building in the selected residential estates was counted using GIS and IKONOS Imagery.

Respondents/households population was a mix of various population segments, such as workers (civil servants - public, private), traders, students, apprentices, and other professionals. The questionnaires focused majorly on information obtained from the (NPC), Ministry of Housing, Housing Corporations, Goggle Earth Imagery and ground truthing operations. Empirical analysis shows that Egbewa, Falegan, and Federal housing estates had a total of 315, 1,079, and 482 buildings respectively. Twenty percent of the total number of building on each of the estates was sampled, giving a total sample size of 375. This forms the sample size for the study. Simple and systematic random sampling techniques were used to select buildings in the study area. The justification for the 20 percent was appropriate bearing in mind the geographical features, development pattern, homogenous, social and economic characteristics of the residents and housing types amongst others factors. The percentage captured all interest groups in the study area. Table 1 shows sampling in the selected residential estates of Ado-Ekiti.

Table 1. Sampling in residential estates of Ado-Ekiti

S/N	Name of Estate	Total no. of Building	20% of buildings (questionnaires administered)
1	Egbewa	315	63
2	Falegan	1,079	216
3	Federal Housing	482	96
	Total	**1,879**	**375**

In each resident; a knock-on-the-door approach was used to initiate contact with participants on information relating to the study. Participants were chosen based on age, using the probability sampling with replacement (PSR) approach in obtaining representative sample. The choice of household heads/representative was restricted to the minimum age of 18. Structured questionnaire was employed to collect data from the study population.

Data were collected at specific periods and places (in residences and offices). The institutional questionnaires were administered during office hours, while questionnaires for residents of housing estates were administered during weekends (saturday and sunday) between 9am and 4pm, when majority of the respondents were at home. They were administered based on participants' convenience, availability and willingness to be interviewed. The questionnaires administration lasted for six weeks. Further relevant information for the study was collected from in-situ observations, photographs, informal interviews and discussions with the respondents.

Data collected were analyzed using percentages frequency distribution tables, figures and binary logistic regression model based on the contingent valuation method. The frequency distribution was used to analyze challenges of electricity supply and the socio-economic characteristics of the respondents. Cronbach's alpha coefficient(α) using the Test-retest method was used to determine the reliability of the research questions.

5 Research Findings

The age distribution of households in the estates (Egbewa and Falegan) indicates that the majority of the respondents were between the age of 42–49 years, representing 47.6%, and 53.7%, respectively, while majority of the respondents in the Federal housing estate were between the age of 34–41 years and 50 years and above representing 25% of respondents respectively. This shows that respondents are matured in responding to the researcher's questions and their opinion can be considered relevant to the research work. Age-related growth is positively associated with household energy expenditure on grid-electricity. Further findings reveal that age's between 34–41 are the main end user of household electricity consumers in the study area.

On Educational status, respondents are well educated and could understand the purpose of the study. The finding reveals that 47.6%, 41.6% and 53.1% of the respondents in Falegan and Federal Housing Estate respectively has a minimum of tertiary education (ND/NCE/HND/BSc), and none was without any form of formal education. In the study area, level of education reflects the nature of employment, as majorities of the respondents were public servant.

People working in public organization in the estates (Egbewa 42.8%, Falegan 50.0% and Federal 42.7%) had the highest percentage because of their proximity to public institutions and agencies. Those Retired (9.7%) came least on the employment status in the study area. Finding from the study revealed that employment status enhances household energy sources for lighting (Miah et al. 2011).

The occupational characteristics revealed an imbalance in types and representations across the estates. Majority of the people in the area were civil servants (Egbawa 41.2%, Falegan 29.17% and Federal housing estates 36.4%). Occupational status of the people reflected the type of buildings, as well as number of electrical appliances they can afford.

Majority of the respondents in Egbewe (47.6%) and Falegan (45.3%) estate earned between ₦80,001-₦100,000 annually, while most respondents (32.2%) in Federal housing estate earn above ₦100,000. The occupation of the people correlates with income and expenditure, and the financial constraints of most of the urban poor households do not encouraged their investment in new modern energy technologies that are accessible and available, thereby creating affordability problems. Unaffordable clean energy may create additional financial burden in adopting them, because many low-income households already live on limited income and have access to 'no-cost' energy sources. Thus, they see additional cost on clean electric power supply as a diversion of their income to electric energy they cannot control in terms of cost. This study is in agreement with Ouedraogo (2006) who reported that income is a major driver of the uptake of modern fuels.

The distribution of the household according to type of housing shows that 4.7% of the sampled households in Egbewa reside in 1-bedroom flat, 6.3% in 2-bedroom flat, 15.8% in 3 bedrooms flat; while 6.3% and 19.0% reside in 4 bedrooms flat and Duplex respectively. In Falegun estate, 0.9% leave in 1-bedroom flat, 23.6% in 2 bedrooms flat, 46.8% in 3 bedrooms flat, 6.9% and 8.3% reside in 4 bedroom flat and duplex respectively. In Federal housing estate 5.2%, reside in 1-bedroom flat, 31.2% in 2-bedroom flat, 46.8% in 3 bedroom flat, 4.1% and 12.4% reside in 4 bedroom flat and duplex respectively. Three (3) bedroom flat constituted the main type of housing design in the three estates. This is because majority of the respondents were married. Marital status of the respondents was a reflection of their housing type, which increases electricity demand.

Household heads are predominantly homeowners, with 74.6% of them being a private house owner in Egbewa estate, and 70.6% in Falegan estate owing a home. Thus it is expected that they would be willing to use alternative modern and improved electricity supply since most of the respondents do not expend money in the payment of house rents.

From Table 2 the Cronbach's Alpha values ranges from 0.800 to 0.853. This inclination shows that the reliability estimates of the instrument are high as they tend towards 1.0, and for a test to be reliable Cronbach's Alpha coeffient must be at least 0.7 (May,

Table 2. Variables employed in the model of reliability and availability

S/n	Variable code	Definition of variables	Cronbach's Alpha (α)	Measurement scale
1	GENDER	Gender	0.831	1 (female), 0 (male)
2	EDUSTA	Education status	0.822	1 (tertiary), 0 (otherwise)
3	EMPLOY	Employment status	0.841	1 (employed), 0 (otherwise)
4	OCCUP	Occupation	0.816	1 (civil servant), 0 (otherwise)
5	INCOME	Monthly income	0.813	1 (₦80,001-₦100,000), 0 (otherwise)
6	H-TYPE	Type of house	0.801	1 (3 bedroom), 0 (otherwise)
7	HD-SIZES	Household size	0.814	1 (4 and above), 0 (less than 4)
8	H-OWN	House Ownership	0.842	1 (owner), 0 (rented)
9	REL	Reliability of public electricity	0.812	1 (Not reliable), 0 (otherwise)
10	AFFORD	Affordability of public electricity	0.822	1 (Not Affordable), 0 (otherwise)
11	CONN	Connection to the national grid	0.820	1(Yes), 0 (otherwise)
12	SOURCE	Source(s) of household energy	0.843	1 (public electricity), 2 (generator), 3 (solar PV). 4 (lumus), 5 (gas)
13	DUR	Duration of electricity supply per day	0.807	1 (less than 3 h), 0 (otherwise)
14	T-DAY	Time of electricity supply	0.819	1 (night), 0 (otherwise)
15	QUALI	Quality of electricity supply	0.818	1 (low quality), 0 (otherwise)
16	METER	Preferred Metering service	0.822	1 (prepaid), 0 (otherwise)
17	OPINION	Opinion on cost of electricity bills	0.817	1 (unreasonable), 0 (otherwise)
18	ALT	Availability of alternative sources	0.817	1 (available), 0 (otherwise)
19	COST	Cost on self-generated electricity	0.818	1 (₦6001-₦9000), 0 (otherwise)

Source: Field Survey, 2018

2001). This approach helped to gain diverse views of participants and developing a good understanding in the research, thus aid the measurement scale for the study (see Table 3).

The field work carried out as depicted with Table 4, duration of electricity supply in the area varied widely. Egbewa, Falegan and Federal housing estates enjoy a maximum of 3–8 h of electricity supply a day on an average (15.8%, 18.9%, and 53.2% respectively) and a minimum of less than 3 h. Relatively, Federal Housing Estate enjoys more supply than Egbewa and Falegan Estates. No household could enjoy electricity supply above 14hrs/day. The Business Head Distribution of BEDC, Ado-Ekiti revealed that duration of electricity supply per resident in Ado-Ekiti is 6 h/day. Information on the frequency of electricity supply shows the severity of poor electricity power supply in Ado-Ekiti, for which this study seek to find out the economic cost. This is because the electricity power supply in Ado-Ekiti is very much erratic, thus needing immediate attention. The findings of this study is in conformity with Oginni, et al. (2017) that availability of electricity supply would encourage entrepreneurs to invest in the nation economy rather than neighboring countries.

Table 3. Hours/duration of electricity supply in Egbewa, Falegan and Federal housing estate

Hours of electricity supply per day	Egbewa Estate (63)		Falegan Estate (216)		Federal Estate (96)		Total	
	Freq.	Percent (%)	Freq.	Percent (%)	Freq.	Percent (%)	Freq.	Percent (%)
Less than 3 h	53	84.1	170	78.8	35	36.4	258	68.8
3–8 h	10	15.8	41	18.9	51	53.2	102	27.2
8–14 h	0	0	5	2.3	10	10.4	15	4
14–20 h	0	0	0	0	0	0	0	0
20–24 h	0	0	0	0	0	0	0	0

Source: Field survey (2018)

From the result in Table 4, despite the poor supply, electricity bill appears to be high in Egbewa estates, as larger percentages (31.2%) of the households spend between ₦6001 to ₦9000 on electricity bill per month. The cross-tabulation further shows that majority of the respondents in Egbawa live in a 3-bedroom flat, and they spend above ₦9000 per month on electricity bill, while respondents that lived in a 1-bedroom bungalow spend between below ₦3000 and ₦3001 - ₦6000. Meaning, the larger the housing occupancy, the more expenses incurred on the electricity billing.

The result derived from Table 5 shows that a larger percentage, approximately 38.8% of the respondents in Falegan Estate, spends between ₦6001 to ₦9000 on electricity bill per month. This can be considered unreasonable as the majority of the respondents in the 3-bedroom bungalow (frequency of 60) are low income earner, while respondents that lived in a 1-bedroom spend below ₦3000. Meaning, the larger the type of housing occupancy, the more the expenses incurred on electricity billing. Further findings reveals that the major electronic appliances and used were incandescent light bulbs, compact

Table 4. Electricity bill per month and type of Housing Occupancy (Egbawa)

Electricity bill per month	Type of housing occupancy					Total
	1-bdrm Bgl	2-bdrm Bgl	3-bdrm Bgl	4-bdrom Bgl	Duplex	
	Freq	Freq	Freq	Freq	Freq	
Below ₦3000	2	3	0	0	0	5
₦3001-₦6000	3	5	4	1	0	13
₦6001-₦9000	0	0	13	9	8	30
Above ₦9000	0	0	8	5	2	5
Total	**5**	**8**	**25**	**15**	**10**	**63**

KEY: Bdrm Bgl = Bedroom Bungalow. Source: Field survey (2018)

florescent lights/tubes, LCD/LED TV set, stereo/radio systems, refrigerators, washing machines, electric cookers while the use of air- conditioner were few.

Table 5. Electricity bill per month and type of housing occupancy (Falegan Estate)

Electricity bill per month	Type of housing occupancy					Total
	1-bdrm Bgl	2-bdrm Bgl	3-bdrm Bgl	4-bdrom Bgl	Duplex	
	Freq	Freq	Freq	Freq	Freq	
Below ₦3000	10	7	5	0	0	22
₦3001-₦6000	0	19	7	28	2	54
₦6001-₦9000	0	1	77	2	4	84
Above ₦9000	0	0	14	17	25	48
Total	**10**	**27**	**103**	**47**	**29**	**216**

KEY: Bdrm Bgl = Bedroom Bungalow. Source: Field survey (2018)

The result of the analysis of electricity bill in Federal housing estate is presented in Table 6. About 46.8% of the household spend above ₦9000 on electricity bill per month. Findings revealed that, the housing occupancy type is the determinant of the electricity bill and not electricity usage/consumption. The electricity bill is believed not to be reasonable. This is because the power supply is erratic and may not even be available over a period of time, like days or even weeks, and respondents are made to pay monthly bills even in the absence of power supply. This corroborates the findings of Azekhumen (2016) which discovered that Nigerians are billed to pay for services not rendered. If electricity is improved and affordable, households will be willing to pay for supply. Further findings revealed that few persons are willing to pay a little above their current bills, while others are not.

Table 6. Electricity bill per month and type of housing occupancy (Federal Housing Estate)

Electricity bill per month	Type of housing occupancy					Total
	1-bdrm Bgl	2-bdrm Bgl	3-bdrm Bgl	4-bdrom Bgl	Duplex	
	Freq	Freq	Freq	Freq	Freq	
Below ₦3000	2	2	0	0	0	4
₦3001-₦6000	0	9	3	1	2	15
₦6001-₦9000	0	1	24	5	2	32
Above ₦9000	0	0	16	8	21	45
Total	**2**	**12**	**43**	**14**	**25**	**96**

KEY: Bdrm Bgl = Bedroom Bungalow. Source: Field survey (2018)

As seen in Fig. 1. 50.5% of the respondents claimed that their electricity bill is very unreasonable (Falagen and Egbewa estates), and they are of the opinion that they do not pay their electricity bill due to its cost. The complaints of households in this category is that marketers in charge of meter reading do not read meters; and that, even where they read the meters, the readings do not reflect the exact electricity consumptions. Consequently, efficiency and stability is essential before majority (population) of the final consumer of electricity will be paying their electricity bills.

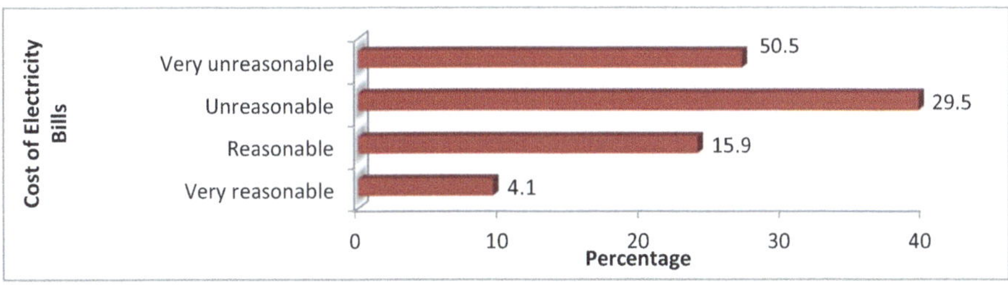

Fig. 1. Opinion on the cost of electricity bills in the study area. *Source: Field survey (2018)*

Findings from the field survey as depicted with Table 7, shows that one of the greatest challenges to the regularity of power supply in the residential neigbourhoods is technical problem. This is evident in the information gathered as respondents in Egbewa (41.2%), Falegan (42.5%) and Federal housing estate (28.1%) attest to this. To a great extent, current economic situation, political, obsolete equipment and private generator sellers are major obstacles to regular electricity power supply (public). The salvaging role of private generators as an alternative source of power supply does not seem to significantly address the problem of electric power insufficiency in Nigeria as it poses its own challenges.

Pearson product moment correlation (PPMC) was used to test hypothesis 1 (Table 8), which states that there is significant relationship between electricity sources and availability of household energy supply. The results show that there existed a medium

Table 7. Challenges to regular electricity power supply in the study area

Challenges	Egbewa	Estate	Falegan	Estate	Federal housing estate	
	Freq	%	Freq	%	Freq %	
Political	10	15.8	21	9.7	16	16.6
Economic	9	14.2	53	24.5	25	26.0
Location of house	2	3.1	5	2.3	6	10.4
Technical problem	26	41.2	92	42.5	27	28.1
Private generator sellers	2	3.1	7	3.2	5	5.2
Obsolete equipment	14	22.2	34	**15.7**	**17**	**17.7**
Total	**63**	**100.0**	**216**	**100.0**	**96**	**100.0**

Source: Field survey (2018)

correlation between the combination of electricity sources and availability of household energy supply in the study area with correlation coefficient of P = 0.000 and 0.006 (two tailed) < 0.01 respectively. Which show there exist a relationship (electricity sources and availability of household energy supply.) in the research sample, thus be given due attention. This implies that availability of household energy supply depends on the available electricity sources.

Table 8. Relationship between electricity sources and availability of household energy supply

		Value	Asymp. Std. Error	Approx. T	Approx. Sig
Interval by Interval	Pearson's R	0.503	0.035	3.615	0.000**
Ordinal by Ordinal	Spearman Correlation	0.670	0.046	3.115	0.006*
No of Valid Cases		611			

** $P \leq 0.01$ level (2-tailed). Source: Field survey (2018)

In Table 9, the R^2 value of 0.402 shows that, only 40.2% of the variation in Y (Availability of electricity) are accounted for by X (Use of public electricity) while 59.8% are due to other factors. For instance, factors such as Connection to public light source (CON), Initial cost of electricity connection (COST), Hours/Duration of electricity supply (HRS), Quality of electricity supply (QUALI), Distance covered before accessing electricity payment centers (DIST), Awareness of electricity tariff increase (Aware), Agreement with periodic increase in electricity tariff (TARIFF), Metering service used (METER), Amount spent on public electricity monthly (AMOUNT), and Electricity bill payment reflection of consumption (BILL) are responsible for the availability of public electricity supply in the study area. However, use of public electricity explains 40.2%

of the variation in availability of electricity. The correlation r = 0.634. The calculated T 47.126 is greater than the critical of 4.46 hence, H_0 is rejected and H1 is accepted.

Due to greater proportion (59.8%) that is not accounted for by X as a result of variation in Y, the erratic nature, poor quality and unreliability of electricity supply led to the continuous increase in the use of self-generation gasoline-powered generating sets. The overall cost of unavailable public electricity supply has caused residents to spend on self-generated electricity (generator) 5–10 times as much as what they spend on grid-electricity (World Bank, 2013). The cost of providing alternative self-generated electricity is high and at the detriment of other household needs together with the adverse effects on human health and the environment. The inadequacy, unreliability and unavailability of public electricity supply/services provision to meet the desire of household energy services needs is a major factor affecting the non-payment of electricity consumed by some of the households. The effect of over-billing of customers owing to the non-provision of meters is a major contentious issue. Metering all customers will overcome the problems associated with the frustration of contentious estimated bills. The findings of this study support the statement by NERC (2013) that metering accounts for 80% of consumer complaints.

Table 9. Regression results of availability and use of public electricity in the study area

Model	Unstandardized coefficients		Standardized coefficients	T	Sig
	B	Std. Error	Beta		
Constant	3.868	0.230		16.833	0.000**
CONN	−0.686	0.113	−0.181	−6.093	0.000**
COST	−0.125	0.039	−0.110	−3.229	0.001**
HRS	0.423	0.027	0.478	15.466	0.000**
QUALI	−0.243	0.040	−0.190	−6.087	0.000**
DIST	−0.009	0.022	−0.013	−0.433	0.665
AWARE	−0.177	0.036	−0.150	−.873	0.000**
TARIFF	−0.234	0.068	−0.105	−3.427	0.001**
METER	−0.051	0.033	−0.047	−1.548	0.122
AMOUNT	−0.051	0.025	−0.069	−2.015	0.044*
BILL	−0.120	0.060	−0.064	−1.986	0.047*
F-ratio	47.126				0.000**
R	0.634				
R^2	0.402				

Dependent variable: Availability of electricity
* $P \leq 0.05$ level (2-tailed)
** $P \leq 0.01$ level (2-tailed)
Source: Field survey, 2018

6 Recommendation and Conclusion

It is evident from the empirical work carried out in this study that households in Ado-Ekiti do not receive adequate electricity supply and are adversely affected by poor electricity supply. To alleviate these challenges, generator was observed to be the predominant alternative source of power supply in the town. The issue of generator usage in households due to public electricity deficit is a challenge to resident's income, which demands active participation of both the government and her citizens to address. This could be through prompt payment of electricity bills, avoidance of vandalism on the part of the citizens, ensuring adequate power generation and adopting healthy maintenance culture of existing facilities on the part of the government. Therefore, this is a need for government to enact laws or policies what will efficiently improve the supply of power by encouraging entrepreneurs and individuals in the maintenance and utilization of energy resources to boost the electricity supply as well as solar energy in the country, this will bridge the gap between demand and supply of electricity in Nigeria. However, research that will encourage innovation, and provide clean, reliable and available electric power supply (energy security) is recommended. It is advisable to review the present energy cost which according to households is too high. Affordability of electricity supply is thus recommended. The study concludes that household income, metering type (prepaid/estimated billing), availability of alternative, occupation, and reliability of current supply is a major effect to households' energy security attainment and Willingness To Pay (WTP) for electricity bill.

References

Ado-Ekiti Local Government Medium Term Fiscal Framework: Budget Review, Risk Analysis, Debt Profile, and Revenue Collection. Ado-Ekiti LGA Annual Report (2016)

Africa Progress Panel: Power people planet: Seizing Africa's energy and climate opportunities: Geneva (2015). https://www.africaprogresspanel.org/publications/policypapers.

Akintan, O.B.: Socio-cultural perceptions of indoor air pollution among rural migrant households in Ado Ekiti, Nigeria. PhD thesis, University of Nottingham (2014)

Azekhumen, E.:Challenges of Energy Fuels in Cities; A Case of Benin Metropolitan City, Nigeria. Ph.D. thesis: University of Wales, Wales, U K (2016)

Azodo, A.P.: Electric power supply, main source and backing: a survey of residentialutilization features. Int. J. Res. Stud. Manage. **3**(2), 87102 (2014)

Choong, C.K., Yusop, Z., Liew, V.K.S.: Export-led growth hypothesis in Malaysia: an investigation using bounds test. Sunway Acad. J. **2**, 13–22 (2005)

Edewede, O.B.: Assessment of Energy Security and its implication in Oredo Local Government Area, Nigeria. Ph.D. thesis, University of Nairobi, Kenya (2016)

Etiosa, U. (ed.): Energy Efficiency Survey in Nigeria: A Guide for Developing Policy and Legislation. Journal of International, Rivers, 1–37 (2009)

Ikeme, J.: Future of Nigeria's Economy: Ignored threats from the global climate changedebacle. De Montfort University, ULeicester, UK, African Economic Analysis (2008)

International Energy Agency [IEA], (2017): Energy Security. https://www.iea.org/topics/energy security. On 18/05/2018

International Energy Agency [IEA], (2016), Energy Technology Perspectives (2016) – TowardsSustainableUrban Energy Systems. OECD/IEA: Paris, France. https://www.iea.org/etp/etp2016.

Joskow, P.: Retail electricity consumption. Rand J. Econ. **37**(4), 180–198 (2008)
Leadership Nigeria Newspapers. BEDC Billings: Ekiti Electricity Consumers Protect (2018). www.leadership.ng/2018/03/14/bedc-electricitybillingAdo-ekiti).
May, T.: Social Research: Issues, Methods and Process, 3rd edition. Open University Press, Buckingham (2001)
Miah, M.D., Foysal, M.A., Koike, M., Kobayashi, H.: Domestic energy-use patternby thehouseholds: a comparison between rural and semi-urban areas of Naokhali inbangladesh. Energy Policy **39**(6), 3757–3765 (2011)
National Population Commission of Nigeria: The 1991 Census: Federal Republic of National (2006)
NERC (Nigerian Electricity Regulatory Commission): Overview of the NigerianElectricity Regulatory Commission. July 14–18 2008 (2008)
Programmes, N.S.E.: The Nigeria Energy Sector. An Overview with a Special Emphasis on Renewable Energy, Energy Efficiency and RuralElectrification (2015)
OECD/IEA. (2011). *Energy for all: Financing access for the poor.* www.worldenergyoutlook.org/weowebsite/2011/weo2011/energy_for_all. 04/05/201
Oginni, O.T., Rominiyi, O.L., Eiche, J.F.: Comparative Study of ResidentialHouseholdEnergy Consumption in Ekiti State. Nigeria. British J. Appl. Sci. Technol. **21**(2), 1–0 (2017)
Ogunleye, O.S.: Urban Mobility in Ekiti State: Options and Transformation*:* A Public Lecture Delivered in World's Habitat Day at Lady Jibowu Hall, Ado-Ekiti (2013)
Orazulike, C.: Energy Crisis: The Bane of Nigeria's Development, Oil/gas Magazine, December 12 (2013)
Ouedraogo, B.: Household energy preferences for cooking in urban Ouagadougou. Burkina Faso, Energy policy **34**(18), 3787–3795 (2006)
Sambo, A.S.: Matching electricity supply with demand in nigeria. Int. Assoc. Energy Econ. **4**, 32–36 (2008)
United Nations Development Programme (UNDP): The Millennium DevelopmentGoals (2001).www.undp.org/mdg, www.unmilleniumproject.org/html
United Nation Energy [UN-Energy]: Background Note*:* Energy: A Brief Discussion On Goals, Targets and Indicators (2014)
Uyigue, E.: Renewable energy and energy efficiency and sustainable development in Nigeria. In: Conference on Promoting Renewable Energy and Energy Efficiency in Nigeria (2007)
World Energy Council [WEC]. The Potential for Regionally Integrated Energy Development in Africa. London, United Kingdom (2013). www.worldenergy.org

Deep Learning for Automatic Parasitemia Identification from Peripheral Blood Smear Images

A. U. Rufai(✉) and J. O. Enikuomehin

Department of Computer Sciences, University of Lagos, Lagos, Nigeria

Abstract. This paper proposes a novel method to identify the presence of malaria parasites in human peripheral blood smear images by transferring knowledge of pre-trained models which include the Frozen VGG-19, and Fine-tuned VGG-19 model which is already pre-trained on a large dataset (ImageNet) with a lot of diverse image categories. A comparative analysis is made between the regular state-of-the-art models which include the vanilla convolutional neural network model, and the deep belief networks. The proposed method has performed significantly better than other state-of-the-art methods with an F-score of 96.00%, a sensitivity of 96.01% and specificity of 96.10%. The results obtained in this study indicates the need for the incorporation of artificial intelligence into the ground rules of the roll-back Malaria programme by state actors in sub-Saharan Africa. Further research would be carried out by transferring knowledge from larger pre-trained models such as the ResNet52 model.

Keywords: Deep Learning · Malware · Gated Recurrent Unit · Convolutional Neural Network

1 Introduction

Protozoan infections cause an incredible burden of malady in each the tropics and climatic zone further as in additional temperate climates. Of all parasitic diseases, protozoal infection causes the foremost deaths globally protozoal infection kills more or less 600 thousand individuals every year, most of them young kids in sub-Saharan Africa (CDC 2020). Hence an immediate large-scale response to diagnosis and treatment is essential in order to minimize the mortality rate over said geographical zones. Considering malaria parasite infection as a case study, malaria is caused by a plasmodium genus protozoan parasite, transmitted through the bite of an infected, mainly pregnant female anopheles mosquito that then corrupts red blood cells, most deaths occur in African children (CDC 2020).

According to the statistics provided (WHO 2018), malaria is highly prevalent worldwide, particularly in tropical areas and is considered critical in sub-Saharan Africa, which includes Nigeria. This elevated rate of malaria diseases and mortality underlines the significance of the Nigerian population of rapid and quickly obtainable malaria therapy. Other protozoan infections that predominantly cause havoc in the human system

J. N. Mojekwu et al. (Eds.): *Sustainable Education and Development*, pp. 480–489, 2021.
https://doi.org/10.1007/978-3-030-68836-3_41

include: *Amoebiasis, Diarrhoea, Trypanosomiasis, Leishmaniasis, Trichomoniasis, Toxoplasmosis* and *Balantidial Dysentery*, although these infections are not as dominant as the afore-mentioned Malaria, there is still a necessity for treatment (WHO 2018).

There are many types of laboratory tests available for diagnosing protozoan infections. The form of test(s) that will be prescribed by a medical doctor will be based on signs and symptoms, any other health problems that may be present, and travel history. Diagnosis can be daunting, so a health care provider may conduct various tests. These protozoa studies fall into three groups, faecal (stool) analysis, previously known as ovary and parasite screening (O&P), endoscopy/colonoscopy and blood testing. Many worm infections, though not all, are often identified by blood testing. Blood tests rummage around for a particular parasite infection; no blood test can look for all parasite diseases. The two types of blood tests that can be performed are serology and blood smear Check for parasites in the blood. It is possible to detect parasitic diseases such as filariasis, malaria, and babesiosis by check at a blood sample under a microscope. This experiment is conducted by putting a drop of blood on a slide of the microscope. The slide will then be microscopically painted and studied. This method is considered the most common diagnostic technique for malaria and the conventional gold standard. Over the coming centuries, the optimistic disposition of the use of technology and artificial intelligence methods in healthcare, automation, and computerization of healthcare facilities and systems has grown significantly in recent years as one of the major research areas.

This optimism is rejuvenated by the latest development of Artificial Intelligence in the non-healthcare industry as such, ground-breaking developments in the areas of Image Recognition, Computer Vision and Natural Language Processing, for instance, by investing billions of dollars in the development of different Image Recognition technologies such as Deep Face on Facebook, FaceNet by Google. Etcetera. This growth is driven by the steady internet-wide acquisition of data, an instance of which are the picture repositories used in past and continuous research and development of image recognition systems and computer vision and artificial intelligence are Google's ResNet, AlexNet, and CIFAR10 datasets.

As a result, countless Artificial Intelligence applications in healthcare were created possible owing to the rapidity of augmented availability of medical data and express growth of vast data analytical techniques, therefore healthcare's data-driven characteristics add up to it a traditional dig for the devotion of AI over many disciplines, from pathology, epidemiology, to drug discovery and diagnosis. At the same time, medical data awareness raises basic questions about trust and privacy. This combination makes healthcare one of the most dangerous, sensitive and possibly one of its interesting areas of AI. Such an element includes diagnosis and laboratory tests involving extremely sensitive and accurate processes to guarantee an unadulterated outcome.

The method involves regular manual microscopy of peripheral blood smears in the field of malaria diagnosis, as the malaria parasite mainly affects human blood RBCs. It is the responsibility of pathologists to analyse RBCs under a light microscope to observe differences in the length, shape and colour of RBCs to detect malaria infection, hence the precision of the diagnosis varies on the pathologists' expertise in the field, including the automated Microscopy Analysis System, the accuracy and consistency of the diagnostic results can be further boosted (Mohammed, 2017).

This study investigated the development of an automated system of microscopy analysis of peripheral blood smear for diagnosis of protozoan related blood infections like malaria. The model detects and classifies infected red blood cell (RBC) at protozoal infected RBC from microscopic images of peripheral blood smear (PBS) films rendered as input to the model using transfer learns that greatly outperformed existing models for parasite detection.

2 Theoretical Framework on Identification of Malaria Parasites

Early research conducted by the World Health Organization implemented the use of Fluorescent Microscopy and the Identification of Malaria parasites using Acridine-Orange Staining Method (Shute and Sodeman 1973). The objectives of which amongst many was to ascertain the accuracy with which malaria parasites could be identified and to determine the advantages of acridine-orange staying over Romanowsky, particularly to making positive detections when the parasite counts were low. They concluded that the acridine-orange staining operation is easy, fast and within the average lab technician's expertise. The fluorescence of malaria parasites is brilliant and while the existence of artifacts has caused occasional misdiagnosis, it has not been deemed sufficiently numerous to constitute a severe handicap to the use of the method.

(Sio et al. 2007) proposed the rule-based segmentation which accurately detects and segment the named cells respective to the rules stated for identifying the features. However, these requires the knowledge about the cell shape, size, colour etc.

(Anggraini et al. 2011) and, (Malihi et al. 2013) proposed the Otsu thresholding which calculates the optimum threshold if the image has a bi-modal histogram. However, the calculation is only possible on images with fully bi-modal data.

(Nasir et al. 2012) and Nanoti et al. (2016) used the K-means clustering, an unsupervised learning method that iteratively assign pixels to K clusters using their characteristic descriptors. The drawback here, is the difficulty in determining the initial value of k, for accurate analysis and difficulty in identifying features from overlapping regions in k-space.

Yang et al. (2017) proposed an adaptive histogram thresholding which worked for a higher percentage of the images provided in contrast to local methods. However, the threshold value is difficult to determine.

Bibin et al. (2017), proposed a novel method for identifying malaria parasites in peripheral human blood smear images using a Deep Belief Learner (DBN). They presented a qualified model based on a DBN to classify in the parasite or non-parasite class 4100 peripheral blood smear images. The proposed DBN was pre-trained using the contrastive divergence method for pre-training to stack restricted Boltzmann machines. They extracted the characteristics from the images to train the DBN and initialize the DBN's visible variables. Then they used a concentrated colour and texture feature as a feature vector. Finally, a backpropagation algorithm that calculates the probability of class labels was used to fine-tune the DBN discriminatively. The optimum size of the DBN architecture used by (Bibin et al. 2017) was "484–600-600-600-600-2", where there are 484 nodes in visible layer and two nodes in the output layer with four hidden layers containing 600 hidden nodes in each layer. The suggested techniques conducted considerably better than the other state-of-the-art techniques with 89.66% F-Score, 97.60% F-score, 97.60% sensitivity, and 95.92% specificity". This is the first application of DBN for the detection of parasite from human peripheral blood smear images.

Mohammed, (2017) developed an image processing system to locate and classify malaria parasites in thin blood smears (Images prepared using the Light Microscope imaging techniques) into one of the four distinct malaria species. In the pre-processing phase, many methods were applied to improve the images. Morphological processing was implemented in the first portion of the scheme to distinguish the RBCs from images of thin blood smear. The algorithm created was able to select the suspected areas and detect the parasite in the pictures, including overlapping cells. The RBCs were hence classified into infected and non-infected cells, calculating the number of RBCs in each image, Afterward, they utilized the feature of standardized cross-correlation to classify the parasite into one of the four species, Their results showed 95% precision for the detection and counting of RBCs and 100% for the identification and classification of the parasite into one of its four kinds compared to manual outcomes.

According to Poostchi et al. (2018), Automated Cell Microscopy System typically uses a series of main processing steps that can be used as guidelines, these steps would be further explored in regards to the vast majority of papers on automatic malaria microscopy ever released.

The aforementioned series of steps include, (1). Acquisition of digital images of blood smears, (2) Image Preprocessing, (3). Red Blood Cell (RBC) detection and segmentation (4). Feature extraction and selection (5). Parasite Identification and Labelling. This section would provide insight into the core of this field, taking a review of articles published per process pipeline.

The variations in this step greatly depend on the type of microscopy used. Most researchers have introduced conventional microscopy technologies because light microscopy is the most prevalent type of malaria diagnosis in resource-poor environments, where automation will also have the greatest effect on health care and the economy. Likewise, other imaging techniques that have been found in research articles for which automated systems have been created.

In (Poostchi et al. 2018), pre-processing is primarily used to enhance image quality and to decrease differences in images that would needlessly complicate the forthcoming processing steps. Three main goals can be recognized: removal of noise, enhancement of contrast, illumination and correction of stain. The most common methods for noise removal were well-established filters, such as mean and median filters, or low-pass Gaussian filtering. Moreover, it is very common to apply morphological operations. In specific, contrast stretching methods and histogram equalization were the most common methods for enhancement in comparison. Colour normalization methods have been implemented for lighting and staining differences, including the common use of gray-scale colours.

Detection and Segmentation of RBC involves a variety of techniques that are used singularly or batch during the detection phase, thresholding techniques, such as Otsu thresholding in conjunction with morphological operations, are the vast majority of these techniques. However, these techniques may not dominate due to their superior results compared to other methods, but due to their comparative simplicity. Other techniques include transforming Hough, which makes assumptions about the form of the blood cell, and clustering of unmonitored k-means pixels. To calculate the right parasitemia, cell segmentation must be precise. In specific, touching cells, however, make it difficult to identify and segment individual cells.

Methods such as watershed and active contours have been introduced to this issue. For Feature Extraction and Selection, the objective is to deduce an empirical and valid description of the appearance of RBCs, both infected and uninfected in thin smears, considering that the parasites have been stained, colour features are natural and used in many cases. Conclusively, the final phase being the Parasite identification and labelling phase, virtually all of the classification techniques common in the last century have been used to diagnose malaria, varying from decision trees and fundamental artificial neural networks to support vector machines to random tree classifiers. Very few papers have created cell discrimination or parasite detection classification techniques specifically. Most of the information about malaria-specific domains reside in segmentation, characteristics, and classification interplay.

The gaps observed in literature include the difficulty in managing variations in feature extraction. Also, colour normalization methods have been implemented for lighting and staining differences, including the common use of gray-scale colours. Detection and Segmentation of RBC involves a variety of techniques that are used singularly or batch during the detection phase, thresholding techniques, such as Otsu thresholding in conjunction with morphological operations, are the vast majority of these techniques. This study seeks to mitigate the difficulty in managing variations in feature extraction.

3 Experiments

The research design for the study is based on quantitative research (experimental research design). Experimental design in the machine learning domain are largely algorithmic. The steps taken in carrying out the experiment are as follows:

Data collection, image acquisition, thin and dense peripheral blood smear (PBS) collection images, grouping into marked information sets recognized by the corresponding image methods, such as prevalent Light Microscope blood images, fluorescent, polarized and binocular blood film images. Pre-processing approaches such as dealing with noise reduction, low image contrast, etc. to be applied to the automatic analysis of digital blood slide images primarily to improve the image standard and reduce variations within images which would unnecessarily complicate subsequent processing steps.

Detection and segmentation of red blood cells: not necessarily an AI-based technique as other reliable methods (mostly thresholding) have been used. This stage is crucial for the model because RBCs are only required for the model, so it is only necessary to identify WBCs and other constituents and not to process, classify and index them further.

Extraction and selection feature Red blood cells have different distinguishing features for both infected and non-infected thin smears, choice of RBC identification factors such as colour features, texture, and morphological features can be conducted using colour auto-correlation plot, coincidence matrix, coincidence level matrix, and regional granulometry techniques respectively.

The Identification and Classification of Parasite phase involves the, Training of Model using various Deep Learning Algorithms as it is a Transfer Learner, a comparison between the two types of learners would be carried out, on deciding which best suits this project, further Training of the transfer learning model, proposed ML algorithms be used as sub learners include: Frozen VGG-19, Activated Pre-Trained VGG-19, Frozen VGG-16, Pretrained VGG-16.

Assessment, assessment, and comparison of the results of trained models in the test dataset classification.

Diagnosis and Parasitemia Medical professionals evaluate the model.

3.1 Dataset Description

The proposed model architectures are implemented in python3 using Keras on TensorFlow, use of numpy for fast maths operations with Data structures, scikit-learn for metrics evaluation, matplotlib for graphing and plotting output vectors and matrices and pandas for data-set manipulation and processing. Developed on Google colab environment with GPU acceleration on a Debian LTS operating system.

Given that the best models developed for malaria parasite detection are all based on the architecture of the Convolutional Neural Network (CNN), which offers precise automated and scalable models of feature engineering and classification. It is therefore a strong foundation on which to capitalize. A custom CNN model is built in this study experiment and compared to the CNN model is built and compared to the CNN model which leverages six pre-trained models. Six pre-trained models are built and compared to the CNN model. That model -transfer functions respectively as an extractor function and a classification system. The principle of deep transfer learning would be implemented in this context as improved models for image recognition and malaria detection, two deep transfer learning techniques would be applied, including the use of pre-trained model. As an extractor function and using a fully graded pre-trained template with fine tuning.

The proposed pre-trained model to be implemented is the VGG-19 deep learning model, developed at Oxford University by the Visual Geometry Group (VGG), The VGG-19 is a pre-trained model on a large dataset (ImageNet) with many different image categories. In view of this, the model should have discovered a solid hierarchy of features that are invariant in terms of the characteristics learned from CNN models in space, rotation, and translation. Having learned a good representation of the features of over a million images, the template can therefore serve as a valuable extractor of fresh images suitable for computer vision issues, just like malaria detection. For one of the VGG models, it will be used as a straightforward feature extractor by freezing all five convolution blocks to ensure that their weights are not changed after each epoch and we applied a fine tuning for the second model while the last two blocks (Block 4 & Block 5) are unfreezed so that their weights are modified after each iteration per batch during the training phase. Also, image augmentation protocols are applied to the training set which involve image transformation operations such as rotation, shearing, translation and zooming to produce new altered versions of existing images.

Prior to the proposed classification phase, Cell segmentation and Detection phase is implemented. Each image is annotated manually with each cell's centre point and some hard-negative examples. The steps taken are as follows:

1. All points within sample radius of a cell centre are sampled as positive samples.
2. An equal number of negative samples are randomly sampled outside the positive radius.
3. All points within sample radius of the hard-negative examples are sampled as negative sample [box_size], is used as input to the network is trained using the negative and positive samples. For each sample, a box of size [box_size], is used as input to the network.
4. Given a new image [box_sized] window is slid through each possible patch in the image, generating a probability map local maxima in the probability map are marked as cell centres.

Hence, two datasets were considered (LHNCBC & BCCD), both datasets covered a large range of RBC samples (infected and healthy) cell images of processed blood samples acquired from patients globally, as curated by medical professionals. The LHNCBC dataset was fine-tuned to individual RBC images which have been processed and segmented from Peripheral blood smear images from the malaria screener research activity (NIH 2019). The BCCD dataset is a small-scale dataset of curated pre-processed and segmented images of Peripheral blood images. The LHNCBC dataset is composed of 27,558 cell images with equal instances of parasitized and uninfected cells. The Level-Set based algorithm that ensures topological flexibility was used to detect and segment the red blood cells.

4 Results

The performance reports of each model for each dataset are given below:

LHNCBC dataset: The Vanilla CNN model ran for only ten epochs with a batch size 64, and achieved a training accuracy of 99.97% and validation accuracy of 95.59%.

The dataset was divided into 60% for training, 10% for validation and 30% for testing. The table below highlights the experimentation results from training the models on the LHNCBC Dataset (Table 1).

Table 1. Test Evaluation results

Model	Experiment	Accuracy	F1 score	Precision	Recall
Vanilla CNN	Trained on 60% of LHNCBC dataset Batch size of 64 and 25 epochs	0.9497	0.9497	0.9497	0.9497
VGG-19 Frozen	...	0.9376	0.9376	0.9379	0.9376
VGG-19 Fine Tuned	...	0.9601	0.9600	0.9610	0.9604

The Frozen VGG-19 model ran with a batch size of 64 and for 15 epochs, it achieved a training accuracy of 93.76% and a validation accuracy of 92.05%.

The Fully activated fine-tuned VGG-19 model ran with an accuracy of 96.00% and a validation accuracy of 95.98%.

The performance reports of each model for each dataset are given below:

LHNCBC dataset: The Vanilla CNN model ran for only ten epochs with a batch size 64, and achieved a training accuracy of 99.97% and validation accuracy of 95.59%.

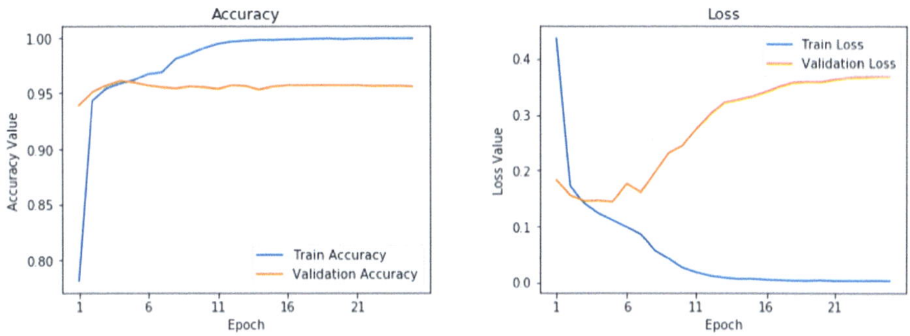

Fig. 1. Vanilla CNN evaluation.

The Frozen VGG-19 model ran with a batch size of 64 and for 15 epochs, it achieved a training accuracy of 93.76% and a validation accuracy of 92.05%.

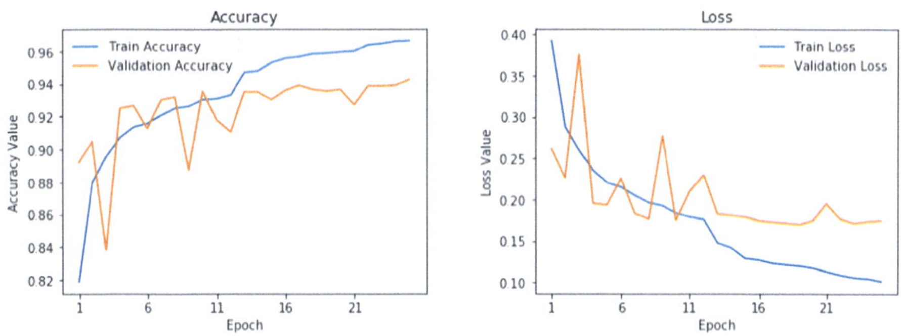

Fig. 2. Frozen VGG-19 (feature extractor) evaluation.

The Fully activated fine-tuned VGG-19 model ran with an accuracy of 96.00% and a validation accuracy of 95.98%.

4.1 Discussion of Results

From the above table of performance results, it is shown clearly that the fine-tuned transfer learning model performs better than the CNN model as well as the Feature Extraction transfer learning model during validation and testing with different sets of the dataset. On the LHNCBC dataset, the CNN model got a validation accuracy of 95.6%

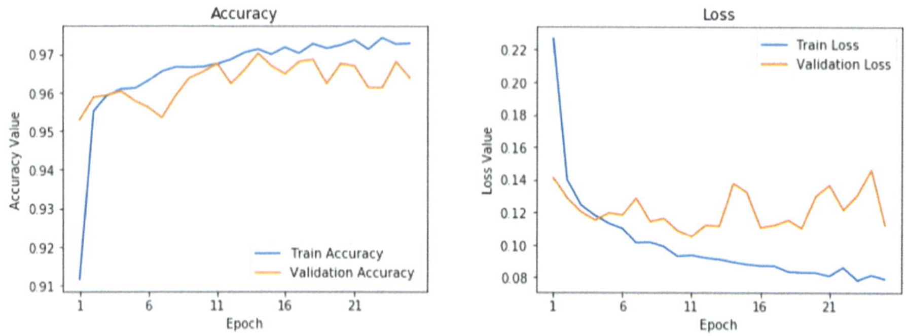

Fig. 3. Fine-tuned Pre-trained VGG-19 evaluation.

which is good, though the model overfitted slightly over the training set as proven with a training accuracy of 99.9%. From evaluation plot in Fig. 1 we can see that the overall improvement of the training process does not progress until after the 5th epoch. But with the VGG-19 feature extractor, after plugin our dense layers at the end of the first 6-layers of the frozen pre-trained VGG ConvNet architecture for classification given a sum total of 28 layers with only 6 trainable layers, the overall training performance was less than that of the regular CNN, with a training accuracy of 96.66% and validation accuracy of 94.30% as indicated in Fig. 2 it shows us that our model is not overfitting as much as the vanilla CNN model. In the 3rd model, we ensured that all layers were trainable, hence acting as a feature extractor and classifier. By fine-tuning the weights of the layers present in the last two blocks of our pre-trained VGG-19 model and implementing image augmentation protocols on just the training set, but the validation set was only scaled, and also reducing the learning rate so as to avoid making large weight updates to the pre-trained layers when fine-tuning it achieved a validation accuracy of nearly 96.5% on 10% of the data per epoch with minimal overfitting and maximum accuracy of 97.29% as observed in Fig. 3 this model out-performed previous models as well as existing models.

5 Conclusion and Future Work

This research work entails using the concept of transfer learning as leverage for building highly effective models for the purpose of parasite identification, using a pre-trained VGG-19 deep learning model, ResNet model which have already been pre-trained on a huge dataset (ImageNet) with a lot of diverse image categories. Based on this fact this the model should have learned a robust hierarchy of features that could hence serve as complete feature extractors, thereby outliving the need for a conventional approach to feature extraction.

In conclusion, it is shown that the transfer learners outperform the regular Neural Networks, vanilla CNN and Deep belief Network models (Bibin et al. 2017). This work was conducted under the scope of an interesting real-world medical imaging case study of malaria detection in this work. Detection of malaria in itself is not a simple process, and the accessibility of the correct staff worldwide is also a severe problem, Hence, we considered providing open-source methods based on AI that can offer us state-of-the-art precision and accuracy in detecting and diagnosing malaria, allowing AI for social benefit. The limitations encountered in this work was the lack of a local runtime environment for training models, the major requirement for training the VGG-19 or ResNet models are GPU Cuda cores or tensor cores which were absent locally.

The study with influence the medical imaging field in the aspect of malaria detection. Governments in sub-Saharan Africa have policies of rolling-back malaria, in line with the United Nations sustainable development goal number 3: good health and well-being. Our work if adopted, will improve on the existing ground rules in medical imaging for malaria detection.

In our future work, we aim to improve on the current transfer learner by training with the ResNet152 & ResNet50 models as a feature extractor and existing deep belief networks as well as other pre-trained models as well as improving on the cell detection frameworks and algorithms using methods discussed in this research work.

References

Anggraini, D., Nugroho, A.S., Pratama, C., Rozi, I.E., Iskandar, A.A., Hartono, R.N.: Automated status identification of microscopic images obtained from malaria thin blood smears. In: Proceedings of the 2011 International Conference on Electrical Engineering and Informatics, pp. 1–6. IEEE (2011). https://doi.org/10.1109/ICEEI.2011.6021762

Bibin, D., Nair, M.S., Punitha, P.: Malaria parasite detection from peripheral blood smear images using deep belief networks. IEEE Access **5**, 9099–9108 (2017)

CDC. Malaria. CDC (2020). https://www.cdc.gov/parasites/malaria/index.html

Malihi, L., Ansari-Asl, K., Behbahani, A.: Malaria parasite detection in giemsa-stained blood cell images. In: 2013 8th Iranian Conference on Machine Vision and Image Processing (MVIP), pp. 360–365. IEEE (2013)

Nanoti, A., Jain, S., Gupta, C., Vyas, G.: Detection of malaria parasite species and life cycle stages using microscopic images of thin blood smear. In: 2016 International Conference on Inventive Computation Technologies (ICICT), vol. 1, pp. 1–6. IEEE, August 2016

Nasir, A.A., Mashor, M.Y., Mohamed, Z.: Segmentation based approach for detection of malaria parasites using moving k-means clustering. In: 2012 IEEE-EMBS Conference on Biomedical Engineering and Sciences, pp. 653–658. IEEE (2012)

NIH. Malaria Datasets, National Library of Medicine (2019). NIH: https://ihlncbc.nlm.nih.gov/publication/pub9932

Poostchi, M., Silamut, K., Maude, R.J., Jaeger, S., Thoma, G.: Image analysis and machine learning for detecting malaria. Transl. Res. **194**, 36–55 (2018)

Shute, G.T., Sodeman, T.M.: Identification of malaria parasites by fluorescence microscopy and acridine orange staining. Bull. World Health Organ. **48**(5), 591 (1973)

Sio, S.W., Sun, W., Kumar, S., Bin, W.Z., Tan, S.S., Ong, S.H., Tan, K.S.: MalariaCount: an image analysis-based program for the accurate determination of parasitemia. J. Microbiol. Methods **68**(1), 11–18 (2007)

WHO (2018). World Malaria report WHO. https://www.who.int/malaria/publications/atoz/9789241549127/en/

Yang, D., Subramanian, G., Duan, J., Gao, S., Bai, L., Chandramohanadas, R., Ai, Y.: A portable image-based cytometer for rapid malaria detection and quantification. PLoS ONE **12**(6), e0179161 (2017)

The Digital Diplomacy (DD) Apparatus and the Conduct of Diplomacy in Tanzania

J. Kajerero[1](✉) and L. S. Mujwahuzi[2]

[1] Department of Political Science and Public Administration, The University of Dodoma, P.O. Box 259, Dodoma, Tanzania
[2] Institute of Development Studies (IDS), The University of Dodoma, P.O. Box 395, Dodoma, Tanzania

Abstract. The main triggering argument for this paper is that although much has been aired on the practice of diplomacy in addressing the response conventional diplomacy to the Digital Diplomacy (DD) apparatus but little has been known regarding the impact of DD apparatus on the conduct of diplomacy in Tanzania, especially the extent to which DD apparatus can help achieve foreign policy objectives. In responding to this puzzle, the paper specifically, examines the status of diplomacy conduct in the study area, and assesses the impact of digital diplomacy apparatus on the conduct of diplomacy. A cross-sectional research design is adopted coupled with purposive sampling technique to obtain data. Quantitative data were descriptively analyzed by using SPSS version 24, while the qualitative data were analyzed through thematic analysis. Under the status of diplomacy in Tanzania, the findings reveal that both offline and digital diplomacy apparatus are used in conducting diplomacy and in accessing diplomatic services. For the impact of DD apparatus it has been concluded that DD has enhanced the ability to shape and frame diplomatic agenda and empower states diplomatic agents and missions. It is recommended that the United Republic of Tanzania has to conduct capacity building training on DD apparatus, installation, and maintenance of wireless technology infrastructure, and give preference to hybrid conduct of diplomacy.

Keywords: Digital diplomacy apparatus · Diplomacy · Foreign Service officers

1 Introduction

Diplomacy is a famous word in the globe especially when it comes to the study of International Relations (IR). Thus, (Aksoyk and Çiçek 2018), view diplomacy as an independent discipline, in addition to being an institution of International Relations included under the rubric of International Relations, which emerged as discipline after the First World War. This definition underscores a key feature of diplomacy that is, basing upon conducting state affairs through negotiations in order to ensure peaceful relations. It is imperative to note that, the quest for conducting state affairs between countries in a diplomatic manner is not a recent phenomenon in international relations. Thus, (Ahonen-Strom 2006) asserts clearly that for a number of centuries, countries have interacted in

J. N. Mojekwu et al. (Eds.): *Sustainable Education and Development*, pp. 490–501, 2021.
https://doi.org/10.1007/978-3-030-68836-3_42

a myriad of ways: engaging in business and trade affairs, peace and security issues; as well as promoting political, economic, cultural or scientific relations. It is from this understanding that diplomacy has existed since the time when states, empires or other centers of power dealt with each other on an official basis (Swiss Federal Department of Foreign Affairs FDFA Manual 2008).

Despite the above historical underpinning of diplomacy, recently, its management and conduct (both bilaterally and multilaterally) is increasingly expanding to embrace ICT's technologies in the conduct of relations between states/countries. As noted by Studemeister (2001), diplomacy has stretched out as it is turned to be everybody's business due to the access and effects of wireless technology more specifically ICT's. This implies that ICT is changing the conduct of diplomacy the same as it changes societies. However, ICT-driven changes only complement the existing institutional arrangements that are already in place by facilitating the conduct of international relations activities between countries. But a more interesting question would be to find out to what extent ICT can facilitate or hinder the achievement of diplomatic objectives of a country. In this context, 'Digital Diplomacy (DD), as one of the digital apparatus under the ICT package for enhancing diplomatic relations between countries will be assessed in a way it impacts the conduct of Diplomacy among countries.

The main triggering argument for this paper is that although much has been aired on the practice of diplomacy in addressing the response conventional diplomacy to the DD apparatus, these include Fitzpatrick (2012),on the power of DD platforms by having an outstanding use for the practice of diplomacy, (Cucos 2012) on the DD as a new apparatus in international relations, complementing the traditional methods of conducting diplomatic relations between and among countries, however, little has been known regarding the status and impact of DD apparatus on the conduct of diplomacy in Tanzania, especially the extent to which DD apparatus can help achieve foreign policy objectives. In responding to this puzzle, the paper specifically, examines two issues which are status of diplomacy conduct in the study area and the impact of digital diplomacy apparatus on the conduct of diplomacy in Tanzania.

This paper is underpinned by Actor-Network Theory (ANT) as it is a helpful tool of investigation and analysis of digital studies. Ziemkendorf (2007) affirms that ANT at times is linked with sociology as drawn from works of a scholar like Bruno Latour and John Law, and that crucial features of ANT are the unbiased capacity of examining both human and human actors both as identical actors in digital networks with aim of achieving common diplomatic goals. In reviewing theoretical and empirical literature much of the theorists and researchers focus much in multi-purpose diplomatic interaction platform. For instance, (Cucos 2012) concentrated on virtual Diplomacy as news way of conducting international affairs while (Ahonen-Strom 2006) focused on Virtual Diplomacy and changing diplomacy actors or structures. (Gichoya 2016) paid attention to Virtual Diplomacy and Inter-State Relations, whereas Grech (2006) center of attention was on Virtual Diplomacy as the Diplomacy of the Digital Age. Further, Martin (2001) focused on Virtual Diplomacy while Smith (1999) shared the Challenges of virtual Diplomacy and Ipu (2013) focused on E-Diplomacy in East Africa. With this regard, this paper required to investigating the impacts of digital diplomacy apparatus following the incorporation Digital Diplomacy apparatus in the practice of modern and contemporary diplomacy as a way of promoting, safeguarding and protecting Tanzania's Foreign Policy objectives. Together with this theoretical frame work, the reviews of the literatures give rise to the following conceptual framework which is a roadmap towards the research which laid foundation for this paper (Fig. 1).

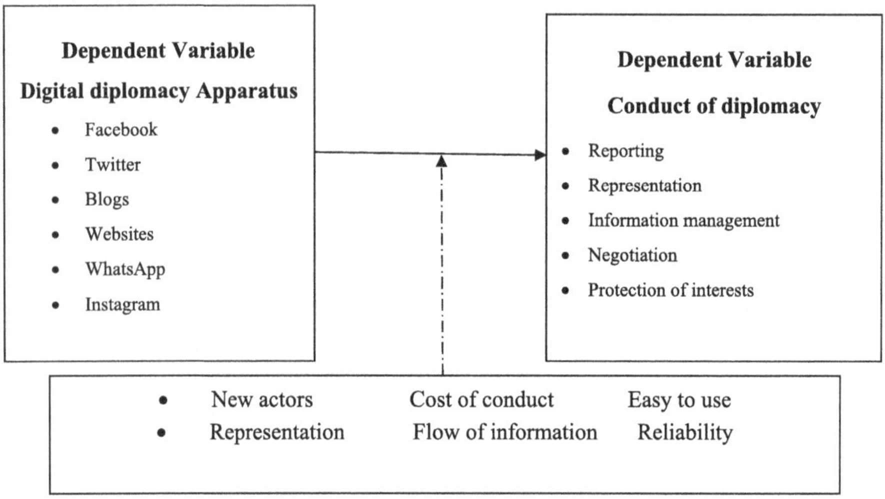

Fig. 1. Conceptual Frame work showing some study variables ***Sources****: Authors construct from the literature (2019).*

2 Methodology

2.1 Research Design

The exploratory research design with a cross-sectional research design was adopted to collect data from the respondents at one point in time. This design was useful because as it helped the researcher to obtain a general picture of representatives at a given minimum in time, this design had a greater degree of accuracy and precision in research because of both dependent and the independent variable could be measured at the time (Deaton 1997).

2.2 Description of the Research Area

This study was conducted in two cities of Tanzania where the diplomatic community resides; these are Dar es Salaam and Dodoma cities. Dar es Salam was preferred because a large number of embassies are located there, while Dodoma is the domicile of the custodian ministry responsible for the conduct, operations, and management of diplomacy in the United Republic of Tanzania (URT).

2.3 The Target Population

The target population in the proposed study comprised of career diplomats (practitioners/FSOs), graduate students who previously pursued diplomatic studies and instructors teaching diplomacy from three higher learning institutions. This population was taken under the assumption that respondents were to cover the objective and answer the research questions as well.

2.4 Sampling Techniques and Sample Size

The manual of (FAO 2015) states that sample design identifies for every possible sample and its probability of being drawn to participate in the research while the Statistics Canada (2014) define sampling as a means of selecting a subset of units from a target population to collect information. In choosing this sample, Dodoma and Dar es Salam cities were selected and used purposively due to the presence of large number of the targeted population that is the diplomatic community. But, to obtain the desired sample size, a simple random sampling technique was used to select three strata then simple random sampling used to select respondents from each stratum. Finally, purposive sampling was used to select the respondents. The size of the sample for this study was 100 respondents from both cities.

3 Data Collection Methods and Apparatus

3.1 Survey Data Collection Method

Kothari (2004) defined survey as the method of gathering information with reference to the concerned phenomenon under research from all the selected samples where the researcher studies the phenomenon which exists in the universe free from his influence. For this study, the survey method employed the questionnaire as a data collection apparatus. The questionnaire focused on investigating the impacts of DD apparatus on the conduct of diplomacy in Tanzania. Information collected from respondents included their experiences and perception on the impacts between DD apparatus and the conduct of diplomacy.

3.2 Interview Data Collection Method

According to Kumar (2011) interview refers to oral/unwritten interchange which may be conducted by face to face interaction or by telephone or by telephone. On the other side Kothari (2004) describes the interview data collection method as the presentation of oral verbal stimuli and reply in terms of oral verbal response. For this study, interviews were used to collect data from key informants, including media personnel, various college instructors and practitioners of diplomacy who have different experience and perceptions on DD apparatus.

3.3 Documentary Review Method

Document review is a way of gathering data by reviewing presented literature. Kumar (2011) defined document review as the data which have been laready collected whereby the required information are extracted so as to serve purpose of study. Documentary review checklist was used in the entire process of reviewing documents as an apparatus for gathering secondary data needed to complement primary data.

3.4 Data Processing, Analysis, and Presentation

(Kothari 2004) defines analysis of data as a process which involves data inspection, data cleaning, data transformation, and modeling data with the goal of discovering useful information, suggesting conclusions, and supporting decision making. Following the coding process and data classification, the analysis was done by a computer software program namely Microsoft Excel and SPSS software and data were descriptively analyzed for the case of quantitative data and the unstructured interviews were analyzed by using thematic and content analysis to identify themes and subthemes from discussions conducted.

4 Results and Discussion

4.1 Status of Diplomacy Conduct

In knowing status of diplomacy conduct in Tanzania, the information captured included experience of both offline and use of DD apparatus, the best mode, and participation in conducting diplomacy using DD apparatus. The information are presented and discussed here under:

4.2 Experience of both Offline and Digital Diplomacy Apparatus

The researcher was interested to know the experience of the respondents in using both offline and digital diplomacy apparatus. The analysis of the data revealed that 90% of the respondents had experience of using both offline and digital diplomacy apparatus, while the minority of the respondents taking 10% of the respondents in study area admitted that they do not have experience in using offline and digital diplomacy apparatus as shown in Table 1. The result favor Hocking & Melissen (2015) argument that hybridity is the norm in the diplomatic context and present media. On the other side, Nirupama (2017) support the adoption of DD apparatus as she considers ignoring the adoption of DD apparatus communication platforms as the threat. Many writers favor DD apparatus to complement conventional diplomacy as these apparatus have been becoming very important and dominant in providing a linkage among diplomatic actors ranging from states to non-states actors and the population in the provision of information and diplomatic services.

Table 1. Experience for both Offline and Digital Diplomacy Apparatus (n = 100)

Experience of both modes	Frequency	Percent
Yes	90	90.0
No	10	10.0
Total	**100**	**100.0**

Source: Field data, 2019

4.3 Best Mode

There are many apparatus for conducting diplomacy in Tanzania, both online mode and offline mode are used to conduct diplomacy in Tanzania. The tablebelow shows the respondents' opinions of which mode of conduct the population considers to be the best. The analysis results show that 27% of the population prefers the use of conventional (offline) mode, 41% of the respondents acknowledged that they prefer using digital apparatus in conducting diplomacy. 32% of the respondents in the study area admitted that they prefer using both conventional (offline) and digital apparatus (online) modes of conducting diplomacy. These results coincides with Hocking and Melissen (2015) who clearly state that DD apparatus are incredibly helpful in the diplomatic area due to complex objectives when it comes to FP management and fundamental changes increasing the day by day. On the other hand, it is admitted that there will be no instant agreement among diplomatic agents on how to use the DD apparatus. Though a large number of respondents support DD apparatus, the use of both modes is good because the weakness of DD apparatus has to be covered by conventional practice with aim of ensuring effectiveness and efficiency in safeguarding and protecting diplomatic objectives. (Cucos 2012) noted that the advancement of DD apparatus has changed the way how international relations actors interact in the international arena. To demonstrate the best mode, Fig. 2 has been used for more illustrative manner.

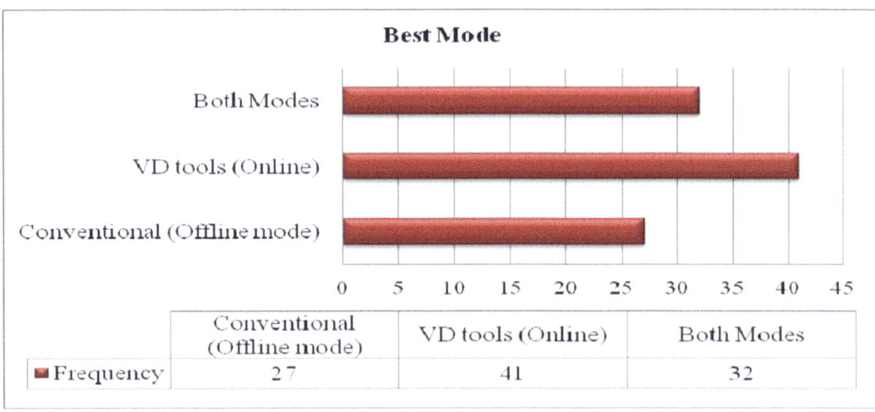

Fig. 2. Best mode (n = 100) Source: Field data, 2019

Data from interviews resemble with the data analyzed from questionnaires as a large number of respondents considers DD apparatus to be the best mode, followed by those who consider both modes to be best and lastly few respondents considered conventional diplomacy to best mode. The interview with one of the Foreign Service officers done on 4thMay 2019 regarding the best mode of conducting diplomacy support revealed the following:

> *"The world is moving and advancing very fast, aspects of communications and transport are not static, establishing, coordinating and monitoring actual (physical) missions is expensive compared to DD apparatus, therefore the use both modes may be a workable solution of ensuring effectiveness and efficiency in safeguarding and protecting diplomatic objectives."*

4.4 Participation in Conducting Diplomacy Using DD Apparatus

The researcher was interested at determining the participation of the respondents in conducting diplomacy using digital diplomacy apparatus. The respondents who participated in conducting diplomacy using DD apparatus were 24 (fresh graduate do not participate in conducting diplomacy) many of them from media industry and foreign services officers categories the findings we that 76% of the respondents in study area admitted that they are not using digital diplomacy apparatus to conduct diplomacy. A significant majority, i.e. 24% of the respondents, acknowledged that they are using digital diplomacy apparatus to conduct diplomacy in Tanzania as shown in Table 2. This implies that, despite the availability of many digital diplomacy apparatus in Tanzania, the majority populations of Tanzania are not utilizing well the availability of digital diplomacy apparatus in conducting diplomacy this might be caused by a large number of respondents to be graduate who pursued diplomacy related subjects.

Table 2. Participation in Conducting Diplomacy Using Digital Diplomacy apparatus (n = 100)

Participation in conducting diplomacy using DD Apparatus	Frequency	Percent
Yes	24	24.0
No	76	76.0
Total	**100**	100.0

Source: Field data, 2019

5 Impacts of Digital Diplomacy Apparatuss on the Conduct of Diplomacy

5.1 Digital Diplomacy Apparatus Improve the Practice of Diplomacy

In order to find the efficiency and effectiveness of digital diplomacy apparatus, respondents were asked to say if digital diplomacy apparatus are appropriate in improving the practice of diplomacy. 97% of respondents admitted that digital diplomacy apparatus improve the practice of diplomacy while only 03% of respondents denied that digital diplomacy apparatus do not improve the practice of diplomacy as shown in Fig. 3. This implies that digital diplomacy apparatus have created new diplomatic functions. Digital diplomacy apparatus have created an interactive diplomatic environment by giving chance to different actors to interact and provide diplomacy services from anywhere throughout the nation and the world in as well. Also, digital diplomacy apparatus are broader compared to conventional diplomacy in terms of both geographical coverage and time-consuming. Alexandru (2015) who exposed that DD apparatus are essential communication instrument for state actor seven real-world variances are playing out on DD apparatus then finish up in hash tag wars between mission and MFA's.

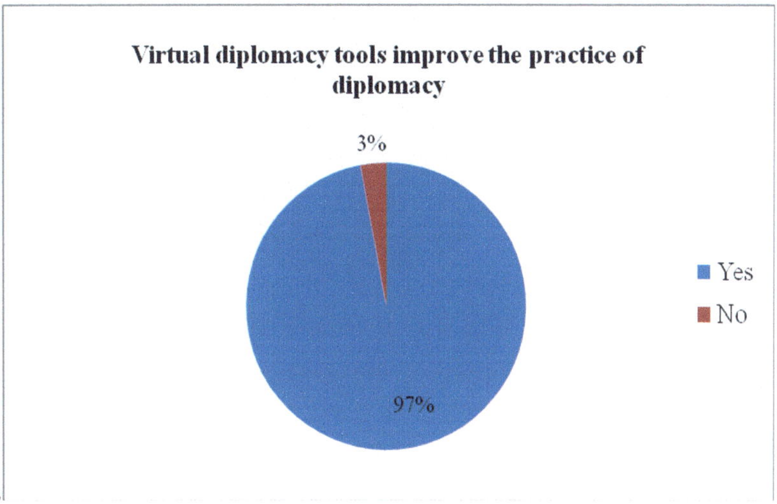

Apparatus

Fig. 3. Digital diplomacy apparatus improve the practice of diplomacy (n = 100) Source: field data

5.2 Digital Diplomacy Apparatus Make Diplomacy Conduct Easier

The study was interested to discover whether digital diplomacy apparatus make diplomacy conduct easier or not. A majority of the respondent (97%) admitted that it is true that digital diplomacy apparatus make diplomacy conduct easier while only 03% said that digital diplomacy apparatus do not make diplomacy conduct easier as shown in Fig. 4. The result matches with Hocking and Melissen (2015) who recognized the rise of networking sites like DD apparatus to be important and increased an important actual time feature on conduct of diplomacy, resulting to both information gathering as well as sharing ultra-fast and often precise. This implies that DD apparatus support the digital representation of actors and supporting documents. DD apparatus are more experimental, recently information is stored in digital form, therefore, DD apparatus simplify the process of accessing stock of information, DD apparatus have made easy to manage states reputation and country branding and easy to coordinate missions abroad; thus, they improve the relations between the ministries of foreign affairs and missions abroad. Therefore, the respondent acknowledged that DD apparatus have made conventional diplomacy conduct easy. On the other side, (Bloodgood and Masson 2018) challenged the results that DD apparatus provide platforms for states put on air national brands but create pathetic national relations. DD apparatus are inappropriate for a successful reply to exogenous tension or diplomatic crises which demand building trust and the slight contact of intentions and resolve, such as trade-related dispute (Ibid).

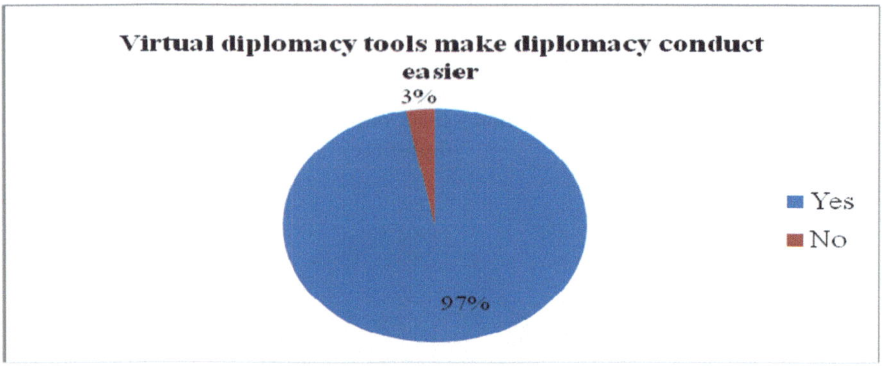

Fig. 4. Digital diplomacy apparatus make diplomacy conduct easier (n = 100) *Source: field data, 2019.*

5.3 Digital Diplomacy Apparatus Make Diplomacy Conduct Viable

The researcher was interested to know if Digital diplomacy apparatus are viable and can be applied. Therefore, the respondents were asked to provide their experience in practicing diplomatic activities by using digital diplomacy apparatus. 98% of the respondents in the study area admitted that it true that digital diplomacy apparatus make diplomacy conduct viable. 02% of the respondents answer that digital diplomacy apparatus do not make diplomacy conduct viable as shown in Fig. 4. The result matches Hocking and Melissen (2015) explanations that DD apparatus add a lot to the capabilities of a diplomatic agent which make diplomatic practice more viable. This implies that DD apparatus are too fast when using DD apparatus makes it easy to frame agenda as it is very flexible, simplify amplification and projection of diplomatic message and DD is not limited to internal procedure of delivering and handling secret messages, confidential reports and instructions. DD apparatus are used in negotiations process which is among the core functions of diplomacy and DD apparatus have simplified diplomatic function simply an observation, collection, and dissemination of information on various aspects ranging from social, political to economic which is a core function of diplomats. These findings contrast those of Adesina (Adenisina 2017) who clearly stated that Digital Diplomacy apparatus have risks which are not limited to information and message leakage, hacking, and secrecy of anonymity of wireless of Internet users. Nirupama (2017) also challenged the viability of Digital Diplomacy apparatus asserted the limitation of Digital Diplomacy apparatus that limits communication due to the largely ignored commentary section of private messaging (Fig. 5).

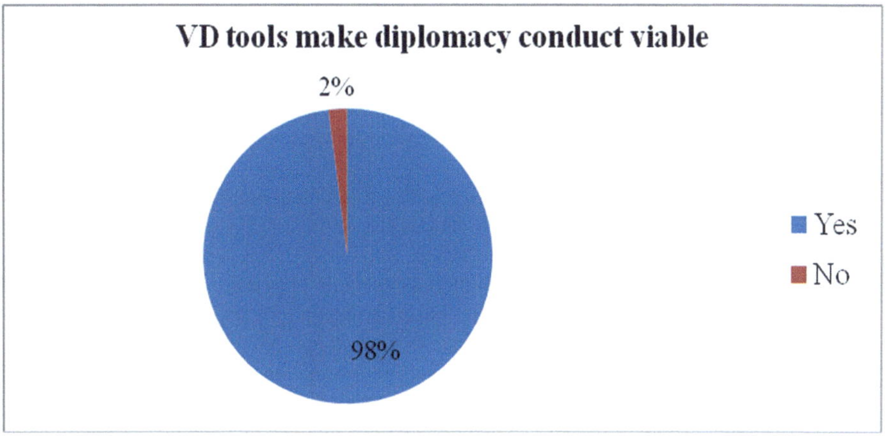

Fig. 5. Digital ddiplomacy apparatus make diplomacy conduct viable (n = 100) Source: field data, 2019

6 Conclusion And Recommendations

Under the status of diplomacy conduct in the study area, it is concluded that the majority of respondents use both offline and online and use Digital Diplomacy to access various services. Digital Diplomacy apparatus support the conduct of conventional diplomacy while making it more open to the public compared to conventional diplomacy alone thus the use both is modes considered to be good so as ensuring effectiveness and efficiency in safeguarding and protecting diplomatic objectives. It is there recommended that The United Republic of Tanzania's (URT) government under the Ministry of Foreign Affairs (MFA) on the use of Digital Diplomacy apparatus and public diplomacy in general to perform diplomatic functions more efficiently and effectively by the Tanzania government. By establishing the capacity building programs, they will be equipped with soft but necessary skills important for them to cope and be capable of utilizing the opportunities available via Digital Diplomacy platforms in diplomacy conduct.

It is further concluded that Digital Diplomacy apparatus have enhanced the ability to shape and frame diplomatic agenda and empower states diplomatic agents and missions while energizing the general public and they are more efficient and cost-effective. Digital Diplomacy apparatus have made easy to manage states reputation and country branding, easy to coordinate Missions abroad, Digital Diplomacy apparatus are too fast and not limited internal procedure for delivering confidential reports, instructions and messages and can be used in the negotiations process. It is there recommended that Digital diplomacy should be implemented not by the ministry concerned but by other government machinery in energizing the diplomatic agenda.

References

Adenisina, O.S.: Foreign policy in an era of digital diplomacy, cogent social sciences. Retrieved-July 8, 2019 from Tandfonline Web site, June 2017. https://www.tandfolline.com/action/showCitformats?doi=10.1080%2f23311886.2017.1297175

Ahonen-Strom, K.: Changing Diplomacy-Actors or structures?: Lund University Publications (pdf). Retrieved from lup.lub.lu.com, 3 February 2006 https://lup.lub.lu.se/luur/download?func=downloadfile&recordold=132581&fileOld=132588 . Accessed 9 July 2019

Alexandru, A.: Twiplomacy 2015 report: Twitter is the channel of choice for digital diplomacy. RetrievedMay 8, 2019 from Digital diplomacy Web site: https://digitaldiplomacy.ro/twiplomacy-2015-report-twitter-is-the-channel-of-choice-for-digital-diplomacy/?lang=en, 2 May 2015

Aksoyk, M., Çiçek, A.S.: Redefining Diplomacy In The 21st century & Examiningthe Characteristics of An Ideal UniversityInternational Relations Departmentmeaksoy@selcuk.edu.trAhmet Servet (2018)

Bloodgood, E., Masson, T.: Diplomacy in the digital era brings both risks and rewards. Retrieved May22, 2019 from Policy options Web site. https://policyoptions.irpp.org/magazines/march-2018/digital-technology-and-the-changing-face-of-diplomacy7 March 2018

Cucos, R.: Virtual diplomacy-a new way of conducting international affairs? The World Bank, Information and Communication Technologies blog Available at. Retrieved July 13, 2019 from World Bank Web site, 2 September 2012: https://www.blogs.worldbank.org/ic4d/virtual-diplomacy-a-new-way-of-conducting-international-affairs.

Deaton, A.: The Analysis of Household Surveys: A Microeconometric Approach to Development Policy. The Johns Hopkins University Press, Baltimore (1997)

FAO. A guide for woodfuel surveys. Retrieved December 12, 2018, from Corporate document repository, May 2015: https://www.fao.org/docrep/005/y3779e/y3779e08.htm

Fitzpatrick, A.: mashable.com. Retrieved June 17, 2019, from mashable, 22 September 2012. https://mashable.com/2012/09/22/social-media-diplomacy/

Gichoya, F.W.: (201). Virtual Diplomacy and Inter-State Relation: A Case Study of Kenya. Nairobi: University of Nairobi- Master Dissertation

Grech, O.M.: Virtual Diplomacy- Diplomacy of the Digital Age. Retrieved on december 18, 2018 from Virtual Diplomacy Web site, 24 March 2006. http:www.virtualdiplomacy.net/pdfdrive

Hocking, B., Melissen, J.: Diplomacy in the Digital Age-Clingendael Report. Netherlands Institute of International Relations, Clingendael (2015)

Kothari, C.R.: Research Methodology; Methods and Technique, 2nd edn. New Delhi: New Age International (P) Limited Publisher (2004)

Kumar, R.: Research Methodology: A Step-by-Step Guide for Beginners. SAGE Publications Ltd., London (2011)

Nicolson, H.: Diplomacy, 3rd edn. Oxford University Press, Oxford (1968)

Nirupama, R.: Diplomacy in the Age of Social Media, Retrieved May 11, 2019, from Speech delivered at UNESCO, Paris, 6 May 2017. https://www.thewire.in/diplomacy/foreign-relations-diplomacy-social-media

Studemeister, S.J.: (2018, 12 13). Virtual Diplomacy: Rethinking Foreign Policy Practice in the Information Age*: Retrieved.* Retrieved December17, 2018 from Research Gate Web site: https://www.researchgate.net/publication/273239088_Virtual_Diplomacy_Rethinking_Foreign_Policy_Practice_in_the_Information_Age

Smith, G.: Challenges of Virtual Diplomacy, United States Institute of Peace, pdf Available at. Retrieved December 13, 2018 from Usip Web site: https://www.usip.org/sites/default/files/challenge_virtual_diplomacy_DDi.pdf

Swiss Federal Department of Foreign Affairs, (FDFA), ABC of Diplomacy, Berne. Retrieved November 29, 2018, from Pdf, 16 May 2008. https://www.eda.admin.ch/dam/eda/en/documents/publications/GlossarezurAussenpolitik/ABC-Diplomatie_en.pdf
Ziemkendorf, M.: Actor-Network Theory. Druck and Binding Publishers, Norderstedt Germany (2007)

Improving "Werewere" (Cucumeropsis *Mannii* N.,) Oil Biodiesel Fuel Characteristics Using Diethyl Ether Additives

L. Atepor(✉)

Department of Mechanical Engineering, Cape Coast Technical University, Box AD 50, Cape Coast, Ghana
lawrence.atepor@cctu.edu.gh

Abstract. Diesel engines are widely used on farms and for generation of electrical power in developing Countries like Ghana and cannot be dispensed with easily without challenges. As the petroleum diesel obtained from fossils that are mainly used in diesel engines are continually depleting accompanied by increasing consumption and prices, there is the need to find alternative fuels to fulfill the energy demand of the world and especially in developing countries. Alternative fuels like biodiesel, are being used as an effective alternative to diesel. The feasibility of biodiesel production from "werewere" (*Cucumeropsis mannii* N., Cucurbitaceae) oil of Ghanaian origin was investigated with respect to its fuel properties. Though biodiesel can replace diesel satisfactorily, problems related to fuel properties persist. In this study an oxygenated additive diethyl ether (DEE) was blended with "werewere" oil biodiesel (WOME) in the ratios of 2%, 4%, 6% and 8% and tested for their properties improvement. These blends were tested for kinematic viscosity and energy content and various fuel properties according to ASTM standards. Qualifying "werewere" biodiesel and the effect of DDE additive on its fuel properties can serve the purpose for developers who work on biodiesel fuels to indicate the fuel suitability for diesel engines. Blending DEE with WOME resulted in a slight decrease in the energy content but improved viscosity, acid value, density and pour point and these became better as the DDE content increases. The drastic improvement in viscosity makes WOME-DEE blend very suitable for use in powering diesel for badly needed energy.

Keywords: "Werewere" biodiesel · Diethyl Ether · Energy Content · Additive · Fuel properties

1 Introduction

Recently Biodiesel has received a great deal of attention because of the advantages associated with its environmental acceptability, availability, economic competitiveness, lower sulfur and aromatic content and classification as a resource for renewable energy. Biodiesel is mostly produced from transesterification of either edible plant oil, non-edible plant oil, waste fish oil or waste meat product oil with either methanol or ethanol.

J. N. Mojekwu et al. (Eds.): *Sustainable Education and Development*, pp. 502–511, 2021.
https://doi.org/10.1007/978-3-030-68836-3_43

The current mandates regarding the use of biodiesel around the world are mostly based on a biodiesel–diesel blend. The additive is the most visible option to introduce the biodiesel as complete alternative fuel for mineral diesel (Ali et al. 2013).

The availability and sustainability of biodiesel feedstocks will be the crucial determinants in the popularization of biodiesel (Pinzi et al. 2009). Opoku-Boahen et al. (2013) researched on Werewere" (*Cucumeropsis mannii* N.) seed oil as a potential feedstock for biodiesel production. "Werewere" (*Cucumeropsis mannii* N.) a member of the Cucurbitaceae family is an important crop in Ghana and most other African countries. It is native to West Africa where it has been in cultivation for many centuries (Akoh and Nwosu 1992 and Dokosi 1998). "Werewere" seeds are small, flat and oval containing a white cotyledon in a thin walled shell with a thick ring around the edges. They are grown in Ghana for their seeds, which are particularly rich in fat. The oil content is the main temptation for possible use as source of oil but it is also self-sustaining as it is widely grown in Ghana. Due to increasing importance of oilseeds in the national economy of Ghana, the high demand for new sources of oil and the availability of this plant in Ghana, the scarcity of scientific studies of "werewere" seed oil, the need to evaluate the physio-chemical properties of *Cucumeropsis mannii* N. seed oil becomes relevant. The use of "Werewere" seed oil for biodiesel can be especially beneficial to the economies of West African countries since the crop is already domestically produced and has the potential of reducing dependency on imported petroleum.

Biodiesel generally has higher cloud, pour point, density, and kinematic viscosity as well as acid value compared to diesel. Density and viscosity are important for various diesel engine performance. According to Opoku-Boahen et al. (2013), the fatty acid compositions of "werewere" seed oil such as linoleic acid 58.8%, oleic acid 15.5%, stearic acid 14.1% and palmitic acid 11.5% are similar to that of some conventional vegetable oils used for biodiesel such as soybean, sunflower, corn and jatropha oils. The biodiesel fuel properties of WOME were comparable to ASTMD 6751 and EN14214 and the other biodiesels prepared from other vegetable oils. The high kinematic viscosity and distillation process results of 15.5 mm^2/s and 50% at 368 °C respectively were however the major drawbacks to the use of WOME as a biodiesel. The authors however concluded that the other parameters determined indicated that WOME has a potential as a biodiesel fuel. The use of fuel with high kinematic viscosity can lead to undesired consequences, such as poor fuel atomization during spraying, engine deposits, wear on fuel pump elements and injectors, and additional energy required to pump the fuel (Alptekin and Canakci 2008 and Satyanarayana and Muraleedharan 2009). The fuel viscosity and energy content has a direct influence on the engine power performance. The biodiesel viscosity is more than that of mineral diesel, therefore using of additive must better the viscosity and energy content of the WOME fuel. Because biodiesel has lower energy content and higher viscosity compared to diesel resulting from its chemical structure, the blending of biodiesel with additive that have less viscosity usually causes the viscosity of the fuel blend to decrease depending on the additive portion. Currently, viscosity and energy content of biodiesels are some of the major technical issues in the use of biodiesel–diesel blends, as it relates to the engine power. Information concerning the viscosity and energy content of "werewere" oil biodiesel and its blending with additives are not available.

Diethyl ether (DEE), an oxygenated additive can be added to diesel/ biodiesel fuels to suppress emissions. The addition of DEE with biodiesel led to the lowering of the viscosity of the biodiesel and the improvement of atomization and energy content leading to better combustion and lowering of combustion temperature (Nagdeote and Deshmukh 2012; Sudhakar and Sivaprakasam 2014 and Jayaprabakar et al. 2017). Pugazhvadivu and Rajagopan (2009) found experimentally that DEE addition was very beneficial in reducing NOx emission when using Pongamia biodiesel and diethyl ether as a fuel. Similarly, (Kannan and Marappan 2010; 2011) in their experimental works agreed that the blending DEE and Thevetia Peruviana biodiesel gives better performance and lesser emissions. (Swaminathan and Sarangan, 2012) stated that fish oil biodiesel (BOF), with 2% blend of DEE gave the maximum percentage of reduction of all emission pollutants and suggested as the best option for running the engine with EGR. None of the previous studies investigates the effect of DEE on WOME fuel properties. Therefore, the first objective of this study was to characterize the properties of the "werewere" oil methyl esters (WOME), including the energy content. The second objective was to investigate the fuel properties of WOME-DEE blends at different ratios for compliance with current mandates. DEE was added in the ratio of 2%, 4%, 6% and 8% to the WOME to improve the fuel properties and meet the fuel standard requirement.

In an earlier study by Opoku-Boahen et al. (2013), it was reported that "werewere" oil biodiesel (WOME) has a potential as a biodiesel fuel. However, the major drawback to the use of WOME as a biodiesel is its very high viscosity value of 15.5 mm^2/s. Kinematic viscosity is the most important property of biodiesel since it affects the operation of fuel injection equipment and that a high viscosity may lead to the formation of soot and engine deposits due to insufficient fuel atomization. Information concerning the viscosity and energy content of "werewere" oil biodiesel and its blending with additives are scarcely available. Hence, this study for the first time investigates the effect of diethyl ether (an additive) on WOME fuel properties at different blend ratios for compliance with current mandates.

2 Materials and Method

The "werewere" seeds were roasted and milled into fine particle size using a blender and sieved to finer seed powder. Lipid extraction and transesterification processes were carried out as described in Opoku-Boahen et al. (2013). The "werewere" oil biodiesel (WOME) and DEE fuel mixture properties were determined following Ali et al. (2013) method and these were done at the Tema Oil Refinery Chemical Laboratory, Tema, Ghana. The DEE was added at small proportions of 2%, 4%, 6% and 8% by volume to WOME, which corresponded to WB-DE2, WB-DE4, WB-DE6 and WB-DE8 fuels, respectively (after Ali et al. 2013).

2.1 Engine Test Equipment

The engine test was carried out in the laboratory using a four-stroke single cylinder victor type air-cooled diesel engine. Table 1 provides the specifications of the diesel engine. Figure 1 depicts the equipment connections for the engine test. The equipment was assembled and procedure followed (Maina 2014). The engine (1) was coupled with a dynamometer (2) to provide brake load, while the engine throttling and dynamometer settings were controlled by a computer (8). A pressure transducer (9) was installed in one of the piston cylinders. Cylinder pressure signals from pressure transducer were amplified by a charge amplifier (11), and connected to the SMETech COMBI-PC indication system (7) for data acquisition.

Table 1. Specification of test engine

Manufacturer	Victor Diesel Engine Company Ltd
Engine	Number 42
Type	Single cylinder, 4 stroke, vertical compression, Air cooled, fixed throttle
Cylinder Bore	80 mm
Torque arm	10 mm
Stroke	100 mm
Swept Volume	0.5 (l)
Fuel	Diesel
Max. Speed	1500 rpm
Brake Power	2.982 KW at 1500 rpm

The data acquisition system was externally triggered 1024 times in one revolution by an incremental crank angle transducer-optical encoder (10). Fuel was introduced from a fuel tank (3) equipped with flow measurement system. During fuel switching, the fuel tank was drained from the engine fuel filter, new fuel was introduced into the tank until the fuel filter was full,and the engine was then started and allowed to run for a few minutes to clear fuel lines and stabilize. AVL ditest MDS 350 mission analyser station designed for diesel engines (5) was used for measuring (CO, CO2, and HC), (THC), and (NOx) respectively and a smoke meter (6) connected before the oxidative converter at the engine exhaust pipe (4).

The fuel properties of the WB-DE2, WB-DE4, WB-DE6 and WB-DE8 blends such as density (ASTM D1298), kinematic viscosity (ASTM D445), flash point (ASTM D93), pour point (ASTM D97), acid value (ASTM D664), cloud point (ASTM D2500) and heating value (EN 14214) were determined according to relevant biodiesel test methods.

3 Results and Discussions

3.1 Analysis of Biodiesel Properties

The measured fuel properties of the WOME are listed in the Table 2 and compared to the biodiesel specifications of ASTM D6751 and EN 14214. The WOME presented satisfactory fuel properties that satisfied most biodiesel specifications except the viscosity value

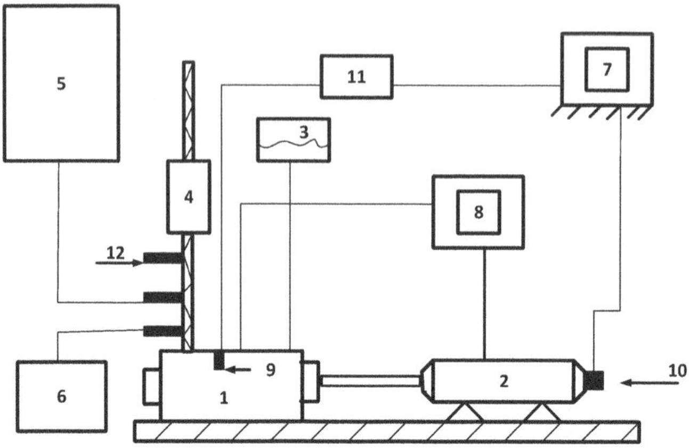

Fig. 1. Experimental Setup. 1-Engine, 2-Dynamometer, 3-Fuel Tank, 4-Exhaust Pipe, 5-Gas Analyzer, 6-Smoke Meter, 7-Computer, 8-Computer, 9-Pressure Transducer, 10-Crank Angle Transducer, 11-Charge Amplifier, 12-Temperature Sensor.

of 14.93 mm^2/s, a property that limited the beneficial use of the WOME as alternative to petroleum diesel.

Diethyl Ether was selected as the additive for oxygenating the fuel based on its economic feasibility, toxicity, fuel blending property, additive solubility, flash point of the blend, viscosity of the blend, solubility of water in the resultant blend, and water partitioning of the additive (after Swaminathan and Sarangan 2012 and Ali et al. 2013). The Diethyl Ether additive was added to the WOME at different volumetric ratios (varied from 0% to 8% in steps of 2% after Ali et al. 2013) to study the variations in the kinematic viscosity, Calorific value and other important fuel properties of the WOME-DEE blends.

Table 2. Fuel properties of WOME compared to the biodiesel specifications.

Property	Unit	WOME	ASTM D6751	EN14213
Density	kg/m^3	890	880	860–900
Cetane N_O.	–	57	47 min	51 min
Flash point	^OC	155	130 min	120 min
Pour point	^OC	−3	–	–
Cloud point	^OC	9.1	–	–
Kinematic				
Viscosity, 40 ^OC	mm^2/s	14.93	1.9–6.0	3.5–5.0
Calorific value	kJ/kg	41200	–	35000 min
Acid value	mg/KOH	0.42	0.5 Max	0.5 max

3.2 Density Results

The density of biodiesel oil is important because it gives indication of the delay between the injection and combustion of the fuel in a diesel engine (ignition quality) and the energy per unit mass (specific gravity). The densities of WOME-DEE blended fuel produced in this research are close to each other and in the range of 890–878.5 kg/m^3 for WOME and WB-DE8 respectively. They fall within the ASTM and EN standards but slightly higher than that of petroleum diesel. Figure 2 shows the variation in density with volumetric percentage of DEE for WOME. The density of the WOME-DEE blend decreases with increase in the volumetric percentage of the DEE, with WB-DE8 having the lowest. The density of the WOME-DEE blends therefore meets the specifications for biodiesel blends listed in the American and European standards.

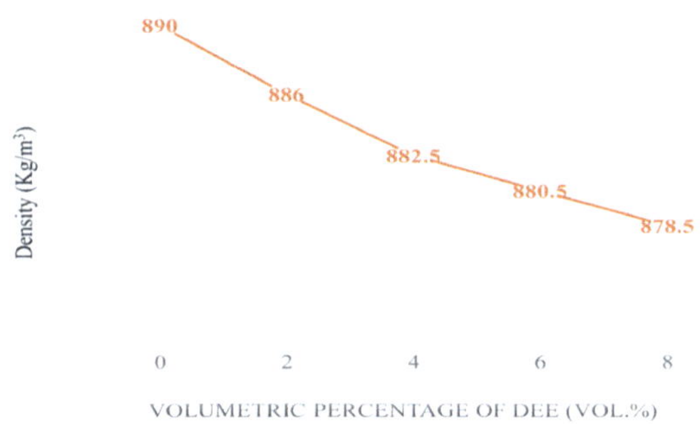

Fig. 2: Variation in density with the volumetric percentage of DEE for WOME

3.3 Pour Point and Cloud Point Results

The Pour Point (PP) is the temperature at which the amount of wax in the solution is sufficient to gel the fuel. Thus, it is the lowest temperature at which the fuel can flow. Adding DEE to WOME from 0% to 8% resulted in decrease in PP from -3 for the pure WOME to -3.6 for the DEE-WOME blend of WB-DE8. The Cloud Point (CP) is the temperature at which a cloud of wax crystals first appears when the fuel is cooled under controlled conditions during a standard test. Adding DEE-WOME from 0% to 2% gave an initial slight decrease in the CP and further increase in the percentage of the DEE in the blend from 2% to 8% resulted in a constant CP value. Thus, further increase in the percentage of DEE in the WB-DE blends did not affect the CP and this is shown in Fig. 3.

3.4 Kinematic Viscosity Results

Viscosity is defined as the resistance of liquid flow. It refers to the thickness of the oil and is determined by measuring the amount of time it takes for a given volume of oil to pass

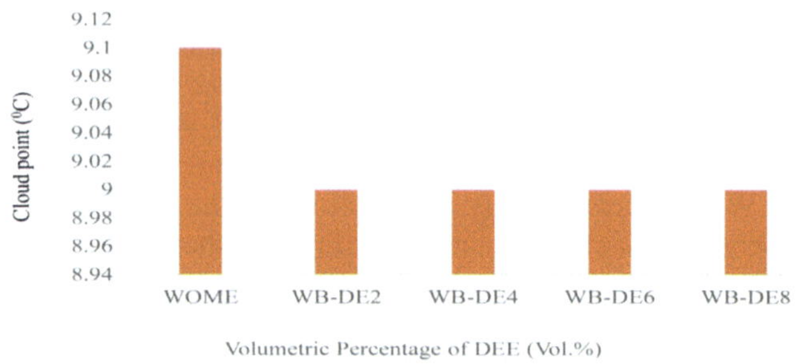

Fig. 3: Variation in CP with the volumetric percentage of DEE for WOME

through an orifice of a specified size. Kinematic viscosity is the most important property of biodiesel since it affects the operation of fuel injection equipment and that a high viscosity may lead to the formation of soot and engine deposits due to insufficient fuel atomization. The variation in viscosity with volumetric percentage of DEE for WOME is shown in Fig. 4. The viscosities of the biodiesels under consideration vary in the range of 3.56, 3.65, 4.0, 4.31 and 14.93 mm^2/s for WB-DE8, WB-DE6, WB-DE4, WB-DE2 and WOME respectively. All blends satisfied the kinematic viscosity specification contained in ASTM D6751 except that of the neat "werewere" biodiesel (WOME) which is significantly higher than the limits of 6.0 and 5.0 for ASTM D6751 and EN14213 respectively.

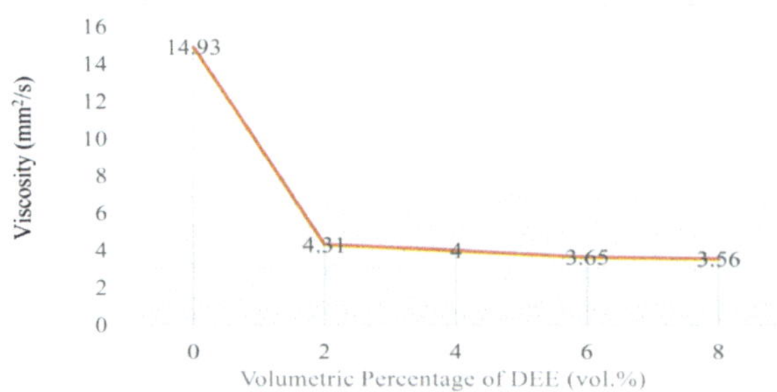

Fig. 4. Variation in Viscosity with the volumetric percentage of DEE for WOME

3.5 Calorific Value Results

The Calorific Value (CV) or Heating Value or Energy value of a biodiesel fuel is the amount of heat released during the combustion of a specified amount of the fuel. The CV is specified in EN 14213 with a minimum of 35000 kJ/kg (Rashid et al. 2009). Figure 5 shows the variation in calorific value with volumetric percentage of DEE for WOME. The results show that the heating value of the WOME-DEE blend decreased slightly

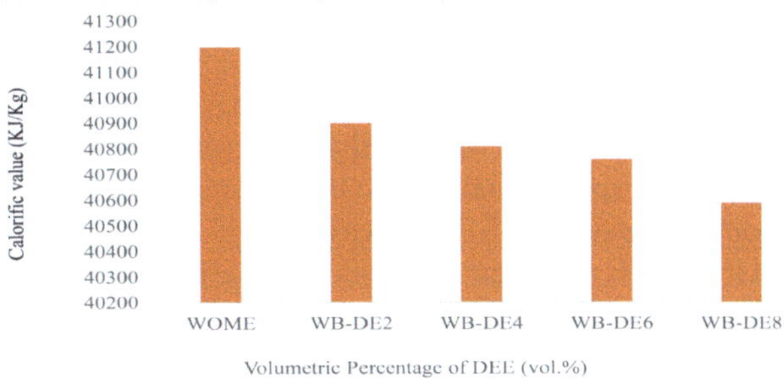

Fig. 5. Variation in CV with the volumetric percentage of DEE for WOME

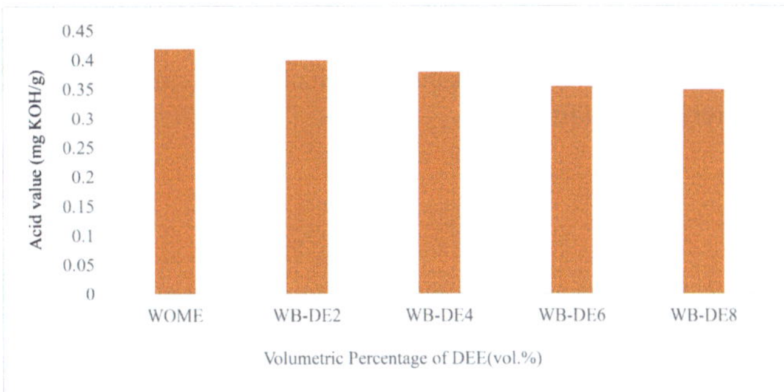

Fig. 6. Variation in AV with the volumetric percentage of DEE for WOME

with increasing volumetric percentage of the DEE with the WB-DE8 having the lowest value of 40590 kJ/kg. The CV of the WOME-DEE blend satisfies the EN 14213 standard for all its blends.

3.6 Acid Value Results

The Acid Value (AV) is a measure of the amount of carboxylic acid groups such as a fatty acid, in the biodiesel and its blends. AV can provide an indication of the level of lubricant degradation while the fuel is in service. Acid value or neutralization number is expressed in mg KOH required to neutralize 1g of fatty acid methyl esters and is set to a maximum value of 0.5 mg KOH/g of the oil in the ASTM D6751 and EN14213 standards. A higher acid value can cause severe corrosion to a fuel supply system and an internal combustion engine. Figure 6 depicts the variation in acid value with volumetric percentage of DEE for WOME. The acid value decreases by an average of 4.45% for each 2% of DDE added to the WOME with the minimum acid value of 0.35 mg KOH/g for the blend WB-DE8. According to Ali et al. (2013) this should be expected, as the DEE dilutes the free fatty acids present in the WOME, resulting in reduction in the AV. Thus, the AV of all the WOME-DEE blends meet the requirement of the ASTM D6751 and EN14213 standards.

4 Conclusion

The objective of this research was to characterize how a major fuel property of kinematic viscosity and other properties changed when diethyl ether were blended with "werewere" oil methyl esters. From the experimental results; the kinematic viscosity of the WOME-DEE blend significantly decreased with the increase of DEE concentration in the blended fuel. The density of the blends also decreased with increase in concentration of the DDE. Similarly, the acid value of the WOME-DEE blends was improved with increasing DDE content. Increasing the percentage of DEE content in WOME resulted in lower temperature performance with a difference of 0.6 ^{O}C between WB-DE8 and pure WOME for the pour point. There was no significant difference for the cloud point between WOME and the WB-DEs. Adding diethyl ether to "werewere" biodiesel exhibited significant and superior reduction in viscosity, slightly better temperature performance, better acid and density values and slightly reduced energy content. The above deductions suggests that "werewere" oil biodiesel can be used to replace petroleum diesel when properly blended with diethyl ether additive.

References

Akoh, C.C., Nwosu, C.V.: Fatty acids composition of melon lipids and phospholipids. J. Am. Oil Chem. Soc. **69**(4), 314–316 (1992)

Ali, O.M., Mamat, R., Faizal, C.K.M.: Effects of diethyl ether additives on palm biodiesel fuel characteristics and low temperature flow properties. Int. J. Adv. Sci. Technol. **52**, 111–120 (2013)

Alptekin, E., Canakci, M.: Determination of the density and the viscosities of biodiesel–diesel fuel blends. Renewable Energy **33**(12), 2623–2630 (2008)

Dokosi, D.O. (1998). *Herbs of Ghana.* Ghana University Press.

Jayaprabakar, J., Anish, M., Beemkumar, N., Mathew, A., Alex George, A.: Effect of diethyl ether blended with neem oil methyl esters in CI engine. Int. J. Ambient Energy **40**(2), 116–118 (2017)

Kannan, T.K., Marappan, R.: Study of performance and emission characteristics of a diesel engine using Thevetia Peruviana biodiesel with diethyl ether blends. Eur. J. Sci. Res. **43**(4), 563–570 (2010)

Kannan, T.K., Marappan, R.: Comparative study of performance and emission characteristics of diesel engine fueled by emulsified biodiesel/diethyl ether blended biodiesel. J. Appl. Sci. **11**(16), 2961–2967 (2011)

Maina, P.: Investigation of fuel properties and engine analysis of Jatropha biodiesel of Kenyan Origin. J. Energy South Africa **25**(2), 107–116 (2014)

Nagdeote, D.D., Deshmukh, M.M.: Experimental study of diethyl ether and ethanol additives with biodiesel-diesel blended fuel engine. Int. J. Emerging Technol. Adv. Eng. ISSN, 2250–2459 (2012)

Opoku-Boahen, Y., Clemente, R., Wubah, D.: Investigation of Cucumeropsis mannii N. seed oil as potential biodiesel feedstock. Int. J. Biol. Chem. Sci. **7**(4), 1767–1776 (2013)

Pinzi, S., Garcia, I.L., Lopez-Gimenez, F.J., Luque de Castro, M.D., Dorado, G., Dorado, M.P.: The ideal vegetable oil-based biodiesel composition: a review of social, economical and technical implications. Energy Fuels **23**(5), 2325–2341 (2009)

Pugazhvadivu, M., Rajagopan, S.: Investigations on a diesel engine fuelled with biodiesel blends and diethyl ether as an additive. Indian J. Sci. Technol. **2**(5), 31–35 (2009)

Rashid, U., Anwar, F., Knothe, G.: Evaluation of biodiesel obtained from cottonseed oil. Fuel Process. Technol. **90**(9), 1157–1163 (2009)

Satyanarayana, M., Muraleedharan, C.: Biodiesel production from vegetable oils: A comparative optimization study. J. Biobased Mater. Bioenergy **3**(4), 335–341 (2009)

Sudhakar, S., Sivaprakasam, S.: Potential of diethyl ether blends with biodiesel in DI diesel engine-an experimental investigation. Int. J. Res. Eng. Adv. Technol. **2**(5), 1–6 (2014)

Swaminathan, C., Sarangan, J.: Performance and exhaust emission characteristics of a CI engine fueled with biodiesel (fish oil) with DEE as additive. Biomass Bioenerg. **39**, 168–174 (2012)

Exploration of the Patterns of Child-Caregivers Interactions Leading to Improved Children's Cognitive Abilities

F. S. Nsolezi[1(✉)] and T. Bali[2]

[1] Department of Psychology, College of Education, The University of Dodoma, 259, Dodoma, Tanzania
[2] Department of Education, Faculty of Humanities and Education, St. John's University of Tanzania, 47, Dodoma, Tanzania

Abstract. It is now a world widely concerns of developing cognitive development of children both at home and at school settings. However, the general patterns of child-caregivers interactions leading to improving cognitive abilities of these children are rarely academically presented. Hence, this paper is presenting the patterns of child caregivers' interactions with regard to children's cognitive abilities. Specifically, this paper aimed at presenting findings on the parents and guardians on the following issues; i) reactions on children's behaviour, ii) engagement on children's activities and plays and iii) support on children's activities and plays, emerged as shared by the respondents. Phenomenology research design was employed in this paper. Qualitative research approach was used; this study was conducted in Bahi local community, the target population comprised of parents and guardians who were living with a pre-primary child aged 2–7. The sample size was 10 (ten) respondents. Data Collection included interviews and observations methods with interview guides and observation checklist tools respectively. The data were analyzed thematically following six stages of qualitative data analysis. It was found that children's activities which are oriented on real life situations were praised and approved comparing to normal activities and plays. It was further found that parents and guardians have own experiences of child-parents/guardians interactions connected to traditional valued meaning of life, hence their engagements were on those activities. Lastly, there was no support for getting children's activities materials; rather children were observed searching and collecting local materials in their surroundings. It can therefore be concluded that, the patterns of child-parent/guardians interactions in the Bahi local community is socially determined basing on norms and values of cultural milieu. It is recommended that community, NGOs, CBOs, to increase the cooperation and trainings so as to increase caregiver-children interactions as an avenue for improving issues pertaining to children's cognitive, social and psychological needs at home.

Keywords: Caregivers · Patterns · Interactions · Cognitive development

J. N. Mojekwu et al. (Eds.): *Sustainable Education and Development*, pp. 512–525, 2021.
https://doi.org/10.1007/978-3-030-68836-3_44

1 Introduction

Child-caregiver interaction is conceptualized as the necessary activities that professional individuals or relatives perform, to support children's cognitive, social, and emotional growth patterns (Maggi et al. 2005; WHO (2004)). It can also be seen as the pre-requisite for the healthy neurophysiological, physical and psychological development of a child (WHO (2004). This means that there is always a responsible person to take care of a child's development. For that reason, Arranz Freijo, Oliva, Olabarrieta, Martin, Manzano, & Richards (2006) describes the practice and behaviours of caregivers including mothers, siblings, fathers and child care providers as necessary support for the children survival, growth and development. Caregivers' behaviours include: involving the child in family activities like cooking, fetching water, tending animals, fetching firewood, cleaning utensils and other house chores; children activities and plays like pretence cooking, making playing dolls and cars, *Mdako, Pilika, Ngwelengwenje, Gololi* (marble) and other children plays and activities. Caregivers' behaviours of involving children in different activities and plays enhance the child's cognitive ability. Therefore, children caregivers need to be aware of the child requirements for development and growth as necessary behaviours for positive interactions.

Available evidence suggests that the family and school have emerged as promising contexts to influence overall growth rate and quality of child development (Arranz Freijo et al. 2006; Child Welfare Information Gateway 2006). The prominence of such contexts is particularly seen during early childhood. According to Evans (1994), early childhood is a critical phase for the child's social, emotional, physical, language, and cognitive development. This is due to the fact that the biological factors [inheritance], ecological experiences [children's relationship with various stakeholders including caregivers], socio-cultural experiences [social interactions and culturally organized activities] as per Awde, (2009) and socio-economic influences in the forms of family income, parental education and occupational status, largely affect child development (Bronfenbrenner 1979; Owen, Ware and Barfoot 2000). It is also accepted that the child's brain and neural pathways development take place during the early childhood period to support and facilitate latter learning and development (Shonkoff and Phillips 2000).

Furthermore, other research findings support the hypothesis that children interacting with older siblings develop a theory of mind skills at an earlier age (Das and Babu 2004; Ruffman et al. 1998). Das and Babu (2004), for instance, found that 2 and 3 year-old-children have a consistent trend to direct questions to their mothers about why people act as they do. This means that such children would direct questions related to their mental states to older siblings, provided that they have better overall knowledge than the younger siblings (Ruffman et al. 1998). In a similar vein, Baumrind (1967), commented on interaction patterns that are results of the following four dimensions in child-caregivers interactions: first, the disciplinary strategies which involve reactions of caregivers on perceived children misbehaviours; second, the warmth and nurturance in which caregivers are involved with children and guide their activities; third, the communication style which can be displayed during children-caregivers' activities and plays; and fourth, the expectations of maturity and control over children.

This paper has become necessary and current due to the fact that child-caregivers' interactions is an increasingly important topic of research in children cognitive development. Due to that, different studies in Tanzania (Mapana 2014; Mtahabwa 2007) as in other parts of the world (Mainela-Arnold et al. 2006; Santrock 2011) indicate the central role that parents play for refining the children's cognitive development. However, many of these studies ignored interaction styles of parents and or guardians with children (Assan and Sarfo 2015; Bornstein and Cheah 2006). Ignoring traditional models of adult-child interactions in the local communities including those in Tanzania (Mapana 2014), resulted into inadequate views and narrow conclusions in pursuit of integrated African perspectives when discussing child's cognitive development (Assan and Sarfo 2015; Dasen 2011). This paper therefore, has explored the patterns of child-caregivers interactions leading to improved children's cognitive abilities by exploring the reactions of parents on children's behaviour, exploring the engagement of parents on children's behaviour and lastly exploring the support provided by parents during children's activities.

The studies by (Awde 2009; Cornell and Prinz (2002); Hennessy et al. 2010; Raikes 2005; Vigil 2002) have shown that child-parent interactions are important. In this regard, the authors have timely contributed to the far and wide held view that child-parents' interactions within the family are inevitable to considerable children's cognitive development. Those literatures have highlighted more on the children's social, language, physical and emotional dimensions of development. Yet, the findings do not explain the child's cognitive development in much detail. Knowing the inevitability of child-parent interactions, additional work is required in this area to better understand the forms of parent-child relationship in the context of cognitive related development. To fill this research gap, the current study focused on the patterns of child-parent/guardian interactions for improving performances of children on cognitive tasks in their respective social-cultural settings beyond what the researchers (Dasen 2011; Gwanfogbe 2011; Mapana 2011; Mwamwenda and Mwamwenda 1989) call the Western experiences.

2 Research Methodology

This paper adopted qualitative research approach as a research paradigm that favours personal interpretations and meanings based on interpretivist or constructivist philosophical perspectives (Conrad and Serlin 2011; Creswell 2013; Maxcy 2003; Silverman 2015; Stake 2010). Consistent to qualitative research approach, phenomenology research design was employed. Phenomenology is a qualitative research design which is used to describe how human beings experience a certain incident (Creswell 2015). Creswell (2015) adds that the design attempts to set aside biases and preconceived assumptions about human experiences, feelings, and responses to a particular situation. The focus was on respondents' perceptions on the patterns of child-parent interactions. Interviews and sometimes observations were used as methods of data collection. Dodoma region and specifically Bahi district was selected because Dodoma is the capital city of Tanzania; this means that it is the emerging city with high political significance in the country. With this significance it was expected that the caregivers would also be involved in changing life styles with varied cultures and that it might influence the child-caregivers interaction patterns. For that reason, it was important to come up with research-based evidences to support the influence of child-caregivers interactions on children performance.

The sample size consisted of parents/guardians of pre-primary school children, in villages of Bahi, Mundemu, Chipanga and Mwitikila divisions. Purposeful sampling technique was used. The study employed semi-structured interviews and observations as methods and interview guides and observation checklist as the tools (Creswell 2013; Merriam 2009). Interview guides were used to access useful views, experiences, ideas and feelings about the patterns of the child-caregivers' interactions and interactive opportunities. The non-participant observation method was employed because it helped to gain insight of a setting, events or behaviour through sighting (Merriam 2009). The researcher used this thematic analysis for making sense of the respondents' perspectives, systematic quotations and views related to research questions (Merriam 2009; Miles and Huberman 1994; Silverman 2015). It was also used for helping in the systematic organization of massive data into manageable units in which the patterns, themes and categories of analysis came from the data (Miles and Huberman 1994). The analysis followed the six stages as stipulated below: familiarization of the data, generating initial coding, searching the themes, reviewing the themes, refining and naming themes and subthemes and report writing.

3 Findings

In connection to the scope of the study, the caregivers were engaged to share their overall experiences on the patterns of child-caregivers interactions. This section reports on the respondents' practices, perceptions of and insights into child-caregivers' interactions. The reactions on children's behaviour, engagement on children's activities and support on children's activities were the specific objectives developed to themes.

3.1 Reactions to Children's Behaviour

While exploring more about the respondents' experiences, perceptions and practices on patterns of child-parent/guardian interactions, it was found that parents and guardians were concerned about children's behaviours. Manzala was one of the more informed respondents who shared her experiences, perceptions and practices. She stated that "Noting and approving impressive behaviour is one of the most important conditions that parents and guardians should practise while nurturing children". As a single mother to three children, Manzala believes in establishing a participative environment as necessary for children to develop basic competences. Despite her demanding schedule, Manzala was keen on what was taking place at home. To exemplify her keenness, she said: "Yesterday, I was stunned by my young children. I was not around when they came back home after school hours. She was convinced that her children had acquired the basic cognitive processes as reflected in their performance. Perhaps, due to this performance, Manzala said:

> *...You know that it is not easy. In these days, parents do not have enough time to orient their children to real life experiences. The parents are busy with the*

> *children's normal life skills such as cooking. This is very bad. So, I had to thank and appreciate my children's good behaviour. My intention was to encourage such good behaviour so that it continues automatically. I told them that I was impressed because it was one of the positive signs of being independent in the future...*

Based on that experience, Manzala was keen to parents' interactions as the base for children's impressive behaviours. Similarly, Sulagwa stressed on the importance of praising and approving children's remarkable behaviours as the cornerstone for good ways of orienting them into real life situations. She said,

> *... Most of the time, I do not spend my day at home. I am old as you can see and I have no one to help me in taking care of these children. For that reason, I situate the participative role to promote good life skills amongst my grandchildren...*

Responding to how her grandchildren coped with her orientation, Sulagwa said, "You know that I have no time. I am used to moving here and there while striving for our survival. So, my grandchildren implement my orientation very well". When asked about how she knew that, Sulagwa said that it was reflected by their way of doing things and how they played after they tight school schedule. Whilst Sulagwa did not mention the kind of plays that her grandchildren were engaged in after school, she undoubtedly substantiated the need to comment and commend children's impressive activities. Responding to the question on how often she guided her grandchildren towards good behaviour, Sulagwa gave detailed explanation. Central to her explanation was her frequent directives to her grandchildren on a daily basis. She said,

> *...As I told you before, I regularly go out to search for food. But before I leave, I direct them to carry out the house chores like fetching water, cooking, cleaning the house and its surroundings. Excitingly, when I go back home in the evening from my day long activities, it is already late. By that time, the food is ready. So, as a responsible grandmother, I praise them and then, we just eat our dinner and go to sleep...*

This kind of response provided an important opportunity for advancing the understanding of interactive patterns of life amongst respondents with their respective children/grandchildren. It can thus be suggested that Sulagwa and Manzala were keen to authenticate and support inspiring behaviours. A similar experience was shared by Majimbi. Rather than speaking directly, Majimbi's experience was based on her neighbours' practices. When asked about how often she approved her five children's impressive behaviour that they had been showing, for instance, she replied that her neighbour had the habit of praising her children. In social gatherings, she used to feel proud of herself before other women due to the fact that her children behaved well. She rarely punished her children. Majimbi's remarks showed awareness of the practices among parents and guardians with regards to admiring children's good behaviours. One of the issues that emerged from these findings is that interactive parents were proud of their children's good behaviour and they were ready to share the pride with other parents in the society. Thus, the respondents' view point of relating impressive behaviours to children seemed to place them at the centre of patterns of child-parent/guardian interactions.

Majimbi's experience for instance, seemed to reveal the concerns of parents who were against unlimited praising of impressive children's behaviours. By citing a child's failure to complete her secondary education, it could be translated that praising should not compromise children's cognitive development. Responding to how she often corrected her children when they responded contrary to her directives, including not going to school, she said, "I normally direct my children to attend school. I usually follow up their progress by contacting their teachers too. I do not praise them if they neglect school. I can even punish them for being careless in their own learning". Majimbi's assertion indicates her dimension that praising unnecessarily may spoil the children's good behaviour. On the contrary, Majimbi viewed children's negligence as a result of lack of parents' and guardians' care on the interactions especially noting and praising them when they show impressive behaviours. This, however, must be done with caution because it might ignore other factors that might contribute to children's delinquency behaviours.

Manvula shared the importance of children's obedience to the orders as a reflection of good patterns of child-parent/guardians interactions. Her conviction was that responsible parents or guardians must leave double instructions on children in order to help their cognitive development. She stated that whenever she left for the shamba work in the morning, she asked her grandchild to fetch water and attend to all other assignments given at school. With this understanding, Manvula seemed to have a correct perception of the connection between home and school works. Interestingly, Manvula was also committed to responsible child-parent interactions. According to her, a responsible parent needs to punish children upon misbehaving. With reference to her grandchild, she stated the following:

> *... Yesterday, when I came back home from my shamba work, it was already late in the evening. To my surprise, I found my grandchild playing with fellow children in the street. I was surprised because that was the time for fetching water as I instructed him in the morning. When I entered the house, I realized that he had neither fetched water nor attended to other domestic chores. I was very angry! For that reason, I asked him to go to bed without taking his dinner because he did not want to work...*

This implied that although the grandparent spent most of her day time out of her family, in order to attend to her caregivers' roles such as securing food for her grandchild; she did not care letting him sleep without eating food. However, the child's failure to fetch water affected the preparation of dinner. Failure to fetch water was a problem, yet denying the children's right to get food was also a problem. Overall, these findings indicate that noting and approving children's behaviours, praising children, ignoring children's misbehaviours and or punishing children for misbehaving emerged as an integral part in defining patterns of child-parent/guardian interactions. Closely related, the respondents shared the following aspect of engagement in children's activities in the same line of discourse.

3.2 Engagement in Children's Activities

Another key concept for explaining patterns of child-parent/guardian interactions was engagement on children activities. All respondents almost shared their experiences on this aspect. Matika, for instance, was concerned with the idea of shared responsibility. She stated that she was living with two children and the other girl and her brother were just left to her by their mother who works in town when they were still little children. To justify this, Matika had the following observation,

> *... I have been taking care of these young grandchildren since they were small kids. Ah! Now, they are grownups and they are going to school. I want them to be good people...*

It is possible that Matika cited the history of her two grandchildren to highlight her potential role in securing their inborn talents including the cognitive aspect. Given her position, Matika looked active and strong-minded in playing her role. She, for example, exposed the fact that she was aged and knew that she could not undertake many activities far from her house. She also added that she felt responsible to ensuring that her grandchildren were competent in the house chores. In this case, the mentioning of house chores might be related to activities such as fetching water, running errands, cleaning utensils and cleaning the house environment. Other activities would include storytelling, pounding, grinding maize, and tending animals, cooking and meals preparations. From the practical view, the grandchildren were as young as five or six years old. Therefore, Matika felt that responsibility to teach them how to perform those household chores with reason. She said that she felt that it was her duty to teach them. She commented that it was important for their life and she believed that even when she is not around they will be able to cook and feed themselves. This combination of grandparent's vow and broad exposure of household chores to the young children has at least two important meanings.

First, it provides support for the theoretical premise that guiding and directing children's way of behaving are important for a child's social and cognitive development. Second, the responsible grandparents would initiate and sustain interactions with grandchildren, something which might also constructively help grandchildren's cognitive development. The said grandparents' contribution would be possible because they are expected to balance the difficulty of the household tasks according to grandchildren's age. Mazengo shared his version on a similar point by responding that:

> *... I frequently train my young children in capturing the necessary requirements for quality life in this social setting. Here, I have cattle. The children I have are my inheritors. My training focuses on orienting them on what it means when they are asked to look after cattle. The logic is that when they grow up, they will be required to do all these activities of taking care of animals alone while guiding the rest of their younger brothers. So, my training is for their life...*

The message from this shared experience is that the children in the studied community were viewed as integral parts of the bigger society. The logic behind the training seemed to focus on helping children to possess the life pre-requisites in the context of the traditional valued household chores. Hence, some parents and guardians followed them closely. Mazengo, for example, noted the following,

> *... I teach them details about animals. The details include identification of pastures, local plants and nourished trees. I also train them how to defend themselves upon experiencing risky situations. I have to make a follow up too, for them to master the essence of the whole exercise. If I fail to teach and make follow up on them about the care of animals then how will they guide others?*

The possible implication is that Mazengo engaged his children in order to help them to excel in life. The key issue emerging from Mazengo's experiences relates specifically to the question of being a good role model for the children. In this way, the children were expected to mature while learning. To insist on the conception, Mazengo remarked:

> *... I have good dreams for these children. I want them to be useful members of this society. But, I am aware of the challenges of 'utandawazi' (globalization). It comes with bad behaviours to such young children like mine. To avoid bad behaviours, I just take my children in the fields to look after cattle, especially in the days which they do not go to school. During evening meals, I try to engage them with folktales to connect them with our history. Here, children from neighbours also join the sittings...*

The shared Mazengo's views are significant in at least major three respects. First, that storytelling was still used as a way to engage children in learning good behaviours. Second, that the parents and guardians directed and guided children's activities. Ilogo was another respondent with informative experiences regarding the engagement with children's activities. She was keen to valued plays and activities in her culture. It was revealed that the children's useless activities were not part of the parents' and guardians' engagement. Regarding useless activities, Ilogo had the following to say,

> *... It is not our custom to engage with children in their childish plays. We do this for our cultural feelings. You know, if I attempt to engage in playing with children, my neighbours might think that I have gone crazy or I am acting like a child. In our village, the children play with their fellow children in the neighbourhood. We support peer culture in which children interact and inspire one another to play in good terms...*

From this perspective, it appeared that the parents and guardians were keen to children's plays. Moreover, parents and guardians were concerned about guiding their children in important and valued activities. In support of the above statement, Ilogo had this to say,

> *... After the daylong activities, I sit, just like other elders in this village, with children to share with them allegories and related inspiring hero stories to bring out moral lessons and values. This tendency of gathering the children is common to us...*

An implication of this experience is the possibility that the Wagogo families believe in stimulating the children's intellect through engaging them in valued activities and inspirational folktales. Thus, it can be reasoned that culturally appropriate activities and plays were given the chance for children to benefit from child-parent/guardian interactions.

3.3 Support on Children's Activities

To get the parents' and guardians' experience on this particular concept, they were asked to share their experiences on the way they supported children's activities. It was noted that the parents and guardians were keen to support children's activities by providing the play materials. This appeared as one of the crucial indicators of quality interactions. In this study, the support on children's activities appeared on provision of basic needs to children and support to their activities and considering these activities as a child's basic needs. The parents and guardians had different perceptions regarding the provision of materials by parents/guardians for these activities. Secelela was one of the important respondents on this aspect. She was very informative during the interview. She was among the grandparents who seemed to be responsible to help her grandchildren to deal with and overcome the variations and realities of daily life. She stated that she considered herself as a member of both extended family and community. She felt that her role was to support these children to acquire the basics of life and avoid societal loneliness. This description suggests that Secelela used to spare her time to support her grandchildren through telling them valued riddles, songs and legends. This particular respondent's practices support the view that grandparents among *Wagogo*, just like in many other African communities, are central mediators of communication values. In this way, the development of grandchildren's cognitive abilities could not be secluded. Furthermore, Secelela did not hide her appreciation to what she considered as the good work done by her neighbours in nurturing and supporting the children to emerge as true heirs of the community.

Considering education as the child's basic needs, Secelela had her own version. She had the following to say,

> *...You know, other elders like me share the broad life experience. It is the school by itself. We have survived through punitive natural environment throughout, something which helped us to accumulate survival knowledge and experience which is important even for these young children...*

Some of the issues emerging from this description relate specifically to the endorsement of traditional education and what it could offer to the present schooling system. In essence, Secelela seemed to suggest that her home-grown knowledge which had been amassed over time is necessary even to the current generation. She was, for instance, seen to adore the efforts by her own neighbours in the way they supported their children to what she called basic education. She said;

> *...I commend my neighbours. I admire them because they are thoughtful in inculcating basic education to their children as I do. I consider education as a basic need when children are trained to be very obedient and respectful to the elders,*

and willing to work hard. Specifically, the daughters here are very obedient and do exactly what their parents ask them to do. This is very basic because it will help them to mature wholly into acceptable adulthood...

This perspective has important implications for conceptualizing the support offered by parents and guardians to children and grandchildren in African contexts. By implication, Secelela reflected education as a child's basic need. Yet, her meaning of education seemed to be more inclusive beyond the current schooling.

Nyemo was another respondent in this study. She looked as an experienced aged grandparent. She had a vast experience on the history of her community. In connection to provision of support and considering education as the child's basic need, Nyemo shared her views based on her own lens. Like Secelela, Nyemo seemed unconvinced of education that fails to assign a great reflection of the valued social aspects and entirety of children's development. She said, "I am concerned with the education of my grandchildren. I do not know what will happen". Looking very sad, she kept quiet for a while before continuing. She said, "I have seen more than five girls from this village that joined secondary education but failed to complete it. They became pregnant! That was not good at all." She added that, "The examination which is exclusive of incorporating valued life practices is not a good way of supporting the children. In my view, it is wastage of resources". Taken together, the parents and guardians seemed to have their own experiences connected to the traditional valued meaning of life. For this reason, their interaction patterns looked more holistic; of which cognitive abilities appeared central. From their descriptions, the respondents' reactions, engagement and supporting of children's behaviours and activities had an interactive essence of the overall local societal cultural practices. In this respect, the child-parent and guardian participation and interaction in communal activities such as keeping cattle, singing, dancing and recounting of tales, legends and puzzles were a matter of necessity. This means that opportunities in the local settings were explored to nurture children's and grandchildren's cognitive abilities and completeness. Thus, the patterns of child-parent and guardian interactions had collective meaning for unity on children's development.

4 Discussion

The patterns of child-parent/guardian interactions were discussed in various dimensions. These dimensions include parents and guardians reactions on children behaviours and engagement in children's plays and activities. Another dimension is in the support provided regarding children's plays and activities.

4.1 Reactions on Children's Behaviours

In accordance with the current study, parents and guardians shared their experiences on children's behaviours. This study found reactions of parents/guardians in the form of noting, approving and praising; to impressive children's behaviours. Other reactions found were punishment for misbehaving children. This means that right from the home settings, the parents and guardians among the Wagogo just like other African communities, keenly help the children to develop cognitive abilities and social liability. This facilitation was reflected when children's impressive behaviours were nurtured positively through noting and praising. This practice seemed to encourage children's confidence in harmony with development of cognitive abilities. Manzala, for instance, praised her young children for acquiring problem-solving ability to cook in her absence. It implies that noting and praising have created supportive family environments for the children to succeed in performing cognitive and practice-related tasks as they developed.

Goldberg (2014), for example, establishes that positive noting, warm approval and praising; underlined by parents and guardians contribute to reasonable children's useful confidence which is a sound base for the development of cognitive abilities. The same idea is shared by Mapana (2011), Booren et al. (2012), Bodrova and Leong (2005) that praising and approving children's initiatives enhances self-esteem which in turn improves cognitive development. Not praising children's good behaviours might be linked to retarding the children's inquisitive mind and hence impairing cognitive development (Vygotsky 1981). Here, parents and guardians need to be attentive to sense and commend the useful children's behaviour when they first become visible during motivating activities such as doing household tasks. This is because the nature of such activities is social and cognitive as well as entertaining (Tchombe 2011).

4.2 AN

The other considerable finding was on parents'/guardians' engagement in children's plays and other activities. This commitment was categorized as parents'/guardians' valued and less valued activities. The valued activities included fetching water, pounding, grinding, cleaning utensils, cooking, looking after animals, story-telling and running errands. These were valued activities because they engaged children in learning and developing the necessary knowledge and skills, which keep them in agreement with their culture (Barry and Zeitlin 2011). Understandably, this finding is important because it requires parents and guardians to engage children in the valued activities in preparing them for the future life while capitalizing on the available time to work on other family activities. There are similarities between the valued activities shared by respondents in this study and those described by Mapana 2011; Nsamenang and Tchombe 2011; Gwanfogbe 2011.

Moreover, the parents and guardians shared the experiences on less valued or cherished activities. Those valued tasks included children's activities and plays such as hide-and-seek. Other plays were *nasaka mke wangu, rede, mdako, gololi, ngwelengwenje, pilika*, football, *isolo, baba na mama* (father and mother). There were also activities like pretence cooking and moulding dolls and cars. Parents and guardians were found to be holding the views that children's activities and plays were just for children's amusement and refreshment. In addition to that, those plays and activities seemed not to have a direct advantage to the family as it is real cooking and other house chores. Perhaps, this was the reason that the parents and guardians appeared to allocate minimal time for engaging in children's activities. This means engaging or letting children do useful activities is vital in helping them to develop the ability in solving complex activities (Lovas 2005) and support their cognitive development. It can thus be concluded that once children are opportune to do their activities and plays with follow-ups they can strengthen their cognitive abilities.

4.3 Support for Children's Activities

It was found that children enjoyed freedom to conduct their own activities at home. Children were also guided to behave in a good manner, followed-up on their activities and exposed to stories to improve their intellectual confidence. Parents and guardians were found to support children by allowing them to capitalize on the local settings to prepare play materials. By implication, there was promising interpretation by parents and guardians that provision of children's play materials in favour of children's cognitive development could be done using the locally available inputs including clay soil and remnants of bottles and pieces of cloths. This experience provides its own interpretation of sustaining children's activities and plays in the settings where parents and guardians are constantly occupied to spend time and meagre financial resources for provision of basic needs like food, clothes and shelter for survival. Interestingly, this kind of children's support seemed to let them learn ways of integrating local knowledge in preparing variety of play materials with different designs, shapes and weight which imply improved performance of cognitive tasks. Further, previous studies have demonstrated that understanding the importance of children's plays and activities is a reason for caregivers' commitments to support them. Studies by researchers such as Bornstein and Putnick 2012; and Mapana 2011 are keen to the idea of providing freedom to learn from their setting in favour of their cognitive performances.

To sum up this particular aspect of support for children's activities amongst the Wagogo, one needs to appreciate their experiences and challenges concurrently. From the findings of this study, it has emerged that the parents and guardians do support children in their own ways. This means that they are aware of the benefits of plays and children's activities. They are also sure of the potentials of the present local settings in terms of permitting the children to explore and learn from wide variety of playing activities (Das and Babu 2004) and elders (Mapana 2011). Basing on this understanding, therefore, it can be reasoned that the parents/guardians supported children's activities (e.g. cooking, fetching water, tending animals, cleaning utensils and other house chores) which engage their cognition.

4.4 Recommendations

The study recommends to the community, NGOs, CBOs, to increase the cooperation and trainings so as to increase caregiver-children interactions as an avenue for improving issues pertaining to children's cognitive, social and psychological needs at home. Through this sharing, parents and guardians may be in a better position of improving home environment so as to ensure positive and encouraging child-caregivers interaction leading to improved child's cognitive development.

5 Conclusion

It is generally concluded that positive child-caregivers interactions create the foundation for pre-primary school children cognitive development. Further, the pattern of child-parent/guardians interactions in the Bahi local community is socially determined basing on norms and values of cultural milieu. Children plays and domestic activities were given time by the parents and guardians though, unknowingly, they were the main corner stone for their cognitive development.

References

Arranz Freijo, B.E., Oliva, A., Olabarrieta, F., Martin, L.J., Manzano, A., Richards, M.P.M.: Quality of family context or sibling status influences on cognitive development. *J. Early Child Dev. Care Routledge*, **178**, 1–12 (2006)

Assan, E.A., Sarfo, J.O.: Piagetian conservation tasks in Ghanaian children: the role of geographical location, gender and age differences. Eur. J. Contemp. Edu. **12**(2), 137–149 (2015)

Awde, N.: The influence of cultural values on the parent-child interaction patterns of families from an Asian background. Arecls **6**, 1–7 (2009)

Baumrind, D.: Child-care practices anteceding three patterns of pre-school behaviour. Genet. Psychol. Monogr. **75**, 43–88 (1967)

Bodrova, E., Leong, D.: The importance of play, why children need to play. Early Child. Today **20**(3), 6–7 (2005)

Booren, L.M., Downer, J.T., Vitiello, V.E.: Observations of children's interactions with teachers, peers, and tasks across pre-school classroom activity settings. Early Edu. Dev. **23**(4), 517–538 (2012)

Bornstein, M.H., Cheah, C.S.L.: The place of "culture and parenting" in an ecological contextual perspective on developmental science. In: Rubin, K.H., Chung, O.B. (eds.) Parental Beliefs, Parenting, and Child Development in Cross-Cultural Perspective, pp. 3–33. Psychology Press, London, UK (2006)

Bornstein, M.H., Putnick, D.L.: Cognitive and socio-emotional care giving in developing countries. J. Child Dev. **83**(1), 46–61 (2012)

Bronfenbrenner, U.: The Ecology of Human Development. Harvard University Press, Cambridge (1979)

Child Welfare Information Gateway: The Importance of Fathers in the Healthy Development of Children, Washington D.C: Department of Health and Human Services, Children's Bureau (2006)

Conrad, C.F., Serlin, R.C.: Inquiry through a keyhole retroduction. In: Conrad, C.F., Serlin, R.C. (eds) The SAGE Handbook for Research in Education: Pursuing ideas as the keystone of exemplary Inquiry. SAGE, California (2011)

Creswell, J.W.: Qualitative Inquiry and Research Design: Choosing among Five Approaches, 3rd edn. SAGE Publications, Thousand Oaks (2013)

Creswell, J.W.: Educational Research: Planning, Conducting and Evaluating Quantitative and Qualitative Research, 5th edn. Pearson, Boston (2015)

Das, S., Babu, N.: Children's acquisition of theory of mind: the role of presence v/s absence of sibling. Psychol. Stud. **9**, 36–44 (2004)

Dasen, P.R.: Culture, cognition and learning. In: Nsamenang, A.B., Tchombe, T.M.S. (eds.) Handbook of African Educational Theories and Practices: A Generative Teacher Education Curriculum, pp. 159–174. Human Development Resource Centre (HDRC), Bamenda (2011)

Evans, L.J.: Child Rearing Practices and Beliefs in Sub-Saharan Africa. Report of a Workshop Held in Windhoek, Namibia, 26–29 Oct 1993. Consultative Group on Early Childhood Care and Development (1994)

Gwanfogbe, M.B.: Africa's triple education heritages: a historical comparison. In: Nsamenang, A.B., Tchombe, T.M.S. (eds.) Handbook of African Educational Theories and Practices: A Generative Teacher Education Curriculum, pp. 39–54. Human Development Resource Centre (HDRC), Bamenda (2011)

Lovas, G.S.: Gender and patterns in emotional availability mother-toddler and father-toddler dyads. Infant Ment. Health J. **26**, 327–353 (2005)

Maggi, S., Irwin, L.G., Siddiqi, A., Poureslami, I., Hertzman, E., Hertzman, C.: Analytic and Strategic Review Paper: International Perspectives on Early Child Development. WHO: Commission on the Social Determinants of Health (2005)

Mainela-Arnold, E., Evans, J.L., Alibali, M.W.: Understanding conservation delays in children with specific language impairment: task representations. J. Speech Lang. Hear. Res. **49**, 1267–1279 (2006)

Mapana, K.: The musical enculturation and education of Wagogo children. Br. J. Music Educ. **28**, 339–351 (2011)

Merriam, S.B.: Qualitative Research: A Guide to Design and Implementation. Jossey-Bass, San Francisco (2009)

Miles, M.B., Huberman, M.A.: Qualitative Data Analysis: An Expanded Sourcebook. Sage, Beverley Hills (1994)

Mtahabwa, L.: Pre-Primary Educational Policy and Practice in Tanzania: Observations from Urban and Rural Pre-Primary Schools. University of Hong Kong, PhD Thesis (2007)

Nsamenang, A.B., Tchombe, T.M.S.: Introduction: generative pedagogy in the context of all cultures can contribute scientific knowledge of universal value. In: Nsamenang, A.B., Tchombe, T.M.S. (eds.) Handbook of African Educational Theories and Practices: A generative Teacher Education Curriculum, pp. 5–20. Human Development Resource Centre (HDRC), Bamenda (2011)

Owen, T.M., Ware, A.M., Barfoot, B.: Caregiver-mother partnership behaviour and the quality of caregiver-child and mother-child interactions. Early Child. Res. Q. **15**(3), 413–428 (2000)

Ruffman, T., Perner, J., Naito, M., Parkin, L., Clements, W.: Older (but not younger) siblings facilitate false belief understanding. Dev. Psychol. **34**, 161–174 (1998)

Santrock, J.W.: Educational Psychology, 5th edn. New York, McGraw-Hill (2011)

Shonkoff, J.P., Phillips, D.A.: From Neurons to Neighbourhoods: The Silence of Early Childhood Development. National Academy Press, Washington, DC (2000)

Silverman, D.: Interpreting Qualitative Data, 5th edn. SAGE, New Cross (2015)

Stake, R.E.: Qualitative research: studying how things work. Can. J. Program Eval. **25**(2), 88–91 (2010)

Tchombe, T.M.S.: Cultural strategies for cognitive enrichment in learning among the Bamiléké of West Region of Cameroon. In: Nsamenang, A.B., Tchombe, T.M.S. (eds.) Handbook of African Educational theories and Practices: A Generative Teacher Education Curriculum, pp. 205–216, Human Development Resource Centre (HDRC), Bamenda (2011)

Vygotsky, L.: Thought and Language. MIT Press, Cambridge (1981)

WHO: The Importance of Caregiver–child Interactions for the Survival and Healthy Development of young Children. Department of Child and Adolescent Health and Development (2004)

Breaking Patriarchal Chains in Nwapa's *Women Are Different and One Is Enough*

H. Thomas[1](✉) and L. S. Mujwahuzi[2]

[1] Department of Foreign Languages and Literature,
The University of Dodoma, P.O. Box 259, Dodoma, Tanzania
[2] Institute of Development Studies (IDS),
The University of Dodoma, P.O. Box 395, Dodoma, Tanzania

Abstract. Patriarchy system has been a long debate in African research community. Many researchers have been portraying patriarchy as a hindrance to women empowerment and thus development. However, the means on how can this system be broken has not been given much attention. Therefore this paper is intending to uncover the said gap by showing how Nwapa's Women are Different and One is Enough is breaking patriarchal chains. The study which gave rise to this paper employed largely qualitative approach that relied on textual interpretation and analysis. The books under review were purposively selected from Nwapa's works. It was found that the means by which patriarchy chains can be broken include changing the mindset or perception of the community about women, breaking traditional chains fettering women, unleashing different potentials of women and alternative lifestyles of women. It is therefore concluded that it is difficult to change the community's perception however, when different capabilities and potentials of women are discovered the mind set can be changed. It was further concluded that women resort to alternative lifestyles such a single parenthood when the traditional marriage which fosters patriarchy including oppression of women does not work. It is recommended that another study to be done closely to examine Nwapa and other writings for the mechanism of breaking patriarchy chains not only in Nigerian community but Africa as whole. Its contribution to knowledge is that African feminist literary scholarship can stand as a weapon in emancipating women from various chains particularly male domination. This broadens the better understanding of women empowerment not from other disciplines but from literature point of view. This empowerment which is manifested in the form of resort to alternative lifestyles uncovers different potentials of women's capabilities such courage, enterprise and initiative spirits.

Keywords: Patriarchy chains · *Women are Different* · *One is Enough*

1 Introduction

Many writers show that traditions try to undermine African women by treating them as inferior and second class citizens because patriarchy and traditional values favour men and also protect their interest. For instance, men are protected under the umbrella of

J. N. Mojekwu et al. (Eds.): *Sustainable Education and Development*, pp. 526–536, 2021.
https://doi.org/10.1007/978-3-030-68836-3_45

patriarchy and traditional values; as a result they use it as a scape goat for humiliating women. The use of the female voice in African women writings is, therefore, an attempt of shedding light on women's experiences in male dominated societies. In the paper presented at the Second African Writers Conference in Stockholm, Aidoo (1998) commented on the present predicament of African women thusly: "For on our continent, millions of women and girls have been and are being prevented from realising their full potential as human beings whether it be the possibility of being writers and artists, doctors and other professionals, athletes or anything else outside the traditional roles assigned to women. It is definite that anything that has to do with African women was all vital pieces of information, the most unknown, the most ignored of all concerns, the most unseen of all the visible and one might as well face it, of everything to do with humanity". In the quotation, Aidoo (1998) wants women to have more than just the female gender constructive roles, that is, domestic activities and domesticity as women can do better than that; they can be doctors, lecturers, writers and so forth. Referring to Aidoo, Katrak (1989) comments that, African women writers challenge the stereotypical representation of womanhood and motherhood imposed on them through the traditions such as dowry, bride-price and polygamy. The women of Africa have been regarded as weak and even reduced to the level of babies as they are not allowed to make their own decisions in their families. In fact, they face heavy burdens of female roles in their families and their communities. Against this backdrop, African women writers try to make women conscious by giving them a voice in their writings. Silku (2002) argues that African women writers have created a language which seek to break the patriarchy chains which undermine women and thus, liberate them from oppressive and humiliative means of colonialism and patriarchy by challenging their male counterparts who for so many years have presented African women as second-class citizens in their texts. In the representation of African women, there are some male African feminists whose contribution to the struggle for the liberation of African women cannot be ignored. These include Ngugi wa Thiong'o, Sembene Ousmane, Chimalum Nwankwo, Cheick Oumar Sissoko and Amilcar Cabral, Nuruddin Farah to mention but a few. Davies & Graves (1986) in their introduction to *Ngambika* agree on the contribution of men when they assert: "Mongo Beti, Ferdinand Oyono, Sembene Ousmane, Henri Lopes and Ahmadou Kourouma have contributed to the promotion of women, convinced that the liberation of Africa is directly connected to the liberation of women".

However, different from the above mentioned authors, this paper seeks to examine Nwapa's *Women are Different (WAD)* and *One is Enough (OIE)* to scrutinise closely Nwapa's subversive writing on how it reverses the values of patriarchy. The specific objective is to examine how Nwapa's portrayal of key female characters in the selected novels breaks patriarchal tendencies and stereotyping hence debunking the entrenched patriarchy taking a Nigerian community as a case study.

2 Theoretical Framework

This paper is underpinned by Feminist literary theory, with a particular focus on African feminism. It is used in understanding and interpreting Nwapa's *Women are Different* and *One is Enough*. Feminists seek to reinstate the marginalised in the face of the dominant patriarchal ideology. Feminist literary theory in a literary work considers the relationship between men and women and their relative roles in the society. Jackson and Jones (1998) argue that the inequalities between women and men are not natural and inevitable. It is simply men's creation. Feminist theorists pay particular attention to the patterns of thought, behaviour, values, and power in the relationship between men and women in a literary work.

3 African Feminist Theory

African feminism is concerned with autonomy and co-operation. Its emphasis is on nature over culture. Davies & Graves (1986) idea of the African feminist critical approach was used in understanding and interpreting the two novels since this paper centers on an African woman writer (Flora Nwapa). The African feminist critical approach considers both textual analysis criticism and contextual analysis criticism. Textual analysis constitutes close reading of texts and contextual analyses of the emotions to which the text appeals, the characters' expressions, the arguments and ideas that the writer presents as well as the style of the author. This paper is guided by the following tenets of African feminism. Firstly, African feminism recognises African societies as ancient societies and, therefore, it is only logical that African women address the problems of women's positions in society historically, so that they are given equal opportunities with men. The second tenet is that African feminism examines African societies for institutions which are of value to women and rejects those which work against women's welfare and the society in general. African feminism in this regard does not import western agendas as it works on African perspectives by questioning the obligatory motherhood and the long established tradition of favouring sons. The third tenet is that African feminism respects African woman's self-reliance and the penchant for cooperative work and social organisation. The final tenet is that the paper deploys African feminist objectively by looking at the women's situation in societies which have undergone a war or national liberation and society reconstruction. Molara Ogundipe-Leslie (1994) says; African women face: oppression from outside, heritage tradition, backwardness of African men, the African race and, lastly, African woman herself. All these goes hand-in-hand with lack of choice in motherhood and marriage, oppression of barren women, female genital mutilation, enforced silence and other kinds of oppression which African women face in various traditions and societies. Therefore, the African feminist theory addresses these issues in a bid to make the conditions of women in Africa known to bring about necessary changes.

4 Methodology

The paper used information from the selected novels of Flora Nwapa that is, *Women are Different* and *One is Enough*, as its primary sources. The information from the texts was obtained through close and textual reading of the texts. In addition, the paper made use of already organised information from different secondary readings of *Women are Different* and *One is Enough*. Also it has included critical readings of books, journals, articles, dissertations, theses in hard and soft online forms related to this paper. The paper primarily focused on the critical examination of *Women are Different* and *One is Enough* to unveil the means of breaking patriarchy chains in those novels and how Nwapa challenges patriarchal values. The critical examination of the texts was done through textual reading and analysis. When analysing the novels, the concentration was on the portrayal of key female characters in relation to patriarchy as well the portrayal of male characters in relation to female characters and how both categories of characters uphold, eschew or rebel against the values of a patriarchal system in Nigerian society.

5 Findings

5.1 Changing the Mindset or Perception of the Community About Women

Both *Women are Different* and *One is Enough* aim to make the Nigerian community and people at large change how they perceive women, their dependence upon men, lack of courage, opportunities and initiatives. The title *Women are Different* attests to how the society perceive and treat women differently when it comes to school and other opportunities as well as in making their own decisions including pursuing their career choices. Generally, women are thought of as second class citizens. Rose is sidelined by her father who does not believe that he has a female child to educate. When explaining the predicament in which Rose finds herself in, the narrator says, "her own mother was dead years ago, and her father was so busy with his work that he had no time to think about his daughter's education" (WAD 7). Rose's father sees her as less important only because she is a girl. Women also tend to think less of fellow women. During a conversation among the four girls, Comfort, Rose, Agnes and Dora about the impending debate titled: 'The education of girls is a waste of money (WAD 12), set to be carried out between their school and Okrika Grammar School Boys. Some of them agree with the motion that educating a girl is a waste of resources: "...Comfort said she believed that their parents were wasting their money educating them. They would eventually marry, have children and forget all they learnt in school...All that mattered to women was getting married and having children and starting a beautiful home" (WAD 12).

However, as the narrative progresses, the narrator begins showing the readers that women are not so different from men's, if at all they are different it is because they experience monthly period and give birth to children, something which men cannot do. Miss Hill says to Dora, "Oh God! This bleeding occurring every month. God, what a life" (WAD 11). The narrator presents different episodes aimed at demystifying different dubious assumptions and misconceptions held about women. For example, the Archdeacon Crowther Memorial Girls' School (ACMGS) fear to take the risk of going to Okrika Grammar School Boys via the water trip even though they have good swimmers simply because boys are socially constructed to be courageous and, therefore, should take the risk (WAD 14). However, this idea falls on deaf ears as the ACMGS students take the initiative by following the Okrika boys through the supposedly dangerous water trip instead of asking them to come. This act of the girls following the boys through the river trip dispels the myth that women cannot dare and thus they cannot embark on a dangerous adventure.

With regard to the perception held about women that they do not have decision or bargain when it comes to love relationships, the narrative shows that women make their own decision in these relationships. Although it is their wish to get married and have a family just like Amaka in *One is Enough* (OIE 1) wishes to and eventually has. In fact, getting married appears to be a wish of every woman (OIE 66). However, when matters get out of hand, Amaka initiates the divorce proceedings and divorces officially Obiora. She tells her mother "You see, Mother, I want to be free, absolutely free" (OIE 84). She goes ahead with her plans and eventually divorces Obiora. Similarly, Dora initiates divorce proceedings and subsequently divorces Chris after he betrays her (WAD 78). Traditionally, it is unheard for a woman to divorce a man. It constitutes a role reversal under patriarchy. However, in the context of the selected novels, women act extraordinarily in hitherto considered to be for men.

Even when it comes to learning, some domains such as Mathematics are traditionally thought to be difficult for women and therefore, they are out of their capabilities. In *Women are Different*, Agnes expresses some difficulty with learning Mathematics but she keeps at it with determination and in the process she makes it: "Maths gave her quite a problem, but she tackled it with vigour and single-mindedness (WAD 61). Although Mathematics poses a big challenge to her, she surmounts it with her unwavering determination and finally she succeeds thus dispelling the notion that Mathematics is a domain for men only.

Traditionally, men are expected to make sexual advances to women. In *Women are Different*, Comfort, a pragmatic girl, tells her friends that she proposes after her schooling to "hook a man, get him to the altar" (WAD 30). To her, a woman can initiate a love relationship if she feels attracted to a man. Again, in *One is Enough*, Amaka is accused of seducing Rev. Father Mclaid with whom she has twins because she is the one who initiates the relationship (OIE 137). In both novels women are not passive in taking initiatives or doing things which were traditionally reserved for men. All these aspects are presented to debunk patriarchy by showing that women are capable of doing things that men can do and, sometimes, outperform them.

6 Breaking Traditional Chains Fettering Women

Both novels portray women in a way aimed at challenging the traditional perceptions and ways of life that have been putting women in shackles, thus making them fail to realise their potentials as human beings. Women are portrayed in different ways such as militant and the people who are the masters of their own or those people who can take their fate into their own hands. They can divorce a man if they find him no longer desirable. They enter into marriages as equals and, sometimes, they take an upper hand in this bargain. Such traits are aimed at challenging patriarchy which entrenched the rule of the father. In this regard, Rose in *Women are Different* detests bribes and during a discussion at school with her friends she expresses her reservation about them and that she can even divorce her husband if it turns out that he takes bribes: "Rose had said that if she knew her husband received a bribe or a gratification, she would ask him to return the bribe; if he refused, she would divorce him (WAD 49). The woman has been presented here as militant, the one who is capable of dictating terms in a marital relationship. This new dimension in the African marriage relationship is a point of departure from patriarchy's man's rule that allow all directions to be given by the man and the woman to remain passively obedient. By painting women in the new light with the bargaining power in their relationship with men, the narrative suggests that women can be good agents of change in the community if they realise their full potentials denied of them by patriarchy as a system for a long time.

To illustrate further the point about women's power to decide or call it off when a marriage relationship does not work, a girl who has been living with her husband and who seems to lavish her with Ovaltine, disappears or desserts the man when he loses his job and, therefore, cannot go on lavishing on her: "What did the bride do? One morning she disappeared" (WAD, 50). Although she goes away, she is brought back to her husband by her father a week later (WAD 51). The narrator presents this humorous and light episode within the narrative to show that modern women demand more transparency from their spouses within the marriages because they have their own expectations about what kind of the relationship with regard to their current life or their future. The example of the girl walking out on her husband appears that simple, childish and thus far-fetched on the surface; however, examined closely, it offers a lesson to men as perpetrators of patriarchy as now women enter the marriage contracts with their own premium or expectations. Thus expect their hopes to be fulfilled and when they are not, they have to be told the truth regarding why they have not been met. This means that they demand for more transparency and truth from their spouses. Traditionally, a husband would hold every idea close to his chest without involving his wife simply because being transparent and telling all the truth would result into rejection, conflict or desertion. Although we are not told explicitly within the narratives of both novels why a number of female characters within a marriage bond never involve their husbands in some of the decisions they to take unilaterally. There are various possibilities for such acts. One, these women know their husbands' egos and thus would probably hurt them if they knew prematurely of what they were doing. As a result, they would stand in the way of their plans from being fully materialised. Two, they want to have some privacy of their own as individuals by pursuing single-handedly some of the things they like the most. Three, they decide to pursue their plans single-handedly when the relationship with their husbands is sour or when the marriage is crumbling.

Agnes, in *Women are Different*, registers herself with Wolsey Hall in England to pursue the Advanced General Certificate of Education Examination without telling her husband (WAD 57). Because her relationship with her husband is rocky as the two do not have much in common (WAD 58). When she finally lets Egemba, her husband, know that she has been attending the evening classes, he does not agree with her. He questions that decision (WAD 58). When he refuses her the permission to go and study, Agnes uses her weapon: she refuses to cook for him. Agnes' act in response to her husband's refusal to allow her to pursue her studies contrasts with what Abbenyi explains that women have traditionally been portrayed as passive, always prepared to do the bidding of their husbands and family, as having no status of their own and, therefore, completely dependent on their husbands (4).

Finally, because her relationship with her husband is poor, she leaves him (WAD 59). Likewise in *One is Enough* Adaobi starts building a "bungalow in Ikeja on the plot of land she bought without saying a word to her husband" (OIE 107). She does this because her relationship with her husband backs a spark. Perhaps, a clue may be provided through the reaction Obiora, Amaka's ex-husband, exhibits when he goes to see her at her mother's place following her delivery of baby twins. The narrative tells us that when he sees Amaka's wealth he is embarrassed: "Amaka's wealth was everywhere for him to see, and it embarrassed him" (OIE 118). His ego has been hurt and flattened because he does not expect to see the woman he no longer lives with to be so much more prosperous economically and materially than he is. He has a patriarchal perspective that a woman cannot make it independent of a man. With this in mind, Mike, Adaobi's husband, psychologically threatened if his wife lets it be known that she has been building such a big house relying solely on her own resources. Therefore, to maintain their marital harmony she keeps that secret to herself.

Even when it comes to faithfulness or lack of it within a marriage or love relationship, women demand more rights and fairness. When men, as husbands, have strayed in their marriages by having extra-marital relationships, and therefore, hurt their spouses' feelings, these women in turn think about having lovers as a form of revenge or simply as a way of releasing their betrayed or unreciprocated feelings. In a conversation between two old friends, Dora and Rose, they muse about how the society has become rotten, especially men who have lost faithfulness in marriage and how women react to this faithfulness. Rose tells Dora: "When I was talking with a group of women the other day, one of them, who was (sic!) a doctorate degree in history and is unmarried, agreed with us that the society was sick. She said very heatedly, "If husbands run round with other men's wives, why should not their wives do the same?" (WAD 101). This quotation should not be taken literally that women have always want to do the same when their spouses or lovers betray them by having love affairs. The general implication here is that women characters are conscious of their rights and position in marriage. They can question and scrutinise the behaviour of their spouses contrary to what happens in a traditional marriage when man has a series of love affairs or marry many women without consulting his first wife. Such a woman played a subordinate role in such a relationship. The liberated women in the novels, can initiate sexual relationship with men whom they are interested in to meet their own plans especially when they want to get a child regardless of whether those men are married or not. Rose tells Dora; "My instinct tells me that if I see anybody who can give me a child, I shall damn all consequences, and go ahead whether he is married or not" (WAD 105). This is a point of departure from the traditional patriarchy where men are the sole decision-makers in almost everything including love matters. Women's changing perspective in the way they perceive and do things including hunting for men with whom they can get children, challenges patriarchy by decentralizing its position.

7 Unleashing Different Potentials of Women

The selected novels also present different potentialities which women are capable of and which further erode the stranglehold of patriarchy. Agnes in *Women are Different* makes it on her own after living with her partner Ayo Dele, without being officially married, dies and after his children attacks her and her children (WAD 62). She now has to stand on her own, including fending for her four children. She forges ahead with life and, eventually, makes it to an executive position with a firm called Levis Production and Research Bureau (WAD 65). Her top executive position gives her a fat salary and enough fringe benefits. Thus maintains her family on her own without having to rely on a husband or lover as the patriarchal tradition demands.

Again, the narrative paints Dora as a hard-working person who supports her lazy husband, Chris. When she builds a house out of the product of her sweat, Chris takes all the credit as a husband and, for that matter, the head of the family (WAD 70). Although Chris cheats on and betrays Dora, she is not discouraged; instead she continues working hard and survives the Biafran war. As a result she emerges out of the conflict prosperous with her five children intact. She regains the family house which Chris had sold by buying it again (WAD 75). She is a female character who shows that women have talents or potentials which can make them survive even in the absence of men or without them completely.

In *One is Enough*, women's potentialities are exposed through Amaka who is oriented much earlier in life not totally to depend upon men for everything. Her mother tells her: "...never depend on your husband. Never slave for him. Have your own business no matter how small..." (OIE 9). This statement lays a future foundation for her life because, when her marriage with Obiora fails, she stands on her own feet without enlisting help from any man because she believes that it is worse if a woman depends financially on a man (OIE 27). She also does not allow Obiora, her husband, to beat her at his whims. In one particular incident, during a quarrel, she hits him with a hammer on his chest, nearly killing him (OIE 29). This incident shows a departure from the rule of patriarchy under which men or husbands can beat their wives at will as in Achebe's *Things Fall Apart* where Okonkwo beats his wife up at the slightest provocation without her hitting back. When she leaves her husband and goes to Lagos, she joins a group of women who are known as humorously by their union as 'Cash Madam Club' which attests to the material affluence (OIE 80). This group consists of highly financially prosperous women most of whom are 'independent' women leading their own lives without husbands. These women constitute 'the new generation of women contractors' (OIE 49) made up of widowed women and those who had left their husbands on their own volition. They are enterprising women who earn a lot of money; therefore, they are independent of men. They are a manifestation of the overt challenge to patriarchy which fosters the idea that women cannot make it on their own without enlisting the aid of men. Hearing of Amaka's success, Obiora wishes to visit her in Lagos because he believes that she can be useful to her now that she is wealthy (OIE 92). This marks a shift of the pendulum with regard to the economic relationship that characterises men and women. Traditionally, a man is supposed to be the only bread-winner in the family to support his wife and children. In the context of the narrative of this novel, on the other hand, in a position to scale lofty height, hence making men envious of them because they are so economically successful that they can support men if they so wish.

8 Alternative Lifestyles of Women

In a bid to break or challenge patriarchy, some women in the narrative of both novels are disenchanted with marriage as an institution which has been known to degrade women in one way or another. With this disillusionment, these women resort to some alternative lifestyles notably a single lifestyle, concubinage and multiple wives marriages. In a conversation, Mama Emeka and Mama Nkem on the inevitable change of the young generation about marriage, Mama Emeka says: "It is a fact; our children will not take what we are taking from our husbands" (WAD 54). Faced with many options in life such as pursuing education or business, some women find that they fail to reconcile both the marriage and education or business pursuit. Due to the demands imposed by both marriage and education/business, sometime and at a certain point women have to choose. In a conversation between Amaka's mother and Obiora's mother, the former talks about the lifestyle that her daughter has decided to pursue, thusly: "Amaka has made it without a husband. She will pull through. Do you think she is going to get on well, do her business well, if she has to look after her husband or her business, she could not have both. The demands of her husband would be too much and she would be unable to cope" (OIE 118).

She further underscores the importance of a woman engaging in business to be free by citing an example of Ayo, Amaka's sister: "Your sister Ayo has passed this stage. She is learning to be like you. She is discovering what is to be independent, she is discovering what is to have wealth, she wouldn't sacrifice that for any man even if he were a top army officer or a millionaire" (OIE 118). Because of the so many demands imposed by the modern life on women, many feel so overwhelmed that they cannot manage the life of a wife and husband with all its demands which more often than not hinge on a patriarchy induced kind of relationship. As a result, they opt for other lifestyles because they treasure their independence so much.

Because they are determined to succeed in whatever they tend to clash with the established order of married life, especially at the handle of husbands who decide what was supposedly best for them. Amaka tells her mother in *One is Enough*: "I have said goodbye to husbands not goodbye to men. They are two different things" (OIE 85). This statement is much in line with African feminism and womanism than it is with the radical feminism as it does not rule out any co-existence with men. The narrator in *One is Enough* says with referring to Amaka: "she wanted a man in her life. All women should have men in their lives. The men could be husbands or lovers" (OIE 66). In other words, women could have husbands, and when their marriages do not work, they can turn to the second option of having a man as a lover. This kind of single life appears to be an option for many of the female characters in both *Women are Different* and *One is Enough*.

Some of these women leave their husbands because they have been hurt psychologically in some of their love or marital encounters they had had before. Therefore, they have learnt to play it safe by not getting completely committed to one person in their love life. One particularly remarkable example is Rose in *Women are Different* goes through a series of love affairs hoping that such love relationships will eventually translate into marriage. When she does get married eventually, Rose is not successful in her marriage (WAD, 82). First, she has had Ernest, her school days lover whom she loses contact with and does not succeed in getting him even when she tries to do so (WAD 79). After realising that there is no way she can locate him, she meets Mark and they become lovers and eventually get married (WAD 81), but her marriage is short-lived because Mark jilts her. After Mark comes Olu, a married man with whom she has a love relationship but which does not last long because his wife discovers the affair and threatens to harm Rose, thus bringing the relationship to an end (WAD 89). When Rose falls in love with Olu, she develops an interest in conceiving, bear a child and starting a single parent family of her own (WAD 87).

Likewise, in *One is Enough* some women define and lead life on their own terms. As rebels against the patriarchal system that oppresses them, they leave their husbands and become attached to some big men in cities as their lovers. Ayo is one of such women. Amaka's mother tells Amaka, her daughter: "Ayo is the only one among you who is like me. She took no nonsense from any man. When her husband came up with his pranks, she left him and got herself 'kept' by a Permanent Secretary whose wife went to the land of the white people to read books…Ayo moved in. In four years she had four children…She is cleverer than all of you. She qualified as a teacher. In the fifth year she was able to make her 'husband' buy her a house in Surulere, and that year the wife returned without anything and my daughter moved out gracefully with her children, into her own home" (OIE 33). The women characters who become disenchanted with marriage resort to single parent families to negate or undermine patriarchy. They get some men who give them children, give them some initial support and then they live life on their own terms as single parents which amounts to what Amaka calls 'absolute freedom' (OIE 84).

9 Conclusion and Contribution to the Body of Knowledge

Women characters break patriarchal chains through different lifestyle because they do not want to be fettered or tied down by the repressive regime of patriarchy which many African men appear to embrace and exercise. They would like to exercise their freedom and, therefore, realise many things they intend to have in life. In *One is Enough* almost all the women, who belong to the Cash Madam Club are now single women who had been married before. They are either divorced, deserted, widowed or have simply left their husbands to make it alone. The significance of this paper lies in its attempt to analyse Nwapa's writings in breaking patriarchal chains. Its contribution to knowledge is that African feminist literary scholarship can stand as a weapon in emancipating women from various chains particularly male domination. This broadens the better understanding of women empowerment not from other disciplines but from literature point of view. This empowerment which is manifested in the form of resort to alternative lifestyles uncovers different potentials of women's capabilities such courage, enterprise and initiative spirits.

References

Aidoo, A.A.: To be an African woman writer: An overview and a detail. Criticism and Ideology: Second African Writers Conference 1986. Ed. Kirsten Holst Petersen. Uppsala, Sweden: Scandinavian Institute of African Studies, pp. 155–172 (1988)

Chinua, A.: Things Fall Apart. Heinemann, Oxford (1958)
Davies, C.B., Graves, A.A.: Ngambika: Studies of Women in African Literature. Africa World Press, Trenton (1986)
Jackson, S., Jones, J. (eds.): Contemporary Feminist Theories. Edinburgh University Press, Edinburgh (1998)
Katrak, K.H.: Decolonizing culture: toward a theory for postcolonial women's texts. Mod. Fiction Stud. **35**(1), 157–179 (1989)
Nfah-Abbenyi, J.M.: Gender in African Women's Writing: Identity, Sexuality, and Difference. Indiana University Press, Bloomington (1997)
Nwapa, F.: One is Enough. Tana P, Nigeria (1986)
Women Are Different. Tana P., Nigeria (1990)
Ogundipe-Leslie, M.: Re-creating ourselves: African women & critical transformations. Africa World Press, Lawrenceville (1994)
Silkü, R.K.: Postcolonial feminist discourse in flora Nwapa's women are different. J. Postcolonial Writ. **40**(1), 125–135 (2002)
Umeh, M.: Emerging Perspectives on Flora Nwapa: Critical and Theoretical Essays. Africa World Press Inc, Trenton (1998)
Umeh, M., Flora, N.: The poetics of economic independence for female empowerment: an interview with Flora Nwapa. Res. Afr. Lit. **26**(2), 22–29 (1995). Website. Site visited on 7 Sept 2012
Uwakweh, P.A.: Debunking patriarchy: the liberational quality of voicing in Tsitsi Dangarembga's "Nervous Conditions". Res. Afr. Lit. **26**(1), 75–84 (1995). Website. Site visited on 15 Oct 2012

Correction to: Characterization of Palm Oil Mill Wastewater: The Case of Small-Scale Mills in Ghana

E. Awere, A. Bonoli, and P. A. Obeng

Correction to: Chapter "Characterization of Palm Oil Mill Wastewater: The Case of Small-Scale Mills in Ghana" in: J. N. Mojekwu et al. (Eds.): *Sustainable Education and Development*, https://doi.org/10.1007/978-3-030-68836-3_29

In the original version of the book, the following change has been made: The title of Chapter 29 has been changed from "Qualitative Assessment of Palm Oil Mill Wastewater from Small-Scale Processing Mills in Ghana" to "Characterization of Palm Oil Mill Wastewater: The Case of Small-Scale Mills in Ghana". The book and the chapter have been updated with the change.

The updated version of this chapter can be found at
https://doi.org/10.1007/978-3-030-68836-3_29

J. N. Mojekwu et al. (Eds.): *Sustainable Education and Development*, p. C1, 2022.
https://doi.org/10.1007/978-3-030-68836-3_46

Author Index

J. N. Mojekwu et al. (Eds.): *Sustainable Education and Development*, pp. 537–538, 2021.
https://doi.org/10.1007/978-3-030-68836-3

The manufacturer's authorised representative in the EU is Springer Nature Customer Service Centre GmbH, Europaplatz 3, 69115 Heidelberg, Germany. If you have any concerns regarding our products, please contact ProductSafety@springernature.com

Printed and bound by CPI Group (UK) Ltd, Croydon, CR0 4YY
30/09/2026
02225692-0014